UK Ambulance Services
Clinical Practice
Guidelines 2016

Edited for JRCALC and AACE by

Simon N Brown, Dhushy Kumar and Mark Millins

on behalf of NASMeD by

Julian Mark and medical director colleagues

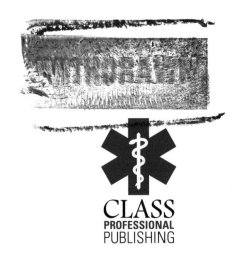

CLASS
PROFESSIONAL
PUBLISHING

© Association of Ambulance Chief Executives (AACE) 2016

Printing history
First edition published 2000, second edition 2004, third edition 2006
Fourth edition published 2013, reprinted 2014, 2015 (twice, Version 1.3)

The content for Reference Edition 1.3 and Pocket Book 1.2 was updated in January 2015.
This edition published 2016, reprinted 2016 (Version 1.4)

The authors and publisher welcome feedback from the users of this book.
Please contact the publisher:
Class Professional Publishing,
The Exchange, Express Park, Bristol Road, Bridgwater TA6 4RR
Telephone: 01278 427 800
Email: post@class.co.uk
Website: www.classprofessional.co.uk

Class Professional Publishing is an imprint of Class Publishing Ltd

A CIP catalogue record for this book is available from the British Library
ISBN 978 1 85959 594 7

Designed and typeset by RefineCatch and DLXML Associates

Edited by Emma Milman

Digital consultancy by Veruschka Selbach

Line illustrations by David Woodroffe

Printed in Slovenia by arrangement with KINT Ljubljana

For free updates, to give feedback and for details of how to order, go to
www.AACEGuidelines.co.uk

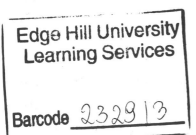

Contents

Disclaimer ii

Foreword vii

Guideline Developers and Contributors viii

Guideline Development Methodology ix

Update Analysis x

List of Abbreviations xviii

Section 1 – General Guidance

Consent in Pre-hospital Care 3

Patient Confidentiality 4

Pain Management in Adults 8

Pain Management in Children 11

Safeguarding Children 16

Sexual Assault 22

Safeguarding Vulnerable Adults 24

End of Life Care 26

Death of a Child Including Sudden Unexpected Death in Infancy, Children and Adolescents (SUDICA) 32

Staff wellbeing and health 35

Section 2 – Resuscitation

Airway and Breathing Management 39

Traumatic Cardiac Arrest 44

Recognition of Life Extinct by Ambulance Clinicians 46

Adult Resuscitation Guidelines:

Basic Life Support 50

Advanced Life Support 52

Foreign Body Airway Obstruction 58

Maternal Resuscitation 60

Child Resuscitation Guidelines:

Basic Life Support 62

Newborn Life Support 66

Advanced Life Support 70

Foreign Body Airway Obstruction 74

Special circumstances 77

Section 3a – Medical: Undifferentiated Complaints

Abdominal Pain 85

Cardiac Rhythm Disturbance 89

Altered Level of Consciousness 92

Dyspnoea 96

Headache 100

Mental Disorder 102

Mental Capacity Act 2005 (England and Wales) 111

Adult:

Medical Emergencies in Adults – Overview 117

Non-Traumatic Chest Pain/Discomfort 122

Children:

Medical Emergencies in Children – Overview 124

Minor Illness in Children 129

Febrile Illness in Children 130

Respiratory Illness in Children 134

Section 3b – Medical: Specific Conditions

Heat Related Illness 137

Hyperventilation Syndrome 140

Hypothermia 143

Sickle Cell Crisis 146

Meningococcal Meningitis and Septicaemia 149

Adult:

Acute Coronary Syndrome 152

Allergic Reactions including Anaphylaxis 155

Asthma 157

Chronic Obstructive Pulmonary Disease 161

Convulsions 165

Gastrointestinal Bleeding 169

Glycaemic Emergencies 172

Heart Failure 176

Implantable Cardioverter Defibrillator 180

Overdose and Poisoning 185

Pulmonary Embolism 194

Stroke/Transient Ischaemic Attack 198

Children:

Allergic Reactions including Anaphylaxis 200

Asthma 202

Convulsions 206

Childhood Gastroenteritis 211

Glycaemic Emergencies 215

Overdose and Poisoning 218

Section 4 – Trauma

Trauma Emergencies Overview (Adults) 223

Trauma Emergencies Overview (Children) 230

Abdominal Trauma 236

Head Injury 238

Limb Trauma 242

Neck and Back Trauma 246

Major Pelvic Trauma 252

Thoracic Trauma 255

Trauma in Pregnancy 260

Burns and Scalds (Adults) 262

Burns and Scalds (Children) 265

Electrical Injuries 268

Immersion and Drowning 271

Section 5 – Obstetrics and Gynaecology

Obstetrics and Gynaecology Emergencies Overview 277
Birth Imminent: Normal Delivery and Delivery 280
Complications
Care of the Newborn 288
Haemorrhage During Pregnancy (including 292
Miscarriage and Ectopic Pregnancy)
Pregnancy-induced Hypertension (including 295
Eclampsia)
Vaginal Bleeding: Gynaecological Causes 298

Section 6 – Drugs

Drugs Overview 303
Adrenaline 308
Amiodarone 310
Aspirin 311
Atropine 312
Benzylpenicillin (Penicillin G) 315
Chlorphenamine 317
Clopidogrel 320
Dexamethasone 321
Diazepam 322
Entonox 326
Furosemide 327
Glucagon (Glucagen) 328
Glucose 10% 330
Glucose 40% Oral Gel 331
Glyceryl Trinitrate (GTN, Suscard) 332
Heparin 333
Hydrocortisone 334
Ibuprofen 338
Ipratropium Bromide (Atrovent) 340
Metoclopramide (Maxolon) 342
Midazolam 343

Patient's Own Buccal Midazolam for Convulsions 345
Misoprostol 346
Morphine Sulphate 347
Naloxone Hydrochloride (Narcan) 351
Ondansetron 355
Oxygen 357
Paracetamol 363
Reteplase 367
Salbutamol 370
0.9% Sodium Chloride 373
Sodium Lactate Compound (Hartmann's/Ringer's 380
Lactate)
Syntometrine 386
Tenecteplase 387
Tetracaine 4% 390
Tranexamic Acid 391
Intravascular Fluid Therapy (Adults) 392
Intravascular Fluid Therapy (Children) 397
Page-for-Age 400

Section 7 – Special Situations

Major Incident Management 437
Chemical, Biological, Radiological, Nuclear and 438
Explosive Incidents
Atropine (CBRNE) 447
Ciprofloxacin (CBRNE) 453
Dicobalt Edetate (CBRNE) 454
Doxycycline (CBRNE) 455
Obidoxime Chloride (CBRNE) 456
Potassium Iodate (CBRNE) 457
Pralidoxime Mesylate (CBRNE) 458
Incapacitating Agents 459

References 465
Index 491

Foreword

Welcome to the 2016 revision of the JRCALC UK Ambulance Service Clinical Practice Guidelines.

These guidelines reflect the extended role of ambulance clinicians in today's NHS. This includes updates in the management of convulsions, sepsis, mental health and major trauma amongst others.

The updated guidelines recognise the changes in urgent and emergency care and a shift towards an increased proportion of the initial assessment of urgent care patients being undertaken by ambulance clinicians.

JRCALC has continued to grow under the AACE banner and has a new streamlined structure enabling continuing responsive updated guidance to be produced in line with advances in practice and care. JRCALC's independent status remains valuable to the pre-hospital community in producing evidence based best practice.

We would like to acknowledge and thank all those who have contributed to these guidelines as well as previous editions as our guidance continues to evolve.

Dhushy Surendra Kumar

Chair, JRCALC

Simon Brown

Chair, JRCALC Guideline Development Groups

AACE is proud to support the publication of the 2016 Ambulance Guidelines as recommended by JRCALC. Building on the very successful format of the 2013 edition, we are pleased to include some significant revisions and areas of new guidance. As we go to print, it is unclear which publishing medium will be the most popular over the next few years. We don't think '2016' will be the last printed volume but we are very aware of the need to meet the varying needs of current practitioners. Whilst commending this book to you, in whichever format you choose to use, we will continue to work with our publishers and other experts to ensure Paramedics and all ambulance clinicians can continue to access the best guidance, in a timely manner and in a format that suits them and the environment in which they are working.

AACE would like to acknowledge the excellent support and expertise received from Class Professional Publishing in managing this project with special thanks to Emma Milman, Lorna Downing and Dick Warner, with whom, it is a pleasure to collaborate.

Steve Irving

Executive Officer, Association of Ambulance Chief Executives

Guideline Developers and Contributors

Editorial Leads

Mark Millins, AACE
Steve Irving, AACE
Dhushy Kumar, JRCALC
Simon Brown, JRCALC
Julian Mark, NASMeD

For JRCLAC

Simon Brown
Charles Deakin
Kim Hinshaw

Dhushy Kumar
Amanda Mansfield
Keith Porter

Julian Sandell
Alison Walker

For NASMeD

Rob Andrews
Marcus Bailey
John Black
Andy Carson
Kyee Han
Brendan Lloyd

Kevin Mackway-Jones
Julian Mark
Andrew McIntyre
David McManus
Rory McCrea
Fionna Moore

David Ratcliffe
Andy Smith
Jim Ward
Bob Winter
Fenella Wrigley

Contributors

Robert Andrews
Richard Appleton
Louis Appleby
Marcus Bailey
Martin Berry
Richard Berry
Mike Brooke
Will Broughton
Daniel Butterworth
Andy Collen
Adele Dean
Lucy Derwin
Steve Dick
Jon Dickson
Kuda Dimbi
Tim Edwards
Ed England
Paul Fell

Mike Jackson
Cathryn James
Paul Jefferies
Andrew Jenkins
Paul Kelly
Jaqui Lindridge
Gregory Lloyd
Graham McClelland
Rory McCrea
Will Murcott
Barry Murphy-Jones
Georgina Murphy-Jones
Ian Mursell
Andy Newton
Martin Parkinson
Dave Partlow
Richard Pilbery
Sue Putman

Gary Richardson
Adrian Robinson
Mike Smyth
Rashid Sohail
Adrian South
Joanne Stonehouse
Clare Sutton
Andrew Swinburn
Rob Taylor
Dahrlene Tough
Matthew Ward
Roger Watson
Kevin Webb
James Wenman
Dave Whitmore
Jason Wiles
Ian Wilmer
Bartholomew Wood

Guideline Development Methodology

The methodology used by JRCALC (Joint Royal Colleges Ambulance Liaison Committee) to develop the UK Ambulance Services Clinical Practice Guidelines is designed to comply with the criteria used by the AGREE II (Appraisal of Guidelines for Research and Evaluation in Europe) instrument. This process is a leading academic tool to identify good quality guidelines: http://www.agreetrust.org/

The purpose of the AGREE II, is to provide a framework to:
● assess the quality of guidelines
● provide a methodological strategy for the development of guidelines
● inform what information and how information ought to be reported in guidelines.

By adopting these principles, guidelines are developed that support safe decision making and high quality patient care.

Guideline Selection

JRCALC, NASMeD (National Ambulance Service Medical Directors) and the ALPG (Ambulance Lead Paramedic Group) will advise on those clinical guidelines which need updating and those clinical conditions which need a new guideline developing. These are then prioritised and assessed with regard to urgency and risk. Clinical topics can be identified through a variety of means including the monitoring of serious incidents within individual UK Ambulance Service Trusts, preventing future death directives issued by coroners and national service reconfiguration e.g. the move to major trauma centres and networks. In addition JRCALC provide extensive clinical expertise and advice on potential new developments to ensure that the guidelines capture latest best practice and future innovations.

Feedback

Is welcome via

JRCALC@AACE.org or www.aaceguidelines.co.uk

Editorial Independence

No external funding has been received for the development of these guidelines and no competing or conflicting interests have been declared by those involved in their development.

The 2016 Clinical Practice Guidelines contain new guidance on end of life care, staff wellbeing and health, special circumstances in resuscitation and the Mental Capacity Act.

The guidelines on resuscitation, convulsions in children, head trauma and mental health have been significantly revised for this edition. Other guidelines in the book have been subject to updates and corrections as required.

Section 2: Resuscitation has been updated to reflect the new guidelines from Resuscitation Council UK which were published in October 2015.

At the time of going to press, the international sepsis guidelines are in review. JRCALC and AACE will publish recommendations on sepsis for ambulance clinicians following the release of the international sepsis guidelines. This is expected to be in 2016, and will be issued as an update to this edition of the 2016 Clinical Practice Guidelines.

As well as revisions which have been made for the 2016 edition, the following update analysis lists corrections which were made to the 2013 Reference Edition following its publication. Version 1.1 was published in 2013, version 1.2 in 2014 and version 1.3 was printed in 2015. Updates have been published on www.aaceguidelines.co.uk and appeared in reprinted 2013 editions.

Section 1

General guidance	Addition/update of guidance and rationale
Consent Statement	● Reference to interprofessional collaboration has been added.
Pain Management in Children	● The Wong Baker FACES Pain Rating Scale is corrected. The pain scale is based on the numbers 0 to 10, not 0 to 5.
Safeguarding Vulnerable Adults	● Reference to the Doctrine of Necessity has been removed and replaced with the Mental Capacity Act.
End of Life Care	● This is a completely new guideline for the 2016 edition. ● Guidance is available on patients who are not in the active stage of dying, care pathways, reversible emergencies, superior vein compression, neutropenic sepsis, a patient-centred approach and pharmacological treatments.
Death of a Child, including Sudden Unexpected Death in Infancy, Children and Adolescents (SUDICA)	● Reference to an advanced directive was changed to an advanced decision.
Staff Wellbeing and Mental Health	● This is a completely new guideline for the 2016 edition. ● Recommendations for ambulance clinicians on maintaining their own mental health and managing stress have been added.

Section 2

All guidelines in this section were significantly revised for the 2016 edition.

Resuscitation	Addition/update of guidance and rationale
Airway and Breathing Management	• The step wise approach to airway management is reinforced. • Tracheal intubation should only be performed in conjunction with waveform capnography. • Guidance on supraglottic airways has been added. • Guidance on tracheal intubation has been added. • A new algorithm on emergency tracheostomy and laryngectomy management has been added.
Traumatic Cardiac Arrest	• Emphasis on the simultaneous and active management of hypovolaemia, hypoaxaemia and tension pneumothorax was added.
Recognition of Life Extinct by Ambulance Clinicians	• Details about when a condition is unconditionally associated with death were revised to provide consistency across all age ranges. Prolonged submersion after which resuscitation should not be attempted has been amended from greater than 1.5 hours to greater than 60 minutes. • A Special Guidance Note with regards to individual chemical exposure was added. • Bullet point added explaining that CPR should only be paused for a 30-second asystole check if all other criteria are met. • Guidance for submersion victims is covered in the new guideline, Special Circumstances. • Guidance for chemical exposure is covered in the new guideline, Special Circumstances.
Basic Life Support (Adult)	• The critical importance of good quality chest compressions has been emphasised. • With the advent of automated external defibrillators (AED) defibrillation is now considered to be the first priority step of Basic Life Support. • Use of a laryngoscope if a foreign body is suspected to be present in the airway. • The adult basic life support sequence algorithm has been updated to reflect the latest Resuscitation Council UK algorithm.
Advanced Life Support (Adult)	• This section has been fully updated to reflect the Resuscitation Council 2015 guidelines. • In ROSC patients post cardiac arrest syndrome is highlighted. • In cases of ROSC following non-traumatic cardiac arrest passive cooling should be considered in line with local guidance. • Interruptions to chest compressions must be kept to less than 5 seconds. • Defibrillation should take precedence over airway or breathing interventions. • Guidance on combative patients and seizure control has been added. • The adult advanced life support sequence algorithm has been updated to reflect the latest Resuscitation Council UK algorithm.

Update Analysis

Resuscitation	Addition/update of guidance and rationale
Maternal Resuscitation	• An emphasis on rapid transport to hospital if there is no response to resuscitative efforts within 4 minutes. • Groups at particular risk of maternal resuscitation are no longer listed. • New guidance for cardiac arrest in pregnancy appear. These relate to hand positions for chest compressions, moving the uterus, tilting the patient's body, placement of defibrillator electrodes, location of IV access, administration of oxygen and transfers to the emergency department.
Basic Life Support (Child)	• The critical importance of good quality chest compressions has been emphasised. • Inflations should be delivered over 1 second as in adult resuscitation. • General principles for children have been added. Children are likely to have severe underlying illness or injury that can only be managed adequately in hospital and it is therefore particularly important not to delay on scene. Call for support from the most senior clinicians available. • Bag-mask ventilation is the recommended first line method for achieving airway control and ventilation in children. • Children become hypothermic easily. It is important to keep them as warm as possible before and during transfer. • The child basic life support sequence algorithm has been updated to reflect the latest Resuscitation Council UK algorithm.
Newborn Life Support	• Guidance on keeping neonates warm has been updated. Skin to skin contact is advised. Cover the baby with dry towels. In the case of pre-term babies, place them in polythene wrapping. Use a hat with newborn babies. • Guidance on the colours, heart rate and breathing patterns to expect in newborn babies have been added. • The newborn life support sequence algorithm has been updated to reflect the latest Resuscitation Council UK algorithm.
Advanced Life Support (Child)	• The priority is to deliver high-quality chest compressions and effective ventilation with high-flow oxygen. ALS procedures must not delay the transfer to hospital. • Supraglottic airways are ideal for most paediatric airways. These should be considered where bag-mask ventilation is not possible. • During CPR, deliver ventilation at a rate of approximately 10 per minute. This should take priority over attaching a defibrillator. • Gaining rapid vascular access in children is often quickest using an intraosseous needle. This should be used in preference to an intravenous cannula unless a suitable site for venous cannulation is immediately apparent. • The child advanced life support sequence algorithm has been updated to reflect the latest Resuscitation Council UK algorithm. • Children in a VF/VT arrest should receive a second half dose of amiodarone. This was amended in Version 1.3.
Foreign Body Airway Obstruction (Child)	• The foreign body airway obstruction in children algorithm has been updated.
Special Circumstances	• New guidance on drowning, chemical exposure, opioid overdose, anaphylaxis and asthma.

Section 3a

Medical – Undifferentiated Complaints	Addition/update of guidance and rationale
Dyspnoea	• An oxygen saturation of less than 94% is now determined as a time critical feature.
Mental Disorder	• This guideline has been significantly revised. • Data on the prevalence of mental disorders has been updated. • Information on the use of tricyclics and antipsychotics is now available. • A breakdown of the different professionals working in mental health along with service providers. • Learning disabilities, dementia, Asperger's, anxiety, self-harm and acute psychosis are covered. • Pathways for referral are suggested. • The IPAP suicide risk assessment tool is recommended for use. • A flowchart tool for dealing with patients with suicidal ideation is included.
Mental Capacity Act	• This new guideline on the Mental Capacity Act has been added
Medical Emergencies in Adults – Overview	• The assessment and management of medical emergencies table was updated to state that endotracheal intubation should only be performed if appropriate and only if capnography is available. • Guidance with regards to ECGs in secondary surveys was extended.
Non-Traumatic Chest Pain/ Discomfort	• An oxygen saturation of less than 94% is now determined as a time critical feature.
Medical Emergencies in Children – Overview	• Endotracheal intubation must only be performed when capnography is available.
Febrile Illness in Children	• An amendment indicating that paracetamol and ibuprofen should not be co-administered was made.

Section 3b

Medical – Specific Conditions	Addition/update of guidance and rationale
Sickle Cell Crisis	● Key point added: in sickle cell crisis and acute chest syndrome, aim for an oxygen saturation of 94–98% or aim for the saturation level that is usual for the individual patient.
Meningococcal Meningitis Septicaemia	● An oxygen saturation of less than 94% is now determined as a time critical feature.
Allergic Reactions Including Anaphylaxis (Adult)	● Amphotericin was incorrectly listed as an antibiotic in the 2013 guidelines. This has been corrected and it is now named as a drug. ● Half doses of adrenaline are no longer recommended for anaphylaxis in patients who are prescribed beta-blockers or tricyclic anti-depressants.
Asthma (Children)	● Administration of adrenaline is recommended for life-threatening asthma in children.
Chronic Obstructive Pulmonary Disease	● The time frame for using bronchodilators was clarified. Oxygen-driven nebulisation should be limited to six minutes.
Convulsions (Adults)	● New guidance on administering midazolam has been added.
Heart Failure	● The assessment and management of acute heart failure algorithm was amended. SpO_2 levels in this algorithm were revised to less than 94%.
Convulsions (Children)	● This guideline has been significantly revised and expanded.
Overdose and Poisoning (Adults)	● A new point was added to the assessment and management table in the chemical exposure box.
Allergic Reactions including Anaphylaxis (Children)	● Amphotericin was incorrectly listed as an antibiotic in the 2013 guidelines. This has been corrected and it is now named as a drug.

Section 4

Trauma	Addition/update of guidance and rationale
Head Injury	• This guideline has been completely revised and extensive additional guidance has been added on Traumatic Brain Injury (TBI). • The formula for calculating Mean Arterial Pressure (MAP) has been updated. • Guidance on head injuries in the elderly has been added. • Evacuation considerations and treatment goals have been added.
Trauma Emergencies Overview (Adults)	• The management of catastrophic haemorrhage algorithm was amended with regards to where the tourniquet should be placed.
Trauma Emergencies Overview (Children)	• The management of catastrophic haemorrhage algorithm was amended with regards to where the tourniquet should be placed. • The airway advice was amended to explain that ambulance clinicians should administer high concentration oxygen via a non-rebreating mask to maintain an oxygen saturation of at least 94%.
Immersion and Drowning	• Refer to the ROLE guidance and do not attempt resuscitation if a person has been submerged for more than 60 minutes. However, if the person has been submerged in ICY COLD water, then a decision may be made to attempt resuscitation in a witnessed submersion time of 90 minutes.

Section 5

Obstetrics and Gynaecology	Addition/update of guidance and rationale
Birth Imminent: Normal delivery and complications	• Guidance for shoulder dystocia was expanded to include gentle traction.
Care of the Newborn	• Reinforcement of the need to transport a new born baby with a blood glucose level of less than 2.5 mmol/l was added. • Further clarity is given around the dose of naloxone in a new born baby with respiratory or central nervous system depression.

Section 6

Drugs	Addition/update of guidance
Adrenaline	● Use of half doses of adrenaline for patients taking beta blockers or tricyclics has been removed.
Atropine	● Dosages for birth and 1 month age groups were updated.
Chlorphenamine	● Emphasis is placed on the use of chlorphenamine in anaphylaxis with the intravenous route being the route of choice. The intramuscular route should only be used when the former is not available.
Dexamethasone	● Dosage table updated to reflect new presentation.
Entonox	● Reference to Nitronox was removed.
Glucose 10%	● A clarifying note was added to explain that neonatal doses are intentionally larger per kilo than those used in older children.
Glyceryl Trinitrate (GTN, Suscard)	● Headache, dizziness and hypotension were added as side effects.
Hydrocortisone	● Reference to the call to hospital time was removed.
Metoclopramide (Maxolon)	● Drug overdose is now listed as a contra-indication for this drug. Previously it was identified as a caution.
Midazolam	● A new guideline appears in the 2016 edition.
Naloxone Hydrochloride	● An additional note was added about the dose of 200 micrograms for the reversal of respiratory and central nervous system.
Paracetamol	● Dosages for children have been updated.
Tenecteplase	● Reference to a second bolus was deleted.
Tetracaine	● In the drugs table, reference to tablets was taken out and replaced with volume.
Intravascular Fluid Therapy (Children)	● This guideline has been revised and updated.

Section 7

Special Situations	Addition/update of guidance and rationale
Chemical, Biological, Radiological, Nuclear and Explosive Incidents	• The general management for an unspecified CBRNE incident algorithm was updated.
Pralidoxime Mesylate	• Mesylate has been added in to the full name of the drug.

List of Abbreviations

The glossary of terms listed below is designed to assist reading ease and is **NOT** provided as a list of short-hand terms. The Joint Royal Colleges Ambulance Liaison Committee reminds the user that abbreviations are not to be used in any clinical documentation.

Term	
AAA	Abdominal Aortic Aneurysm
ACPO	Association of Chief Police Officers
ACS	Acute Coronary Syndrome
AED	Automated External Defibrillation
ALS	Advanced Life Support
AMHP	Approved Mental Health Professional
APGAR	**A** – Appearance **P** – Pulse rate **G** – Grimace or response to stimulation **A** – Activity or muscle tone **R** – Respiration
ARDS	Acute Respiratory Distress Syndrome
ATP	Anti-Tachycardia Pacing
AVPU	**A** – Alert **V** – Responds to voice **P** – Responds to pain **U** – Unresponsive
bd	Twice daily
BLS	Basic Life Support
BM	Stick Measures blood sugar
BP	Blood Pressure
BR	Breech
BVM	Bag-Valve-Mask
CBRNE	Chemical, Biological, Radiological, Nuclear and Explosive
CBRT	Capillary bed refill time
CD	Controlled Drug
CEW	Controlled Electrical Weapon
CHD	Coronary Heart Disease
CNS	Central Nervous System
CO	Carbon monoxide
CO_2	Carbon dioxide
COPD	Chronic Obstructive Pulmonary Disease
CPAP	Continuous Positive Airway Pressure
CPP	Cerebral Perfusion Pressure
CPR	Cardiopulmonary Resuscitation
CRT	Capillary Refill Time
CRT	Cardiac Resynchronisation Therapy

Term	
CSE	Convulsive (tonic-clonic) status epilepticus
CT	Computerised Tomography
CVA	Cerebo Vascular Accident
DIC	Disseminated Intravascular Coagulation
DKA	Diabetic Ketoacidosis
DM	Diabetes Mellitus
DNA	Deoxyribonucleic Acid
DNAR	Do Not Attempt Resuscitation Order
DNACPR	Do Not Attempt Cardiopulmonary Resuscitation Order
DPA	Data Protection Act
DVT	Deep Vein Thrombosis
E	Ecstasy
EC	Enteric Coated
ECG	Electrocardiograph
ED	Emergency Department
EDD	Estimated Date of Delivery
EMS	Emergency Medical Services
ET	Endotracheal
ETA	Expected Time of Arrival
FC	Febrile Convulsions
g	Grams
GCS	Glasgow Coma Scale
GI	Gastrointestinal
GP	General Practitioner
GTN	Glyceryl Trinitrate
HIV	Human Immunodeficiency Virus
IBS	Irritable Bowel Syndrome
ICD	Implantable Cardioverter Defibrillator
ICP	Intracranial Pressure
IHD	Ischemic Heart Disease
IM	Intramuscular
IO	Intraosseous
IV	Intravenous
JRCALC	Joint Royal Colleges Ambulance Liaison Committee

JVP	Jugular Venous Pressure
kg	Kilogram
LBBB	Left Bundle Branch Block
LMA	Laryngeal Mask Airway
LMP	Last Menstrual Period
LOC	Level of Consciousness
LSD	Lysergic Acid Diethylamide
LVF	Left Ventricular Failure
MAOI	Monoamine Oxidase Inhibitor antidepressant
MAP	Mean Arterial Pressure
mcg	Microgram
MDMA	Methylene Dioxymethamphetamine
mg	Milligram
MI	Myocardial Infarction
ml	Millilitre
mmHG	Millimetres of Mercury
mmol	Millimoles
mmol/l	Millimoles per Litre
MOI	Mechanisms of Injury
MSC	**M** – Motor **S** – Sensation **C** – Circulation
Neb	Nebulisation
NiPPV	Non-invasive Positive Pressure Ventilation
NPA	Nasopharyngeal Airway
NPIS	National Poisons Information Service
NSAID	Non-Steroidal Anti-inflammatory Drug
O₂	Oxygen
OPA	Oropharyngeal Airway
P	Parity
PCO₂	Measure of the Partial Pressure of Carbon Dioxide
PE	Pulmonary Embolism
PEA	Pulseless Electrical Activity
PEF	Peak Expiratory Flow
PHTLS	Pre-hospital Trauma Life Support
PIH	Pregnancy-induced Hypertension

PO	Pulmonary Oedema
POM	Prescription Only Medicine
PPCI	Primary Percutaneous Coronary Intervention
PPE	Personal Protective Equipment
pr	Per Rectum
prn	When required medication
RAID	Rapid, Assessment, Interface and Discharge
ROLE	Recognition Of Life Extinct
ROSC	Return of Spontaneous Circulation
RTC	Road Traffic Collision
RVP	Rendezvous Point(s)
SAD	Supraglottic Airway Device
SaO₂	Oxygen Saturation Of Arterial Blood
SBP	Systolic Blood Pressure
SC	Subcutaneous
SCI	Spinal Cord Injury
SpO₂	Oxygen Saturation Measured With Pulse Oximeter
SSA	Senior Scientific Authority
SSRIs	Selective Serotonin Re-Uptake Inhibitors
STEMI	ST Segment Elevation Myocardial Infarction
STEP	Safety Triggers For Emergency Personnel
SUDI	Sudden Unexpected Death in Infancy
SUDICA	Sudden Unexpected Death in Infancy, Children and Adolescents
SVT	Supraventricular Tachycardia
TBI	Traumatic Brain injury
TBSA	Total Body Surface Area
TIA	Transient Ischaemic Attack
TLoC	Transient loss of conciousness
UTI	Urinary Tract Infection
VAS	Visual Analogue Scale
VF	Ventricular Fibrillation
VT	Ventricular Tachycardia
VTE	Venous Thromboembolism

1

General Guidance

General Guidance

Consent in Pre-hospital Care 3

Patient Confidentiality 4

Pain Management in Adults 8

Pain Management in Children 11

Safeguarding Children 16

Sexual Assault 22

Safeguarding Vulnerable Adults 24

End of Life Care 26

Death of a Child Including Sudden
Unexpected Death in Infancy, Children
and Adolescents (SUDICA) 32

Staff wellbeing and health 35

Consent in Pre-hospital Care

The laws and guidance that relate to consent to assessment, treatment, care and other interventions are different in the countries and/or jurisdictions that constitute the United Kingdom.

Therefore, these guidelines do not offer guidance on obtaining consent beyond the general advice in this statement. The Joint Royal Colleges Ambulance Liaison Committee (JRCALC) advises strongly that readers should seek specific guidance on consent from their Ambulance Services, Trusts or other relevant employers.

JRCALC advises that obtaining consent in ways that are lawful in the jurisdiction in which each reader works is fundamental to meeting patients' legal and ethical rights in determining what happens to them and to their own bodies. Therefore, it is important to ensure that you have legally valid consent to conduct assessments, treatments and other interventions, and provide care. Consent must be obtained from each patient or their legally valid representative (defined according to the law in the relevant country or jurisdiction) prior to conducting examinations, treatment, or providing care.

In pre-hospital situations, it is not uncommon for patients to refuse assessment, care or treatment. Although patients may refuse, there may be, depending on the circumstances, continuing moral duties and legal responsibilities for ambulance clinicians to provide further intervention, particularly if life-threatening risk is involved. Again, ambulance clinicians are advised to obtain advice from their employers about circumstances of this nature so the actions they take are appropriate to the legal jurisdiction in which they are working.

When communicating with other health care professionals, discussion should include information about the patient's consent.

Patient Confidentiality

1. Introduction [1–7]

Health professionals have a duty of confidentiality regarding patient information. They also have a priority, which is to ensure that all relevant information about their patients, their assessments, examinations and advice is recorded clearly and accurately, and passed to other staff whenever it is necessary for provision of ongoing care.

Sometimes, aspects of legislation relating to these issues appear to conflict with each other. This guideline provides a brief overview of the relevant legislation under the following headings:

- Patient Identifiable Information.
- Data Protection Act 1998 (DPA).
- NHS Policy.
- Protecting Patient Information.
- Patients' Rights of Access to Personal Health Records.
- Disclosure to Other Bodies and Organisations.
- Research.
- Consent.

2. Patient Identifiable Information [1–2, 7–11]

Patient Identifiable Information is any information that may be used to identify a patient directly or indirectly. It may include:

- Patient's name, address, postcode or date of birth.
- Any image or audiotape of the patient.
- Any other data or information that has the potential, however remote, to identify a patient (e.g. rare diseases, drug regimes, statistical analysis of small groups).
- Patients' record numbers.
- Combinations of any of the items here that may increase the risk of a breach of confidentiality, that include all verbal, written and electronic disclosure, whether formal or incidental.

3. Data Protection Act [1, 12–14]

The main principles of the DPA should be read in conjunction with this guideline. This Act describes processes for obtaining, recording, holding, using and sharing information:

- Patients must be informed and give consent to any sharing of their personal information. Exceptions to this general rule may exist (see sections on Disclosure and Consent).
- Only the minimum amount of data should be collected and used to achieve the agreed purpose.
- Information can only be retained for as long as it is needed to achieve its purpose.
- Strict rules apply to sharing information and with whom it may be shared.

4. NHS Policy [1–4]

All NHS employees must be aware of, and respect a patient's right to confidentiality. A disciplinary offence may have been committed for any behaviour contrary to their organisation's policy or the *NHS Code of Practice: Confidentiality* (in Scotland, the *NHS COP on Protecting Patient Confidentiality*). Ambulance clinicians should be aware of how to gain access to training, support or information, which they may need, and be able to show that they are making every reasonable effort to comply with the relevant standards.

5. Protecting Patient Information [6, 15]

There are five essential steps that all ambulance clinicians should take to ensure that they comply with the relevant standards of confidentiality. They are listed below:

5.1 Record information given by, and about, patients concisely and accurately. [1–2]

- Inaccurate clinical records about patients may contain false information that has been created by, for example, omissions, errors, unfounded comments or speculation. This breaches DPA standards. It also brings the professional integrity of ambulance clinicians and their employing organisations into question. Any comments and opinions, whether verbal, written or electronic, must be justifiable and accurate.

5.2 Keep patient information physically secure. [7, 13, 16]

- Ambulance services have particular difficulties in ensuring that information is not shared accidentally with the public. Not only must patients be treated confidentially, but the information gained must not be disclosed to anyone else unless to do so genuinely promotes patient care. (Comments to the public must be guarded). Information given to other clinicians when handing over patients' care should not be overheard or shared with people who are not directly involved in each patient's care. Patients' records, either electronic or written, must be protected against unwarranted viewing: thus, patients' clinical records must be shielded from the view of other people, stored securely after case closure, and only handed over to staff who are entrusted with ongoing care of particular patients or other authorised personnel who have legitimate reasons for possessing the information. Personal health data must be destroyed in an approved manner and according to each organisation's policies when they have served their function. Discussions of each patient must not disclose personal information unless there is genuine and provable health benefit.

- Leaders of healthcare and health information systems believe that electronic health information systems, which include computer-based patient records, can improve healthcare. Achieving this goal, requires systems to be in place that: protect the privacy of individual persons and data about patients; provide appropriate access; and use data security measures that are adequate. Sound policies and practices relating to handling confidential information must be in place prior to deploying health information systems. Strong and enforceable policies on privacy and security of confidential and patient identifiable information must shape the development and implementation of these systems.

5.3 Follow guidance before disclosing any patient information [3–4]

- It is not sufficient for ambulance clinicians to understand the basic principles of confidentiality alone. They must also understand and comply with their employing organisations' requirements for information-sharing. Similarly, it is the responsibility of each service to ensure that policies for data-sharing are produced, communicated, monitored, updated and reviewed. There must be a Data Protection Officer, Information Governance Manager, and/or a Caldicott Guardian available to advise ambulance clinicians if they have any doubts about sharing information.

5.4 Conform to best practice [1, 14–16]

- All grades of ambulance clinicians come into contact with the public and other NHS clinicians. Any temptation for ambulance clinicians to share information unnecessarily with other people who are known to them must be avoided, and the responsibility lies firmly with the holder of the data, both personally and in respect of employing organisations. Commitment to best practice should be applied to all information in any form about patients (e.g. patients' records, electronic data, surface mail, email, faxes, telephone calls, conversations that may be overheard, and private comments to friends or colleagues).

- If, for any reason, ambulance staff discover that personal data has been lost or has the potential for being viewed by anyone not authorised to view it, they have a duty to immediately:
  - take every action possible to recover the data and/or protect them, and
  - to inform immediately an officer in their employing organisation who has responsibility for data (or their immediate supervisor) that such an event has occurred
  - record the event.

5.5 Anonymise information where possible [3, 5]

- Information about patients is said to be anonymised when items such as those listed in section 2 are removed. It means that patients cannot be identified by any receiver of the information and any possibility of recognition is extremely small.

- Ambulance clinicians are advised to anonymise confidential data about patients wherever possible and reasonable. If information is recorded, retained or transmitted in any way, it should be anonymised unless to do so would frustrate any genuine reasons for its collection/storage that create identifiable benefits to patients' health.

6. Patients' Rights of Access to Personal Health Records [2, 11]

Patients have a right to see, and obtain a copy of, personal health information held about them. This right in law includes any legally appointed representative and those persons who have parental responsibility for children who are patients. Children also have this right provided they have the capability to understand the information. Services have the right to charge for this information; and there are guidelines on the processes that are to be followed.

- There are exceptions to the rights of patients to see their personal health information. The information is subject to legal restrictions if it could identify someone else and if that information cannot be removed from the record. Also, a request can be refused if there is substantial opinion that access to the information could cause serious harm to a particular patient or to someone else's physical or mental well-being. These instances are extremely rare in ambulance service operations. If there were to be doubt about whether exceptions such as these do exist, staff should consult the Caldicott Guardian, Information Governance Manager or Data Protection Officer and agreement should be reached with each patient's lead-clinician.

- Notwithstanding the exceptions noted here, clinicians should make every effort to support each patient's right to gain access to their personal health information. It is a requirement that this information should be received by a patient who requests it within 40 days of their request. Services should have clear written procedures in place to deal with these requests.

7. Disclosure to Other Bodies and Organisations [2–3, 14, 16–17]

7.1 Police

- The police have the right of access to personal information (name, address, etc.) in their investigation, detection and prevention of any crime. They also have the right of access to confidential health information (type of illness or injury, etc.) in their investigation, detection or prevention of a serious crime (e.g. rape, arson, terrorism, murder, etc.).

- They have no right to expect to receive information when criminality, crew safety or public safety are not involved. Generalised information regarding attendance at an incident may be passed to the police through locally agreed procedures, when details of the location of an incident and what is involved **may** be disclosed – but passage of personal or confidential health data **may not.**

7.2 Local authorities

- A local authority officer may require any person holding health, financial or other records relating to a person whom the officer knows or believes to be an adult at risk to give the records, or copies of them, to the officer, for the purposes of enabling or assisting the authority to decide whether it needs to do anything in order to protect an adult at risk from harm.

7.3 Secretary of State (by proxy)

- The Secretary of State's '**security management functions**' in relation to the health service mean that his powers to take action for the purpose of protecting and improving the security of health service providers (and persons employed by them) includes releasing documents for the purpose of preventing, detecting or investigating fraud, corruption or other unlawful activities.

7.4 Fire service and other emergency services

- There is no right of access for emergency service personnel other than the police to patients' personal health information. Situations may occur in which ambulance clinicians feel that such disclosure would be in the best interests of a particular patient, or that, by not disclosing it, other emergency workers could be put at risk. Ambulance clinicians should be fully aware of their obligations towards their patients' confidentiality. Avoidable breaches of confidentiality occur when colleagues and authorities (such as the police and persons in a judicial context) ask for information. On these occasions ambulance clinicians should follow the best practice advice given in the relevant section of the NHS Code of Practice on Protecting Patient Confidentiality; otherwise, access to information should be governed by formal documented requests and consideration by the Data Protection Officer, Information Governance Manager and/or the Caldicott Guardian.

7.5 The media

- There is no basis for disclosure of confidential or patient identifiable information to the media. Services may receive requests for information in special circumstances (e.g. requests for updates on celebrity patients or following large incidents, and when responding to press statements – public interest exemption). In instances such as these the explicit consent of the persons about whom information is sought should be gained and recorded prior to any disclosure. Occasionally, services or ambulance clinicians can be criticised in the press by patients or by someone else with whom a patient has a relationship. Criticism of this nature may contain inaccurate or misleading details of behaviour, diagnosis, or treatment. Services or ambulance clinicians should always seek advice from professional bodies on how to respond (if at all) to press criticism and about any legal redress that may be available. Although these instances may cause frustration or distress, they do not relieve anyone of their duty to respect the confidentiality of any patient.

7.6 For commercial purposes

- Ambulance services are not registered to use information for primarily commercial purposes. If such use was permitted, each patient would have to give explicit consent for information given by, or about them to be used within the express commercial setting and each patient should be given an opt-out facility. This includes all intended purposes of all parties to the agreement and lists of all persons/groups who would have access to the data. Due to the nature of commercial enterprise, this consent must be explicit (expressly and actively given) as opposed to implied (acceptance without voicing an objection).

8. Research [3]

All data for research should be anonymised wherever possible. If anonymisation would be contrary to the aims of the research, prior consent must be gained. Formal research guidelines exist for the use of health-related data and they must be adhered to.

9. Consent [2, 18–19]

Consent and patients' confidentiality are inextricably linked. In essence, each patient is said to be the owner of their own personal, non-anonymised patient information and/or data. Therefore, each patient should give approval before information provided by, or about them, is used by other people. There are exceptions to this general rule:

- There may be legal requirements to disclose data without consent (e.g. due to persons having **notifiable diseases**). Even then, however, each patient must be informed that this situation has arisen.

- When there is a risk to a patient's well-being by not informing other professionals without consent (e.g. where a child or vulnerable adult, an adult without capacity, or a patient who is being treated using powers given by the Mental Health Act, may be in need of protection) and informing the relevant authorities would appear to be to the patient's wider benefit.

- Inability to consent (e.g. some children, adults who lack capacity or patients who are seriously ill or injured and who could reasonably be expected to give consent if it were otherwise possible to do so). Even in circumstances such as these, information must be used cautiously and anonymised when possible. A proxy, guardian or parent should be consulted if such a person is available.

- Use of personal information without consent may be justified if it is in the **public interest** to do so. This may occur to prevent or detect a serious crime, for example.

In all of the instances that are described here, the advice of the service's Caldicott Guardian, Information Governance Manager and/or Data Protection Officer should be sought prior to using or releasing any personal health information or data. Each service must advise their own ambulance clinicians in relation to consent, and this advice must be studied by ambulance clinicians.

KEY POINTS

Patient Confidentiality

- Health professionals have a duty of confidentiality regarding information about or that may identify patients. They also have a priority to ensure that all relevant information is recorded clearly and accurately, and passed to others when this is necessary for providing ongoing care.

- Inaccurate clinical records may contain false information about patients, which is created by, for example, omissions, errors, unfounded comments or speculation. Any comments or opinions, whether verbal, written or electronic, must be justifiable and accurate.

- Data Protection Officers, Information Governance Managers and Caldicott Guardians are available to advise and assist ambulance clinicians of the ambulance services.

- Consent and confidentiality of information that is held about patients are inextricably linked. In essence, patients are the owners of personal, non-anonymised information that is provided by, or about them, and they, therefore, are required to give approval before it is used by other people.

- Ensure you are aware of the rules in your service regarding patients' confidentiality and follow them – but remember that ongoing care of patients should never be compromised in their application.

Further Reading

The principles within the following documents have significant impact on patient confidentiality issues, and should be considered essential reading.

1. Health and Care Professions Council. Standards of conduct, performance and ethics: Your duties as a registrant.
2. Confidentiality: NHS Code of Practice (NHS Scotland Code of Practice on Protecting Patient Confidentiality).
3. Data Protection Act 1998.

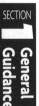
Pain Management in Adults

1. Introduction

Pain is one of the commonest symptoms in patients presenting to ambulance services.

Control of pain is important not only for humanitarian reasons but also because it may prevent deterioration of the patient and allow better assessment. Analgesia should be administered as soon as clinically possible after arriving on scene although this can be done en-route so as not to delay time-critical patients.

There is no reason to delay relief of pain because of uncertainty with the definitive diagnosis. It does not affect later diagnostic efficacy.

Many studies have demonstrated the inadequacy of pre-hospital pain relief and that time to pain relief is reduced by pre-hospital administration of analgesia.

Pain is a multi-dimensional construct (see below).

> **Pain consists of several elements:**
> - Treatment of the underlying condition.
> - Non-pharmacological methods including:
>   - psychological support and explanation
>   - physical methods e.g. splinting.
> - Pharmacological treatment.
>
> **Pain relief will depend on:**
> - Cause, site, severity and nature of the pain.
> - Age of the patient.
> - Experience/knowledge of the clinician.
> - Distance from receiving unit.
> - Available resources.

2. Assessment

An assessment should be made of the requirements of the individual. Pain is a complex experience that is shaped by gender, cultural, environmental and social factors, as well as prior pain experience. Thus the experience of pain, including assessment and tolerance levels, is unique to the individual.

It is important to remember that the pain a patient experiences cannot be objectively validated in the same way as other vital signs. Attempts to estimate the patient's pain should be resisted, as this may lead to an underestimation of the patient's experience. Several studies have shown that there is a poor correlation between the patient's pain rating and that of the healthcare professional, with the latter often underestimating the patient's pain.

Instead, ambulance clinicians need to seek and accept the patient's self-report of their pain. This is reinforced by a popular and useful definition of pain: 'pain is whatever the experiencing person says it is, existing whenever he/she says it does'.

Pain scoring

All patients in pain should have their pain assessed using the mnemonic **SOCRATES** for its:

- site
- onset
- character
- radiates
- associated symptoms
- time/duration
- exacerbating or relieving factors
- severity.

All patients with pain should have a pain severity score undertaken. It has been recognised that pain scoring increases awareness of pain, reveals previously unrecognised pain and improves analgesic administration.

There are a variety of methods of scoring pain using numerical (analogue) rating scales and simple scoring systems. JRCALC recommend that a simple 0–10 point verbal scale (0 = 'no pain' and 10 = 'the worst pain imaginable') will be the most suitable method in most pre-hospital situations.

This should be undertaken on all patients who are in pain and should be repeated after each intervention (the timing of the repeat score depends on the expected time for the analgesic to have an effect). The absolute value is used in combination with the patient assessment to determine the type of analgesia and route of administration that is most appropriate. The trend in the scores is more important than the absolute value in assessing efficacy of treatment. Scoring will not be possible in all circumstances (e.g. cognitively impaired individuals, communication difficulties, altered level of consciousness) and in these circumstances behavioural cues will be more important in assessing pain.

3. Management

Analgesia should normally be introduced in an incremental way, considering timeliness, effectiveness and potential adverse events, and titrating to effect. However, it may be apparent from the assessment that it is appropriate to start with stronger analgesia (e.g. in apparent myocardial infarction or fractured long bones). Entonox should be supplied until the other drugs have had time to take effect and if the patient is still in pain, other analgesics administered. Administering analgesia in this step-wise, incremental, titratable manner, utilising a balanced analgesic approach, minimises the amount of potent analgesia that is required whilst still obtaining good analgesic effect with fewer side effects.

Any pain relief must be accompanied by careful explanation of the patient's condition and the pain relief methods being used.

Patients with chronic pain, including those receiving palliative care, may experience breakthrough pain despite their usual drug regime. They may require large doses of analgesics to have significant effect. If possible, contact should be made with the team caring for the patient.

4. Treating the Cause

Many conditions produce pain and it is vital to treat the cause of the pain, including underlying conditions. This will also help relieve the pain in many situations (e.g. giving GTN in cardiac pain or oxygen in sickle cell crisis).

NOTE: Most commonly, a patient requires a combination of pharmacological and non-pharmacological methods of pain relief (refer to Tables 1.1–1.3 and Figure 1.1). For example, entonox, morphine or ketamine may be required to enable a splint to be applied.

Pain Management in Adults

Table 1.1 – NON-PHARMACOLOGICAL METHODS OF PAIN RELIEF

Psychological

Fear and anxiety worsen pain; reassurance and explanation can go a long way towards alleviation of pain.

Distraction is a potent analgesic, commonly used in children, but may also apply to adults; simple conversation is the simplest form of distraction. It is important to keep the patient as comfortable as possible (e.g. warm).

Dressings

Burns dressings that may cool, such as those specifically designed for the task or cling film, can alleviate the pain. Burns should not be cooled for more than 20 minutes total time and care should be taken with large burns to prevent the development of hypothermia. However, analgesia should also be provided at the earliest opportunity.

Splintage

Simple splintage of fractures provides pain relief as well as minimising ongoing tissue damage, bleeding and other complications.

Table 1.2 – PHARMACOLOGICAL METHODS OF PAIN RELIEF (refer to specific drug protocols)

Inhalational analgesia

Entonox (50% nitrous oxide, 50% oxygen) is a good analgesic for adults who are able to self-administer and who can rapidly be taught to operate the demand valve. It is rapidly acting but has a very short half-life, so the analgesic effect wears off rapidly when inhalation is stopped. It can be used as the first analgesic whilst other pain relief is instituted. It can also be used as part of a balanced analgesic approach (several agents working at different sites to enable effective analgesia with fewer side effects), particularly during painful procedures such as splint application and patient movement.

Oral analgesia

Paracetamol and ibuprofen may be used in isolation or together for the management of mild to moderate pain when used in appropriate dosages. It is important to assess the presence of contra-indications to all drugs including simple analgesics. Non-steroidal anti-inflammatory drugs are responsible for large numbers of adverse events, because of their gastrointestinal and renal side effects and their effects on asthmatics. Some ambulance services may also choose to add a paracetamol/codeine combination and/or other opioid based oral analgesics (e.g. tramadol) to their formulary.

Parenteral and enteral analgesia

Morphine is approved for administration by paramedics. However, opioids are not as effective (especially when used in isolation) for the management of musculoskeletal type pain and may well lead to significant side effects before achieving adequate analgesia for skin and musculoskeletal pain and therefore other agents such as IV paracetamol should be considered (see medication sheets). As with other opioids morphine is reversed by naloxone. When administering opioids, facilities for maintaining airway, breathing, circulation and naloxone **MUST** be available. If clinically significant sedation or respiratory depression occurs following the administration of opioids the patient's ventilations should be assisted. Decisions to reverse the opioid's effect using an opioid antagonist such as naloxone should be made cautiously as this will return the patient to their pre-opioid pain level and may lead to even more sympathetic stimulation with associated cardiovascular and endocrine detrimental effects (e.g. hyperglycaemia).

The intravenous route has the advantage of rapid onset and the dose can be easily titrated against analgesic effect. In certain patients the intramuscular/subcutaneous routes may be used effectively and may be most appropriate for patient specific protocols for groups of patients such as end of life and sickle cell disease. Intraosseous pain relief should only be considered in very specific circumstances and local Trust guidelines should be followed.

Oral morphine is useful for less severe pain but has the disadvantage of delayed onset, some unpredictability of absorption and having to be given in a set dose. It has the advantage of avoiding the need for intravenous access. It is widely used for patients with mild/moderate pain from injuries such as forearm fractures and hip fractures. Those with severe pain are best treated with an intravenous preparation, augmented with entonox and other agents if required. In the event of break-through pain with palliative care, advice should be sought from the patient's care team whenever possible. Opioids are often required in sickle cell disease (a review is under way to look at the optimal analgesic treatment in sickle cell disease). There is limited evidence to suggest that metoclopramide is effective in relieving the nausea induced by opioids in hospital situations but this has not been evaluated in the pre-hospital environment where motion sickness may also contribute, however, other anti-emetic agents should be utilised when required and available (e.g. ondansetron).

Intranasal opioids (morphine, diamorphine and fentanyl)

Intranasal opioids are not currently approved for administration by paramedics. Although it has been suggested that they may be useful in the pre-hospital environment and are sometimes used by doctors, legal restrictions on the administration of opioids by paramedics have to be addressed before this will be possible. Intranasal opioid analgesia is becoming used more frequently in hospital and has the advantage of potent, rapid action without needing parenteral administration; however it may be logistically more difficult in the pre-hospital context.

Topical analgesia

In vulnerable adults or needle phobic adults, where venepuncture may be required in a non-urgent situation, tetracaine 4% gel/amethocaine can be applied to the skin overlying a suitable vein and the area covered with an occlusive dressing. Such an application takes about 30–40 minutes to work.

Methods of Pain Management which Require Appropriately Trained Pre-hospital Practitioners

These methods are included because it is necessary to know what can be done to reduce pain before hospital, if time and logistics allow. An appropriately trained practitioner should be called early to the scene if it is thought that such assistance may be necessary. Hospital personnel may not all have these skills.

Table 1.3 – METHODS THAT REQUIRE APPROPRIATELY TRAINED PRACTITIONERS

Ketamine analgesia/anaesthesia

Ketamine is particularly useful in entrapments where a person can be extricated with combined analgesic and sedative effects.

Ketamine is a parenteral analgesic, with a relatively small opioid action, that at higher doses is a general anaesthetic agent. It is particularly useful in serious trauma because it is less likely to significantly depress blood pressure, or respiration compared to other agents. Adults may experience unpleasant emergence phenomena if used in moderate to higher analgesic or anaesthetic dosages. Ketamine produces salivation so careful airway management is important, although unnecessary interference should be avoided as laryngospasm may occasionally occur. Atropine may be used with care concurrently to minimise hypersalivation.

Regional anaesthesia

There is limited room for regional nerve blocks because of the environment and the need to transport the patient to hospital in a timely manner. However, they can be effective in certain circumstances of severe pain and do not induce drowsiness or disorientation. Femoral nerve blocks may be useful and provide good analgesia for a lower limb injury such as a fractured femur. Clinicians undertaking regional anaesthesia must be suitably trained, prepared and experienced including the management of local anaesthetic toxicity.

KEY POINTS

Pain Management in Adults

- Pain should be treated as early as possible in all patients unless there is an exceptional specific reason not to.
- Pain relief does not affect later diagnosis.
- A balanced analgesic approach to pain management consists of treating the cause wherever possible, and analgesia involving psychological, physical and pharmacological interventions (more than one agent, when possible, in smaller and titrated doses to achieve better analgesia with fewer side effects by acting at different areas involving the pain pathways).
- Balanced analgesia remains the objective and should be tailored according to both patient and practitioner variables.
- All patients should have a pain score before and after each intervention.

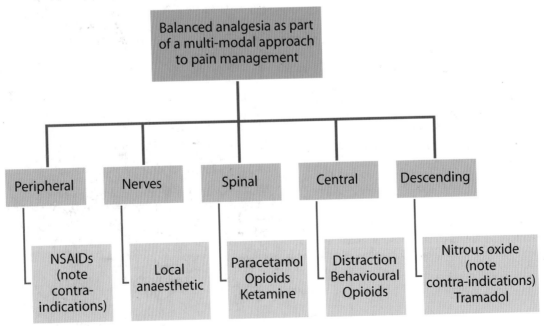

Figure 1.1 – Balanced approach to analgesia.

Pain Management in Children [20]

1. Introduction

All children in pain need analgesia, regardless of age or situation, and when appropriate, analgesia should be administered as soon as clinically possible after arriving on scene although this can be done en-route so as not to delay time-critical patients. There is no reason to delay relief of pain because of uncertainty with the definitive diagnosis.

Pain is one of the commonest symptoms in patients presenting to ambulance services.

Control of pain is important not only for humanitarian reasons but also because it may prevent deterioration of the child and allow better assessment.

There is no excuse for leaving a child in pain because of lack of necessary skills in the clinician. If necessary, suitable expertise should be sought to provide pain relief.

Pain is a multi-dimensional construct (see below).

Pain consists of several elements:

- Treatment of the underlying condition.
- Non-pharmacological methods including:
  - psychological support and explanation
  - physical methods e.g. splinting
- Pharmacological treatment.

Pain relief will depend on:

- Cause, site, severity and nature of the pain.
- Age of child.
- Experience/knowledge of the clinician.
- Distance from receiving unit.
- Available resources.

---

2. Assessment

An assessment should be made of the requirements of the child. Pain is a complex experience that is shaped by gender, cultural, environmental, social and personal factors, as well as prior pain experience. Thus the experience of pain is unique to the individual.

It is important to remember that the pain a child experiences cannot be objectively validated in the same way as other vital signs. Attempts to estimate the child's pain should be resisted, as this may lead to an underestimation of the child's experience. Several studies have shown that there is a poor correlation between the patient's pain rating and that of the health professionals, with the latter often underestimating the patient's pain.

Instead, ambulance clinicians need to seek and accept the child's self-report of their pain. This is reinforced by a popular and useful definition of pain: 'pain is whatever the experiencing person says it is, existing whenever they say it does'.

All children in pain should have their pain assessed for its location, nature, severity and duration. Any factors related to, or that exacerbate or improve, the pain should also be assessed.

Pain scoring

There is no validated method of pain scoring for children in the pre-hospital environment. It is suggested that, pending this, a method that has been validated in the paediatric emergency department (ED) setting is used. The Wong–Baker 'faces' (scoring 0 = no hurt, 1–2 = hurts little bit, 3–4 = hurts little more, 5–6 = hurts even more, 7–8 = hurts whole lot, 9–10 = hurts worst) (**refer to Appendix 1**) are useful for younger children. The FLACC scale is useful for preverbal children and may also be used for older children if needed (**refer to Appendix 2**).

The trend in the scores is more important than the absolute value in assessing efficacy of treatment. Scoring will not be possible in all circumstances (e.g. cognitively impaired individuals, and those with communication difficulties or altered level of consciousness) and in these circumstances behavioural cues will be more important in assessing pain.

3. Management

Analgesia should normally be introduced in an incremental way with each agent being titrated to effect, considering timeliness, effectiveness and potential adverse events. Utilising a balanced analgesic approach will often allow improved efficacy with reduced side effects. Generally this should always include the non-pharmacological methods of treatment as a starting point and background to all pharmacological therapy (refer to Tables 1.4–1.7).

However, it may be apparent from the assessment that it is appropriate to start with stronger analgesia because of the child's condition; for example, a child with bilateral fractured femurs is likely to require vascular access to provide circulatory replacement and will be in severe pain. It would, therefore, be inappropriate to only try paracetamol and ibuprofen and wait for them to work. Other agents including inhaled (entonox) and intravenous/transmucosal agents as part of a balanced analgesic approach would be indicated at an early stage (this may include paracetamol, opioids and ketamine when appropriate). This along with non-pharmacological methods of pain control would provide the best possible analgesia with a lower risk of side effects. However, in a child with a small superficial burn one might try paracetamol with or without ibuprofen and along with non-pharmacological methods, this may be adequate. The child will still require regular re-assessment and a change of approach if needed.

Entonox should be given using an appropriate technique until the other drugs have had time to take effect, and if the child is still in pain. Administering analgesia in this step-wise, incremental way minimises the amount of potent analgesia that is required while still achieving adequate analgesia with fewer side effects.

Any pain relief must be accompanied by careful explanation, involving the child, where possible, and the carer. Include details of the child's condition, the pain relief methods being used, and any possible side effects.

Pain Management in Children

Table 1.4 – NON-PHARMACOLOGICAL METHODS OF PAIN RELIEF

Psychological

Fear and anxiety worsen pain and a child-friendly environment (e.g. removing equipment which may cause fear and having toys or child-friendly pictures around) may go a long way towards alleviation of pain as may keeping the patient comfortable (e.g. warm).

The presence of a parent has been shown to reduce the unpleasantness of hospital emergency procedures more than any other single factor and there is no reason why this should not be true in the pre-hospital setting.

Distraction (toys, stories, games etc.) is a potent analgesic – whatever is to hand may be used, but there is no substitute for forward planning.

Dressings

Burns dressings that may cool, such as those specifically designed for the task or cling film, can alleviate the pain in the burnt or scalded child. Burns should not be cooled for more than 20 minutes total time and care should be taken with large burns to prevent the development of hypothermia.

Splintage

Simple splintage of fractures provides pain relief as well as minimising ongoing tissue trauma, bleeding and other complications.

NOTE: These should be part of all other methods of pain relief.

Table 1.5 – PHARMACOLOGICAL METHODS OF PAIN RELIEF (refer to specific drug protocols)

Topical analgesia

It is no longer acceptable to consider the pre-hospital portion of the child's treatment in isolation, although the pre-hospital context must be taken into account with regards to prioritising of care, skill-sets and time-line. The child is on a pathway of care, from the pre-hospital scene to the most appropriate setting within definitive care. Care that can be improved by one sector (e.g. pre-hospital) to enhance the quality of another (e.g. hospital cannulation) should be provided. Local anaesthetic agents such as **tetracaine gel 4%/amethocaine** can be applied to the skin overlying a suitable vein and the area covered with an occlusive dressing if it is thought likely that the child will require venepuncture on arrival in hospital. Such an application may take about 30–40 minutes to work.

Oral analgesia

Paracetamol and **ibuprofen** may be used in isolation or together for the management of mild to moderate pain as long as appropriate dosages of both are utilised.

Oral morphine solution may also prove very effective in the child with moderate to severe pain such as a fractured forearm (although in isolation this is not the ideal class of drug for musculoskeletal pain), but has the disadvantage of delayed onset, some unpredictability of absorption and having to be given in a set dose. It has the advantage of avoiding the need for intravenous access. Those with severe pain are best treated with an intravenous preparation, augmented with entonox if required.

Inhalational analgesia

Entonox (50% nitrous oxide, 50% oxygen) is a good analgesic for children who are able to self-administer and who can rapidly be taught to operate the demand valve. It is rapid acting but has a very short half-life, so the analgesic effect wears off rapidly when inhalation is stopped. It can be used as the first analgesic whilst other pain relief is instituted. It can also be used in conjunction with morphine, particularly during painful procedures such as splint application and patient movement. Quite young children can use the system providing they can be taught to operate the demand valve, and the child's fear of the noise of the gas flow and the mask can be overcome. Flavoured (e.g. bubblegum) clear masks may help the child overcome the fear.

Parenteral and enteral analgesia

Morphine remains an important component for balanced analgesia and can be administered intravenously, intraosseously, and orally (refer to morphine drug guidelines). Opioid analgesics should be given intravenously rather than intramuscularly to avoid erratic absorption when possible. When used in isolation for musculoskeletal pain, there may be an increased risk of side effects before achieving adequate analgesia, emphasising the need for a balanced analgesic approach. Therefore other agents such as IV paracetamol should be considered (see medication sheets).

As with the other opioids, morphine is reversed by naloxone. When administering opioids to children, ability to maintain airway/breathing/circulation and naloxone **MUST** be available and the required dose calculated in case urgent reversal is necessary. If clinically significant sedation or respiratory depression occurs following the administration of opioids, the child's ventilation should be assisted. Decisions to reverse the opioid effects using an opioid antagonist such as naloxone should be made cautiously as this may return the child to their pre-opioid pain level depending on dosage of naloxone given, which should therefore be titrated to desired effect.

Intranasal opioids (morphine, diamorphine and fentanyl) are not currently approved for paramedic administration. Intranasal opioid analgesia is becoming used more frequently in hospital and has the advantage of potent, rapid action without needing parenteral administration. However, it is fairly difficult to prepare the appropriate dose and concentration in the pre-hospital context.

In certain patients the subcutaneous routes may be used effectively, and these may be most appropriate for patient specific protocols for groups of patients such as end of life and sickle cell disease. In the event of break-through pain with palliative care, advice should be sought from the patient's care team whenever possible.

There is no evidence that metoclopramide is effective in relieving nausea induced by opioids. Children have a significant risk of dystonic reactions with metoclopramide and therefore it is not advised in these circumstances.

Other anti-emetics (e.g. ondansetron) can be used for opioid-induced nausea and vomiting.

4. Pain Relief which Requires Appropriately Trained Practitioners

These methods are included because it is necessary to know what can be done to reduce pain in children before hospital, if time and logistics allow. A suitably licensed and trained pre-hospital practitioner should be called early to the scene if it is thought that such assistance may be necessary. Hospital personnel may not all have these skills.

Table 1.6 – PAIN RELIEF WHICH REQUIRES APPROPRIATELY TRAINED PRACTITIONERS

Ketamine analgesia/anaesthesia

Ketamine is particularly useful in entrapments where a child can be extricated with combined analgesic and sedative effects. At present only doctors and suitably trained and authorised paramedics may carry ketamine.

Ketamine has a predominantly non-opioid mechanism of action. At higher doses it can be used as a general anaesthetic agent. It is particularly useful in serious trauma because it may not significantly depress blood pressure or respiration depending on the particular patient (acute and chronic comorbidity) and the time since injury.

Older children in particular may experience unpleasant emergence phenomena but these tend to be less common in the young especially if appropriate analgesic doses are utilised and titrated to effect. Ketamine in higher doses (not often a problem with appropriate analgesic doses titrated to effect) produces salivation so careful airway management is important, although unnecessary interference should be avoided as laryngospasm may occasionally occur. Atropine may be used with care concurrently to minimise hypersalivation.

Regional anaesthesia

There is very limited room for regional nerve blocks because of the environment and the need to transport the child to hospital in a timely manner. However, they can be effective in certain circumstances of severe pain and do not induce drowsiness or disorientation. Femoral nerve blocks may be useful and provide good analgesia for a fractured femur. Clinicians undertaking regional anaesthesia must be suitably trained, prepared, experienced and fully understand and have the mechanism to treat local anaesthetic toxicity in the pre-hospital environment.

Table 1.7 – PRE-HOSPITAL ANALGESIC DRUGS USED IN CHILDREN

Drug	Topical	Pain severity	Advantages	Disadvantages
Tetracaine 4% gel	Topical	N/A	Reduces pain of venepuncture	Takes about 30–40 minutes to work
Paracetamol	Oral (the rectal route is no longer recommended for analgesia)	Mild–moderate (may be opioid sparing when used for more severe pain as better efficacy for musculoskeletal pain than opioids alone)	Readily accessable and well tolerated orally. Well accepted antipyretic	Slow action when given orally. Inadequate and unpredictable plasma levels if given rectally
Ibuprofen	Oral (other IV NSAIDs are available but currently not available for paramedic use)	Mild–moderate (may be opioid sparing when used for more severe pain as better efficacy for musculoskeletal pain than opioids alone)	Moderately good analgesic, antipyretic and anti-inflammatory	Slow action. May cause bronchospasm in asthmatics. Caution in trauma and patients with regards to platelet and renal function
Entonox	Inhaled	Mild–moderate (may be opioid sparing when used for more severe pain as better efficacy for musculoskeletal pain than opioids alone)	Quick, dose self-regulating. Relative contra-indications are important	Fear of mask. Understanding, coordination and cooperation required. (Demand valves for younger children becoming more available. Cannot use free-flow if not scavenging in confined space, e.g. ambulance.)
Oral morphine	Oral	Moderate	Good analgesic for minor/moderate pain particularly of a visceral nature	May need to adjust dose of IV morphine if given subsequently. Reduced oral bioavailability. Slow action
Morphine	Intravenous Intraosseous	Severe	Rapid onset. Reversed with naloxone (although requires care). Some euphoria	Not ideal as solo agent when used for musculoskeletal pain. Need access. Respiratory depression, vomiting. Controlled drug
Diamorphine[a]	Intranasal Intravenous Intraosseous	Moderate–severe pain particularly of visceral nature	Intranasal – quick and effective although logistically difficult in pre-hospital practice. Best efficacy if used with other agents (e.g. paracetamol)	As for morphine if given IV. More euphoria. Intranasal not currently approved for paramedics
Ketamine[a]	Intravenous Intramuscular Oral	Severe pain from either musculoskeletal or visceral aetiologies (excluding acute coronary syndromes)	Can be increased to general anaesthesia in experienced hands. Less respiratory and cardiovascular depression than other strong analgesic/anaesthetic drugs. Concerns re. raised ICP less clinically relevant than previously thought	Emergence phenomena, salivation, occasional laryngospasm (usually with higher doses, therefore small doses 0.1 mg/kg/dose for analgesia and titrate to effect). Comes in three different concentrations which may lead to confusion

[a] Currently not approved for general paramedic administration; doctor and suitably trained and authorised paramedic administration only.

Pain Management in Children

- All children in pain need analgesia.
- The method of pain relief used will depend on the cause, site, severity, nature of the pain and age of child.
- Analgesia should be introduced incrementally and titrated to effect.
- Pain scoring faces and the FLACC scale are useful for use with young children.
- A balanced analgesic approach to pain management consists of treating the cause wherever possible, and analgesia involving psychological, physical and pharmacological interventions (more than one agent, when possible, in smaller and titrated doses to achieve better analgesia with fewer side effects by acting at different areas involving the pain pathways).
- Balanced analgesia remains the objective and should be tailored according to both patient and practitioner variables.

APPENDIX 1 – The Wong–Baker FACES Pain Rating Scale

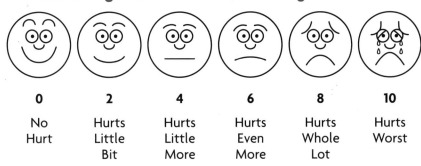

0	2	4	6	8	10
No Hurt	Hurts Little Bit	Hurts Little More	Hurts Even More	Hurts Whole Lot	Hurts Worst

This rating scale is recommended for persons aged three years and older.

Instructions: Point to each face using the words to describe the pain intensity. Ask the child to choose the face that best describes their own pain and record the appropriate number.

Explain to the child that each face is for a person who feels happy because he has no pain (hurt) or sad because he has some or a lot of pain.

Face 0 is very happy because he doesn't hurt at all.
Face 2 hurts just a little bit.
Face 4 hurts a little more.
Face 6 hurts even more.
Face 8 hurts a whole lot.
Face 10 hurts as much as you can imagine, although you don't have to be crying to feel this bad.

Ask the child to choose the face that best describes how they are feeling.

From Hockenberry MJ, Wilson D, Winkelstein ML: Wong's Essentials of Pediatric Nursing, ed. 7, St. Louis, 2005, p. 1259. Used with permission. Copyright, Mosby.

APPENDIX 2 – The FLACC Scale

The **Face, Legs, Activity, Cry, Consolability scale** or **FLACC scale** is a measurement used to assess pain for children up to the age of seven years or individuals who are unable to communicate their pain. The scale is scored on a range of 0–10 with 0 representing no pain. The scale has five criteria which are each assigned a score of 0, 1 or 2.

Table 1.8 – THE FLACC SCALE

Criteria	Score - 0	Score - 1	Score - 2
Face	No particular expression or smile	Occasional grimace or frown, withdrawn, uninterested	Frequent to constant quivering chin, clenched jaw
Legs	Normal position or relaxed	Uneasy, restless, tense	Kicking, or legs drawn up
Activity	Lying quietly, normal position, moves easily	Squirming, shifting back and forth, tense	Arched, rigid or jerking
Cry	No cry (awake or asleep)	Moans or whimpers, occasional complaint	Crying steadily, screams or sobs, frequent complaints
Consolability	Content, relaxed	Reassured by occasional touching, hugging or being talked to, distractible	Difficult to console or comfort

1. Introduction

- Safeguarding, promoting welfare and protecting children from significant harm is reliant on effective joint working between agencies and professionals.

- **Duty of care** – as a healthcare worker who may come into contact with children, you have a duty to report concerns about abuse. If you do not report the abuse you may be putting the victim at greater risk. You may also discourage them from disclosing again, as they may feel they were not believed. This may put other people at risk.

- All partners who work with children including local authorities, police, health service, courts, professionals, the voluntary sector and individual members of local communities share the responsibility for safeguarding and promoting the welfare of children and young people. It is vital that all partners are aware of, and appreciate, the role that each of them plays in this area – for further information on the roles and responsibilities of each partner refer to *Working Together to Safeguard Children 2010*.

- Social services and the police have statutory authority and a responsibility to investigate allegations or suspicions about child abuse.

- Ambulance clinicians are often the first professionals on scene and therefore may identify initial concerns regarding a child's welfare and be able to alert social care, the police, the GP, or other appropriate health professional, in line with locally agreed procedures. Accurate recording of events/actions may be crucial to subsequent enquiries.

- The role of the Ambulance Service is not to investigate suspicions but to ensure that any suspicion is passed to the appropriate agency (e.g. social care or the police). Ambulance clinicians need to be aware of child abuse issues and the aim of this guideline is to:

  - Ensure all staff are aware of, and can recognise, cases of suspected child abuse, or children at risk of significant harm and provide guidance enabling operational and control staff to assess and report cases of suspected child abuse.
  - Ensure that all staff involved in a case of suspected abuse are aware of the possible outcome and of any subsequent actions.
  - Further information on local procedures can be obtained from the named professional for safeguarding within individual Ambulance Trusts. The contact details for the named professional for safeguarding can be obtained from ambulance control.

2. Significant Harm

All children have the right:

- To be protected from significant harm/ill-treatment.[a]
- To be protected from impairment of their health[b] and development.[c]
- To grow up in circumstances consistent with the provision of safe and effective care.

The maltreatment of children, physically, emotionally, sexually or through neglect can have a major impact on their health, well-being and development.

There are no absolute criteria on which to rely when judging what constitutes significant harm. In some cases a single traumatic event may constitute significant harm, but more generally it is a compilation of significant events, both acute and long-standing, which interrupt, change, or damage the child's physical and psychological development. Considerations include:

- The degree and extent of physical harm.
- The duration and frequency of abuse and neglect.
- The extent of premeditation.
- The degree of threat, coercion, sadism, and bizarre or unusual elements.
- In order to understand and identify significant harm, consider:
  - the nature of harm, in terms of maltreatment or failure to provide adequate care
  - the impact on the child's health and development
  - the child's development within the context of the family and wider environment
  - any special needs, such as a medical condition, communication impairment or disability, that may affect the child's development and care within the family and the capacity of parents to meet adequately the child's needs.
- Abuse and neglect are forms of maltreatment and children may suffer as a result of a deliberate act, or failure on the part of a parent or carer to act to prevent harm – descriptions of abuse and neglect are detailed in Table 1.10.
- Children may be abused in a family or in an institutional or community setting, by those known to them or, more rarely, by a stranger.
- Children in a care setting can be subject to exploitation (e.g. for prostitution).

Children in need

- Children are defined as being 'in need' when:
  - they are unlikely to reach or maintain a satisfactory level of health or development
  - their health and development will be significantly impaired, without the provision of services (section 17 (10) of the Children Act 1989)
  - they have a disability.
- Local authorities have a duty to safeguard and promote the welfare of children in need.

3. Recognition of Abuse

Ambulance clinicians may receive information or make observations which suggest that a child has been abused or is at risk of harm, for example:

- The nature of the illness/injury.
- The account given for the illness/injury may be inconsistent with what is observed.

---

[a] Harm means ill-treatment or the impairment of health or development, including, for example, impairment suffered from seeing or hearing the ill-treatment of another. Ill-treatment includes sexual abuse and forms of ill-treatment which are not physical.

[b] Health means physical or mental health.

[c] Development means physical, intellectual, emotional, social or behavioural development.

- Observation of hazards in the home.
- Child(ren) has been locked in a room.
- Signs of distress shown by other children in the home.
- Observations regarding the condition of other children or adults in the household (e.g. an environment where domestic violence has taken place). In the case of domestic dispute between adults, the presence of children in the household creates a need to notify even if the child(ren) was not injured.
- Parents or carers who seek medical care from a number of sources.

Non-accidental injury

- When assessing an injury in any child, you should be aware of the possibility of the injury being non-accidental and you should consider this possibility in every case, even if you promptly dismiss the idea.
- For an injury to be accidental it should have a clear, credible and acceptable history and the findings should be consistent with the history and with the development and abilities of the child.

Suspicions of abuse should be raised by:

- Any injury in a non-mobile baby.
- Accidents/injuries in unusual places (e.g. the buttocks, trunk, inner thighs).
- Extensive injuries or signs of both recent and old injuries.
- Small deep burns in unusual places.
- Repeated burns and scalds.
- 'Glove and stocking' burns.
- Poor state of clothing, cleanliness and/or nutrition.
- Delayed reporting of the injury.
- Inappropriate sexual knowledge for the child's age.
- Overt sexual approaches to other children or adults.
- Fear of particular people or situations (e.g. bath time or bedtime).
- Drug and alcohol abuse.
- Suicide attempts and self-injury.
- Running away and fire-setting.
- Environmental factors and family situations (e.g. domestic violence, drug or alcohol abuse, learning disabilities).

The following symptoms should give cause for concern and further assessment:

- Soreness, discharge or unexplained bleeding in the genital area.
- Chronic vaginal infections.
- Bruising, grazes or bites to the genital or breast area.
- Sexually transmitted diseases.
- Pregnancy, especially when the identity of the father is vague.

When assessing an injured child, you should use your clinical knowledge regarding what level of accidental injury would be appropriate for their stage of development. Although stages of development vary (e.g. children may crawl or walk at different ages), injuries can broadly be divided between mobile and non-mobile children.

Non-mobile Babies

- Any injury in a non-mobile baby must be considered carefully and have a credible explanation if it is to be considered accidental.
- Healthy babies do not bruise or break their bones easily. They do not bruise themselves with their fists or toys, bruise themselves by lying against the bars of a cot, or acquire bruises on the legs when they are held for a nappy change.
- Bruising on the ears, face, neck, trunk and buttocks is particularly suspicious. A torn frenulum (behind the upper lip) is rarely accidental in babies, and bleeding from the mouth of a baby should always be regarded as suspicious.

Fractures

- Fractures may not be obvious on observation and the baby may present only with crying on handling. Often a fracture will not be diagnosed until an X-ray is performed. Fractures in babies are seldom caused by 'rough handling' or putting their legs through the bars of the cot. Babies rarely fracture their skull after a fall from a bed or a chair. Fractures in non-mobile infants should be assessed by an experienced paediatrician to exclude non-accidental injury (refer to Table 1.9 for types of fractures).

Table 1.9 – TYPES OF BONE FRACTURES

Greenstick

The bones bend rather than break. This is a very common accidental injury in children.

Transverse

The break goes across the bone and occurs when there is a direct blow or a direct force on the end of the bone (e.g. a fall on the hand may break the forearm bones or the distal humerus).

Spiral or oblique

A fracture line which goes right around the bone or obliquely across it is due to a twisting force, which may be a feature in non-accidental injuries.

Metaphyseal

Occur at the extreme ends of the bone and are usually only confirmed radiologically. These are caused by a strong twisting force.

Skull

These must be consistent with the history and explanation given. Complex (branched), depressed or fractures at the back of the skull are suspect of abuse.

Rib

These do not occur accidentally, except in a severe crushing injury. Any other cause is highly suspicious of non-accidental injury.

Shaking injuries

- When small babies are shaken violently their head and limb movements cannot be controlled, causing brain damage and haemorrhage within the skull.

- Finger bruising on the chest may indicate that a baby has been held tightly and shaken. These babies usually present with collapse or respiratory problems and the diagnosis is only made on further detailed assessment.

Burns and scalds

- See below.

Mobile Babies and Toddlers

Bruising

- It is normal for toddlers to have accidental bruises on the shins, elbows and forehead. Bruises in unusual areas such as the back, upper arms and abdomen do not tend to occur accidentally.

- Bruising caused by a hand slap leaves a characteristic pattern of 'stripes' representing the imprint of fingers. Forceful gripping leaves small round bruises corresponding to the position of the fingertips. 'Tramline' bruising is caused by a belt or stick and shows as lines of bruising with a white patch in-between. Bites result in small bruises forming part or all of a circle.

Burns and scalds

- Burns are caused by the application to the skin of dry heat and the depth of the burn will depend on the temperature of the object and the length of time it is in contact with the skin.

- Abusive burns are frequently small and deep, and may show the outline of the object (e.g. the soleplate of an iron), whereas accidental burns rarely do so because the child will pull away in response to pain.

- Cigarette burns are not common. They are round, deep and have a red flare around a flat brown crust. These burns usually leave a scar.

- Scalds are caused by steam or hot liquids. Accidental scalds may be extensive but show splash marks unlike the sharp edges of damage done when the child is dunked in hot water (although splash marks may also feature in a non-accidental burn indicating that the child had tried to escape hot water). The glove and stocking pattern of burns on the arms and legs is typical of non-accidental injury. The head, face, neck, shoulders and front of the chest are the areas affected when a child pulls over a kettle accidentally.

Fractures

- Children's bones tend to bend rather than break and require considerable force to damage them. There are various kinds of fractures (refer to Table 1.9), depending on the direction and strength of the force which caused them.

- Unless there is an obvious bony deformity, bony injuries may not be apparent on initial clinical assessment. A clear history and appreciation of the mechanism of injury are crucial parts of the initial assessment and must be clearly documented.

Deliberate poisoning and attempted suffocation

- These are very difficult to assess and may need a period of close observation in hospital. Deliberate poisoning, such as might be found in a child in whom illness is fabricated or induced by carers with parenting responsibilities (factitious or induced illness), may be suspected when a child has repeated puzzling illnesses, usually of sudden onset. The signs include unusual drowsiness, apnoeic attacks, vomiting, diarrhoea and fits.

Older Children and Adolescents

- If the injury is accidental, older children will give a very clear and detailed account of how it happened. The detail will be missing if they have been told what to say.

- Overdosing and other self-harm injuries must be taken seriously in this age group, as they may indicate sexual or other abuse (such as exploitation).

Who is Vulnerable to Abuse?

Although any child can potentially be a victim of abuse, there are some groups of children who may be particularly vulnerable. Factors which may put a child at increased risk of harm include both child and parental factors (adapted from Child Protection Companion, RCPCH 2006).

Child factors:

- Prematurity.
- Feeding difficulties.
- Disability (including learning difficulties).
- Severe physical illnesses or sensory impairments.
- Children with special needs, for example, those who are deaf or autistic. These children may demonstrate challenging behaviour, which may or may not be as a result of abuse.
- Chronic illness.
- Children who are looked after.

Parental factors:

- Parental unavailability for whatever reason increases the risk to the child of all forms of abuse, especially neglect and emotional abuse. Specific consideration of the effects of the parent's problem on the children must be made, whatever the circumstances of presentation. Sources of stress within families may have a negative impact on a child's health, development or well-being, either directly or because they affect the capacity of parents to respond to their child's needs. Sources of stress may include social exclusion, domestic violence, unstable mental illness of a parent or carer, or drug and alcohol misuse. Parents who appear overanxious about their child when there is no sign of illness or injury may be signalling their inability to cope.

- Parental factors which might have a negative impact on parenting capacity include:
  - learning difficulties
  - mental health problems
  - substance abuse
  - domestic violence

- chronic ill health
- physical disability
- unemployment or poverty
- homelessness/frequent moves
- social isolation
- young, unsupported parents
- parents with poor role models of their own.

4. Special Circumstances

Individuals who pose a risk to children

- Once an individual has been sentenced and identified as presenting a risk of harm to children, agencies have a responsibility to work collaboratively to monitor and manage the risk of harm to others.

- Where an offender is given a community sentence, Offender Managers or Youth Offending Team workers will monitor the individual's risk of harm to others and their behaviour, and liaise with partner agencies as appropriate.

- Multi-Agency Public Protection Arrangements (MAPPA) should be in place to enable agencies to work together within a statutory framework for managing risk of harm to the public.

Disabled children

- Abuse may be difficult to separate from symptoms of disability (e.g. increase in seizures in a child with epilepsy if anticonvulsants are withheld). Induced and fabricated illness may be even more difficult to recognise because the child may have coexistent diagnoses. Important points to remember about abuse of disabled children are:

  - it may be more common than abuse of non-disabled children but evidence for this is poor
  - it may be under reported
  - children may have difficulty communicating their abuse
  - abuse may compound pre-existing disability, or be the cause of the disability
  - all forms of abuse are seen including neglect and sexual abuse
  - it is easy to fail to recognise abuse in disabled children by making too many allowances for the disability as a cause of problems
  - be aware that professionals can be drawn into collusion with families.

- These children are at risk of achieving poor outcomes. Ambulance clinicians need to be aware of the role they can play in recognition of these children, identifying their particular needs and preventing significant harm. In the current multicultural society of the United Kingdom, it is important to recognise that there may be children and families in need of skilled interpreters. You should also recognise the differences that may exist in child-rearing practices in minority groups.

Special circumstances for consideration

  - **Children and young people living away from home** – it has been estimated that 4% of foster carers/placements are abusive to children. Many looked-after children and young people that live independently have been abused or neglected prior to going into care. This is a particular group where assessment may be made more difficult, because of

pre-existing symptoms and behaviour. There should be a low threshold in seeking advice from experienced professionals in these circumstances (e.g. designated/named professional).

  - **Asylum-seeking children or refugees, both with families and unaccompanied** – the importance of having skilled interpreters in assessment of these children cannot be over-emphasised. The children's behaviour on entering the country may already have been influenced by previous experience. It is important to remember their general health needs and the families will need help in accessing services.

  - **Children with troubled parent(s)** (see also **Parental factors**, p. 18) – these include children of substance misusing parents, children living with domestic violence, children whose parents have chronic mental or physical health problems, children whose parents have a learning disability, children with a parent in prison. Effects on the child are profound and include fearfulness, withdrawal, anxious behaviour, lack of self-confidence and social skills, difficulties in forming relationships, sleep disturbance, non-attendance at school, aggression, bullying, post-traumatic stress disorder, behaviour suggestive of ADHD.

The following children may also have unmet health needs – low immunisation levels, poor dental health and non-attendance at clinic appointments.

  - **Children in the armed forces** – extra strains are placed upon the families engendered by frequent moves, frequent changes of school, separation of parents by the nature of the job and separation from immediate support from family and friends.

  - **Children of travelling families** – are subjected to the same problems because of frequent moves. They may also suffer from poor health, poor access to primary healthcare and vaccinations, in addition to poor living conditions.

  - **Runaway children and prostitution** – many runaway children may already have been the subject of abuse and are at risk of exploitation and prostitution. Children of troubled families are more likely to be involved in prostitution than other groups. They also are at risk of child trafficking for sexual exploitation.

  - **Children as young carers** – neglect and emotional abuse may be part and parcel of the difficulties of taking on parental responsibilities and a caring role at a young age. Young carers lose out on normal childhood experiences (e.g. school attendance, peer groups).

5. Procedure

If physical, sexual, or emotional abuse or neglect is suspected, follow local procedures; information can be obtained from the named professional for safeguarding within individual Ambulance Trusts. Ambulance clinicians may obtain contact information from ambulance control.

5.1 If the child is the patient

- The first priority is the health and safety of the child. Ambulance clinicians should follow the usual **ABCDE** and **<C>ABCDE** assessment (**refer to medical and trauma overview guidelines**). Children with significant injury should be transferred to further care without delay.

- Where a child is thought to be at immediate risk, they should be referred to the police as an emergency by contacting ambulance control for a 999 response.

In all circumstances:

- Limit questions to those of routine history taking, asking questions only in relation to the injury or for clarification of what is being said. It is important to stop questioning when your suspicions are clarified. Unnecessary questioning or probing may affect the credibility of subsequent evidence.

- Accept the explanations given and do not make any suggestions to the child as to how an injury or incident may have happened.

- Care must be taken not to directly accuse parents or carers of abuse as this may result in a refusal to transfer to further care and place the child at further risk. However, you should always work in partnership with parents as far as possible, and inform them of your concerns and the need to share these with the statutory agencies, unless to do so would put the child or others at greater risk of harm. Professional judgement is crucial as to what information should be shared with parents.

- Any allegation of abuse by a child is an important indicator and should always be taken seriously – it is important to listen to the 'voice of the child' and what they are saying. Do not ask probing questions.

- Adult responses can influence how able a child feels to reveal the full extent of the abuse. Listen and react appropriately to instil confidence. It is important to note that children may only tell a small part of their experience initially.

- It is important to make an accurate record of events and actions. Write down exactly what you have been told. The child's first language may not be English and care must be taken not to use family members or carers as interpreters in cases of suspected abuse. Take note of any inconsistency in history and any delay in calling for assistance.

- On arrival inform the receiving staff and the most senior member of nursing staff on duty of your concerns or suspicions. When reporting suspected abuse, the emphasis must be on shared professional responsibility and immediate communication.

- Complete safeguarding documentation/report as per local procedures; complete in private if possible. Follow local/Trust protocols/guidelines.

- Ambulance clinicians must report suspected child abuse to the relevant statutory bodies (e.g. social care

and the police), but they do not have a statutory duty to investigate it.

- Where a practitioner feels that their concerns have not been taken up, they have a duty to escalate their concerns to a higher level by discussing this with their line manager, a more experienced colleague or named/designated doctor or nurse.

5.2 If the child is not the patient

- If the circumstances are suspicious, the ambulance clinician(s) should consider the implications of leaving the child.

- If the child is accompanying another person (e.g. a parent/carer) who is being conveyed, the ambulance clinician(s) should inform ED staff of their concerns.

- If no one is transferred to hospital, follow local/Trust protocols/guidelines and inform them of the incident/concerns at the earliest opportunity.

- Complete safeguarding documentation/report as per local procedures; complete in private if possible. Follow local/Trust protocols/guidelines.

5.3 Allegations against ambulance staff

- An allegation made by a child against a member of ambulance staff is no different to an allegation made against any other healthcare professional and the appropriate procedures should be followed, that is a referral to social care or the police. In other words, a child protection inquiry must follow such allegations.

- The member of staff who is alleged to have abused the child will have to report the allegation to his line manager who should follow employment procedures, that is suspend the member of staff while investigations are conducted. There should be close liaison between the police doing the investigation and the line manager who should be guided by the police as to how much information about the inquiry should be relayed to the member of staff. There will also need to be a support system in place for the member of staff.

Further Reading

The National Service Framework for Children, Young People and Maternity Services, which sets out a ten-year plan to stimulate long-term and sustained improvement in children's health and well-being.

There are many other documents which are important to inform strategy and delivery of services. These are referenced on the Government's website http://www.dcsf.gov.uk/everychildmatters/.

KEY POINTS

Safeguarding children

- **The safety and welfare of the child is paramount.**
- **There is a duty to report concerns. Staff should not investigate suspicions themselves.**
- **Be aware of the special circumstances that the child is in which may increase the risk of abuse.**
- **Police should be involved where there may be an immediate risk to the child.**
- **Staff should document the circumstances, giving rise to their concern as soon as possible.**

Table 1.10 – EXAMPLES OF TYPES OF ABUSE AND NEGLECT

Emotional abuse

The persistent emotional maltreatment of a child so as to cause severe and persistent adverse effects on the child's emotional development. It may:

- Involve conveying to children that they are worthless or unloved, inadequate, or valued only insofar as they meet the needs of another person.
- Involve not giving the child opportunities to express their views, deliberately silencing them or 'making fun' of what they say or how they communicate.
- Feature age or developmentally inappropriate expectations being imposed on children (e.g. interactions that are beyond the child's developmental capability), as well as overprotection and limitation of exploration and learning, or preventing the child participating in normal social interaction.
- Involve seeing or hearing the ill-treatment of another.
- Involve serious bullying (including cyberbullying), causing children frequently to feel frightened or in danger, or the exploitation or corruption of children. Some level of emotional abuse is involved in all types of maltreatment of a child, though it may occur alone.

Emotional abuse alone can be difficult to recognise as the child may be physically well cared-for and the home in good condition. Some factors which may indicate emotional abuse are:

- If the child is constantly denigrated before others.
- If the child is constantly given the impression that the parents are disappointed in them.
- If the child is blamed for things that go wrong or is told they may be unloved/sent away.
- If the parent does not offer any love or attention (e.g. leaves them alone for a long time).
- If the parent is obsessive about cleanliness, tidiness etc.
- If the parent has unrealistic expectations of the child (e.g. educational achievement/toilet training).
- If the child is either bullying others or being bullied themselves.
- If there is an atmosphere of domestic violence, adults with mental health problems or a history of drug or alcohol abuse.

Sexual abuse

Sexual abuse involves forcing or enticing a child or young person to take part in sexual activities, not necessarily involving a high level of violence, whether or not the child is aware of what is happening.

Both girls and boys of all age groups are at risk. The sexual abuse of a child is often planned and chronic. A large proportion of sexually abused children have no physical signs, and it is therefore necessary to be alert to behavioural and emotional factors that may indicate abuse. Although some children are abused by strangers, most are abused by someone known to them. Some are abused by other children, including siblings, who may also be at risk of abuse. The majority of abusers are male, although occasionally women abuse children sexually or cooperate with men in the abusing behaviour.

The activities may involve physical contact, including assault by penetration (e.g. rape or oral sex) or non-penetrative acts such as masturbation, kissing, rubbing and touching outside of clothing. They may include non-contact activities, such as involving children in looking at, or in the production of, sexual images, watching sexual activities, encouraging children to behave in sexually inappropriate ways, or grooming a child in preparation for abuse (including via the internet).

Physical abuse

Physical abuse may involve hitting, shaking, throwing, poisoning, burning or scalding, suffocating, or otherwise causing physical harm. Physical harm may also be caused when a parent or carer fabricates the symptoms of, or deliberately induces ill-health; this situation is commonly described using terms such as 'factitious or induced illness'.

Neglect

Neglect is more difficult to recognise and define than physical abuse, but its effects can be life-long. Impairment of growth, intelligence, physical ability and life expectancy are only a few of the effects of neglect in childhood.

The persistent failure to meet a child's basic physical and/or psychological needs is likely to result in the serious impairment of the child's health or development.

A neglected or abused infant may show signs of poor attachment. They may lack the sense of security to explore, and appear unhappy and whining. There may be little sign of attachment behaviour, and the child may move aimlessly round a room or creep quietly into corners.

Neglect may occur during pregnancy as a result of maternal substance abuse. Once a child is born, neglect may involve a parent or carer failing to:

- Provide adequate food, clothing and shelter (including exclusion from home or abandonment).
- Protect a child from physical and emotional harm or danger.
- Ensure adequate supervision (including the use of inadequate care-givers).
- Ensure access to appropriate medical care or treatment.
- Respond to the child's basic emotional needs.

In pre-school and school-age children, indicators of neglect may include poor attention span, aggressive behaviour and poor cooperative play. Indiscriminate friendly behaviour to unknown adults is often a feature of children who are deprived of emotional affection. Other signs include repetitive rocking or other self-stimulating behaviour. Personal hygiene may be poor because of physical neglect, and this may lead to rejection by peers.

Sexual Assault [30–39]

1. Introduction

- Sexual assault is extremely distressing; managing such cases demands sensitive, non-judgemental medical and emotional care and an awareness of the forensic requirements.

- Patients are likely to be very distressed about the events surrounding sexual assault. They may not want to involve anybody else, and may not consent to disclosure of information to other parties such as the police. Do not judge, or give the appearance of judging the patient. Be kind and considerate, and allow the patient space, and as much choice about options for their treatment as possible. They may feel worthless, guilty and humiliated; dominant and controlling behaviour will intensify these feelings.

- Alcohol and drugs such as rohypnol may also be involved.

- It may be appropriate for the patient to be accompanied by another person. The patient may be anxious when left alone with a person of the same sex as the assailant. On the other hand, they may be reassured by the presence of a professional person. The wishes of the patient must be considered and attempts made to reassure them and make them feel safe.

- **Further care** – it is important to encourage all victims of sexual assault to attend a specialised unit for forensic examination, and inform the police. Both will be able to provide physical, medical and emotional support.

- In cases of sexual assault in vulnerable adults and children **refer to suspected abuse of vulnerable adults and recognition of abuse and safeguarding children**.

2. Incidence

- Sexual assault affects approximately 23% of women, 3% of men, 21% of girls and 11% of boys. Rape affects 5% of women and 0.4% of men. In 2009/10 there were approximately 20,000 sexual assaults and 14,000 rapes against women, reported to the police in England and Wales. However, many assaults go unreported.

- One-fifth of all rapes reported to the police involved children under the age of 16 years. Child sexual abuse is more likely in missing children, looked-after children, children with a disability and those whose family experience domestic violence.

3. Severity and Outcome

The severity of the assault can vary from sexual touching to sustaining life-threatening injuries. The outcome of the assault can lead to long-term psychological and physical effects.

4. Pathophysiology

- **Sexual assault** is touching another person in a sexual way without consent.

- **Serious sexual assault** is penetration of the vagina or anus with a part of the body or anything else without consent.

- **Rape** is penetration of the vagina, anus or mouth with a penis without consent.

5. Assessment and Management

For the assessment and management of sexual assault refer to Table 1.11.

KEY POINTS

Sexual Assault
- Sexual assault may be concurrent with other injuries which will need treating.
- Treatment should avoid disturbing evidence where possible.
- Leave the investigation to the police.
- Accommodate patient wishes where possible.
- Police may have special facilities for managing patients.

Table 1.11 – ASSESSMENT and MANAGEMENT of:

Sexual Assault

ASSESSMENT	MANAGEMENT
● Assess ABCD	If any of the following **TIME CRITICAL** features present **major ABCD problems:** ● Start correcting **A** and **B** problems. ● Undertake a **TIME CRITICAL** transfer to nearest receiving hospital. ● Continue patient management en-route. ● Provide an alert/information call.
● Assess	● Limit questions to those identifying the need for medical treatment, but allow the patient to talk and document what is said – it is not appropriate to probe for details of the assault and could affect the outcome of criminal investigations. ● Manage according to condition. ● Acute injury – **refer to trauma emergencies overview**. ● Acute illness – **refer to medical emergencies overview**. ● It may be appropriate to delay assessment for non-urgent injuries until transfer to specialised unit for forensic examination to avoid further distress and disturbing the evidence.
● Approach	● Sensitive and respectful manner. ● Call police promptly – so the scene may be secured. ● If possible ensure privacy. ● Consider cultural/religious issues. ● Where possible accommodate patient's requests. ● Where possible avoid disturbing the scene. ● Where possible avoid being alone with the patient.
● Forensic examination	Forensic examination will focus specifically on the areas affected, including wounds, mouth, anus and vagina and other areas where the patient has been kissed, licked or bitten, as these areas may well be contaminated with the assailant's DNA; therefore patients should not: ● Wash (shower/bathe) or brush their teeth. ● Change clothes, throw away or destroy clothes. ● Urinate. The police will want to collect early evidence samples including a urine sample to screen for the presence of drugs as some drugs have a very short half-life. ● A mouth swab and mouth wash may also be requested by the police. ● Defecate. ● Smoke. ● Drink/eat. ● If a blanket is required for modesty or warmth a single-use blanket should be used and kept with the patient – the blanket needs to be retained in order to analyse cross-contamination. ● If the patient is not wrapped in a single-use blanket, place a sterile sheet or single-use blanket under the patient where they sit or lie and retain for forensic examination. ● Avoid cleaning any wounds unless clinically absolutely necessary – if possible keep 'washings'. ● If required, lightly apply dry dressings – retain any used dressing and swabs for forensic examination; also keep the sterile packets in which they were contained in order to examine cross-contamination. NB All of these recommendations are vital to conserve evidence for a successful prosecution of the offender; **BUT** the need for this approach must be conveyed with great sensitivity to the patient who may well want to wash and change.
● Transfer[a]	● Encourage all patients to attend further care and to inform the police. ● Transfer patients to further care according to local guideline. ● Many services no longer employ 'courtesy calls'. Follow local procedures around information provided prior to arrival / shared with triage nurse. ● Hand over to an appropriate member of staff and not in a public area. ● Where a patient is competent and refuses hospital treatment, advise them to seek further medical attention. They may need post-exposure prophylaxis, vaccination, and/or contraception, all of which can be provided confidentially.
● Documentation	Complete the clinical record in great detail contemporaneously: ● Document only facts not personal opinion. ● Document what the patient says. ● Clinical findings with relevant timings. ● Ambulance identification number. ● A police statement may be required later.

[a] In some areas arrangements exist for patients to be examined and interviewed in police or other facilities.

1. Introduction

- All vulnerable adults have the right to be protected from harm. Safeguarding vulnerable adults from significant harm is reliant on effective joint working and communication between responsible agencies and professionals.

- This guidance is for the management of people aged 18 years or over; for those under the age of 18 years **refer to the Safeguarding Children guideline**.

- **Duty of care** – as a healthcare worker who may come into contact with vulnerable adults, there is a duty to report concerns about abuse. Not reporting abuse may put the person at greater risk. It may also discourage people from disclosing again, as they may feel they were not believed and this may put others at risk.

- Ambulance clinicians are often the first professionals on scene and therefore may identify initial concerns regarding abuse. The role of the Ambulance Service is not to investigate suspicions but to ensure that any suspicion is passed to the appropriate agency (e.g. social care or the police) in line with locally agreed procedures.

- Ambulance clinicians need to be aware of issues and local policies and procedures related to the abuse of vulnerable adults. The aim of this guideline is to assist ambulance clinicians to recognise and report cases of suspected abuse of a vulnerable adult.

- The principles of adult protection differ from those of child protection, in that adults have the right to take risks and may choose to live at risk if they have the capacity to make such a decision. Their wishes should not be overruled without full consideration. For example, older people are not 'confused'; similarly, people with learning disabilities or mental health problems may have the capacity to make some decisions about their lives, but not others.

- All Local Authorities should have Inter-Agency Adult Protection Procedures which comply with the 'No Secrets' guidance and many authorities will also have an Inter-Agency Adult Protection Committee / Safeguarding Adults Board. In addition, the Care Quality Commission is responsible for the standard of care provided in nursing homes, residential care homes and by domiciliary care agencies.

2. Incidence

The National Adult Social Care Intelligence Service survey of councils in England with responsibility for adult social services found that the majority of referrals were:

- In the 18–64 age group.
- For women.
- For people with physical disabilities.
- Regarding physical abuse.
- Undertaken in the person's own home.
- Reported by social care staff.

However, not all councils reported data; in those that did, some data were incomplete. Also it is likely that abuse of vulnerable adults is underreported.

3. Assessment

- Abuse can be perpetrated by a range of people (refer to Table 1.12) and take a number of forms (refer to Table 1.13). Abuse can be a single or repeated act that can result in significant harm.

- A vulnerable adult is defined as a person '*who is or may be in need of community care services by reason of mental or other disability, age or illness; and who is or may be unable to take care of him or herself, or unable to protect him or herself against significant harm or exploitation*'.

- Abuse is the '*violation of an individual's human and civil rights by any other person or persons*'.

When assessing the seriousness of abuse consider the:

- **Vulnerability** of the individual.
- **Nature and extent** of the abuse.
- **Length of time** it has been occurring.
- **Impact** on the individual.
- Risk of **repeated or increasingly serious** acts involving this or other vulnerable adults.

Table 1.12 – POTENTIAL SOURCES OF ABUSE

- Spouse, relatives and family members
- Professional staff
- Paid care workers
- Volunteers
- Other service users
- Neighbours
- Friends and associates
- People who deliberately exploit vulnerable people
- Strangers

Table 1.13 – TYPES OF ABUSE

Physical
- Hitting
- Slapping
- Pushing
- Kicking
- Misuse of medication
- Restraint or inappropriate sanctions

Sexual
- Rape
- Sexual assault
- Sexual acts to which the vulnerable adult has not consented or could not consent or was pressured into consenting

Psychological
- Emotional abuse
- Threats of harm or abandonment
- Deprivation of contact
- Humiliation
- Blaming

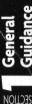

Table 1.13 – TYPES OF ABUSE *continued*

Psychological *continued*

- Controlling
- Intimidation
- Coercion
- Harassment
- Verbal abuse
- Isolation
- Withdrawal from services or supportive networks

Financial/material

- Theft
- Fraud
- Exploitation
- Pressure in connection with wills, property, inheritance or financial transactions
- Misuse or misappropriation of property, possessions or benefits

Neglect

- Ignoring medical or physical care needs
- Failure to provide access to appropriate health, social care or educational services
- Withholding of the necessities of life, such as medication, adequate nutrition and heating

Discriminatory

- Racist
- Sexist
- Based on a person's disability
- Harassment
- Slurs or similar treatment

4. Management

- The first priority is the health and safety of the patient. Ambulance clinicians should follow the usual **ABCDE** and **<C>ABCDE** assessment – **refer to medical and trauma overview guidelines**.

- If the ambulance clinicians are concerned that the abuser may be present, the ambulance clinicians should not let the person(s) know they are suspicious, as this may result in a refusal to attend hospital or a situation where a vulnerable adult may be placed at further risk.

- Any inconsistency in history and any delay in calling for assistance should be noted. A patient who is frightened may be reluctant to say what may be the cause of their injury/condition, especially if the person responsible for the abuse is present.

- If necessary, ask appropriate questions of those present to clarify the situation, but avoid unnecessary questioning or probing, as this may affect the credibility of subsequent evidence.

- Accurate recording of events/actions/information may be crucial to subsequent inquiries. It may be helpful to make a note of the person's body language.

- It is important to ascertain the wishes of the patient and to take into account whether or not they want to be conveyed to hospital. However, the decision not to convey a patient to hospital is one that must be fully considered. In some cases the ambulance clinician may consider that the patient clearly does not have the capacity to make a judgement with respect to their need for medical care, and may decide to act under the Mental Capacity Act (if there is risk to life or limb), or make alternative arrangements for the patient if their condition requires less immediate treatment (e.g. a general practitioner visit the following day).

- If the patient needs to be transferred to further care, and another person tries to prevent this, crews may need to consider whether to involve the police; inform ambulance control about the situation.

- Report concerns to the appropriate agency, that is local social services and/or police.

- If the patient is transferred to further care, inform a senior member of the receiving staff of the concerns regarding possible abuse. Be careful not to alert the alleged abuser or place the vulnerable adult at risk of further abuse or intimidation.

- If the patient is not transferred to further care or if the ambulance clinicians have concerns about someone else in the household or on the premises, they should contact ambulance control and inform them of their concerns.

- Inform the appropriate clinical manager as per local/ Trust guidelines.

- Complete documentation/report as per local procedures; complete in private if possible.

NB The patient may not be the person at risk of harm; it may be a person in the household or someone accompanying the patient.

Further information – on local procedures can be obtained from the named professional for safeguarding within individual Ambulance Trusts. The contact details can be obtained from ambulance control.

KEY POINTS

Safeguarding Vulnerable Adults

- **Vulnerable adults have a right to be protected.**
- **Abuse can take a number of forms.**
- **Concerns of suspected abuse must be reported to the appropriate agency, that is local social services and/or police.**
- **Ambulance clinicians must document the circumstances giving rise to concern as soon as possible.**
- **The wishes of the patient should be taken into account where possible.**
- **Ambulance clinicians should not investigate allegations.**

1. Introduction

Approximately 1% of the population of the UK die each year, which is about half a million people and around 75% of these deaths are expected [71–73]. This presents an opportunity to plan for an individual's death; to improve the quality of life remaining, to support those close to the patient, to provide symptom control and establish preferences for care as an illness progresses.

End of life care is considered for those who have advanced, progressive or incurable illnesses. In addition to cancers this encompasses organ failure and conditions such as: COPD, renal failure, advanced dementia, heart failure and motor neurone disease.

End of life care applies to those who are expected to be in their last year of life but as illness trajectories differ for each condition this can refer to the last few years of life, months, weeks or days [74].

Ambulance clinicians frequently come into contact with patients who are approaching their end of life, facilitating planned transfers or providing an emergency response to a sudden crisis.

Due to an aging population and an expected 17% increase in annual deaths by 2030 [75] there will be an increasing demand for high quality end of life care; this will be reflected in the workload of ambulance services.

Unlike conventional areas of pre-hospital care, such as cardiac arrest and trauma, which aim to save life and rely on algorithms and clear parameters; end of life care seeks to provide supportive care using a holistic approach tailored to each individual. This presents unique challenges to ambulance clinicians. Most commonly there is no pre-existing relationship with the patient, no knowledge of their condition or treatment preferences and, based on limited information, time critical decisions have to be made [76].

It is essential that expert advice and assistance is sought when managing end of life care situations.

People at the end of life may have contact with ambulance services on several occasions, for example, when a complication occurs, which creates a sudden health crisis, or for an unrelated event such as a fall. Be aware of the underlying condition(s) and any advance care planning decisions that may be in place when administering care.

Increasingly, calls to ambulance services, for example, for a person with COPD who is experiencing more difficulty breathing, may indicate that the condition is deteriorating. Here, ambulance clinicians may be the first point of contact for the person; they need to be able to recognise signs, signals and clues that suggest that it may be time to initiate discussions about end of life care and relay this information on to the person's GP, hospital, other health professionals or organisations so that appropriate action can be taken.

2. Severity and Outcome

The focus in managing end of life care situations should always be to enable a person to achieve care according to their needs and wishes [77].

For those who are nearing the terminal phase of illness the aspirational outcome would be for that person to have a 'good death'; to die in a place of their choosing, with dignity and respect, without pain, in a calm and familiar atmosphere, surrounded by loved ones [72, 78].

Not all clinical presentations are during the end stages of disease or should be managed with supportive care alone.

Several acute presentations are reversible and require urgent treatment and transfer to the Emergency Department, in order to improve an individual's prognosis or quality of life.

3. Management – Patients Who Are Not Expected to Die Within 72 Hours

Establish the patient's wishes for their care, including their desire for interventions and place of care.

If the patient does not have the capacity for decision making, establish if an advanced care plan exists.

Consult with family members and carers but remember the patient's best interests take precedence.

Access personalised care plans and follow directions where appropriate.

If not in the active stage of dying determine:

● If there is a reversible cause for symptoms and manage as per guidance below.

● If the patient's symptoms can be managed in their home environment or if hospital/hospice admission is required.

● If the patient has psychological, emotional or spiritual needs that would benefit from specialist support.

● If the patient requires additional social support at home or if hospital admission is necessary: Are family members exhausted? Can they manage to provide care? Is physical equipment required to support care at home?

Care pathways

Unless the patient clearly requires urgent hospital conveyance for a reversible condition seek specialist advice to support decision making:

● Be aware of any advance care plans, especially for palliative patients and those with long term conditions such as COPD and dementia.

● Be prepared to ask the person/carer about possible end of life care planning and related issues.

● Contact palliative care team using contact details in personalised care plan.

● Contact GP or District Nurse if not under specialist care.

● Contact local palliative care pathways (e.g. rapid response teams or hospice at home services).

● Consider contacting a religious leader if appropriate.

● Consider referral to social services if appropriate.

Reversible emergencies

Metastatic spinal cord compression

Background

Spinal cord compression due to direct pressure or collapse of a vertebral body due to spinal metastases can result in vascular injury, cord necrosis and neurological disability [79]. Patients with lung, prostate and breast cancer are at the greatest risk, with the thoracic spine most commonly affected [80, 81].

Signs and symptoms [82]:

- Pain in thoracic or cervical spine and/or progressive, severe lumbar spinal pain.
- Pain aggravated by straining (passing stools, coughing or sneezing) or nocturnal pain preventing sleep.
- Limb weakness.
- Difficulty walking.
- Sensory loss or bladder or bowel dysfunction.
- Localised spinal tenderness.

Management

1. If any of the following time critical features present:
   - Major ABCD problems
   - Neurological deficit in lower limbs
   Undertake a time critical transfer to nearest Emergency Department.
   Provide patient management en-route
   Provide an alert/information call.
2. Measure and record pain score.
   Offer analgesia, **refer to Pain Management guidelines**.
3. Position supine with neutral spine alignment for patients with severe pain, neurological symptoms or signs of compression [82].

   (Note – there are no clear guidelines and a lack of evidence to advise the correct position for patients – adopt NICE guidelines as in pre-hospital phase it seems prudent to manage as if spine unstable until MRI can confirm.)
4. Transfer to the nearest Emergency Department or to a specialist unit if advised by expert team.

Superior vena cava compression

Background

Occlusion of the superior vena cava due to either external compression or internal obstruction. Most commonly caused by a tumour of the bronchus or lymphomas, cancers of the breast, colon or oesophagus.

Severity of symptoms varies depending on the degree of obstruction but reflects the underlying venous congestion, laryngeal and cerebral oedema [83].

Signs and symptoms [84]

- Facial, neck, arm swelling, worse on lying or bending over.
- Dilated veins on neck, chest, arms.
- Dyspnoea.
- Cough or hoarseness.
- Headache.
- Dizziness, confusion or lethargy.

Management

1. If any of the following time critical features present:
   - Major ABC problems
   - Stridor or severe difficulty in breathing
   Start correcting A and B problems
   Undertake a time critical transfer to nearest Emergency Department.

Provide patient management en-route
Provide an alert/information call.
2. Sit patient upright or elevate head.
3. If the patient is hypoxaemic, administer supplemental oxygen and aim for a target saturation within the ranger 94–98% – **refer to oxygen guideline**. [83, 85–89]

   (Note – Points 2 and 3 provide symptomatic relief.)
4. Transfer to the nearest Emergency Department or to a specialist unit if advised by expert team.

Neutropenic sepsis

Background

Neutropenic sepsis is a potentially fatal complication of treatments for cancer, such as chemotherapy or radiotherapy. Such treatments can suppress the ability of bone marrow to respond to infection [83, 89].

Signs and symptoms

- Patient having treatment for cancer.
- Minor illness or feels unwell.
- Raised temperature.
- Classic signs of sepsis may be absent, a high index of suspicion is required.

Management

1. Treat suspected neutropenic sepsis as an acute medical emergency.
2. Manage as per sepsis guidelines.
3. Identify patient alert card and contact oncology unit.
4. Transfer to the nearest Emergency Department or to a specialist unit if advised by expert team.

Care in the last few days of life

A point comes when the person enters the 'dying phase'. Ambulance services are frequently called upon at this stage. This may be for planned transport, such as the rapid transfer of a person from hospital or hospice to their preferred place of death.

Ambulance services are also frequently called during the dying phase because of an unexpected complication, or a sudden deterioration in condition. Good call-handling procedures can help ascertain and pass on to ambulance clinicians what outcome the person or carer wants and expects from ambulance services – to make the person comfortable, for example, and avoid unwanted hospital admission or attempts at resuscitation.

Families and carers may sometimes wish for ambulance services to be called even where the persons themselves have indicated a preference to die at home or in their usual care setting such as a care home.

At the scene, the focus must at all times be on providing the patient with the care and treatment that is in their best interests. Families and carers can be valuable sources of knowledge and expertise on this and should be kept informed. Ambulance clinicians must at the same time be alert to the possibility of differing views and/or resistance to following an agreed care plan or stated preference among families and carers, including GPs, and be prepared to deal with these. Be aware that an ambulance can be called because of an unexpected complication or a sudden deterioration, often by distressed relatives and carers.

- Focus on care and treatment that is in the patient's best interests.
- Try and establish the wishes of the patient but be aware of differing views or resistance to follow an agreed care plan among families and carers.
- Seek clinical decision support or follow the care pathway.
- Recognise the signs that a patient is at the end of life and that lifesaving skills, interventions and clinical observations may not be appropriate.

Signs that a patient is at the very end of life

It can sometimes be difficult to decide when someone is in the last few days or hours, however, some of the signs below may become noticeable.

- Abnormal clinical observations.
- Breathing may become irregular and may stop for short periods.
- Reduced conscious levels; sleeping more and at times being difficult to waken.
- Impaired vision and may develop a fixed stare.
- Confusion about time or may not recognise familiar persons.
- Restlessness, pulling at the bed linen and have visions of persons or things that are not present.
- Loss of appetite.
- Loss of control of urine or bowels. The amount of urine will decrease or stop as death approaches.
- Occasionally after death there may be a 'last sigh' or gurgling sound. There is no need to become alarmed about this, as it is the normal pattern.
- Secretions collect at the back of the throat that sound like a rattle.
- Cool arms and legs as the circulation slows down. Their face may become pale, their feet and legs a purple-blue mottled appearance.

Care at and after death

Ambulance clinicians will often be at the scene at or shortly after the point of death. There may be occasions where it is clear that the patient is in the final stages of dying. If all reversible causes have been considered, then supportive care for the patient and the relatives/carers may be all that is required. **Refer to the Recognition of Life Extinct guideline.**

Pain management in end of life care

1. Introduction

Providing adequate pain management at the end of life is a right of the dying patient and the duty of all clinicians. This provides one of the most challenging tasks that the clinician will face and requires a treatment of the 'whole person' as well as the pain by adopting a biopsychosocial approach.

Pain is persistent in approximately 70% of patients with advanced cancer, and 65% in patients with a non-malignant disease. However, due to the longevity and nature of the dying process it is likely that most end of life patients will feel pain at some stage. In 10% of patients the pain is described as 'difficult' and may require a more indepth investigation and pain management programme.

Most end of life patients are under the management of a pain specialist/clinic who has the responsibility of monitoring for changes in pain intensity and character and adjusting the management strategy accordingly. For those not under the guidance of a pain specialist/clinic, it is advisable for the clinician to make a referral or to make contact with a doctor so that a long term plan to manage the pain can be sought.

35% of patients in the last week of life describe their pain as 'severe' or 'intolerable' and should be treated as a medical emergency where the challenge is to provide aggressive pain management in order to alleviate suffering.

Be aware that not all people in the last days of life experience pain. If pain is identified, manage it promptly and effectively, and identify and treat any reversible causes of pain, such as urinary retention.

2. Aims

The aim of a good pain management programme is to keep patients as pain-free when both resting at home and when performing everyday activities. This is achieved through good pharmacological and non-pharmacological treatments as well as providing advice and education to the patient, their family, and to the carers.

Many end of life patients live with a degree of persistent pain for which they may already be receiving treatment. This is termed 'background pain'. If a new pain or an increase in the severity of the background pain occurs, then this should be treated as a new condition and assessed as such. An increase in severity of background pain or a new pain is termed as 'breakthrough' or 'breakout' pain.

The three principles in providing end of life pain relief:

1. Pain can be controlled in most patients by using the WHO step-care approach.
2. Acute or escalating pain is a medical emergency requiring a prompt response.
3. Addiction is not an issue in patients with a terminal illness.

3. Assessment

Pain is a complex, subjective and dynamic phenomenon which is affected by the emotional context in which it is endured. In line with current JRCALC guidelines set out in the guidelines 'Pain Management in Adults' and 'Pain Management in Children', clinicians should pay particular attention to any psychological and sociological factors. Wherever possible a patient self-assessment strategy should be used and only substituted when the patient is unable to do so. A patient centred approach should take into account the patients needs and preferences so that they may be able to make an informed decision about their care. For this good communication and understanding is essential.

Medical assessment: It is important to be more thorough when assessing end of life patients as there may be other underlying issues that need addressing. As well as the usual assessments carried out in line with clinical training and local protocols, it is advisable to also check for pressure sores and dressings as these may be in need of attention. If the patient is catheterised, it may be worth asking if it is fitted comfortably and causing any issues. If possible advise the patient to maintain a degree of movement as this helps to prevent muscle atrophy, joint stiffness and other diseases caused by a sedentary lifestyle.

Sociological assessment: A sociological assessment builds upon the premise that no illness is suffered in isolation, in fact, the assumption is that people will rationalise what is happening to them within a social model and create a social construction that is based on their relationships, past experience and language. The sociological assessment should look at how the individual makes sense of the illness and the physical and social interactions that are affected as a result. This 'individualism' of the disease combined with the social factors cannot, and does not, fit into the biomedical model which lends its intellect mainly to the giving of drugs to treat a specific dysfunction. If left untreated, the sociological aspect of dying will affect both the medical and psychological states of the patient.

Psychological assessment: For many end of life patients the dying process will lead to various psychological problems, especially disorders such as depression and anxiety. These have long since been known to accompany chronic pain and long-term illness, with research showing that increased pain perception contributes to the variables seen in the development of the symptomatology of psychological disorders.

The general assumption is that pain perception, alongside cognitive behavioural traits, both play important parts in the symptomatology of chronic pain, and therefore patients suffering from more intense, more frequent, and longerlasting painful episodes are more likely to suffer severe depression.

A lack of treatment will only serve to increase the level of depression, which acts as a vicious circle that is degenerative in nature and contributes, or even exacerbates, the psychological problems encountered.

4. Patient centred approach

A patient centred approach places the patient in charge of their care and offers them more powers to choose and make decisions for themselves. This should provide them with a greater sense of comfort and self-control but also reduce the amount of calls made to the emergency services. A patient centred approach should educate and inform the patient how best to manage their pain. Good advice includes:

- Where pain is continuous take pain relief on a regular basis not 'as required'.
- Pain is easier to prevent than to relieve.
- Where additional pain is felt through everyday activities then additional pain medication should be taken prior to such activities.
- Recommed that 'anticipatory' or 'just in case' medication be available and that these pain medications are adequate for need.
- Take pain relief medications as often as prescribed as they do other medications (poor compliance is common in pain management).

5. Pharmacological Treatment

Where pain is intense and opioids are already prescribed morphine should be the first line treatment for breakthrough pain. This should be administered in line with local protocols and as part of a multi-modal pain management strategy (i.e. to be administered alongside other analgesics like NSAIDs or paracetamol). Where the new pain is not intense the WHO analgesic ladder should be followed.

Step 1 – (<3/10) non opioid +/- adjuvant

Step 2 – (3–6/10) opioid for mild to moderate pain +/- non opioid +/- adjuvant

Step 3 – (>6/10) opioid for moderate to severe pain +/- non opioid +/- adjuvant

The use of intramuscular and subcutaneous morphine is often used in end of life patients not wishing to attend hospital. It is still important when using morphine to titrate to effect so as to achieve a stable and satisfactory level of pain relief without the unwanted adverse effects. The use of intravenous paracetamol may also be used by the clinician and has shown to be good at relieving symptoms of bone pain (a pain which does not respond well to morphine).

Note:

- Do not dilute the morphine as more than 1 ml of fluid injected into the site of administration is not recommended.
- Effects of IM/SC morphine are prevalent after 15–20 minutes.
- It is important to check for prior paracetamol and opioid use before administration to avoid overdosing the patient.
- Paracetamol should be infused over a 15 minute period.

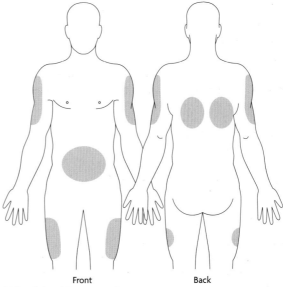

Front   Back

1. The deltoid (upper arm)
2. The abdomen (avoid the umbilicus)
3. The thigh
4. The scapula

Figure 1.3 – Sites for injection of intramuscular and subcutaneous administrations.

End of Life Care

Table 1.14 – END OF LIFE CARE DOSAGES

DRUG	AGE/WEIGHT	MAXIMUM DOSE	ADDITIONAL COMMENTS
IM/SC morphine	All patients up to 85 yrs	5 mg	As a general principle dosage usually starts from 2.5 mg to 5 mg in opioid naïve patients. If already on opioids then treatment for breakthrough pain is 1/6th of the daily dose.
IM/SC morphine	60 yrs – 85 yrs	2.5 mg	Give reduced dosages in the opioid naive elderly.
IM/SC morphine	>85 yrs	2 mg	Extra caution required for this age group.
IV paracetamol	<10 kg	7.5 mg/kg	Maximum daily dose of 25 mg/kg.
IV paracetamol	>10 kg <50 kg	15 mg/kg	Maximum daily dose of 60 mg/kg.
IV paracetamol	>50 kg	1 g	Maximum daily dose of 4 g.

- The minimum dose of paracetamol should not be less than 4 hours apart (6 hours in renal impairment).
- After any drug has been administered it is good practice to inform the patients' own GP or palliative team.
- Be cautious if patient is on a syringe driver. In such cases contact the patient's doctor prior to the administration of any analgesic.

6. Non-pharmacological treatment

- Non-pharmacological treatment of end of life pain involves addressing many different issues.
- *Patient position* – As many palliative patients spend long lengths of time in the same position it may be possible to help reduce levels of pain through movement and pillow placement. Always be aware of pressure sores and treat if required.
- *Psychological, social, and spiritual concerns* – Although the clinicians' time with the patient is limited, studies have shown that addressing these areas will help to provide comfort for the patient. The mental state is very important and will impact on pain levels if left untreated.
- *A good bed-side manner* – Calm and reassurance may be all that the patient needs in some circumstances and this plays a big role in caring for end of life patients.

7. Patients' own medications

Many more palliative/end of life patients are being cared for at home for their final days with the express wishes to remain at home. As part of their end of life care plan they may have 'anticipatory' or 'just in case' medications. Only administer the medications via the prescribed route and ensure all documentation is completed.

Clinicians are permitted to administer these medications provided:

- The clinician is competent in the method of administration.
- A signed Patient Specific Medication (PSM) chart is present and authorised by an independent prescriber.
- The clinician has access to the relevant paperwork supplied with the 'just in case' medication providing

the necessary information of each drug's indication, dosage, adverse effects, signs and treatments for overdose.

8. Managing breathlessness

Identify and treat reversible causes of breathlessness in the dying person, for example pulmonary oedema or pleural effusion.

Consider non-pharmacological management of breathlessness in a person in the last days of life. Do not routinely start oxygen to manage breathlessness. Only offer oxygen therapy to people known or clinically suspected to have symptomatic hypoxaemia.

Medications to manage breathlessness may include:

- an opioid.
- a benzodiazepine.
- a combination of an opioid and benzodiazepine.

See the section on patients' own medication also.

9. Managing nausea and vomiting

Consider likely causes of nausea or vomiting in the dying person. These may include:

- certain medicines that can cause or contribute to nausea and vomiting.
- recent chemotherapy or radiotherapy.
- psychological causes.
- biochemical causes, for example hypercalcaemia.
- raised intracranial pressure.
- gastrointestinal motility disorder.
- ileus or bowel obstruction.

Discuss the options for treating nausea and vomiting with the dying person and those important to them. Consider non-pharmacological methods for treating nausea and vomiting. For people in the last days of life with obstructive bowel disorders who have nausea or vomiting, medications used include:

- hyoscine butylbromide.
- octreotide.

See the section on patients' own medication also.

10. Managing anxiety, delirium and agitation

Explore the possible causes of anxiety or delirium, with or without agitation, with the dying person and those important to them. Be aware that agitation in isolation is sometimes associated with other unrelieved symptoms or bodily needs, for example unrelieved pain, a full bladder or rectum.

Consider non-pharmacological management of agitation, anxiety and delirium in a person in the last days of life.

Consider any reversible causes of agitation, anxiety or delirium, for example, psychological causes or certain metabolic disorders such as renal failure or hyponatraemia.

Medications used include:

- benzodiazepine to manage anxiety or agitation, e.g. lorazepam and midazolam.

- an antipsychotic medicine to manage delirium or agitation.

Seek specialist advice if the diagnosis of agitation or delirium is uncertain, if the agitation or delirium does not respond to antipsychotic treatment or if treatment causes unwanted sedation.

See the section on patients' own medication also.

11. Managing noisy respiratory secretions

These can be associated with the disease process, or as a result of excessive weakness in the patient, and an inability to maintain their own airway through normal physiological procedures such as coughing.

Assess for the likely causes of noisy respiratory secretions in people in the last days of life. Establish whether the noise has an impact on the dying person or those important to them. The noise associated with respiratory secretions can be a source of distress for carers. Ambulance clinicians may need to provide additional explanation and reassurance and although the noise can be distressing, it is unlikely to cause discomfort. Repositioning the patient can be effective in managing secretions. Suctioning is not usually used or recommended.

Be prepared to talk about any fears or concerns the patient or carers may have.

Consider non-pharmacological measures to manage noisy respiratory or pharyngeal secretions, to reduce any distress in people at the end of life.

Medications include:

- atropine.

- glycopyrronium bromide.

- hyoscine butylbromide.

- hyoscine hydrobromide.

See the section on patients' own medication also.

Key points

- **Providing adequate pain management at the end of life is a right of the dying patient and the duty of all clinicians.**
- **Acute or escalating pain is a medical emergency requiring a prompt response.**
- **Wherever possible a patient self-assessment strategy should be used and only substituted when the patient is unable to do so.**
- **Pain is easier to prevent than to relieve.**
- **Where pain is intense and opioids are already prescribed morphine should be the first line treatment for breakthrough pain.**
- **All treatments should use the principle of biopsychsocial model.**

1. Introduction

- Being called to a death of an infant, child or adolescent is one of the most difficult experiences that an ambulance clinician will encounter. They are usually the first professionals to arrive at the scene, and, at the same time as making difficult judgements about resuscitation, they have to deal with the devastating initial shock of the parents/carers.

- Despite the recent fall in incidence,[a] sudden unexpected death in infancy (SUDI) remains the largest single cause of death in infants aged one month to one year. SUDI can also occasionally occur in children older than one year of age.

- In 50% of SUDI a specific cause for the death is found, either from a careful investigation of the circumstances or from post-mortem findings.

- The vast majority of SUDI occur from natural causes. 10% of SUDI are thought to arise from some form of maltreatment by their parents/carers and so a joint paediatric and police investigation is required for **all** SUDIs. When informed of a SUDI, ambulance control should notify the police Child Abuse Investigation Team to initiate this process.

- This document draws on national experiences and is in accord with the recommendations of the Kennedy Report.

2. Multi-Agency Approach

The Kennedy Report requires a multi-agency approach to the management of SUDI, in which all the professionals involved keep each other informed and collaborate.

Objectives

The main objectives for ambulance clinicians when called to a child death are:

- Resuscitation (**refer to Paediatric Basic (BLS) and Advanced Life Support (ALS) guidelines**) should be attempted in all cases, unless there is a condition unequivocally associated with death or a valid advance decision (**refer to Recognition of Life Extinct (ROLE) guideline**).

- Detecting a pulse in a sick infant can be extremely difficult so the absence of peripheral pulses is not a reliable indication of death. Similarly, a sick infant may have marked peripheral cyanosis and cold extremities (**refer to paediatric medical and trauma emergencies guidelines**).

- It is better for parents/carers to know that resuscitation was attempted but failed, than to be left feeling that something that might have saved their infant was not done.

- Once resuscitation has been initiated, the infant should be transported at once to the nearest suitable emergency department, with resuscitation continuing en-route.

Care of the family

- The initial response of professionals (and you will probably be the first on the scene) will affect the family profoundly.

- Having experienced this hugely distressing event, parents/carers exhibit a variety of reactions (e.g. overwhelming grief, anger, confusion, disbelief or guilt). Be prepared to deal with any of these feelings with sympathy and sensitivity, remembering some reactions may be directed at you as a manifestation of their distress.

- Think before you speak. Chance remarks may cause offence and may be remembered indefinitely (e.g. 'I'm sorry he looks so awful').

- Avoid any criticism of the parents/carers, either direct or implied.

- Ask the child's name and use it when referring to them (do not refer to the child as 'it').

- If possible, do not put children in body bags. It is known that relatives do not perceive very traumatic events in the way that unrelated onlookers might and it is important they are allowed to see, touch and hold their loved one.

- Explain what you are doing at every stage.

- Allow the parents/carers to hold the child if they so wish (unless there are obvious indications of trauma), as long as it does not interfere with clinical care.

- The parents/carers will need to accompany you when you take the infant to hospital. If appropriate, offer to take one or both in the ambulance. Alternatively ensure that they have other means of transport, and that they know where to go.

- If they have no telephone, offer to help in contacting a relative or friend who can give immediate support, such as looking after other children or making sure the premises are secure.

Document

- Time arrived on scene.

- The situation in which you find the infant (e.g. position in cot, bedding, proximity to others, room temperature, etc).

- A brief description from the parents/carers of the events that led up to them finding the dead child (e.g. when last seen alive, health at that time, position when found, etc). The police and community paediatrician will go through these events in greater detail, but the parent/carer's initial statement to you may be particularly valuable in the investigation.

- Write all this information down as soon as you have the opportunity, giving times and other details as precisely as possible.

Communication with other agencies

- After you have arrived at the house and confirmed that the infant is dead or moribund, the police child abuse investigation team must be informed (see your locally agreed procedure – Figure 1.2 shows South Central's Child Death Procedures flowchart, as an example).

- In unexpected child deaths, advise the parents/carers that the death will be reported to the Coroner, and that they will be interviewed by the Coroner's Officer and the police in due course.

---

[a] The national 'Reduce the Risk' campaign of 1991 advocating infants sleep on their backs produced a dramatic reduction (70%) in sudden infant deaths.

- Share the information you have collected with the police and with relevant health professionals.

Transferring the infant

- The infant should be taken to the nearest appropriate emergency department, not direct to a mortuary. This should apply even when the infant has clearly been dead for some time and a doctor has certified death at home (it will on occasions be necessary to remind a doctor that taking the infant to a hospital is now the preferred procedure, as recommended by Kennedy).

- The main reasons for taking the infant to the hospital rather than the mortuary are that at hospital an immediate examination can be made by a paediatrician, early samples can be taken for laboratory tests, parents/carers can talk with the paediatricians and other local support services can be contacted.

- Pre-alert the emergency department of your arrival, asking them to be ready to take over resuscitation if this is ongoing.

Support for ambulance clinicians

- The death of a child is very distressing for all those involved, and opportunities for debriefing or counselling should be available for ambulance clinicians.

- Follow local procedures for post critical incident debriefing local guidelines/processes.

- Some clinicians will feel ongoing distress. This is normal but should be recognised and other forms of therapy, from informal support from colleagues, to formal counselling, may be required.

- As part of the ambulance service safeguarding processes, information from local paediatricians and ambulance service safeguarding leads will be available if required for further discussion

- Unsuccessful resuscitation attempts on children weigh heavily on many people's shoulders and it is very important to remember that the vast majority of children who arrest outside hospital will die, whoever is there, or whatever is done – less than 10% of paediatric out-of-hospital cardiac arrests survive. Such outcomes are almost never the fault of those attempting resuscitation who will have done everything possible to help that child.

Conclusion

- Findings from the Foundation for the Study of Infant Deaths have shown that parents/carers regard the actions and attitudes of ambulance clinicians to them as really important and speak very highly of the way both they and their child were treated.

- Your role is not only essential for immediate practical reasons but also has a great influence on how the family deals with the death long after the initial crisis is over.

Further Reading

http://www.dcsf.gov.uk/everychildmatters/
. A guide to inter-agency working to safeguard and promote the welfare of children.

Children Act 2004.

KEY POINTS

Death of a Child (Including Sudden Unexpected Death in Infancy, Children and Adolescents)

- A child death is one of the most emotionally traumatic and challenging events that an ambulance clinician will encounter.
- Resuscitation should always be attempted unless there is a condition unequivocally associated with death or a valid advance decision.
- Communication and empathy are essential, and the family must be treated with compassion and sensitivity throughout.
- Ensure the family is aware of where you are taking their infant/child.
- Collect information pertaining to the situation in which you find the child, a history of events and any significant past medical history.
- Follow agreed protocols with regards to inter-agency communication and informing the police.
- In unexpected deaths, when appropriate explain to the family that the death will be reported to the Coroner and that they will be interviewed by the Coroner's Officer and the police in due course.

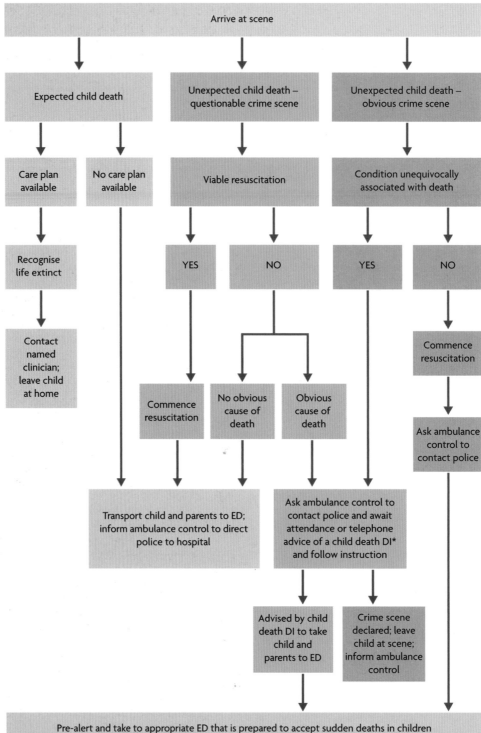

Conditions unequivocally associated with death in children younger than 18 years:

1. Massive cranial and cerebral destruction

2. Hemicorporectomy or similar massive injury

3. Decomposition/putrefaction

4. Incineration

NB The Royal College of Paediatrics and Child Health is starting a review of the whole SUDICA process and its advice will be passed on to all pre-hospital clinicians in due course. In the meantime the presence of rigor mortis and hypostasis should not preclude resuscitation in children unless there is other substantial evidence to suggest that they are clearly beyond help.

***Child Death Detective Inspector** – A Detective Inspector who is trained in the management of child death incidents to ensure the multi-agency investigation is commenced and evidence gathered to ascertain the full facts of the child's death.

Figure 1.2 – Example of a local child death procedure from South Central Ambulance Service – reproduced with kind permission.

Staff wellbeing and health

The importance of staff wellbeing should not be underestimated. The responsibility of all clinicians to pay attention to their own health is paramount if we are to deliver the highest quality of care and service to patients. The value of good sleep, rest, nutrition, relaxation and the need to spend time with family, friends and undertake out of work pursuits has a measurable value to any individual's wellbeing, and, therefore, the care they provide.

Even the most resilient individuals are subject to experiences that can affect their ability to work to their full potential. Despite our best efforts, personal loss and grief, injury and illness, financial difficulties, relationship breakdown, professional demands, long hours and shifts can cause the mental wellness of any individual to be tried. This is in addition to regular exposure to difficult, unpleasant and testing experiences at work that add to the demands put upon all emergency service workers.

Stress and anxiety

Stress and anxiety are common in the workplace and, to an extent, are a normal state that many find motivating. However, the effects of stress can cause people to feel unable to cope and left unchecked, stress can sometimes affect the way in which we think, react, feel and behave. Common signs of stress include:

- Disturbed sleep
- Anxiety
- Irritability
- Poor diet
- Overuse of prescription medication
- Excessive drinking
- Illicit drug use
- Low self esteem
- An inability to relax or repetitive and persistent thoughts and concerns.

Stress can also cause physical symptoms including:

- Headaches
- Nausea
- Dizziness
- Muscle pain, weakness and tension
- Fatigue.

Constantly experiencing stress and failing to deal with it effectively can lead to more enduring and debilitating mental health issues such as low mood and depression. Similarly, experiencing significantly stressful situations and events can lead to post traumatic stress disorders. Furthermore experiencing ongoing poor mental wellbeing significantly increases the risk of self-harm and suicide, even in those considered to be the most resilient.

It is important to remember that any member of the emergency services in any role is at an increased risk of experiencing poor mental health, significantly more so than members of the general public. There are several steps that are widely recognised as being beneficial to maintaining and improving mental well-being which can be used with great effect.

1) Good physical health

Regular exercise, getting enough sleep, having a good and balanced diet, avoiding using too much medication or alcohol to feel better or aid sleep, and ideally finding time for yourself, away from work, for relaxation and rest have obvious and ongoing benefits.

2) Keep on learning

There is research to suggest that learning new skills of any and all types can greatly benefit self-confidence, reduce stress and improve social connections. Continued learning does not have to be career related, it could just be for pleasure.

3) Helping others

Working for the emergency services is very much about public service. However the benefits of going the extra mile for someone has several benefits. Mental wellbeing is closely associated with feeling positive. As well as building relationships and strengthening bonds, going out of your way for someone can offer a sense of reward, increased self-confidence and satisfaction. There are many ways in which this could be done from helping friends, colleagues, neighbours and family to volunteer work.

4) Self-awareness

Mindfulness is the concept that we have a more positive outlook if we take the time to pay attention to thoughts, feelings, sights, smells, sounds and experiences we are subject to or encounter. Especially in a job where the need to focus is paramount, taking the time to appreciate areas of daily life that are pleasant and fulfilling and being more aware of the positive aspects of our lives is believed to be beneficial in achieving and maintaining good mental health.

5) Relationships

The importance of building good relationships with friends, family and work colleagues is well documented. Strong social and family bonds can have a very positive effect on any individual and can have a tangible value. Indeed we can often spend more time with work colleagues than with our own family. Bearing this in mind, good quality relationships at work can afford an opportunity for sharing experiences good and bad, whilst allowing work colleagues to offer support, advice or simply an opportunity to reduce stress and improve knowledge by talking and sharing experiences. This type of relationship can be viewed as a two way street and could be seen as not only a chance to remain positive and maintain good mental health, but also as an opportunity to spot when others may be struggling with their mental well-being and allow us to suggest further action and assistance.

When working in an environment such as the ambulance service, which can be very different to virtually any other type of career, it is worth remembering that anyone can experience a change in their mental health for many different reasons. Much work has been done in recent years to reduce the stigma attached to mental health problems and it is important that this is echoed within the ambulance service as well as outwardly.

Should you or someone you know experience a change in mood that is persistent or that cannot easily be fixed, or should you or someone you know experience thoughts of hopelessness, self-harm, suicide or any of the issues

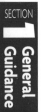
Staff wellbeing and health

mentioned, then there are many sources of help and advice you can turn to where free, confidential, impartial and instant help can be obtained. Many people have or will experience poor mental health. It is not a reflection of personal strength and should not be seen as failure. Seeking out or offering help is always a positive step and usually has the desired positive outcome.

2

Resuscitation

Resuscitation

Airway and Breathing Management   39

Traumatic Cardiac Arrest   44

Recognition of Life Extinct by
Ambulance Clinicians   46

Adult Resuscitation Guidelines:

Basic Life Support (Adult)   50

Advanced Life Support (Adult)   52

Foreign Body Airway Obstruction
(Adult)   58

Maternal Resuscitation   60

Child Resuscitation Guidelines:

Basic Life Support (Child)   62

Newborn Life Support   66

Advanced Life Support (Child)   70

Foreign Body Airway Obstruction
(Child)   74

Special Circumstances   77

1. Introduction

- Airway obstruction (partial or complete) is life-threatening and needs rapid intervention.

- Use a step-wise approach to airway management, commencing with simple airway adjuncts, progressing to supraglottic airways (i-Gel/laryngeal mask airway (LMA)), then tracheal intubation (if trained and equipped) and finally a cricothyroidotomy, only if the preceding step provides inadequate oxygenation and ventilation.

- Spinal immobilisation must be started at the same time as airway control (but does not take priority over airway control). **Refer to neck and trauma guideline**.

- Assessment of breathing includes both airway patency and respiratory effort (refer to Figure 2.1 and 2.2).

2. Airway Sizes

- Table 2.1 provides a guide for airway sizes in children and adults.

3. Supraglottic Airways

- There are several different SADs (i-Gel, laryngeal mask airway) but all sit above the larynx, covering the vocal cords and are simpler and quicker to insert than a tracheal tube. They can be inserted with minimal interruption to chest compressions. SADs are a good alternative to bag-mask ventilation and are associated with less aspiration of gastric contents.

- An air leak from around the laryngeal cuff is common when using these devices. If the chest wall can be seen to be moving, ventilation is generally adequate.

4. Tracheal Intubation

- The tracheal tube is the most challenging of all airway devices to insert successfully and requires both adequate initial training and ongoing practice. Practitioners of this skill must ensure that they have appropriate skills to undertake it safely. There is no evidence that outcome is any better following tracheal intubation compared with any other type of airway.

- When tracheal intubation is undertaken, be absolutely certain that the tube is in the trachea and not the oesophagus. Use a combination of visualisation of the tube entering the trachea, auscultation over both axillae and epigastrium, observation of chest wall movement and waveform capnography to confirm correct position.

- Secure the tracheal tube immediately after insertion (adult males – 23–25 cm, adult females – 22–24 cm at the lips).

- Avoid hypoxaemia during intubation - pre-oxygenate the lungs before and between short intubation attempts. During CPR, aim to minimise the interruptions to chest compressions for tube placement to less than 5 seconds.

5. Capnography

- Capnography (measurement of exhaled (end-tidal) carbon dioxide - $EtCO_2$) assists in confirmation and continuous monitoring of tracheal tube placement, can provide feedback on the quality of CPR and can provide an early indication of return of spontaneous circulation. Waveform capnography is a real-time waveform display of $EtCO_2$ and is more accurate and reliable than a paper indicator.

- Tracheal intubation and subsequent monitoring must only be performed using waveform capnography. Recorded values must be documented on the patient record.

- In the absence of waveform capnography, a supraglottic airway device (SAD) should be used when advanced airway management is indicated. $EtCO_2$ can be monitored with a SAD and can be useful in providing positive feedback on quality of CPR. Any decision to terminate resuscitation should not be based on either the presence or absence of $EtCO_2$ alone.

2 Resuscitation

SECTION

Airway and Breathing Management

Table 2.1 – AIRWAY SIZES BY TYPE

Age	Oropharyngeal	Tracheal tube	LMA	i-Gel
		Airway Size by Tube Type		
Birth	000	Diameter: 3.0 mm Length: 10 cm	1.0	1.0
1 month	00	Diameter: 3.0 mm Length: 10 cm	1.0	1.0
3 months	00	Diameter: 3.5 mm Length: 11 cm	1.5	1.5
6 months	00	Diameter: 4.0 mm Length: 12 cm	1.5	1.5
9 months	00	Diameter: 4.0 mm Length: 12 cm	1.5	1.5
12 months	00 OR 0	Diameter: 4.5 mm Length: 13 cm	1.5	1.5 OR 2.0
18 months	00 OR 0	Diameter: 4.5 mm Length: 13 cm	2.0	1.5 OR 2.0
2 years	0 OR 1	Diameter: 5.0 mm Length: 14 cm	2.0	1.5 OR 2.0
3 years	1	Diameter: 5.0 mm Length: 14 cm	2.0	2.0
4 years	1	Diameter: 5.0 mm Length: 15 cm	2.0	2.0
5 years	1	Diameter: 5.5 mm Length: 15 cm	2.0	2.0
6 years	1	Diameter: 6.0 mm Length: 16 cm	2.5	2.0
7 years	1 OR 2	Diameter: 6.0 mm Length: 16 cm	2.5	2.0
8 years	1 OR 2	Diameter: 6.5 mm Length: 17 cm	2.5	2.5
9 years	1 OR 2	Diameter: 6.5 mm Length: 17 cm	2.5	2.5
10 years	2 OR 3	Diameter: 7.0 mm Length: 18 cm	3.0	2.5 OR 3.0
11 years	2 OR 3	Diameter: 7.0 mm Length: 18 cm	3.0	2.5 OR 3.0
Adult >70kg	4 OR 5	Female diameter: 7.0–8.0 mm length: 22–24 cm Male diameter: 8.0–9.0 mm length: 23–25 cm	4.0 OR 5.0	4.0 OR 5.0

This table is an indicative guide only. Individual manufacturer's sizes may vary.

Airway and Breathing Management

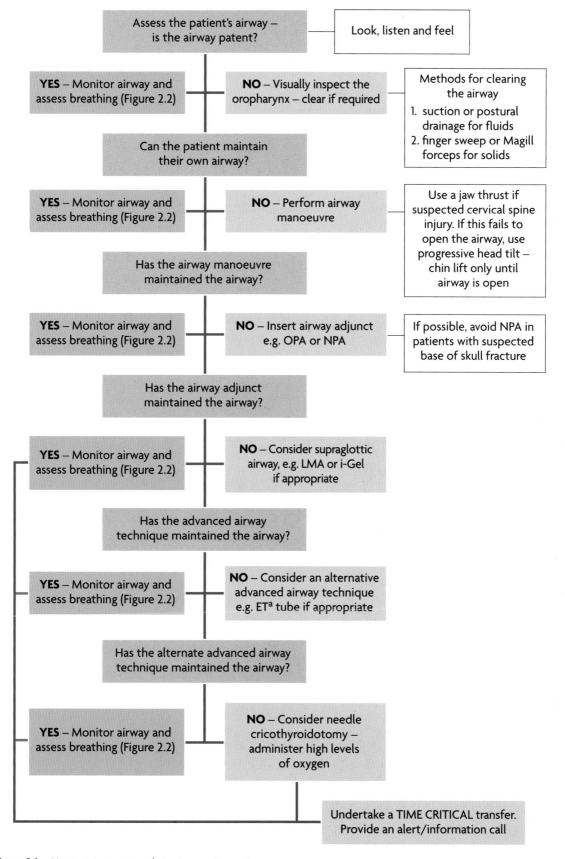

Assess the patient's airway – is the airway patent? — Look, listen and feel

YES – Monitor airway and assess breathing (Figure 2.2)

NO – Visually inspect the oropharynx – clear if required

Methods for clearing the airway
1. suction or postural drainage for fluids
2. finger sweep or Magill forceps for solids

Can the patient maintain their own airway?

YES – Monitor airway and assess breathing (Figure 2.2)

NO – Perform airway manoeuvre

Use a jaw thrust if suspected cervical spine injury. If this fails to open the airway, use progressive head tilt – chin lift only until airway is open

Has the airway manoeuvre maintained the airway?

YES – Monitor airway and assess breathing (Figure 2.2)

NO – Insert airway adjunct e.g. OPA or NPA

If possible, avoid NPA in patients with suspected base of skull fracture

Has the airway adjunct maintained the airway?

YES – Monitor airway and assess breathing (Figure 2.2)

NO – Consider supraglottic airway, e.g. LMA or i-Gel if appropriate

Has the advanced airway technique maintained the airway?

YES – Monitor airway and assess breathing (Figure 2.2)

NO – Consider an alternative advanced airway technique e.g. ET[a] tube if appropriate

Has the alternate advanced airway technique maintained the airway?

YES – Monitor airway and assess breathing (Figure 2.2)

NO – Consider needle cricothyroidotomy – administer high levels of oxygen

Undertake a TIME CRITICAL transfer. Provide an alert/information call

Figure 2.1 – Airway assessment and management overview.

[a] Capnography assists in confirmation and continuous monitoring of tracheal tube placement, can provide feedback on the quality of CPR and can provide an early indication of return of spontaneous circulation. The use of capnography is mandatory to assist in identifying correct tracheal tube placement, although it should be used in conjunction with visualisation of the tracheal tube entering the cords and auscultation. In the absence of a capnograph, a supraglottic airway device (SAD) should be used when advanced airway management is indicated. $EtCO_2$ can be monitored with a SAD and can be useful in providing positive feedback on quality of CPR. Any decision to terminate resuscitation should not be based on either the presence or absence of $EtCO_2$ alone. Note: A capnograph is a device that measures CO_2 withboth a numerical and waveform display.

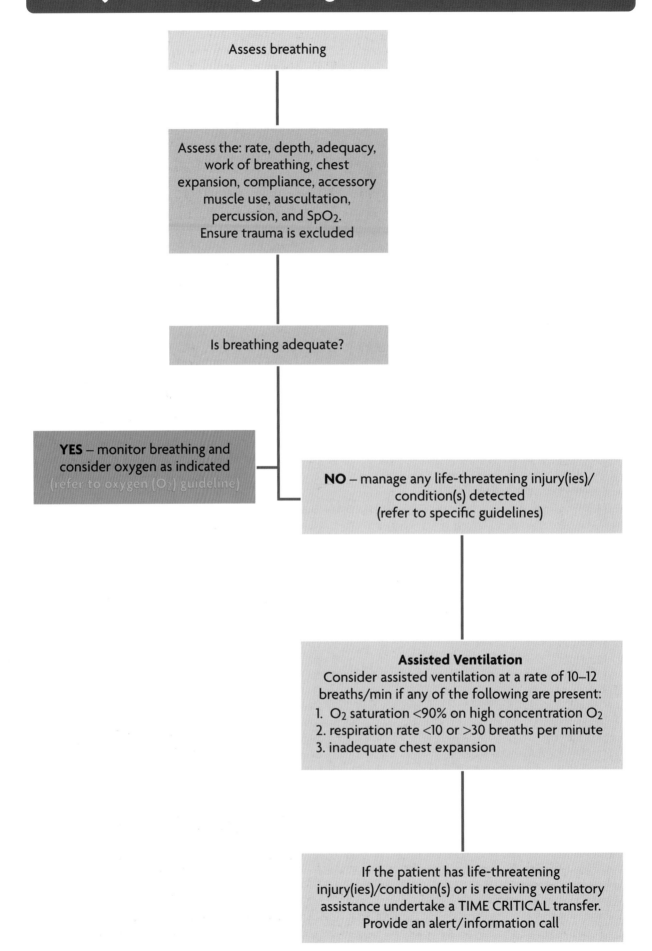

Figure 2.2 – Breathing assessment and management overview.

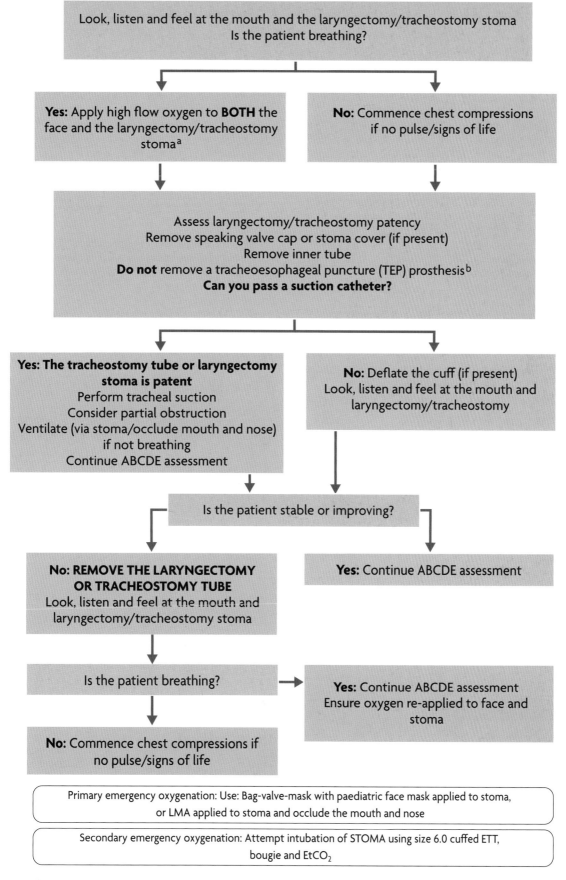

Look, listen and feel at the mouth and the laryngectomy/tracheostomy stoma
Is the patient breathing?

Yes: Apply high flow oxygen to **BOTH** the face and the laryngectomy/tracheostomy stoma[a]

No: Commence chest compressions if no pulse/signs of life

Assess laryngectomy/tracheostomy patency
Remove speaking valve cap or stoma cover (if present)
Remove inner tube
Do not remove a tracheoesophageal puncture (TEP) prosthesis[b]
Can you pass a suction catheter?

Yes: The tracheostomy tube or laryngectomy stoma is patent
Perform tracheal suction
Consider partial obstruction
Ventilate (via stoma/occlude mouth and nose) if not breathing
Continue ABCDE assessment

No: Deflate the cuff (if present)
Look, listen and feel at the mouth and laryngectomy/tracheostomy

Is the patient stable or improving?

No: REMOVE THE LARYNGECTOMY OR TRACHEOSTOMY TUBE
Look, listen and feel at the mouth and laryngectomy/tracheostomy stoma

Yes: Continue ABCDE assessment

Is the patient breathing?

Yes: Continue ABCDE assessment
Ensure oxygen re-applied to face and stoma

No: Commence chest compressions if no pulse/signs of life

Primary emergency oxygenation: Use: Bag-valve-mask with paediatric face mask applied to stoma, or LMA applied to stoma and occlude the mouth and nose

Secondary emergency oxygenation: Attempt intubation of STOMA using size 6.0 cuffed ETT, bougie and EtCO$_2$

[a] Applying oxygen to the face and stoma is the default emergency action for all patients with a laryngectomy/tracheostomy.
[b] A tracheoesophageal puncture (TEP) prosthesis is sited between the trachea and the oesophagus to allow oesophageal speech following a total laryngectomy.

Figure 2.3 – Emergency tracheostomy and laryngectomy management.

2 Resuscitation SECTION

1. Introduction

- Traumatic cardiac arrest is a very different condition from the more usual cardiac arrest which is often related to ischaemic heart disease.

- Management of traumatic cardiac arrest must be directed towards identifying and treating the underlying cause of the arrest or resuscitation is unlikely to be successful. This may require practitioners with advanced clinical skills, who should be mobilised to the incident as soon as possible.

- Traumatic cardiac arrest may develop as a result of:
  i. Hypoxia caused by treatable issues such as airway obstruction (e.g. facial injury or decreased level of consciousness) or breathing problems (e.g. pneumothorax).
  ii. Hypoperfusion caused by compromise of the heart (e.g. stab wound causing cardiac tamponade) or hypovolaemia (either internal or external haemorrhage).

2. Assessment and Management

For the assessment and management of traumatic cardiac arrest refer to Table 2.2.

[Further related reading includes 104, 105–106, 107–108]

3. Reversible Causes of Traumatic Cardiac Arrest

- The 4 Hs and 4Ts approach will highlight the common causes of treatable traumatic cardiac arrest:

  - Hypovolaemia
  - Hypoxia (Oxygenation)
  - Hypothermia
  - Hyperkalaemia
  - Tension pneumothorax
  - Tamponade
  - Toxins
  - Thromboembolism

- Patients with traumatic cardiac arrest commonly have one or more injuries resulting in severe hypovolaemia, critical hypoxaemia, tamponade or tension pneumothorax, either in isolation or concurrently. Each of these conditions needs to be addressed simultaneously and active management commenced.

4. Pre-hospital Fluids

- In traumatic cardiac arrest where hypovolaemia may be a contributing factor, commence fluid infusion as soon as IV/IO access is established.

  - In adults, give fluid in 250 ml boluses only until a radial pulse is palpable. In patients with penetrating chest trauma, titrate fluid to achieve a carotid pulse.
  - In patients who have arrested from hypovolaemia, large volumes (2–3 l) of fluid (preferably blood) may be needed to achieve ROSC. Assess the patient for signs of spontaneous circulation after each 250 ml bolus of fluid is infused.
  - In children, titrate 5 ml/kg fluid boluses as needed until clinical signs improve (e.g. RR, HR, capillary refill, conscious level).*

*NB Hypotensive resuscitation practices (as used in adult trauma) should not be used in children. Due to their physiological reserves, children maintain their systolic blood pressures in the face of major blood loss, with hypotension only occurring at a very late stage. Significant cardiovascular compromise and even cardiac arrest may occur if volume resuscitation were to be delayed until a child had reached such an advanced state of hypovolaemia.

5. Tranexamic Acid

- Give adult trauma patients with suspected haemorrhage a single dose of tranexamic acid 1g IV/IO over 10 min.

- Following IV fluid resuscitation, tranexamic acid should be given to children with catastrophic haemorrhage following major trauma (refer to tranexamic acid guideline).

KEY POINTS

Traumatic Cardiac Arrest

- **Traumatic cardiac arrest is different from cardiac arrest due to primary cardiac disease.**
- **Assessment and management should follow the trauma guideline, treating problems as they are found.**
- **Once a decision to start resuscitation is taken, full ALS-based resuscitation for at least 20 minutes should be performed, aiming to rapidly identify and correct all reversible causes.**
- **If there is no response to resuscitation after 20 minutes of ALS, having treated all reversible causes, further effort is futile. However, resuscitation of children and pregnant women should be continued to hospital.**
- **Patients who have suffered cardiac arrest due to penetrating trauma should have full ALS-based-resuscitation continued with a minimal on scene time and a time critical transfer to hospital undertaken.**
- **The ROLE procedure should be followed if resuscitation is terminated.**

Table 2.2 – ASSESSMENT and MANAGEMENT of:

Traumatic Cardiac Arrest

ASSESSMENT	MANAGEMENT
● Assess potential cause(s)	Manage by applying standard trauma management principles (**refer to trauma emergencies guideline**). Any problem should be dealt with adequately before moving on to the next: **<C>** Control any **CATASTROPHIC HAEMORRHAGE** (extreme bleeding likely to cause death in minutes) by assessing for the presence of **LIFE-THREATENING EXTERNAL BLEEDING** and control with compression, elevation, tourniquet and haemostatic dressings as appropriate (**refer to trauma emergencies overview guideline**). **A** – Airway obstruction; ensure the airway is open and clear. **B** – Impaired breathing; search for and manage a sucking chest wound or a tension pneumothorax (**refer to thoracic trauma guideline**). Support and assist ventilation (refer to airway and breathing management guideline). **C** – Hypovolaemia as a result of major blood loss; apply external haemorrhage control and obtain vascular access while transferring without delay to definitive treatment. **D** – Major head injury (**refer to head trauma guideline**) or spinal cord injury (**refer to neck and back trauma guideline**) impairing ventilation through central nervous system (CNS) depression or loss of neuromuscular function.
● Commencing CPR	● Resuscitation should be commenced in all patients, irrespective of whether the arrest was witnessed, unless the patient is clearly beyond help (non-survivable injury, rigor mortis, decomposition etc). Once resuscitation is commenced, full ALS-based resuscitation (refer to advanced life support guidelines) should be attempted for an appropriate duration (see below). ● In paediatric traumatic cardiac arrest, CPR should always be commenced unless the child has unsurvivable injuries and ROLE is appropriate (refer to ROLE guideline). ● In penetrating traumatic cardiac arrest, patients **must** be transferred **rapidly** to hospital because surgical intervention is often needed to treat the cause of the arrest. In these patients, a 'scoop and run' policy is appropriate. **Do not stay on scene to resuscitate a patient with penetrating injury**. ● If a patient has not responded after 20 minutes of advanced life support (ALS) and reversible causes have been identified and corrected, then resuscitation can be terminated (see below).
● Terminating CPR	● Termination of resuscitation in a patient who has suffered a traumatic cardiac arrest (blunt) should be considered if the patient has not responded (i.e. the patient is apnoeic, pulseless, and without organised cardiac electrical activity) to 20 minutes of ALS, providing all reversible causes have been treated. Patients in cardiac arrest due to penetrating trauma can only have all reversible causes treated in hospital and a **TIME CRITICAL** transfer of these patients should be undertaken. ● The only exceptions to this are pregnancy (when the patient should be rapidly transferred to hospital to deliver the infant), in the presence of hypothermia and with trauma involving children. In this latter case, follow paediatric resuscitation guidelines and undertake a **TIME CRITICAL** transfer to a hospital Emergency Department with ongoing resuscitation. ● After stopping resuscitation, the Recognition of Life Extinct by Ambulance Clinicians (ROLE) procedure should be followed (refer to ROLE guideline) and the police informed.

1. Introduction

In patients with cardiopulmonary arrest, vigorous resuscitation attempts must be undertaken and continued whenever there is a chance of survival.

Nevertheless, it is possible to identify patients in whom there is absolutely no chance of survival, and where resuscitation would be both futile and distressing for relatives, friends and healthcare personnel and where time and resources would be wasted undertaking such measures.

The views of an attending general practitioner (GP), ambulance doctor or relevant third party should be considered when possible.

2. Conditions Unequivocally Associated with Death where Resuscitation should not be Attempted

All the conditions, listed below, are unequivocally associated with death in **ALL** age groups (see below for further details):

1. decapitation
2. massive cranial and cerebral destruction
3. hemicorporectomy or similar massive injury
4. decomposition/putrefaction
5. incineration
6. hypostasis
7. rigor mortis.

In the newborn, fetal maceration is unequivocally associated with death.

Further Details

Decapitation: Self-evidently incompatible with life.

Massive cranial and cerebral destruction: Where the injuries are considered by the ambulance clinician to be incompatible with life.

Hemicorporectomy or similar massive injury: Where the injuries are considered by the ambulance clinician to be incompatible with life.

Decomposition/putrefaction: Where tissue damage indicates that the patient has been dead for some hours, days or longer.

Incineration: The presence of full thickness burns with charring of greater than 95% of the body surface.

Hypostasis: The pooling of blood in congested vessels in the dependent part of the body in the position in which it lies after death (**See Guidance Note 1**).

Rigor mortis: The stiffness occurring after death from the post mortem breakdown of enzymes in the muscle fibres (**See Guidance Note 2**).

In all other cases resuscitation must be commenced and the facts pertaining to the arrest must be established.

Following arrival and the recognition of an absent pulse and apnoea (in the presence of a patent airway), chest compression and ventilations should be commenced whilst the facts of the collapse are ascertained.

3. In the Following Conditions, Resuscitation can be Discontinued

- The presence of a DNACPR (Do Not Attempt Cardio-Pulmonary Resuscitation) order or an Advanced Decision that states the wish of the patient not to undergo attempted resuscitation (see 3b below).

- A patient in the final stages of a terminal illness where death is imminent and unavoidable and CPR would not be successful, but for whom no formal DNACPR decision has been made.

- There would be no realistic chance that CPR would be successful if **ALL** the following exist together:
  - 15 minutes since the onset of cardiac arrest
  - no bystander CPR prior to arrival of the ambulance
  - the absence of any of the exclusion factors on the flowchart (refer to Figure 2.3)
  - asystole for >30 seconds on the ECG monitor screen.

- CPR should only be paused for a 30 second asystole check if all other criteria are met.

- Submersion for longer than 60 minutes (NB submersion **NOT** immersion) (**See Drowning**).

Whenever possible a confirmatory ECG, demonstrating asystole, should be documented as evidence of death. In this situation a 3 or 4 electrode system using limbs alone will cause minimum disturbance to the deceased. If a paper ECG trace cannot be taken, it is permissible to make a diagnosis of asystole from the screen alone (NB due caution must be applied in respect of electrode contact, gain and, where possible, using more than one ECG lead). The use of the flow chart shown in Figure 2.3 is recommended.

If there is a realistic chance that CPR could be successful, then resuscitation must continue to establish the patient's response to Advanced Life Support interventions. If the patient does not respond despite full ALS intervention and is asystolic after 20 minutes, then the resuscitation attempt may be discontinued.

Removal of advanced airways and/or indwelling cannulae should be in accordance with local protocol.

4. Do not Attempt Resuscitation (DNACPR)/Advanced Decision to Refuse Treatment

Ambulance clinicians should initiate resuscitation unless:

1. A formal DNACPR order is in place, either written and handed to the ambulance clinician or verbally received and recorded by ambulance control from the patient's attendant requesting the ambulance providing that:
   a. the order is seen and corroborated by the ambulance clinician on arrival.
   b. the decision to resuscitate relates to the condition for which the DNACPR order is in force: resuscitation should not be withheld for coincidental conditions.

2. The patient is in the final stages of a terminal illness where death is imminent and unavoidable and CPR

would not be successful, but for whom no formal DNACPR decision has been made.

3. An Advanced Decision has been accepted by the treating physician (patient's GP or hospital consultant) as a DNACPR order. This should be communicated to ambulance control and logged against the patient's address.

   a. Patients may have an Advanced Decision although it is not legally necessary for the refusal to be made in writing or formally witnessed. This specifies how they would like to be treated in the case of future incapacity. Case law is now clear that an advance refusal of treatment that is valid, and applicable to subsequent circumstances in which the patient lacks capacity, is legally binding. An advance refusal is valid if made voluntarily by an appropriately informed person with capacity. Staff should respect the wishes stated in such a document.

   b. In an out-of-hospital emergency environment, there may be situations where there is doubt about the validity of an advance refusal or DNACPR order. If staff are **NOT** satisfied that the patient had made a prior and specific request to refuse treatment, they should continue to provide all clinical care in the normal way.

5. Action to be Taken after Death has been Established

For guidance on the actions to be taken following verification of death refer to Figure 2.4.

Complete documentation – including all decisions regarding do not attempt resuscitation (DNAR) / advanced decision to refuse treatment.

It is necessary for a medical practitioner to attend to confirm the fact of death. Moreover, the new GP Contract contains no obligation for a GP to do so when requested to attend by ambulance control.

Services should be encouraged, in conjunction with their Coroner's service (or Procurator Fiscal in Scotland), to develop a local procedure for handling the body once death has been verified by ambulance personnel.

A locally approved leaflet should be adopted for handing to bereaved relatives.

GUIDANCE NOTE 1

Initially, hypostatic staining may appear as small round patches looking rather like bruises, but later these coalesce to merge as the familiar pattern. Above the hypostatic engorgement there is obvious pallor of the skin. The presence of hypostasis is diagnostic of death – the appearance is not present in a live patient. In extremely cold conditions, hypostasis may be bright red in colour, and in carbon monoxide poisoning it is characteristically 'cherry red' in appearance.

GUIDANCE NOTE 2

Rigor mortis occurs first in the small muscles of the face, next in the arms, then in the legs (30 minutes to 3 hours). Children will show a more rapid onset of rigor. The recognition of rigor mortis can be made difficult where, rarely, death has occurred from tetanus or strychnine poisoning.

In some, rigidity never develops (infants, cachectic individuals and the aged) whilst in others it may become apparent more rapidly (in conditions in which muscle glycogen is depleted): exertion (which includes struggling), strychnine poisoning, local heat (e.g. from a fire, hot room or direct sunlight).

Rigor should not be confused with cadaveric spasm (sometimes referred to as instant rigor mortis) which develops immediately after death without preceding flaccidity following intense physical and/or emotional activity. Examples include: death by drowning or a fall from a height. In contrast with true rigor mortis, only one group of muscles is affected and **NOT** the whole body. Rigor mortis will develop subsequently.

KEY POINTS

Recognition of Life Extinct by Ambulance Clinicians

- Ambulance clinicians are increasingly called upon to diagnose death and initiate the appropriate responses to death.

- In patients with cardiopulmonary arrest, vigorous resuscitation efforts must be made whenever there is a chance of survival, however remote.

- Some conditions are incompatible with recovery and in these cases resuscitation need not be attempted.

- In some situations, once the facts of the patient/ situation/etc are known, resuscitation efforts can be discontinued.

- Patients can and do make anticipatory decisions NOT to be resuscitated. An Advanced Decision or DNAR, if verifiable, must be respected.

- These guidelines should be read in conjunction with local policies and procedures.

- Rigor mortis can appear quickly following a child death and resuscitation should always be attempted unless there is a condition unequivocally associated with death.

Recognition of Life Extinct by Ambulance Clinicians

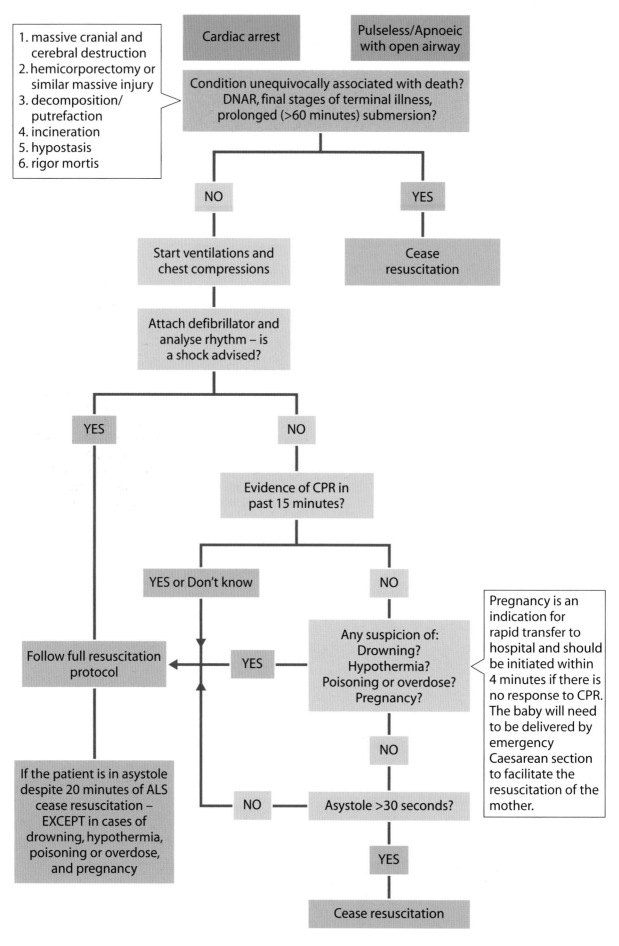

1. massive cranial and cerebral destruction
2. hemicorporectomy or similar massive injury
3. decomposition/putrefaction
4. incineration
5. hypostasis
6. rigor mortis

Cardiac arrest

Pulseless/Apnoeic with open airway

Condition unequivocally associated with death? DNAR, final stages of terminal illness, prolonged (>60 minutes) submersion?

NO

YES

Start ventilations and chest compressions

Cease resuscitation

Attach defibrillator and analyse rhythm – is a shock advised?

YES

NO

Evidence of CPR in past 15 minutes?

YES or Don't know

NO

Follow full resuscitation protocol

YES

Any suspicion of: Drowning? Hypothermia? Poisoning or overdose? Pregnancy?

Pregnancy is an indication for rapid transfer to hospital and should be initiated within 4 minutes if there is no response to CPR. The baby will need to be delivered by emergency Caesarean section to facilitate the resuscitation of the mother.

NO

If the patient is in asystole despite 20 minutes of ALS cease resuscitation – EXCEPT in cases of drowning, hypothermia, poisoning or overdose, and pregnancy

NO

Asystole >30 seconds?

YES

Cease resuscitation

Figure 2.3 – Recognition of life extinct by ambulance clinicians algorithm.

SECTION **2** Resuscitation

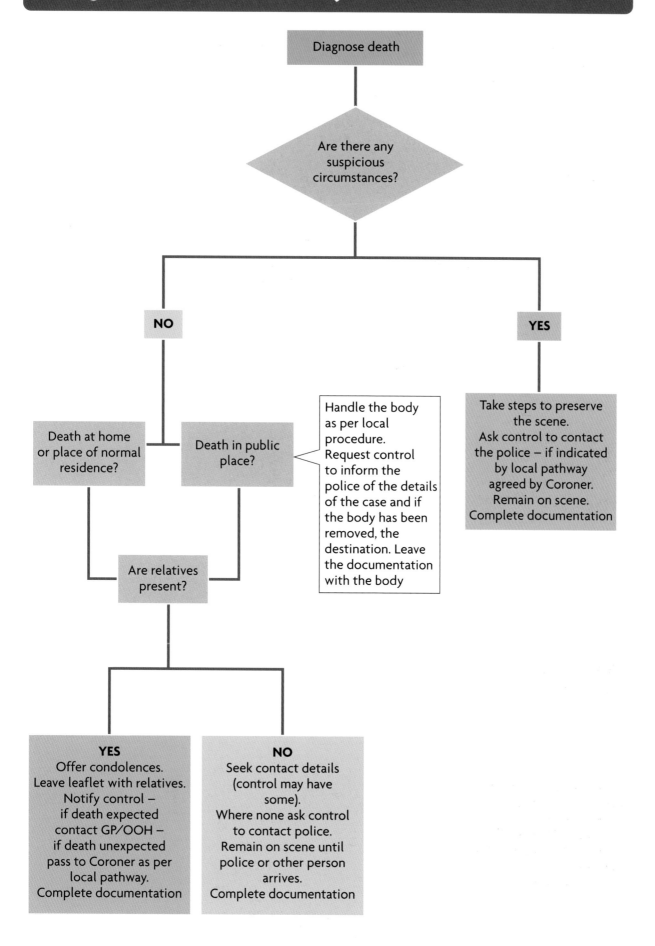

Figure 2.4 – Action to be taken after verification of fact of death.

Diagnose death

Are there any suspicious circumstances?

NO

YES

Death at home or place of normal residence?

Death in public place?

Handle the body as per local procedure. Request control to inform the police of the details of the case and if the body has been removed, the destination. Leave the documentation with the body

Take steps to preserve the scene. Ask control to contact the police – if indicated by local pathway agreed by Coroner. Remain on scene. Complete documentation

Are relatives present?

YES
Offer condolences. Leave leaflet with relatives. Notify control – if death expected contact GP/OOH – if death unexpected pass to Coroner as per local pathway. Complete documentation

NO
Seek contact details (control may have some). Where none ask control to contact police. Remain on scene until police or other person arrives. Complete documentation

1. Introduction

- Basic life support (BLS) refers to maintaining airway patency, and supporting breathing and circulation without the use of equipment other than a protective device, usually a facemask or shield. In the pre-hospital environment, BLS includes the use of a bag-valve-mask and oropharyngeal airway.

- With the advent of automated external defibrillators (AED) that are simple to use with little training, defibrillation is now considered part of BLS.

2. Assessment and Management

- For the assessment and management of adult basic life support refer to Table 2.3 and the adult basic life support sequence detailed in Figure 2.5.

Table 2.3 – ASSESSMENT and MANAGEMENT of:

Basic Life Support (Adult)

This sequence is for a single ambulance clinician; however, when more than one clinician is present, tasks can be shared and undertaken simultaneously.

ASSESSMENT	MANAGEMENT
● Assess safety	● Ensure that you, the patient and any bystanders are safe.
● Check responsiveness	● Gently shake the patient by the shoulders and ask loudly: '**Are you all right?**'
– The **responsive** patient	● Take history and make assessment of what is wrong, with further action determined accordingly.
– The **unresponsive** patient	● Obtain further resources if appropriate. ● Turn the patient onto their back and then open the airway using head tilt and chin lift. Look in the mouth. If a foreign body or debris is visible, attempt to remove it with a finger sweep, forceps or suction as appropriate. Consider the use of a laryngoscope and forceps if FBAO is suspected. ● When there is a risk of back or neck injury, establish a clear upper airway by using jaw thrust or chin lift in combination with manual in-line stabilisation of the head and neck by an assistant (if available). If life-threatening airway obstruction persists despite effective application of jaw thrust or chin lift, add head tilt a small amount at a time until the airway is open; establishing a patent airway takes priority over concerns about a potential back or neck injury.
● Keeping the airway open	● Look, listen and feel for normal breathing, taking no more than 10 seconds to determine if the patient is breathing normally. If you have any doubt whether breathing is normal, act as if it is **NOT** normal. ● Agonal breathing (occasional irregular gasps, slow, laboured noisy breathing) is common in the early stages of cardiac arrest. It is a sign of cardiac arrest and should not be confused as a sign of life/circulation.
● If the patient is breathing normally	● Turn into the recovery position. ● Undertake assessment, monitoring and transport accordingly. ● Re-assess regularly.
● If the patient is not breathing normally	● It may be difficult to be certain that there is no pulse. ● If there are no signs of life (lack of movement, normal breathing, or coughing), or there is doubt, start chest compressions at a rate of 100–120 compressions per minute. ● Compression depth should be 5–6 cm. Allow the chest to recoil completely after each compression. Take approximately the same amount of time for each compression and relaxation. Minimise interruptions to chest compression. Do not rely on a palpable pulse (carotid, femoral, or radial) as a gauge of effective blood flow.
● Combine chest compression with rescue breaths	● After 30 compressions, open the airway again and provide 2 ventilations with the most appropriate equipment available, using an inspiratory time of 1 second with adequate volume to produce normal chest expansion. Each time compressions are resumed the ambulance clinician should place their hands without delay in the centre of the chest. ● Add high flow oxygen as soon as possible. ● Continue chest compressions and ventilation in a ratio of 30:2. ● Stop to recheck only if the patient starts breathing normally; otherwise do not interrupt chest compressions and ventilation. ● Performing chest compressions is tiring; try to change the person doing chest compressions every 2 minutes; ensure the minimum of delay during the changeover. Once the airway is secure (e.g. after supraglottic airway insertion) continue chest compressions uninterrupted at a rate of 100–120 per minute (except for defibrillation or further assessment as indicated). ● Ventilate gently, 8–10 times per minute. Avoid hyperventilation. ● If attempts at ventilation do not make the chest rise as in normal breathing, then before the next attempt at ventilation: – check the patient's mouth and remove any obstruction – recheck that the airway position is optimal with adequate head tilt/chin lift or jaw thrust – do not attempt more than 2 breaths each time before returning to chest compressions.

Basic Life Support (Adult)

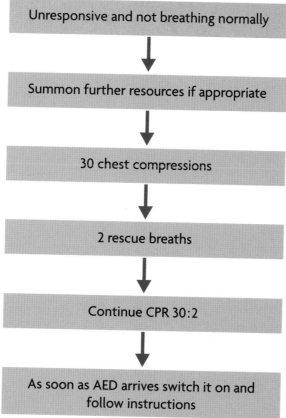

Figure 2.5 – Adult basic life support sequence – Modified from the Resuscitation Council (UK) Guidelines 2015 (www.resus.org.uk).

3. Additional Information

CPR in confined spaces

Over-the-head CPR and straddle CPR may be considered for resuscitation in confined spaces.

Use of the automated external defibrillator (AED)

1. Make sure you, the patient and any bystanders are safe.

2. If you do not have an AED with you, perform CPR until an AED arrives.

3. As soon as an AED is available:

   - switch on the defibrillator and attach the electrode pads. If more than one ambulance clinician is present, CPR should be continued while this is done
   - follow the spoken/visual directions

   - ensure nobody touches the patient while the AED is analysing the rhythm.

4a. If a shock is indicated, continue compression as AED is charging if possible:

   - ensure nobody touches the patient
   - push the shock button as directed
   - continue as directed by the voice/visual prompts.

4b. If no shock is indicated:

   - immediately resume CPR using a ratio of 30 compressions to 2 rescue breaths
   - continue as directed by voice/visual prompts.

5. Continue to follow AED prompts until:

   - the patient starts to breathe normally
   - ALS is started
   - you are exhausted.

KEY POINTS

Basic Life Support (Adult)

- High quality, uninterrupted basic life support is a key determinant of survival from cardiac arrest.
- Agonal breathing is common in the early stages of cardiac arrest and should not be confused as a sign of life/circulation.
- If there are no signs of life, start chest compressions at a rate of 100–120 per minute using a ratio of 30 compressions to 2 breaths.
- Once the airway is secure, chest compressions should be uninterrupted, with ventilations given 8–10 times per minute; avoid hyperventilation.
- As soon as an AED is available switch it on, attach the electrode pads and follow the voice/visual prompts. Use of an AED takes priority over all other aspects of resuscitation.

1. Introduction

The heart rhythms associated with cardiac arrest are divided into two groups:

1. **shockable rhythms** – ventricular fibrillation and pulseless ventricular tachycardia (VF/VT)
2. **non-shockable rhythms** – asystole and pulseless electrical activity (PEA).

- The principal difference in the management of these two groups is the need for attempted defibrillation in VF/VT. Subsequent actions including chest compressions, airway management and ventilation, venous access, administration of adrenaline and the management of reversible factors, are common to both groups.

- The interventions that unequivocally improve survival are early defibrillation and effective basic life support. Attention should focus therefore on early defibrillation and high quality, uninterrupted cardiopulmonary resuscitation (CPR).

- A solo responder should not interrupt chest compressions for any reason other than to deliver 2 breaths or defibrillate the patient. Intravenous (IV) access, drug delivery and advanced airway management require two or more responders. While these procedures are performed, interruptions to chest compressions must be less than 5 secs and kept to an absolute minimum.

- High quality, uninterrupted chest compressions are crucial in achieving improved survival. Chest compressions at the correct rate (100–120/min) and depth (5–6 cm) with complete relaxation should commence immediately and continue while the defibrillator is charging; only pausing to assess the rhythm or deliver the shock (as appropriate) before recommencing the compressions.

- When attending as a solo responder, immediate assessment of the rhythm and defibrillation (when indicated), should take precedence over airway or breathing interventions. Immediate defibrillation should always be performed in patients where a shockable rhythm is identified on the ECG, irrespective of the amplitude.

- IV access should be established as soon as an appropriately trained responder is able to do so. If IV access is not possible after two attempts, intraosseous access should be considered.

2. Assessment and Management

For assessment and management of cardiac arrest refer to Table 2.4 and Figure 2.6. For the care of patients following Return of Spontaneous Circulation (ROSC) refer to Table 2.5 and Figure 2.7.

Table 2.4 – ASSESSMENT and MANAGEMENT of:

Advanced Life Support (Adult)

ASSESSMENT	MANAGEMENT
Having confirmed cardiac arrest	• Request further resources. • Start CPR beginning with chest compressions. Ventilate with high flow oxygen. • As soon as the defibrillator arrives, diagnose the rhythm by applying self-adhesive pads to the chest and attempt defibrillation as appropriate.
1. SHOCKABLE RHYTHMS (VF/PULSELESS VT)	• Attempt defibrillation (1 shock – 150–200 J biphasic). • Immediately resume chest compressions (30:2) without re-assessing the rhythm or feeling for a pulse. • Continue CPR for 2 minutes, and then pause briefly to check the monitor.
If VF/VT persists	• Give a further (2nd) shock (150–360 J biphasic). • Resume CPR immediately and continue for 2 minutes. • Pause briefly to check the monitor. • If VF/VT persists, give a further (3rd) shock (150–360 J biphasic). • As soon as CPR has resumed, give adrenaline 1 mg 1:10,000 IV. Give 300 mg amiodarone IV while continuing CPR for a further 2 minutes. • Pause briefly to check the monitor. • If VF/VT persists, give a further (4th) shock (150–360 J biphasic). • Resume CPR immediately and continue for 2 minutes. • Pause briefly to check the monitor. • If VF/VT persists give a further (5th) shock (150–360 J biphasic). • Resume CPR immediately and give adrenaline 1 mg 1:10,000 IV and an additional 150 mg amiodarone IV while continuing CPR for a further 2 minutes. • Give adrenaline 1 mg 1:10,000 IV immediately after alternate shocks (i.e. approximately every 3–5 minutes). • Give further shocks after each 2 minute period of CPR and after confirming that VF/VT persists.
If organised electrical activity is seen, check for a pulse	• If a pulse is present, start post-resuscitation care. • If no pulse is present, continue CPR and switch to the non-shockable algorithm.
If asystole is seen	• Continue CPR and change to follow the non-shockable algorithm.

Table 2.4 – ASSESSMENT and MANAGEMENT of:

Advanced Life Support (Adult) *continued*

2. NON-SHOCKABLE RHYTHMS (ASYSTOLE AND PEA)	If these rhythms are identified: ● Start CPR 30:2 and give adrenaline 1 mg as soon as IV/IO access is achieved. ● If asystole is displayed, without stopping CPR, check the leads are attached correctly. ● Secure the airway as soon as possible, to enable continuous chest compressions without pausing for ventilation. ● After 2 minutes CPR 30:2 recheck the rhythm. If asystole is present or there has been no change in ECG appearance, resume CPR immediately. ● If VF / VT present, change to the shockable rhythm algorithm. ● If an organised rhythm is present, attempt to palpate a central pulse. High levels of end-tidal CO_2 may also indicate ROSC. ● If a pulse is present, begin post-resuscitation care. ● If no pulse is present (or there is any doubt) continue CPR. Give adrenaline 1 mg IV every 3–5 minutes (alternate loops). ● If signs of life return during CPR, check the rhythm and attempt to palpate a pulse.
3. POTENTIALLY REVERSIBLE CAUSES Potential causes or aggravating factors for which specific treatment exists must be considered during any cardiac arrest. For ease of memory these are presented as 4 Hs and 4 Ts	Assess the 4Hs and 4Ts according to their initial letter. Those amenable to treatment include: 1. **Hypoxia** – ensure adequate chest expansion and breath sounds. Verify tracheal tube placement, using waveform capnography. 2. **Hypovolaemia** – PEA caused by hypovolaemia is usually due to haemorrhage from trauma, gastrointestinal bleeding or rupture of an aortic aneurysm. Intravascular volume should be restored rapidly with IV fluid. Rapid transport to definitive surgical care is essential. 3. **Hypothermia – refer to hypothermia and immersion incident guidelines**. 4. **Hyperkalaemia** and other electrolyte disorders are unlikely to be apparent in the pre-hospital arena or respond to treatment. Consider early removal to hospital. 1. **Tension pneumothorax** – the diagnosis is made clinically; decompress as soon as possible by needle thoracocentesis. 2. **Cardiac tamponade** – is difficult to diagnose as the typical signs (high venous pressure, hypotension) are masked by cardiac arrest. Cardiac arrest after penetrating chest trauma is highly suggestive of cardiac tamponade. These patients should be transported to hospital immediately without any delay on scene as pericardiocentesis or thoracotomy cannot routinely be performed outside hospital. 3. **Toxins** – only rarely will an antidote be available outside hospital, and in most cases supportive treatment will be the priority. 4. **Thromboembolism** – massive pulmonary embolism is a common cause but diagnosis in the field is difficult once cardiac arrest has occurred. Specific treatments (e.g. thrombolytic drugs) are not available to ambulance personnel in the UK at present.
4. THE WITNESSED, MONITORED ARREST	**If a patient who is being monitored has a witnessed arrest:** ● Confirm cardiac arrest; request further resources if appropriate. ● If the rhythm is VF/VT and a defibrillator is not immediately available, consider a precordial thump. ● If the rhythm is VF/VT and a defibrillator is immediately available, give a shock first and immediately commence CPR; treat any recurrence of VF/pulseless VT following the shockable rhythm algorithm. ● Where the arrest is witnessed but unmonitored, using self-adhesive defibrillation pads will allow assessment of the rhythm more quickly than attaching ECG electrodes.

Table 2.5 – ASSESSMENT and MANAGEMENT of:

Return of Spontaneous Circulation (ROSC)

Following ROSC some patients may suffer post-cardiac-arrest syndrome, the severity of which will depend on the duration and cause of the cardiac arrest. Post-cardiac-arrest syndrome often complicates the post-resuscitation phase and comprises:

- **Brain injury:** coma, seizures, myoclonus, varying degrees of neurocognitive dysfunction and brain death; this may be exacerbated by microcirculatory failure, impaired autoregulation, hypercarbia, hyperoxia, pyrexia, hyper/hypoglycaemia and seizures.
- **Myocardial dysfunction:** this is common after cardiac arrest but usually improves in the following weeks.
- **The systemic ischaemia/reperfusion response:** the whole body ischaemia/reperfusion that occurs with resuscitation from cardiac arrest activates immunological and coagulation pathways contributing to an inflammatory response and multiple organ failure.
- **Persistence of the precipitating pathology.**

For the care of patients following ROSC see below.

ASSESSMENT	MANAGEMENT
● Return of Spontaneous Circulation	● Transfer the patient directly to the nearest appropriate hospital in accordance with local protocols relating to PPCI. ● Early recurrence of VF is common, so ensure continuous monitoring in order to deliver further shocks if appropriate. ● Continue patient management en-route – see below. ● Provide an alert/information call.
● Oxygen	● Measure oxygen saturation. ● Maintain oxygen saturations of 94–98%.
● Ventilation	● Use of an automatic ventilator is preferable to manual ventilation. ● Monitor ventilation rate and volume. ● Monitor end-tidal CO_2 (NB Readings may be low because of reduced cardiac output rather than hyperventilation. Normal range = 4.6–6 kPa).
● Circulation	● Following ROSC, patients are usually haemodynamically unstable, often hypotensive and may have further arrhythmias. Aim for a systolic blood pressure of 90–100 mmHg. A 250 ml IV/IO bolus of 0.9% saline is appropriate should the patient be hypotensive, repeated as necessary. ● In the event of symptomatic bradycardia, give atropine 0.6-1.0 mg IV. If ineffective, consider external pacing. ● In the event of severe hypotension despite fluids and correction of arrhythmias, consider boluses of adrenaline (1:1,000)/IV, carefully titrated against blood pressure as per local protocol. This should be undertaken only in the setting of robust governance where telephone medical support is available.
● ECG	● Undertake a 12-lead ECG.
● Blood glucose level	● Measure blood glucose level. ● If the patient is hypoglycaemic (BM <4.0 mmol) **refer to glycaemic emergencies guideline**.
● Combative patient	● Following ROSC, patients may be cerebrally irritated and combative. Exclude hypoglycaemia and hypoxaemia. These patients may benefit from formal anaesthetic management, but incremental doses of IV diazepam or midazolam may be indicated, with appropriate telephone medical support if advanced medical care is not available on scene.
● Seizure control	● Seizures that do not self-terminate within a few minutes may be treated with a benzodiazepine, titrated to effect. The administration of diazepam or midazolam is carried out in line with UK Clinical Practice (JRCALC) or local service clinical guidelines.
● Cooling	● In cases of non-traumatic cardiac arrest in patients that have not regained consciousness, allow passive cooling in line with local protocols.

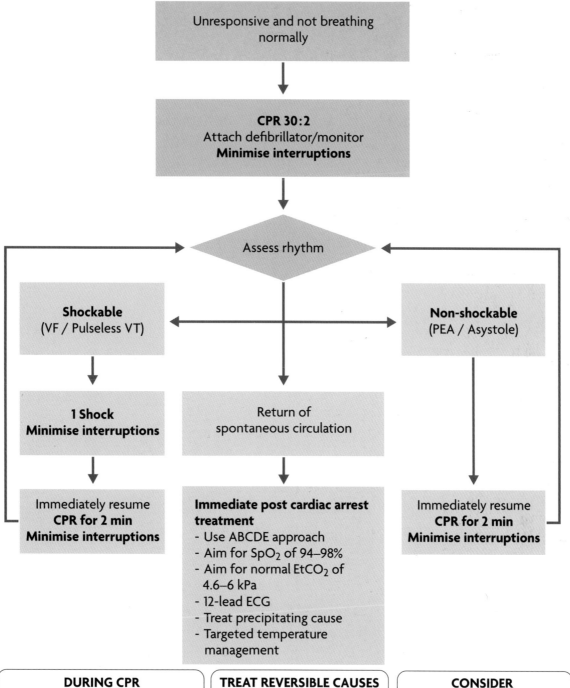

Unresponsive and not breathing normally

↓

CPR 30:2
Attach defibrillator/monitor
Minimise interruptions

↓

Assess rhythm

Shockable
(VF / Pulseless VT)

Non-shockable
(PEA / Asystole)

1 Shock
Minimise interruptions

Return of spontaneous circulation

↓

Immediately resume
CPR for 2 min
Minimise interruptions

Immediate post cardiac arrest treatment
- Use ABCDE approach
- Aim for SpO_2 of 94–98%
- Aim for normal $EtCO_2$ of 4.6–6 kPa
- 12-lead ECG
- Treat precipitating cause
- Targeted temperature management

Immediately resume
CPR for 2 min
Minimise interruptions

DURING CPR	**TREAT REVERSIBLE CAUSES**	**CONSIDER**
• Ensure high-quality chest compressions. • Minimise interruptions to compressions. • Give oxygen. • Use waveform capnography. • Continuous compressions when advanced airway in place. • Vascular access (intravenous or intraosseous). • Give adrenaline every 3–5 min. • Give amiodarone after 3 shocks.	• **H**ypoxia. • **H**ypovolaemia. • **H**ypo/hyperkalaemia/ metabolic. • **H**ypothermia. • **T**hrombosis – coronary or pulmonary. • **T**ension pneumothorax. • **T**amponade – cardiac. • **T**oxins.	• Ultrasound imaging. • Follow local protocols for chest compressions. Where available consider mechanical chest compressions. • Transfer for coronary angiography and percutaneous coronary intervention.

Figure 2.6 – Advanced life support algorithm – modified from the Resuscitation Council (UK) Guidelines 2015 algorithm (www.resus.org.uk).

Advanced Life Support (Adult)

Return of Spontaneous Circulation (ROSC)

Transfer

- Transfer the patient to the nearest appropriate hospital according to local protocols
- Early recurrence of VF is common so monitor continuously – further shocks may be indicated.
- Provide an alert / information call.
- Continue patient management en-route. Address 4 Hs and 4Ts, according to local guidelines. Keep the patient flat during removal to vehicle

Oxygen saturations

Monitor oxygen saturation.

Maintain oxygen saturations between 94% and 98%

Ventilation

Monitor ventilation rate and volume.

Monitor end-tidal CO_2.

(NB Readings may be low because of reduced cardiac output rather than hyperventilation – normal range = 4.6–6 kPa, 35–45 mmHg)

ECG

Undertake a 12-lead ECG

Blood glucose level

Measure blood glucose level – if patient is hypoglycaemic (BM<4.0 mmol) refer to glycaemic emergencies guideline

Body temperature

In unconscious, non-traumatic cardiac arrest patients, ensure that body temperature does not become elevated and allow passive cooling in line with local guidelines.

Figure 2.7 – Assessment and management of Return of Spontaneous Circulation (ROSC).

KEY POINTS

Advanced Life Support (Adult)

- Begin good quality, uninterrupted chest compressions immediately. Attempt defibrillation as soon as a defibrillator is available.

- For shockable rhythms defibrillate and resume chest compressions (30:2) for 2 minutes without re-assessing the rhythm or feeling for a pulse; then check rhythm, if VF/VT persists follow ALS algorithm.

- Start initial defibrillation at 150–200 J. When using a manual defibrillator, consider escalating the energy level with subsequent shocks for refractory or recurrent VF/VT.

- Give adrenaline 1 mg 1:10,000 and amiodarone 300 mg immediately after the 3rd shock.

- Give amiodarone 300 mg IV/IO after three episodes of VF/VT, irrespective of whether these are sequential or intermittent.

- For non-shockable rhythms start CPR at a ratio of 30:2 and give adrenaline 1 mg 1:10,000 as soon as intravascular access is achieved.

- Give adrenaline every second cycle (3–5 minutes).

- Always consider reversible features (4Hs and 4Ts) and correct if possible.

- In most patients where ROSC is not achieved on scene, despite appropriate ALS and treatment of any potentially reversible causes, little is to be gained from transferring these patients to hospital. The exception is patients with penetrating trauma, where rapid transfer to hospital is vital.

2 Resuscitation

SECTION

Foreign Body Airway Obstruction (Adult) [102, 113, 110]

1. Introduction

- Foreign body airway obstruction is an uncommon but potentially treatable cause of accidental death.
- In adults, food is the commonest cause of obstruction.
- Most cases occur when eating and are therefore usually witnessed. The signs and symptoms vary, depending on the degree of airway obstruction (refer to Table 2.6).

2. Assessment and Management

- For the assessment and management of adult foreign body airway obstruction, refer to Table 2.7 and Figure 2.8.

Table 2.6 – GENERAL SIGNS OF FOREIGN BODY AIRWAY OBSTRUCTION

- Attack usually occurs while eating
- Patient may clutch their neck

Mild airway obstruction	Severe airway obstruction
- In response to question – **'Are you choking?'** - The patient speaks and answers **'Yes'**.	- In response to question – **'Are you choking?'** - The patient is unable to speak and may respond by nodding.
Other signs – the patient is able to: – speak – cough – breathe.	**Other signs:** – patient unable to breathe – breathing sounds wheezy – attempts at coughing are silent – patient may be unconscious.

Table 2.7 – ASSESSMENT and MANAGEMENT of:

Foreign Body Airway Obstruction (FBAO)

ASSESSMENT - Assess for severity of obstruction (refer to Table 2.6)	MANAGEMENT
- Mild airway obstruction	- Encourage the patient to cough but do nothing else. - Monitor carefully. - Rapid transport to hospital.
- Severe airway obstruction – conscious patient	- Give up to 5 back blows – after each back blow check to see if the obstruction has been relieved. - If 5 back blows do not relieve the airway obstruction, give up to 5 abdominal thrusts. - If 5 abdominal thrusts do not relieve the obstruction, continue alternating 5 back blows with 5 abdominal thrusts.
- Severe airway obstruction – unconscious patient	- If the patient is unconscious or becomes unconscious, begin basic life support – refer to adult BLS guidance. - During CPR the patient's mouth should be quickly checked for any foreign body that has been partly expelled each time the airway is opened.
- If these measures fail and the airway remains obstructed	- Attempt to visualise the vocal cords with a laryngoscope. - Remove any visible foreign material with forceps or suction. - If this fails or is not possible, and you are trained in the technique, perform needle cricothyroidotomy.
Additional information	- Chest thrusts/compressions generate a higher airway pressure than back blows. - Avoid blind finger sweeps. Manually remove solid material in the airway only if it can be seen. - Following successful treatment for FBAO, foreign material may remain in the upper or lower respiratory tract and cause complications later. Patients with a persistent cough, difficulty swallowing or the sensation of an object being stuck in the throat must be assessed further. - Abdominal thrusts can cause serious internal injuries and all patients so treated must be assessed for injury in hospital.

Foreign Body Airway Obstruction (Adult)

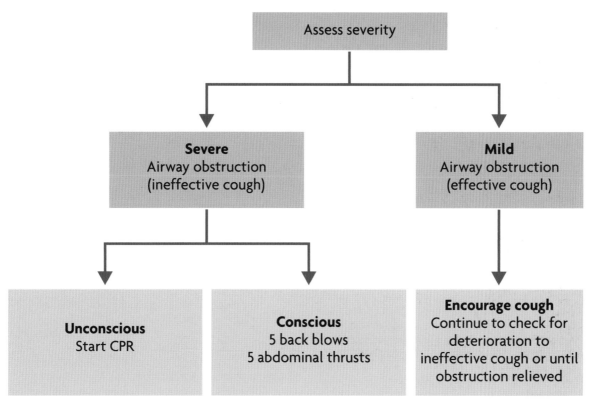

Assess severity

Severe
Airway obstruction
(ineffective cough)

Mild
Airway obstruction
(effective cough)

Unconscious
Start CPR

Conscious
5 back blows
5 abdominal thrusts

Encourage cough
Continue to check for
deterioration to
ineffective cough or until
obstruction relieved

Figure 2.8 – Adult foreign body airway obstruction algorithm – modified from the Resuscitation Council (UK) Guidelines 2015 (www.resus.org.uk).

KEY POINTS

Foreign Body Airway Obstruction (FBAO) (Adult)

- Potentially treatable cause of death; often occurs while eating.
- Asking the patient 'Are you choking?' can aid diagnosis.
- Back blows and abdominal thrusts may relieve the obstruction; check after each manoeuvre to see if obstruction is relieved.
- Abdominal thrusts can cause internal injuries and patients should be assessed in hospital.
- Avoid blind finger sweeps; manually remove solid material in the airway ONLY if it can be seen.

Maternal Resuscitation [101–103, 112, 114]

Introduction

- It is important to recognise that there are two patients.
- Effective resuscitation of the mother will provide effective resuscitation of the fetus.
- Resuscitation priority is the mother.

1. Cardiac Arrest

Undertake a TIME CRITICAL transfer as soon as ventilation is achieved and CPR commenced.

1.1 Introduction

- The approach to resuscitating an obstetric patient is the same as that of any adult in cardiac arrest; but in the third trimester, additional measures must be undertaken to maximise the efficacy of resuscitation.
- Because the fetus can tolerate significant levels of hypoxia, resuscitation should be initiated immediately and **NOT** terminated in pre-hospital care, even in cases where the mother's condition is, or appears non-survivable or unequivocally associated with death, as this will maximise the chances of both maternal and fetal survival.

1.2 Pathophysiology

- Cardiac arrest in pregnancy is very rarely due to a primary cardiac cause. Common causes of sudden maternal death include haemorrhage, embolism (thromboembolic and amniotic fluid), hypertensive disorders of pregnancy, abortion and genital tract sepsis.
- There are a number of physiological and anatomical changes during pregnancy that may influence the management of the obstetric patient (**refer to obstetrics and gynaecology overview guideline**).

1.3 Modifications for cardiac arrest in pregnancy

For the assessment and management of cardiac arrest during pregnancy refer to Table 2.8.

Key points are listed below:

- Start resuscitation according to standard ALS guidelines.
- The hand position for chest compressions may need to be slightly higher (2–3 cm) on the sternum for patients with advanced pregnancy (e.g. >28 weeks).
- Manually displace the uterus to the left to minimise inferior vena cava compression.
- Add left lateral tilt (15–30°) only if this is feasible. The patient's body will need to be supported on a firm surface to enable effective chest compressions. The angle of tilt used still needs to permit high quality chest compressions.
- Defibrillation energy levels are as recommended for standard defibrillation. If left lateral tilt and large breasts make it difficult to place an apical defibrillator electrode, use an antero-posterior or bi-axillary electrode position.
- Establish IV access as soon as possible, preferably at a level above the diaphragm.
- Identify and correct the cause of the arrest using 4 Hs and 4 Ts as appropriate.
- Administer supplemental oxygen and aim for a saturation of 94–98% (refer to oxygen guideline).
- Undertake a **TIME CRITICAL** transfer to nearest suitable receiving hospital; provide an alert/information call. Ask to have an **OBSTETRICIAN ON STANDBY IN THE EMERGENCY DEPARTMENT** for an emergency Caesarean section if the mother has suffered cardiorespiratory collapse (in this situation delivering the fetus **MAY** facilitate maternal resuscitation).

Table 2.8 – ASSESSMENT and MANAGEMENT of:

Cardiac Arrest

ASSESSMENT	MANAGEMENT
- Undertake a primary survey ABCDE - At 20 weeks, the uterine fundus will be at or above the umbilicus	- Manage as per standard advanced life support (refer to ALS guideline). - Assess and exclude treatable causes including hypovolaemia, sepsis and anaphylactic shock.
	- **Caution** – ventilation with a bag-valve-mask may lead to regurgitation and aspiration. A supraglottic airway may reduce the risk of gastric aspiration and make ventilation of the lungs easier (refer to airway and breathing management guideline). - If no response to CPR after 4 minutes, undertake a **TIME CRITICAL** transfer to nearest suitable receiving hospital; provide an alert/information call – ask to have an **OBSTETRICIAN ON STANDBY IN THE EMERGENCY DEPARTMENT** for an emergency Caesarean section (in this situation delivering the fetus **MAY** facilitate maternal resuscitation).
	- For pregnant women at 20 weeks or more, use manual uterine displacement (to the left side) or otherwise apply left lateral tilt (15–30°) to remove compression of the inferior vena cava. - The angle of tilt needs to allow good quality chest compressions (**refer to obstetrics and gynaecology overview**).
	- Aim to establish intravascular access using a **LARGE BORE** cannula, attempt IO access if rapid IV cannulation is not possible. - Transfer to hospital without delay.

Maternal Resuscitation

KEY POINTS

Maternal Resuscitation

- Do not withhold or terminate maternal resuscitation.
- ALWAYS manage patients >20 weeks gestation with manual displacement of the uterus to the left, and when possible, left lateral tilt (15–30°).
- Gastric regurgitation is more likely; be ready with suction, consider supraglottic airway insertion to reduce gastric insufflation.
- Insert at least one LARGE BORE IV cannula.
- Cardiac arrest is commonly caused by pulmonary or amniotic fluid embolism.
- Due to physiological changes of pregnancy, patients may initially compensate for hypovolaemia.
- If the patient is unstable, ask to have an OBSTETRICIAN ON STANDBY IN THE EMERGENCY DEPARTMENT.

SECTION 2 Resuscitation

Basic Life Support (Child) [90]

1. Introduction

- The following sequence is that followed by those with a duty to respond to paediatric emergencies – refer to Table 2.10 and/or Figure 2.9.

Age definitions

- An infant is a child under one year old.
- A child is between one year and puberty.

NB These guidelines are not intended to apply to the resuscitation of the newborn (refer to neonatal resuscitation guideline). In this chapter, the term 'child' includes infants, unless specified otherwise.

General principles

- Children are likely to have severe underlying illness or injury that can only be managed adequately in hospital and it is therefore particularly important not to delay on scene.

- As most cardiorespiratory arrests in children are due to respiratory insufficiency, paediatric resuscitation priorities focus on reoxygenating the child.
- Call for support from the most senior clinicians available.

Airway management

- Bag-valve-mask ventilation is the recommended first line method for achieving airway control and ventilation in children.

Hypothermia

- Children become hypothermic easily because of their large surface area to volume ratio. It is important to keep them as warm as possible before, and during, transfer.

[Further related reading includes 104, 106]

Table 2.10 – ASSESSMENT and MANAGEMENT of:

Basic Life Support (Child)

The following sequence is that followed by those with a duty to respond to paediatric emergencies (also refer to Figure 2.9)

ASSESSMENT	MANAGEMENT
● Assess safety	● Ensure that you, the child and any bystanders are safe.
● Check responsiveness	● Gently stimulate the child and ask loudly 'Are you all right?' – **DO NOT** shake infants, or children with suspected cervical spinal injuries.
● If the child responds (by answering or moving)	● Leave the child in the position found (provided the child is not in further danger). ● Check the child's condition. ● Summon help if necessary. ● Re-assess the child regularly.

● If the child does not respond	● Summon additional resources if required.
	● Open the child's airway by tilting the head and lifting the chin:
	  – place your hand on the forehead and gently tilt the head back
	  – at the same time, with your fingertip(s) under the point of the child's chin, lift the chin. Do not push on the soft tissues under the chin as this may block the airway.
	  – if you still have difficulty in opening the airway, try the jaw thrust method: place the first two fingers of each hand behind each side of the child's mandible (jaw bone) and push the jaw forward. Both methods may be easier if the child is turned carefully onto their back.
	● When there is a risk of back or neck injury, establish a clear upper airway by using jaw thrust or chin lift alone, in combination with manual in-line stabilisation of the head and neck by an assistant (if available).
	● If life-threatening airway obstruction persists despite effective application of jaw thrust or chin lift, add head tilt a small amount at a time until the airway is open; **establishing a patent airway takes priority over concerns about a potential back or neck injury**.

● Keeping the airway open	● Look, listen and feel for normal breathing by putting your face close to the child's face and looking along the chest:
	  – look for chest movements
	  – listen at the child's nose and mouth for breath sounds
	  – feel for air movement on your cheek.
	● Look, listen and feel for no more than 10 seconds before deciding that breathing is absent.

a. If the child **IS** breathing normally	● Turn the child onto their side into the **RECOVERY POSITION** (see below) taking appropriate precautions if there is any possibility of injury to the spine. ● Check for continued breathing.
b. If the child is **NOT** breathing or is making agonal gasps (infrequent, irregular breaths)	● Carefully remove any obvious airway obstruction. ● Turn the child carefully on to their back, taking appropriate precautions if there is any possibility of injury to the spine. ● Give 5 initial rescue breaths. ● While performing rescue breaths, observe for signs of life (any gasp or cough response).

Table 2.10 – ASSESSMENT and MANAGEMENT of:

Basic Life Support (Child) *continued*

The following sequence is that followed by those with a duty to respond to paediatric emergencies (also refer to Figure 2.9)

ASSESSMENT	MANAGEMENT
	Rescue breaths for an INFANT: ● Ensure a neutral position of the head and apply chin lift. ● Use a bag-valve-mask device if available (with a mask appropriate to the size of the child) and inflate the chest steadily over 1 second, watching for chest rise. ● Maintaining head tilt and chin lift, watch the chest fall as air comes out. ● Repeat this sequence 5 times. ● Identify effectiveness by observing the child's chest rise and fall in a similar fashion to the movement produced by a normal breath. **Rescue breaths for an INFANT if no bag-valve-mask is available:** ● Ensure a neutral position of the head and apply chin lift. ● Take a breath and cover the mouth and nose of the infant with your mouth, making sure you have a good seal. ● In an older infant, if the mouth and nose cannot be covered, seal either the infant's nose or mouth with your mouth (if the nose is used, close the lips to prevent air escape). ● Blow steadily into the child's mouth and nose over 1 second, sufficient to make the chest visibly rise. ● Maintain head tilt and chin lift, take your mouth away from the child and watch for the chest to fall as air comes out. ● Take another breath and repeat this sequence 5 times. ● Identify effectiveness by seeing that the child's chest has risen and fallen in a similar fashion to the movement produced by a normal breath.	**Rescue breaths for a CHILD >1 year of age:** ● Ensure head tilted and chin lifted. ● Use a bag-valve-mask device if available (with a mask appropriate to the size of the child) and inflate the chest steadily over 1 second, watching for chest rise. ● Maintaining head tilt and chin lift, watch the chest fall as air comes out. ● Repeat this sequence 5 times. ● Identify effectiveness by observing the child's chest rise and fall in a similar fashion to the movement produced by a normal breath. **Rescue breaths for a CHILD >1 year of age if no bag-valve-mask is available:** ● Ensure head tilted and chin lifted. ● Pinch the soft part of the nose closed with the index finger and thumb, with the hand on the forehead. ● Open the mouth a little, but maintain chin lift. ● Take a breath and place your lips around the mouth, making sure that you have a good seal. ● Blow steadily into the mouth over 1 second, watching for chest rise. ● Maintain head tilt and chin lift, take your mouth away from the child and watch for the chest fall as air comes out. ● Take another breath and repeat this sequence 5 times. ● Identify effectiveness by seeing that the child's chest has risen and fallen in a similar fashion to the movement produced by a normal breath.
● If you have difficulty achieving an effective breath, the airway may be obstructed	● Open the child's mouth and remove any visible obstruction. ● **DO NOT** perform a blind finger sweep. ● Ensure that there is adequate head tilt and chin lift but also that the neck is not over extended. ● If head tilt and chin lift has not opened the airway, try the jaw thrust method. ● Make up to 5 attempts to achieve effective breaths. ● If still unsuccessful, move on to chest compressions.

● Assess the child's circulation	● Take no more than 10 seconds to look for signs of life. This includes any movement, coughing, or normal breathing (not agonal gasps – these are infrequent, irregular breaths).
	 ● Check the pulse but ensure you take no more than 10 seconds to do this:
	   – in a child over one year – feel for the carotid pulse in the neck
	   – in an infant – feel for the brachial pulse on the inner aspect of the upper arm
	   – if you are not sure if there is a pulse, **assume there is NO pulse**.

a. If you are confident that you can detect signs of a circulation within 10 seconds	● Continue rescue breathing, until the child starts breathing effectively on their own. ● If the child remains unconscious, turn them on to their side (into the recovery position), taking appropriate precautions if there is any chance of injury to the neck or spine. ● Re-assess the child frequently.

Basic Life Support (Child)

Table 2.10 – ASSESSMENT and MANAGEMENT of:

Basic Life Support (Child) *continued*

The following sequence is that followed by those with a duty to respond to paediatric emergencies (also refer to Figure 2.9)

ASSESSMENT	MANAGEMENT
b. If there are: no signs of a circulation OR no pulse OR a slow pulse (less than 60/min with poor perfusion) OR you are not sure	• Start chest compressions. • Combine rescue breathing and chest compressions.
For all children, compress the lower half of the sternum	• Avoid compressing the upper abdomen by locating the xiphisternum (i.e. find the angle where the lowest ribs join in the midline) and compressing the sternum one finger's breadth above this point. • Compressions should be sufficient to depress the sternum by at least 1/3rd of the depth of the chest. (Approx 4 cm for an infant and 5 cm for a child). • Release the pressure, and then repeat at a rate of 100–120 per minute. • After 15 compressions, tilt the head, lift the chin and give 2 effective breaths. • Continue compressions and breaths in a ratio of 15:2. • Lone rescuers may use a ratio of 30:2, particularly if they are having difficulty with the transition between compression and ventilation. • The best method for compression varies slightly between infants and children (see below).
• Chest compressions in infants	• The lone rescuer should compress the sternum with the tips of two fingers. • If there are two or more rescuers, use the encircling technique: – place both thumbs flat side by side on the lower half of the sternum (as above) with the tips pointing towards the infant's head – spread the rest of both hands with the fingers together to encircle the lower part of the infant's rib cage with the tips of the fingers supporting the infant's back – press down on the lower sternum with the two thumbs to depress it at least 1/3 of the depth of the infant's chest.
• Chest compression in children	• Place the heel of one hand over the lower half of the sternum (as above). • Lift the fingers to ensure that pressure is not applied over the child's ribs. • Position yourself vertically above the child's chest and, with your arm straight, compress the sternum to depress it by at least one-third of the depth of the chest. • In larger children or for small rescuers, this may be achieved most easily by using both hands with the fingers interlocked.
• Continue resuscitation until	• The child shows signs of life (normal respiration, pulse, movement). • You become exhausted.
	Additional Information **RECOVERY POSITION** An unconscious child with a clear airway that is breathing spontaneously should be turned onto their side into the recovery position: • The child should be placed in as near a true lateral position as possible with their mouth dependent to allow free drainage of fluid. • A small pillow or a rolled-up blanket placed behind their back may be used to maintain an infant/small child in a stable position. • It is important to avoid any pressure on the chest that impairs breathing. • It should be possible to turn a child onto their side and to return them back easily and safely, taking into consideration the possibility of cervical spine injury. • The airway should be accessible and easily observed. • The adult recovery position is suitable for use in children.

Basic Life Support (Child)

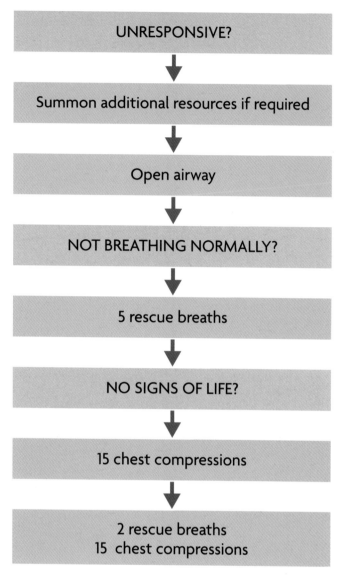

UNRESPONSIVE?

↓

Summon additional resources if required

↓

Open airway

↓

NOT BREATHING NORMALLY?

↓

5 rescue breaths

↓

NO SIGNS OF LIFE?

↓

15 chest compressions

↓

2 rescue breaths
15 chest compressions

Figure 2.9 – Child basic life support sequence algorithm – modified from the Resuscitation Council (UK) Guidelines 2015 algorithm (www.resus.org.uk).

KEY POINTS

Basic Life Support (Child)

- If the child is not breathing, carefully remove any obvious airway obstruction but DO NOT perform blind finger sweeps.

- Give 5 initial rescue breaths using a bag-valve-mask device, watching for chest rise. (Use 'Mouth-to-mouth-and-nose'/'Mouth-to-mouth' if BVM unavailable.)

- The duration of rescue breaths is about 1 second (comparable with adult practice).

- If there are:
  - no signs of life
  - or an absent or slow pulse (<60 bpm with poor perfusion)
  - or you are not sure, start chest compressions at a rate of 100–120 per minute.

- Continue alternating compressions and breaths in a ratio of 15:2.

1. Introduction

- Passage through the birth canal is a hypoxic experience for the fetus since placental respiratory exchange is prevented for the 50–75 seconds duration of the average contraction. Most babies tolerate this well, but those few that do not may require help to establish normal breathing at delivery.

- The newborn life support guideline provides this help and comprises the following elements:

  1. drying and covering the baby to conserve heat
  2. assessing the need for any intervention
  3. opening the airway
  4. lung aeration
  5. rescue breathing
  6. chest compression.

2. Physiology

- In the face of in utero hypoxia, the breathing centre in the fetal brain becomes depressed and spontaneous breathing ceases. The fetus can maintain an effective circulation during periods of hypoxia, so the most urgent requirement for any asphyxiated baby at birth is aeration of the lungs. Then, provided the circulation has remained intact, oxygenated blood will be conveyed from the lungs to the heart and onwards to the brain. The breathing centre should then recover and the baby will breathe spontaneously.

- Merely aerating the lungs is sufficient in the majority of cases. Where cardiac function has deteriorated to an extent that the circulation is inadequate, a brief period of chest compression may be needed.

- In a very small number of cases, lung aeration and chest compression will not be sufficient – the outlook in this group is poor.

3. Sequence of Actions (refer to Figure 2.10)

Keep the baby warm

- Babies are small and born wet. They become cold very easily, particularly if they are allowed to remain wet and exposed.

- Dry the term or near-term infant, remove the wet towels, and cover the infant with a dry towel.

- Significantly preterm infants and those requiring resuscitation are best placed, without drying, into polyethylene wrapping. Food grade plastic bags can be useful for this.

- In infants of all gestations, the head should be covered with an appropriately sized hat.

- Babies who do not need resuscitation may be moved with the mother, and skin-to-skin contact with the baby and mother covered will help to keep the baby warm.

4. Assessment and Management

For the assessment of newborns and management of cardiorespiratory problems refer to Table 2.11 and Figure 2.10.

- A healthy baby will be born blue but will have a good tone, will cry within a few seconds of delivery, will have a good heart rate (normally 120–150 per minute), and will become pink within the first 90 seconds or so.

- A less healthy baby will be born blue, will have less good tone, may have a slow heart rate (less than 100 per minute) and may not establish adequate breathing by 90–120 seconds.

- An ill (very hypoxic) baby will be born pale and floppy, not breathing and with a very slow heart rate.

[Further related reading includes 115]

KEY POINTS

Newborn Life Support

- **Passage through the birth canal is a hypoxic experience and some babies may require help to establish normal breathing at delivery.**

- **Babies become cold very easily; dry the baby, remove any wet towels and replace with dry ones. Once in the ambulance keep the compartment as warm as possible.**

- **Ensure the airway is open by placing the baby on their back with the head in a neutral position.**

- **If the baby is very floppy it may be necessary to apply a chin lift or jaw thrust.**

- **If the baby is not breathing adequately by about 90 seconds give 5 inflation breaths.**

- **If chest compressions are necessary compress the chest quickly and firmly at a ratio of 3:1 compressions to inflations.**

- **Use a two thumbs, encircling technique.**

SECTION 2 Resuscitation

Newborn Life Support

Table 2.11 – ASSESSMENT and MANAGEMENT of:

Newborn Life Support

ASSESSMENT	MANAGEMENT
● In all cases	● Ensure the ambient temperature is as high as possible. ● Clamp and cut the cord. ● Dry the baby. ● Remove wet towels and cover the baby with dry towels.

● Assess	● **Colour.**
	● **Tone.**
	● **Breathing rate.**
	● **Heart rate:**
	   – assess heart rate by listening with a stethoscope (feeling for a peripheral pulse is not reliable)
	   – in noisy or very cold environments, palpating the pulse at the umbilical cord may be an alternative and may save unwrapping the baby (this is only reliable when the pulse is >100 bpm)
	   – attach a pulse oximeter. NB Attaching to the wrist using an infant probe can give an accurate heart rate in approximately 90 seconds.

● Re-assess breathing and heart rate, every 30 seconds ● Decide whether help is required (and likely to be available) and whether rapid evacuation to hospital is indicated. If transferring to hospital follow pre-alert procedure	● An increase in heart rate is usually the first clinical sign of improvement. ● Once the baby is in the ambulance, the patient compartment should be kept as warm as possible (especially if pre-term) even if uncomfortable for the mother and attendant.
Airway	The airway must be open for a baby to breathe effectively: ● Place the baby on their back with the head in a neutral position, that is neither flexed nor extended. ● If the baby is very floppy, a chin lift or jaw thrust may be necessary.
Breathing ● If the baby is not breathing adequately by approximately 90 seconds	● Give 5 inflation breaths – use a 500 ml bag-valve-mask device. NB Until birth the baby's lungs have been filled with fluid; aeration of the lungs in these circumstances is likely to require sustained application of pressures of about 30 cm of water for 2–3 seconds. These are known as **inflation breaths**. Bag–valve-mask devices should incorporate a safety device that allows this pressure to be generated, yet prevents higher pressures that might damage the lungs.
Heart rate ● If the heart rate increases ● If the heart rate increases but the baby does not start breathing ● If the heart rate does not increase following inflation breaths	● Assume that lung aeration has been successful. ● Continue to provide regular breaths (**ventilation breaths**) at a rate of about 30–40 per minute until the baby starts to breathe on their own. NB Ventilation breaths do not need as long an inspiratory time as inflation breaths (approximately 1 second). Continue to monitor the heart rate. If the rate should drop to <100 bpm it suggests insufficient ventilation. In this situation, increase the rate of inflation or use a longer inspiratory time. ● Either lung aeration has not been adequate or the baby requires more than lung aeration alone. It is most likely that you have not aerated the lungs effectively. If the heart rate does not increase and the chest does not move with each inflation, you have not aerated the lungs; in this situation consider: 1. Is the head in the neutral position? 2. Do you need jaw thrust? 3. Do you need a longer inflation time? 4. Do you need help with the airway from a second person? 5. Is there obstruction in the oropharynx (laryngoscope and suction)? 6. Do you need an oropharyngeal airway? ● Check the baby's head is in the neutral position; that breaths are at the correct pressure and applied for the correct time and the chest moves with each breath. ● If the chest still does not move, consider an obstruction in the oropharynx that may be removable under direct vision.

2 Resuscitation
SECTION

Table 2.11 – ASSESSMENT and MANAGEMENT of:

Newborn Life Support *continued*

ASSESSMENT	MANAGEMENT
• If after 5 inflation breaths the heart rate remains slow (<60 bpm), or the heart beat is absent despite good passive chest movements in response to inflations	• Start chest compressions.
• If the baby is not vigorous at birth or does not respond very rapidly to bag-valve-mask ventilation	• **TIME CRITICAL** transfer. • Provide an alert/information call.
• If the mother has received morphine or any other opiate within the previous four hours and the baby does not breathe adequately	• Administer **naloxone** intramuscularly (refer to naloxone drug guideline) and provide respiratory support until it takes effect.
Circulation • If chest compressions are necessary	• Ensure that the lungs have been successfully aerated. • In newborns, encircle the lower chest with both hands in such a way that the two thumbs can compress the lower third of the sternum, at a point just below an imaginary line joining the nipples, with the fingers over the spine at the back. • Compress the chest quickly and firmly in such a way as to reduce the antero-posterior diameter of the chest by a third. • **The ratio of compressions to inflations in newborn resuscitation is 3:1.** • ECG complexes do not indicate the presence of a cardiac output and should not be the sole means of monitoring the infant.
Meconium	• Attempting to aspirate meconium from a baby's mouth and nose while their head is still on the perineum does not prevent meconium aspiration and is not recommended. • Attempts to aspirate meconium from a vigorous baby's airway after birth will not prevent meconium aspiration and are not recommended. • If a baby is born through thick meconium and is unresponsive at birth, the oropharynx should be inspected and cleared of meconium. The larynx and trachea should also be cleared if a suitable laryngoscope is available. This should not, however, unduly delay initial attempts to inflate the lungs.
	Additional information • Commence resuscitation with air. Introduce supplemental **oxygen** if there is not a rapid improvement in the baby's condition. • For **uncompromised** term and pre-term infants, delay cord clamping at least one minute from the complete delivery of the infant.

SECTION **2** Resuscitation

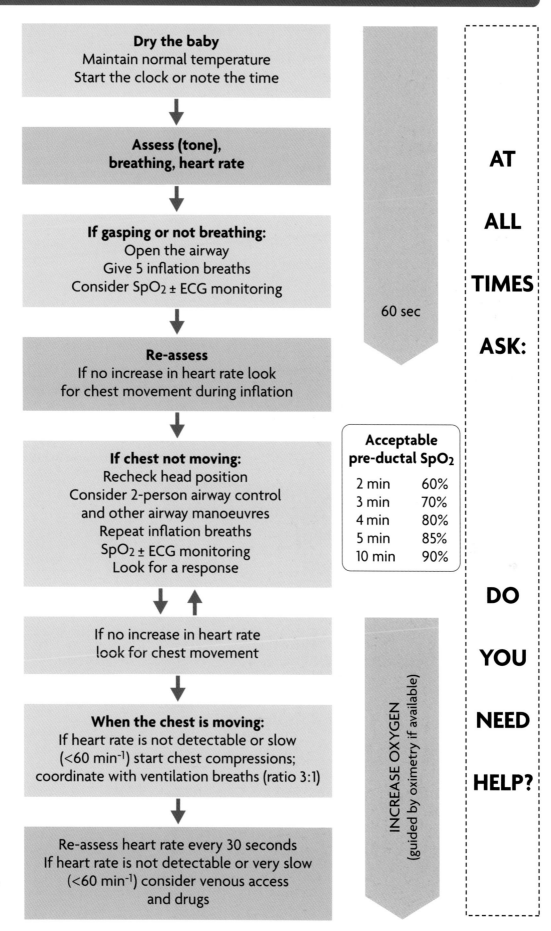

Figure 2.10 – Newborn life support algorithm – modified from the Resuscitation Council (UK) Guidelines 2015 algorithm (www.resus.org.uk).

Advanced Life Support (Child) [90, 103]

1. Introduction

Paediatric resuscitation practices have been simplified to minimise the differences between the adult and paediatric protocols.

Age definitions:

- an infant is a child under one year old.
- a child is between one year and puberty.

NB These guidelines are not intended to apply to the resuscitation of newborn (refer to neonatal resuscitation guideline). In this chapter, the term 'child' includes infants, unless specified otherwise.

General principles

- ALS procedures (e.g. establishing vascular access) must not delay the transfer of the child to hospital – continue good quality BLS as the priority. Attempt ALS procedures en-route, if practical.

Airway management

- Supraglottic airways may provide a useful alternative when bag-valve-mask ventilation is not possible.
- Tracheal intubation is seldom indicated unless an individual with appropriate skills is able to perform the procedure. Even then, the benefits must be weighed up carefully, as it may prolong the time on scene.

Breathing

- During CPR, deliver ventilation at a rate of approximately 10 per minute.
- Once the airway has been secured, then continuous compressions should be performed without pausing for ventilation.
- Following return of spontaneous circulation (ROSC), ventilate gently at a rate of 12–20 breaths per minute (as over inflation of the lungs can cause increased intrathoracic pressure, which has a detrimental effect on venous return and hence cardiac output).

Defibrillation

- For single responders, opening the airway and providing effective ventilation takes priority over attaching a defibrillator.

Vascular access

- Gaining rapid vascular access in children is often quickest using an intraosseous needle. This should be used in preference to an intravenous cannula unless a suitable site for venous cannulation is immediately apparent.

2. Assessment and Management

For children requiring advanced life support, follow the assessment and management guidance in Table 2.12 and Figure 2.11.

[Further related reading includes 105, 116]

Table 2.12 – ASSESSMENT and MANAGEMENT of:

Advanced Life Support (Child)

ASSESSMENT	MANAGEMENT
1. Establish basic life support 2. Oxygenate, ventilate, and start chest compressions	● Refer to basic life support (child) guideline. ● Ensure a patent airway by using an airway manoeuvre as described in the BLS (child) guideline. An adjunct such as an oropharyngeal airway may be needed. ● Provide ventilation, initially by bag and mask, using high flow oxygen. ● Provide compressions (100–120 /min) and ventilations (10 /min) at a ratio of 15 compressions to 2 ventilations. ● If bag-valve-mask ventilation is not possible, and if the clinician is trained, an i-Gel or similar supraglottic airway can be used. ● Once the airway has been secured then continuous compressions should be performed, taking care to ensure that ventilations remain effective.
3. Attach a defibrillator or monitor	● Assess and monitor the cardiac rhythm. ● Place one defibrillator pad on the chest wall just below the right clavicle and the other in the left mid-axillary line. ● Use paediatric pads for defibrillation of children under 8 years and infants. If these are not available, adult electrodes placed in an antero-posterior orientation will suffice. In paediatric practice manual defibrillators are preferred to Automated External Defibrillators (AEDs), but when an AED is the only defibrillator available, it is preferable to use the AED to analyse the rhythm and deliver a shock if prompted to do so, rather than withholding defibrilation. ● ECG monitoring electrodes should be placed in the conventional positions.
4. Check for signs of circulation and assess rhythm	**Look for signs of life** (e.g. moving, responsiveness, coughing, and normal breathing). **Assess the rhythm on the monitor:** ● Non-shockable (i.e. Asystole or Pulseless Electrical Activity (PEA)). ● Shockable (Ventricular Fibrillation (VF) or Pulseless Ventricular Tachycardia (VT)).
5. Non-shockable (Asystole, Pulseless Electrical Activity (PEA))	Asystole and PEA are the commonest paediatric cardiac arrest rhythms. Perform continuous CPR: ● Ventilate with high flow **oxygen**. ● If ventilating with a bag-valve-mask device, give 15 chest compressions to 2 ventilations for all ages.

Table 2.12 – ASSESSMENT and MANAGEMENT of:

Advanced Life Support (Child) *continued*

● Administer adrenaline	● Obtain circulatory access. ● Insert a peripheral venous cannula. If venous access is not readily attainable, give early consideration to intraosseous access. ● Give **adrenaline** 10 micrograms/kg (0.1 ml/kg of 1 in 10,000 solution) IV/IO (**see adrenaline guideline**).
● Continue CPR	
● Repeat the cycle	● Give 10 micrograms/kg of **adrenaline** (**see adrenaline guideline**) every 3–5 minutes. (Administer 10 micrograms/kg for all subsequent doses). ● Continue effective chest compressions and ventilation without interruption, at a ventilatory rate of approximately 10 per minute and a compression rate of 100–120 per minute.
● Consider and correct reversible causes: **4Hs 4Ts**	1. Hypoxia 1. Tension pneumothorax 2. Hypovolaemia 2. Tamponade 3. Hyper/hypokalaemia 3. Toxic/therapeutic disturbance 4. Hypothermia 4. Thromboembolism
6. Shockable (VF/pulseless VT) These rhythms are less common in paediatric practice but more likely when there has been a witnessed and sudden collapse or in children with underlying cardiac disease	**Defibrillate the heart:** ● Give 1 shock of 4 Joules/kg if using a manual defibrillator, rounding the shock up as necessary to the machine settings. If using an AED in a child over the age of eight years, use the adult shock energy – paediatric attenuation is not required. If using an AED in a child under the age of eight years, use a machine with paediatric attenuation (according to the manufacturer's instructions) when available. ● An AED should not routinely be attached to infants unless they have a history of cardiac problems. Where an infant is found to have a shockable rhythm, use a manual defibrillator to administer 4 Joules/kg. (In infants, if a manual defibrillator is not available, a paediatric attenuated AED may be used.) ● If no paediatric attenuated AED is available, use the adult shock energy with adult pads at all ages. ● **Resume CPR:** without re-assessing the rhythm or feeling for a pulse, resume CPR immediately, starting with chest compressions. ● **Continue CPR for 2 minutes.**
● Then pause briefly to check the monitor	**If still VF/pulseless VT:** ● Give a 2nd shock at 4 Joules/kg **as for the 1st shock (see start of step 6)**. ● **Resume CPR immediately after the 2nd shock**.
● Consider and correct reversible causes	● **4Hs 4Ts** (see above.) ● Continue CPR for 2 minutes.
● Pause briefly to check the monitor	**If still VF/pulseless VT:** ● Give a 3rd shock followed by **adrenaline** 10 micrograms/kg PLUS an intravenous or intraosseous bolus of **amiodarone** 5 milligrams/kg (refer to amiodarone guideline for further information). ● Resume CPR immediately and continue for another 2 minutes.
● Pause briefly to check the monitor	**If still VF/pulseless VT:** ● Give a 4th shock. ● Resume CPR, and continue giving shocks every 2 minutes, minimising the breaks in chest compressions as much as possible. ● Give **adrenaline** after every other shock (i.e. every 3–5 minutes) and a second dose of amiodarone following the 5th shock (refer to amiodarone guideline for further information) until ROSC.
● After each 2 minutes of uninterrupted CPR, pause briefly to assess the rhythm	**If still in VF/VT:** ● Continue CPR with the shockable rhythm (VF/VT) sequence. **If asystole:** ● Continue CPR and switch to the non-shockable (asystole/PEA) sequence as above.
● **If an organised rhythm appears at any time, check for a central pulse**	● If there is return of a spontaneous circulation (**ROSC**) begin post-resuscitation care. ● If there is **NO** pulse, and there are no other signs of life, or you are not sure, continue CPR as for the non-shockable sequence as above.

Advanced Life Support (Child)

KEY POINTS

Advanced Life Support (Child)

- Changes in guidelines have been made for simplification and to minimise the difference between the paediatric and adult protocols.
- The priority is to deliver high-quality chest compressions and effective ventilation with high-flow oxygen.
- Supraglottic airways are ideal for most paediatric airways. Intubation is rarely indicated and should only be undertaken by those with appropriate skills and only when waveform capnography is available.

Automated External Defibrillators (AEDs)

- If using an AED in a child <8 years, paediatric pads should be used whenever possible.
- If adult pads are all that is available, they may be used for all ages or the child/infant will die (an anterior-posterior pad position may be necessary in small children/infants).

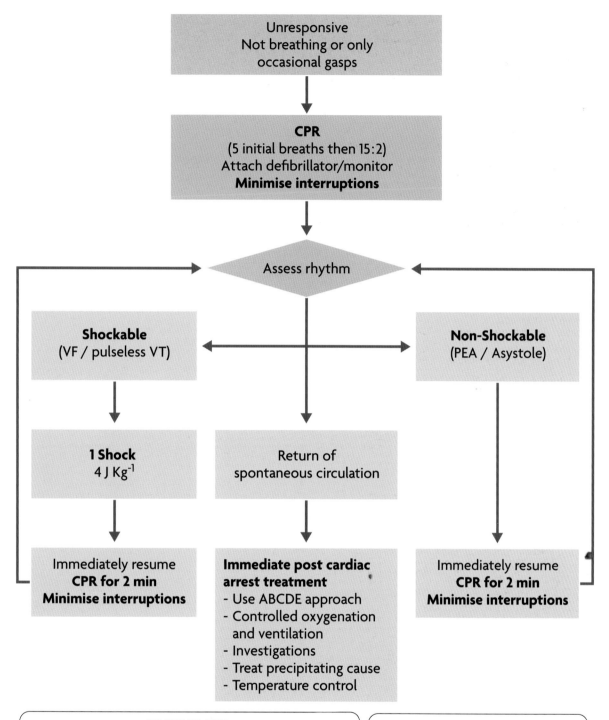

Unresponsive
Not breathing or only
occasional gasps

CPR
(5 initial breaths then 15:2)
Attach defibrillator/monitor
Minimise interruptions

Assess rhythm

Shockable
(VF / pulseless VT)

Non-Shockable
(PEA / Asystole)

1 Shock
4 J Kg⁻¹

Return of
spontaneous circulation

Immediately resume
CPR for 2 min
Minimise interruptions

Immediate post cardiac
arrest treatment
- Use ABCDE approach
- Controlled oxygenation
  and ventilation
- Investigations
- Treat precipitating cause
- Temperature control

Immediately resume
CPR for 2 min
Minimise interruptions

DURING CPR	**REVERSIBLE CAUSES**
• Ensure high-quality CPR: rate, depth, recoil.	• **H**ypoxia.
• Plan actions before interrupting CPR.	• **H**ypovolaemia.
• Administer oxygen.	• **H**ypo/hyperkalaemia/ metabolic.
• Vascular access (intravenous, intraosseous).	• **H**ypothermia.
• Give adrenaline every 3–5 min.	• **T**hrombosis (coronary or pulmonary)
• Consider advanced airway and capnography.	• **T**ension pneumothorax.
• Continuous chest compressions when advanced airway in place.	• **T**amponade (cardiac).
• Correct reversible causes.	• **T**oxic/therapeutic disturbances.
• Consider amiodarone after 3 and 5 shocks.	

Figure 2.11 – Advanced life support algorithm – modified from the Resuscitation Council (UK) Guidelines 2015 (www.resus.org.uk).

1. Introduction

The majority of choking events in infants and children occur during play or whilst eating when a carer is usually present.

Events are frequently witnessed and interventions are usually initiated when the child is conscious.

Foreign body airway obstruction (FBAO) is characterised by the sudden onset of respiratory distress associated with coughing, gagging or stridor (refer to Table 2.13).

Table 2.13 – GENERAL SIGNS OF FOREIGN BODY AIRWAY OBSTRUCTION

- Witnessed episode.
- Coughing or choking.
- Sudden onset.
- Recent history of playing with or eating small objects.

Ineffective coughing
- Quiet or silent cough.
- Unable to vocalise.
- Unable to breathe.
- Cyanosis.
- Decreasing level of consciousness.

Effective coughing
- Crying or verbal response to questions.
- Loud cough.
- Able to breathe before coughing.
- Fully responsive.

Similar signs and symptoms may also be associated with other causes of airway obstruction such as laryngitis or epiglottitis, which require different management.

General management principles

When a foreign body enters the airway, the child reacts immediately by coughing in an attempt to expel it.

A spontaneous cough is likely to be more effective and safer than any manoeuvre a rescuer might perform.

If coughing is absent or ineffective and the object completely obstructs the airway, the child will rapidly become asphyxiated.

Active interventions to relieve FBAO are only required when coughing becomes ineffective, but when required they should be commenced confidently and rapidly.

2. Assessment and Management

For the assessment and management of foreign body airway obstruction refer to Table 2.14 and Figure 2.12.

NOTES ON TECHNIQUES

BACK BLOWS – infant:

- Support the infant in a head-down, prone position, to allow gravity to assist the removal of the foreign body.
- A seated or kneeling rescuer should be able to support the infant safely across their lap.
- Support the infant's head by placing the thumb of one hand at the angle of the lower jaw, with one or two fingers from the same hand at the same point on the other side of the jaw.
- Do not compress the soft tissues under the infant's jaw, as this will exacerbate the airway obstruction.
- Deliver up to 5 sharp back blows with the heel of one hand in the middle of the back between the shoulder blades, aiming to relieve the obstruction with each blow rather than to give all 5.

BACK BLOWS – child over 1 year of age:

- Back blows are more effective if the child is positioned head down.
- A small child may be placed across the rescuer's lap as with an infant. If this is not possible, support the child in a forward-leaning position and deliver the back blows from behind.

CHEST and ABDOMINAL THRUSTS

- If back blows fail to dislodge the object and the child is still conscious, use chest thrusts for infants or abdominal thrusts in older children.
- Abdominal thrusts **must not** be used in infants.

Chest thrusts for infants:

- Turn the infant into a head-down, supine position (this can be safely achieved by placing the free arm along the infant's back and encircling the occiput with the hand).
- Support the infant down your arm, which is placed down (or across) your thigh.
- Identify the landmark for chest compression (lower sternum, approximately a finger's breadth above the xiphisternum).
- Deliver 5 chest thrusts (if required).
- These are similar to external chest compressions but sharper in nature and delivered at a slower rate.

Abdominal thrusts for children over 1 year:

- Stand or kneel behind the child. Place your arms under the child's arms and encircle their torso.
- Clench your fist and place it between the umbilicus and the xiphisternum. Grasp this hand with the other hand and pull sharply inwards and upwards.
- Repeat up to 5 times (if required).
- Ensure that pressure is not applied to xiphoid process or lower rib cage (may result in abdominal trauma).

RE-ASSESSMENT

Following chest or abdominal thrusts, re-assess the child:

- If object has not been expelled and victim is still conscious, continue the sequence of back blows and chest (for infant) or abdominal (for children) thrusts.
- Do not leave the child at this stage. Arrange transfer to hospital.
- If the object is expelled successfully, assess the child's clinical condition. It is possible that part of the object may remain in the respiratory tract and cause complications.
- Abdominal thrusts may cause internal injuries and all victims so treated should be assessed further.

[Further related reading includes 104, 106]

Foreign Body Airway Obstruction (Child)

Table 2.14 – ASSESSMENT and MANAGEMENT of:

Foreign Body Airway Obstruction (Child)

Resuscitation

2
SECTION

ASSESSMENT	MANAGEMENT
Assess safety Assess for severity of obstruction refer to Table 2.13	● Do not place yourself in danger and consider the safest action to manage the choking child.
● Effective coughing	● Encourage the child to cough but do nothing else. ● Monitor continuously. ● Transport rapidly to hospital.
● Ineffective coughing or cough becoming ineffective	● Summon help if appropriate. ● Determine the child's conscious level.
CONSCIOUS CHILD ● Conscious child with ineffective coughing or cough becoming ineffective	● Give back blows. ● If back blows do not relieve the FBAO, give chest thrusts (infants) or abdominal thrusts (children). These manoeuvres increase intrathoracic pressure and may dislodge the foreign body. ● Alternate these until the obstruction is relieved or the child loses consciousness.
UNCONSCIOUS CHILD ● If the child is or becomes unconscious:	● Place them on a firm, flat surface. **Open the airway:** ● Open the mouth and look for any obvious object. ● If one is seen and you think you can grasp it easily, make an attempt to remove it with a single finger sweep. ● **DO NOT** attempt blind or repeated finger sweeps – these can cause injury and impact the object more deeply into the pharynx. **Attempt ventilation** ● Open the airway and make 5 attempts to ventilate the lungs. ● Assess the effectiveness of each ventilation. ● If the chest does not rise, reposition the head before making the next attempt.
● Commence CPR if there is no response to 5 attempts at ventilation (moving, coughing, spontaneous breaths). Proceed to chest compressions without further assessment of the circulation	**Commence CPR** ● Follow the sequence for single rescuer CPR for approximately 1 minute. ● Start with compressions. ● When the airway is opened for attempted ventilation, look to see if the foreign body can be seen in the mouth. ● If an object is seen, attempt to remove it with a single finger sweep. ● If it appears that the obstruction has been relieved, open and check the airway as above. ● Perform ventilations if the child is not breathing. ● If the child regains consciousness and exhibits spontaneous effective breathing, place them in the recovery position. Monitor breathing and conscious level and transfer to hospital.

KEY POINTS

Foreign Body Airway Obstruction (Child)
● FBAO is a potentially treatable cause of death that often occurs whilst playing or eating.

● It is characterised by the sudden onset of respiratory distress.

● If the child is coughing effectively, encourage them to continue to cough.

● If coughing is ineffective, back blows should initially be given.

● If coughing is ineffective and back blows have failed to relieve the FBAO, use chest thrusts in infants and abdominal thrusts in children.

● Abdominal thrusts may cause internal injury – such patients require further hospital assessment.

● Avoid blind finger sweeps.

Foreign Body Airway Obstruction (Child)

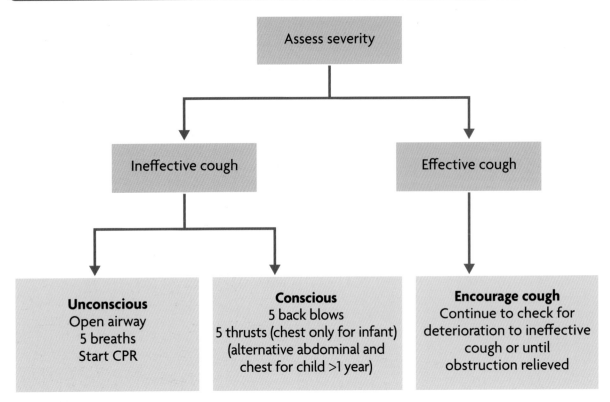

Figure 2.12 – Foreign body airway obstruction in children – modified from the Resuscitation Council (UK) Guidelines 2015 algorithm (www.resus.org.uk).

1. Drowning

1. Introduction

- In the UK, there are approximately 350 accidental deaths from drowning each year. Drowning is commonest in males aged 20–30, and occurs mostly in inland waters (e.g. lakes, rivers) and during summer months.

- Should the water temperature be very cold, it will rapidly cool the blood in the pulmonary circulation, which in turn selectively cools the brain for as long as a viable cardiac output continues, providing some degree of protection when cardiac arrest occurs. For this mechanism to be effective, the water temperature has to be near freezing, and usually, the body mass relatively small. Hence the majority of the accounts of successful resuscitation after submersion pertain to small children being rescued from 'icy cold water'.

2. General principles

- Cardiac arrest from drowning is due to hypoxia. The priority in managing these patients is therefore high quality basic life support and supplementary oxygen.

- The chances of a drowning victim sustaining a spinal injury are very low. Spinal precautions are unnecessary unless there is a history of diving in shallow water, or signs of severe injury after water-slide use, water-skiing, kite-surfing or watercraft racing. No more than 0.5% of these patients have a cervical spine injury and rescue takes precedence over cervical spine protection. If the victim is pulseless and apnoeic, remove them from the water as quickly as possible while attempting to limit neck flexion and extension. If concerns exist about cervical spine injury in the non-arrest patient, limit cervical spine flexion and extension as much as possible and use a scoop stretcher for immobilisation and transfer.

- Hypovolaemia after prolonged immersion can cause cardiovascular collapse/arrest on removal from water, especially if the victim is upright as they are removed from the water. Aim to keep the victim in a horizontal position during and after retrieval from the water.

3. Water rescue

- Whenever possible, bystanders should attempt to save the drowning victim without entry into the water. Talking to the victim, reaching with a rescue aid (e.g. stick or clothing) or throwing a rope or buoyant rescue aid may be effective if the victim is close to dry land.

- Rescue can present significant risk to the rescuer, but a sensible risk assessment is necessary to ensure that potentially survivable victims are rescued promptly.

- If entry into the water is essential, take a buoyant rescue aid, flotation device or boat. It is safer to enter the water with two rescuers than alone.

- Submersion durations of less than 10 min are associated with a very high chance of a good outcome, and submersion durations of more than 25 min are associated with a low chance of good outcome.

- In the UK, combined emergency services guidance recommends review of search and rescue efforts at 30 and 60 min from when the emergency services arrive on scene (Figure 2.13). Extended rescue efforts up to 90 min may be appropriate for children or those submerged in icy cold water, although the protective effects of extreme hypothermia are unlikely to be sufficient in the UK where water is insufficiently cold to cool rapidly and provide neuroprotection.

- Additionally, it would seem prudent that resuscitative efforts **should** be made on:
  - All those where there is a possibility of their being able to breathe from a pocket of air while underwater.
  - Anyone showing any signs of life on initial rescue.
  - Those whose airway has been only intermittently submerged for the duration of their immersion (e.g. those wearing lifejackets but in whom the airway is being intermittently submerged, provided the body still has a reasonably fresh appearance).

4. Resuscitation after water rescue

- Check for a response by opening the airway and checking for signs of life. The drowning victim rescued from the water within a few minutes of submersion is likely to exhibit abnormal (agonal) breathing. Do not confuse this with normal breathing.

- Give 5 initial rescue breaths, supplemented with oxygen.

- If the victim has not responded to initial ventilations, place them on a firm surface before starting chest compressions.

- Massive amounts of foam caused by mixing moving air with water and lung surfactant can sometimes come out of the mouth of victims. If this occurs, consider inserting an advanced airway (e.g. i-Gel, LMA, tracheal tube).

- Follow standard ALS protocols.

- Consider the early use of a mechanical chest compression device when a prolonged resuscitation attempt is to be undertaken.

- Hypothermia is common after drowning. If the victim's core body temperature is <30 °C, limit defibrillation attempts to three (delivered at maximum defibrillator output), and withhold IV drugs until the core body temperature increases >30 °C. Withhold adrenaline, and amiodarone until the patient has been warmed to >30 °C. Between 30 °C and 35 °C, the intervals between drug doses should be doubled when compared with normothermia intervals. Above >35 °C, standard drug protocols should be used. Pre-hospital rewarming is of limited effectiveness in unconscious patients, but use of heating blankets and a warm ambient environment should be considered.

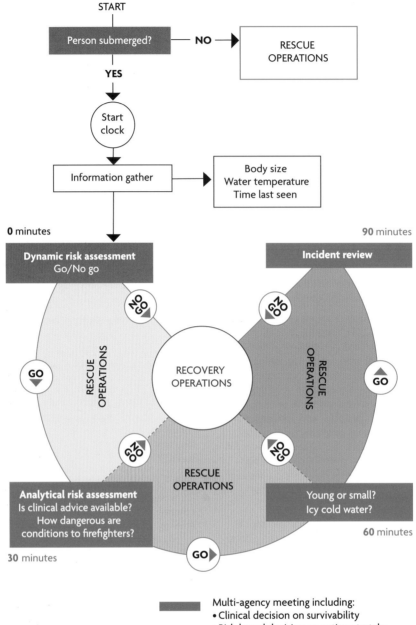

Figure 2.13 – UK risk assessment for submersion

(Reproduced with permission from National Operational Guidance on Water Rescue and Flooding.)

KEY POINTS – Drowning

- Cardiac arrest from drowning is due to hypoxia. The priority in managing these patients is therefore high quality basic life support and supplementary oxygen.

- The chances of a drowning victim sustaining a spinal injury are very low. If the victim is pulseless and apnoeic, remove them from the water as quickly as possible while attempting to limit neck flexion and extension.

- Hypovolaemia after prolonged immersion can cause cardiovascular collapse/arrest on removal from water, especially if the victim is upright. Aim to keep the victim in a horizontal position during and after retrieval from the water.

- Foam from the lungs may make airway management difficult. Consider early use of an advanced airway.

- Survival, although uncommon, is possible up to 90 minutes, particularly in children submerged in icy cold water.

SECTION **2** Resuscitation

Special circumstances

2. Individual Chemical Exposure

(previously referred to as chemical suicide)

1. Background

- There have been an increasing number of incidents of individual chemical exposure in the UK, often occurring in the confines of the victim's vehicle, which may or may not have warnings posted on the outside. There are a variety of different agents now commonly used in attempted chemical suicide, including:

  - hydrogen sulphide (made by mixing a combination of household chemicals)
  - aluminium phosphide (from rat poison)
  - cyanide salts
  - helium gas (from a cylinder for blowing up balloons)
  - nitrogen gas
  - carbon monoxide (e.g. by lighting a disposable barbecue in a confined space).

2. Hydrogen suphide

- Hydrogen sulphide is a colourless gas characterised by a rotten egg smell. It affects the body in three different ways: it causes paralysis and asphyxiation, and acts as a chemical irritant to the eyes and respiratory system. It can be fatal in just a few breaths. The same gas is responsible for deaths in agricultural incidents involving slurry tanks. In addition to claiming the suicide victim, ambulance personnel and bystanders can be exposed to significant risk, even when the scene has been vented, as the victim's body and clothes may emit dangerous gases for a considerable period of time afterwards. However, this risk can be minimised by moving the body into an open space so that the gas does not collect.

3. Rescue principles

- If attending a victim of chemical suicide, a dynamic risk assessment should be made regarding possible identification of the hazard, ease of access to the patient, and starting ventilation of the scene. If there is concern about exposure to poisonous gases, then no attempt should be made to access the patient until specialist help such as the Fire Service, Hazardous Area Response Team (HART) or Special Operations Response Team (SORT) are on scene with respiratory protection. These teams will be able to manage the incident, and make arrangements for the removal of the patient so that a formal clinical assessment can be made as to whether any resuscitation attempt would be likely to be successful, or if Recognition Of Life Extinct (ROLE) is more appropriate.

4. ROLE

- Once ROLE has been performed, then the body is the responsibility of the police. Under no circumstances should a victim of chemical suicide be taken to the Emergency Department, due to the risk of continued emissions of dangerous gases. If, by agreement, the body is removed by specialist ambulance teams to a mortuary, then the nature of the chemical must have been determined and appropriate arrangements should have been made to ensure the safety of mortuary staff.

KEY POINTS – Individual chemical exposure

- **Deliberate exposure to noxious gases is becoming more common. Some agents present a significant risk to the rescuer.**
- **If there is concern about exposure to poisonous gases, then no attempt should be made to access the patient until specialist help (e.g. Hazardous Area Response Team (HART)) is on scene with respiratory protection.**

3. Opioid Overdose

1. Introduction

- Opioid overdose may cause respiratory depression to such an extent that respiratory arrest occurs, leading to hypoxia-induced cardiac arrest.
- Common opioids include heroin (diamorphine), morphine and codeine.
- Naloxone reverses the respiratory depressant effects of opioids and may therefore be of benefit in patients with cardiac arrest (or peri-arrest) due to these drugs.

2. Naloxone administration

- In known opioid overdose associated with respiratory depression, respiratory arrest or to help diagnose suspected opioid overdose, the usual initial adult dosage of naloxone hydrochloride is 400 micrograms IV, given at 2–3 min intervals and titrated to response.
- If no response is observed after a total of 10 mg IV naloxone, consider a non-opioid related drug or other process.
- If the IV route is not available, naloxone may be given by IM, IO, SC or intranasal routes. Additional doses may be necessary if the patient's level of consciousness falls, or if the patient's respiratory rate decreases again, because the half-life of naloxone can be shorter than the opioid causing the respiratory depression.
- Only give as much as is necessary to achieve an adequate respiratory rate, as an excessive dose, particularly in chronic opioid users, can cause agitation and occasionally seizures.

KEY POINTS – Opioid overdose

- **Opioid overdose may cause respiratory depression to such an extent that respiratory arrest occurs, leading to hypoxia-induced cardiac arrest.**
- **Reversal of the effects of opioids may be of benefit in these patients.**
- **Initial naloxone dose is 400 micrograms IV in adults, repeated as necessary to a maximum of 10 mg, or as indicated on Page-for-Age**

4. Anaphylaxis

1. Introduction

- Anaphylaxis is an exaggerated immune response to a specific allergen. Common allergens include peanuts, bee stings and latex.

- It may occur in individuals with a known allergy, or may be a new reaction to an unknown allergen.

- Anaphylaxis may cause a prominent rash over the trunk and face, facial swelling and bronchoconstriction (similar to asthma). A low blood pressure is common and in severe cases, anaphylaxis may rapidly progress to cardiac arrest.

- Anaphylaxis and risk of death is increased in those with pre-existing asthma.

- The most important drug for the treatment of anaphylaxis is adrenaline. It reverses peripheral vasodilation and reduces oedema. It dilates the bronchial airways, increases the force of myocardial contraction, and suppresses release of histamine and other inflammatory mediators.

- Adrenaline is most effective when given early after the onset of the reaction.

2. Risk factors

- Known allergy to a specific allergen
- Asthma

3. Diagnosis

Symptoms

- Generalised rash, itching.
- Swollen lips, tongue, eyes.
- Breathlessness, wheeze.
- Fainting.
- Crampy abdominal pain.
- Nausea and vomiting.

Signs

- Reduced peak expiratory flow.
- Hypoxaemia.
- Hypotension.

4. Treatment

- Remove the trigger (if possible, e.g. remove bee sting).

- Give *immediate* IM adrenaline 0.5 mg in adults, or as indicated on Page-for-Age, to prevent cardiorespiratory arrest. Repeat every 5 minutes until the patient begins to improve.

- Lie the patient flat, elevate the legs and give high flow oxygen.

- Establish IV access and titrate IV fluids according to blood pressure.

- Follow standard ALS guidelines for the resuscitation of patients with cardiac arrest and known or suspected anaphylaxis, including IV adrenaline.

- If IV or IO access cannot be established rapidly, give IM adrenaline if cardiorespiratory arrest has occurred recently.

- Treat bronchospasm as for asthma.

- Give an antihistamine to block the effects of histamine released during anaphylaxis (chlorphenamine 10 mg IV over 1 min in adults, or as indicated on Page-for-Age).

- If severe or life-threatening, give hydrocortisone (200 mg IV over 2 mins in adults, or as indicated on Page-for-Age) to reduce the immune response.

KEY POINTS – Anaphylaxis

- **Anaphylaxis occurs rapidly and may result in life-threatening airway obstruction, bronchospasm and wheeze.**
- **Identify and remove the allergen when possible.**
- **Rapid administration of adrenaline (IM) may prevent cardiac arrest.**
- **If cardiac arrest occurs, follow standard ALS guidelines.**

5. Asthma

1. Introduction

- Asthma is a chronic inflammatory condition of the bronchial tree. Acute exacerbations result in constriction of the airways to cause wheeze and difficulty breathing.

- Bronchoconstriction seen in anaphylaxis may present as an acute asthmatic attack. Consider anaphylaxis as a possible diagnosis in a patient who presents with an acute asthmatic attack.

- Cardiac arrest associated with asthma occurs due to:
  - Severe bronchospasm and mucous plugging leading to severe hypoxia.
  - Cardiac arrhythmias caused by hypoxia.
  - High pressure within the chest reducing venous return and blood pressure.
  - Tension pneumothorax (often bilateral).

- Patients may deteriorate rapidly. Early treatment is vital to prevent cardiac arrest, which has a very high mortality.

2. Risk factors

- Previous hospitalisation or emergency care for asthma in the past year
- Poor compliance with therapy

Food allergy in a patient with asthma.

3. Diagnosis

- *See Table 2.15*

4. Treatment

Acute severe asthma

- Administer high flow oxygen.

- Administer nebulised salbutamol using an oxygen-driven nebuliser.

- If no improvement, administer ipratropium bromide by nebuliser.

- If severe or life-threatening, give hydrocortisone (100 mg IV over 2 minutes in adults, or as indicated on Page-for-Age) to reduce the immune response.

- Exclude unilateral or bilateral pneumothorax and treat as appropriate.

- If asthma is life-threatening, give adrenaline 0.5 mg IM early.

If cardiac arrest occurs:

- Follow standard ALS guidelines for the resuscitation of patients with cardiac arrest associated with asthma.

- If IV or IO access cannot be established rapidly, give IM adrenaline if cardiorespiratory arrest has occurred recently.

- When the appropriate skills are available, intubate the trachea to enable ventilation of stiff lungs and avoid gastric insufflation.

- Identify and treat tension pneumothorax with needle decompression as appropriate.

KEY POINTS – Asthma

- **Acute asthma may rapidly deteriorate to a life-threatening emergency.**

- **Rapid treatment is key to preventing cardiac arrest.**

- **For life-threatening asthma, high flow oxygen, nebulised salbutamol and adrenaline 0.5 mg IM must be administered immediately.**

- **Rapid transfer of patients to hospital is vital before deterioration results in cardiac arrest.**

- **In those who do suffer a cardiac arrest, follow standard ALS guidelines.**

- **High airway pressures often make ventilation difficult. Tracheal intubation may assist ventilation if appropriate skills are available.**

Table 2.15 – Symptoms and signs of asthma, according to severity

Life-threatening asthma	Any one of the following in a patient with severe asthma:	
	Clinical signs	**Measurements**
	Altered conscious level	PEF < 33% best or predicted
	Exhaustion	SpO_2 < 92%
	Arrhythmia	PaO_2 < 8 kPa (60 mmHg)
	Cyanosis	'Normal' $PaCO_2$ 4.6–6.0 kPa; 35–45 mmHg)
	Silent chest	
	Poor expiratory effort	
Acute severe asthma	Any one of: • PEF 33–50% best or predicted • respiratory rate ≥ 25 min^{-1} • heart rate ≥ 110 min^{-1} • inability to complete sentences in one breath	

3

Medical

3a
Undifferentiated
Complaints

Abdominal Pain   85

Cardiac Rhythm Disturbance   89

Altered Level of Consciousness   92

Dyspnoea   96

Headache   100

Mental Disorder   102

Mental Capacity Act 2005 (England
and Wales)   111

Adults:

Medical Emergencies in Adults –
Overview   117

Non-Traumatic Chest Pain/Discomfort   122

Children:

Medical Emergencies in Children –
Overview   124

Minor Illness in Children   129

Febrile Illness in Children   130

Respiratory Illness in Children   134

3b
Specific
Conditions

Heat Related Illness   137

Hyperventilation Syndrome   140

Hypothermia   143

Sickle Cell Crisis   146

Meningococcal Meningitis and
Septicaemia   149

Adults:

Acute Coronary Syndrome   152

Allergic Reactions including
Anaphylaxis   155

Asthma   157

Chronic Obstructive Pulmonary
Disease   161

Convulsions   165

Gastrointestinal Bleeding   169

Glycaemic Emergencies   172

Heart Failure   176

Implantable Cardioverter Defibrillator   180

Overdose and Poisoning   185

Pulmonary Embolism   194

Stroke/Transient Ischaemic Attack   198

Children:

Allergic Reactions including
Anaphylaxis   200

Asthma   202

Convulsions   206

Childhood Gastroenteritis   211

Glycaemic Emergencies   215

Overdose and Poisoning   218

Abdominal Pain [117–144]

1. Introduction

- Abdominal pain is a common presenting symptom to ambulance services. The specific cause can be difficult to identify in pre-hospital care and a definitive diagnosis may require in-hospital investigations.

- The nature, location and pattern of the pain together with associated symptoms, may indicate a possible cause (refer to Table 3.1). It is important to consider life-threatening causes.

- The elderly, alcoholics and immunosuppressed patients may have atypical presentations.

- Abdominal pain can arise from both acute and chronic abdominal conditions:

  - **Acute conditions:** e.g. appendicitis, cholecystitis, intestinal obstruction, ureteric colic, gastritis, perforated peptic ulcer, gastroenteritis, pancreatitis, diverticular disease, leaking or ruptured abdominal aortic aneurysms and gynaecological disorders.
  - **Chronic conditions:** e.g. irritable bowel syndrome (IBS), inflammatory bowel syndromes (ulcerative colitis and Crohn's disease), gastric and duodenal ulcers and intra-abdominal malignancy.

Table 3.1

Common Cause of Abdominal Pain

CONDITION	CHARACTERISTICS OF PAIN	ASSOCIATED SYMPTOMS
Leaking or Ruptured Abdominal Aortic Aneurysms (AAA) Consider AAA in patients >50 years who present with the symptoms listed. Most deaths occur in the elderly.	• Sudden severe abdominal pain or backache. • Renal colic type pain – a new diagnosis of renal colic in a patient over 50 years of age raises the concern of abdominal aortic aneurysm even in the absence of a palpable mass. NB Given that <25% of all AAA patients present with classic signs and symptoms, there is a risk of misdiagnosis.	• Collapse. • Hypotension with bilateral lower limb ischaemia or mottling (a late sign). • History of smoking. • Hypertension and hypercholesterolaemia.
Appendicitis Frequently misdiagnosed. Approximately one-third of women of childbearing age with appendicitis are considered as having pelvic inflammatory disease or UTI.	• A constant pain, increasing in intensity often starting in the peri umbilical area. • The pain may settle in the right lower quadrant; but the location may vary in the early stages. • There is rebound tenderness in the right iliac fossa and coughing and walking may exacerbate the pain. • Older patients may present with generalised pain, distension, and decreased bowel sounds.	• Nausea. • Vomiting. • Loss of appetite. • Constipation. • Increased temperature >37.5˚C. • Diarrhoea.
Acute cholecystitis Accounts for approximately 30% of patients attending ED for acute abdominal pain.	• A sharp pain in the right upper quadrant of the abdomen. • May experience right shoulder-tip pain. • The pain is worse when breathing deeply and on palpation of the right upper quadrant.	• Nausea and vomiting. • Increased temperature >38˚C. • History of fat intolerance.
Intestinal obstruction A partial or complete obstruction of the small or large intestine.	• Abdominal pain that is cramping in nature.	• Abdominal distension. • Nausea and vomiting. • Absolute constipation (late stage).
Urinary tract pathology Infection arising from the kidneys, ureters, bladder and/or urethra. Urinary tract obstruction.	• Pain in the lower abdomen and/or back. • Cramping.	• Pain/burning sensation when urinating, • Needing to urinate frequently. • Urinary frequency and nocturia. • Nausea and vomiting. • Cloudy/bloody urine with a malodour. • If the infection involves the kidneys the patient may have increased temperature >38˚C, and fatigue. • Rigors may be present.
Gastritis An inflammation of the gastric lining can be caused by medication (aspirin, non-steroidal anti-inflammatory drugs), alcohol, *Helicobacter pylori* or stress.	• Upper abdominal pain. • Lower/central chest pain/epigastric pain.	• Nausea and vomiting. • Loss of appetite. • Haematemesis.

Abdominal Pain

Table 3.1

Common Cause of Abdominal Pain *continued*

ASSESSMENT	MANAGEMENT	
Peptic ulcer An erosion of the lining of the stomach or small intestine forming an ulcer.	● Central burning abdominal pain. ● Back pain. ● Perforation may lead to abrupt onset epigastric pain.	● Nausea and vomiting – haematemesis. ● Fatigue. ● Weight loss.
Gastroenteritis Common infection of the stomach or bowel caused by viruses or bacteria.	● Abdominal pain and cramps.	● Nausea and vomiting. ● Diarrhoea. ● Fatigue. ● Weight loss.
Acute pancreatitis Inflammation of the pancreas.	● Constant pain in the upper left quadrant or middle of the abdomen. ● The pain may radiate to the patient's back.	● Abdominal tenderness. ● Hypotension. ● Nausea and vomiting. ● Dehydration. ● Shock. ● History of alcohol abuse or gallstones.
Diverticular disease Inflammation of diverticula in the large intestine.	● Abdominal pain in the lower left quadrant.	● Nausea and vomiting. ● Altered bowel habit. ● Bloating. ● Increased temperature >38°C.
Ectopic pregnancy Pregnancy not implanted in the uterus. It affects 1 pregnancy in 80 and accounts for 13% of all pregnancy-related deaths.	● Pain in the lower abdomen, pelvic area or back. NB Patients may present atypically but pain is almost always present.	● Nausea. ● Missed last menstrual period (though can occur before this). ● History of pelvic inflammatory disease. ● Previous ectopic pregnancy. If the pregnancy ruptures patients may report: ● Severe lower abdominal pain. ● Shoulder tip pain. ● Feeling faint/collapse.
Pelvic inflammatory disease A common cause of abdominal pain in females but rarely presents as an acute collapse.	● Pain in the lower abdomen, pelvic area or back. ● Abdominal tenderness.	● Vaginal discharge. ● Nausea. ● Fever
Intussusception Most commonly found in infants; another peak in incidence occurs at 6 years of age. An inward telescoping of the intestine that may cause an obstruction.	● Intermittent colicky pain associated with bouts of screaming and drawing legs up.	● Vomiting. ● 'Currant jelly stool' – blood and mucus.

SECTION **3** Medical Undifferentiated Complaints

Abdominal Pain

Table 3.2 – ASSESSMENT and MANAGEMENT of:

Abdominal Pain

ASSESSMENT	MANAGEMENT
● Assess ABCD	● If any of the following **TIME CRITICAL** features present: – major **ABCD** problems – suspected leaking or ruptured aortic aneurysm – ectopic pregnancy – sepsis resulting from perforation – traumatic disruption of abdominal organs, e.g. liver, spleen, then: ● Start correcting **A** and **B** and undertake a **TIME CRITICAL** transfer to nearest appropriate receiving hospital – for patients with suspected leaking or ruptured aortic aneurysm follow local care pathway. ● Provide an alert/information call. ● Continue patient management en-route.
	NB For indigestion type pain have a high index of suspicion that it may be cardiac in origin.
● History of pain	Ascertain the: ● Site of pain and whether it radiates to other areas. ● Onset of pain and whether this is a new pain. ● Character of the pain, e.g. constant or intermittent; improving or worsening. ● Radiates – does pain radiate elsewhere? ● Associated symptoms, e.g. nausea, vomiting, dizziness. ● Timing – how long have they been in pain? ● Abnormal or absent bowel sounds may indicate the presence of a serious condition. Medical history: ● Previous abdominal surgery. ● Current drug treatment if any. ● Recent travel. ● Presence of similar symptoms in others.
● Associated symptoms/ conditions	● Altered bowel habit. ● Nausea and vomiting – haematemesis/malaena may indicate gastrointestinal pathology – **refer to gastrointestinal bleeding guideline.** ● Vaginal bleeding/pregnancy/previous ectopic pregnancy – **refer to relevant obstetric, gynaecology guidelines.** ● Burning on urination. ● Menstrual and sexual history in females of childbearing age (is there any possibility of prenancy?). NB For details of signs and symptoms of specific conditions refer to Table 3.1.
● Oxygen	If oxygen is indicated refer to oxygen therapy guideline.
● ECG	● Undertake a 12-lead ECG for elderly patients and those with cardiac risk factors presenting with upper abdominal pain.
● Fluid	● If fluid resuscitation is indicated refer to intravascular fluid therapy guideline.
● Pain management	● Measure the patient's reported pain. ● If analgesia is required refer to **pain management guideline.** NB Opiate administration does not affect later clinical management.
● Transfer to further care	● Transfer to further care (consider most appropriate centre). ● Transfer all children <1 year with bile stained (green) vomit. ● A new diagnosis of renal colic in a patient over 50 years of age raises the concern of abdominal aortic aneurysm even in the absence of a palpable mass. ● Provide an alert/information call as indicated. ● Continue patient management en-route.

2. Severity and Outcome

- The most common diagnosis of patients presenting to emergency departments (ED) with abdominal pain is non-specific abdominal pain, followed by renal colic.

- Many cases are relatively minor in nature (e.g. constipation, urinary tract infection (UTI)); however, 25% of patients contacting the ambulance service with abdominal pain have serious underlying conditions.

- In patients >65 years there is a 6–8 times higher mortality rate due to atypical clinical presentations and the presence of comorbidities.

3. Incidence

Abdominal pain is a common presenting complaint accounting for 10% of attendances to ED. In patients >65 years it is the main complaint in up to 13% of admissions to ED. Of those patients who present by ambulance, approximately 50% are admitted for further investigation and observation.

4. Pathophysiology

Abdominal pain can be localised and referred, due to overlapping innervations of the organs contained in the abdomen (e.g. small and large intestines).

5. Assessment and Management

For the assessment and management of abdominal pain refer to Table 3.2.

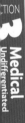

KEY POINTS

Abdominal Pain

- The most important diagnoses to consider are those that are life-threatening, either as the result of internal haemorrhage or perforation of a viscus and sepsis.

- For indigestion type pain have a high index of suspicion that it may be cardiac in origin. Obtain 12-lead ECG for elderly patients and patients with cardiac risks presenting with upper abdominal pain.

- If a patient is in pain, adequate analgesia should be given.

- A precise diagnosis of the cause of abdominal pain is often impossible without access to tests and investigations in hospital.

Cardiac Rhythm Disturbance [101, 103, 112, 145]

1. Introduction

- Cardiac arrhythmia is a common complication of acute myocardial ischaemia or infarction and may precede cardiac arrest or complicate the early post-resuscitation period.

- Rhythm disturbance may also present in many other ways and be unrelated to coronary heart disease.

- The management of disorders of cardiac rhythm is a specialised subject, often requiring detailed investigation and management strategies that are not available outside hospital.

- Diagnosis of the precise rhythm disturbance may be complicated and the selection of optimal treatment difficult. Very often, expert advice will be required, yet this expertise is rarely immediately available in the emergency situation.

2. Principles of Treatment

- Management is determined by the condition of the patient as well as the nature of the rhythm. Manage the patient using the standard ABCDE approach.

- In all cases follow the oxygen guideline and aim for a target saturation within the range of 94–98%.

- Gain venous access.

- Always take a defibrillator to any patient with suspected cardiac rhythm disturbance.

- Establish cardiac rhythm monitoring as soon as possible.

Document the arrhythmia. This should be done with a 12-lead ECG whenever possible. If only a 3-lead ECG is available, lead II provides the best waveform for arrhythmia analysis.

- Provide a printout for the hospital and, if possible, archive the record electronically so that further copies can be available at a later time if needed. Repeat the recording if the rhythm should change at any time. Record the ECG rhythm during any intervention (vagotonic procedures or the administration of drugs).

- If patients are not acutely ill there may be time to seek appropriate advice.

- The presence of adverse signs or symptoms will dictate the need for urgent treatment. The following adverse factors indicate a patient who is unstable because of the arrhythmia:

  - evidence of low cardiac output: pallor, sweating, cold clammy extremities, impaired consciousness or hypotension (SBP <90 mmHg)
  - excessive tachycardia, defined as a heart rate of >150 bpm
  - excessive bradycardia, defined as a heart rate of <40 bpm
  - heart failure implies the arrhythmia is compromising left ventricular function. This may cause breathlessness, confusion and hypotension or other features of reduced cardiac output
  - ischaemic chest pain implies that the arrhythmia (particularly tachyarrhythmia) is producing myocardial ischaemia. It is particularly important if there is underlying coronary disease or structural

heart disease in which ischaemia is likely to lead to life-threatening complications including cardiac arrest.

3. Bradycardia

Introduction

- A bradycardia is defined as a ventricular rate <60 bpm, but it is important to recognise patients with a relative bradycardia in whom the rate is inappropriately slow for their haemodynamic state.

4. Risk of Asystole

Assessment and management

For the assessment and management of bradycardia and risk of asystole refer to Table 3.3.

5. Tachycardia

Introduction

- These guidelines are intended for the treatment of patients who maintain a cardiac output in the presence of the tachycardia.

- Pulseless ventricular tachycardia is treated according to the cardiac arrest algorithm for the treatment of pulseless VT/VF.

- Broad complex tachycardia.

- Narrow complex tachycardia.

Assessment and management

For the assessment and management of tachycardia, broad complex tachycardia and narrow complex tachycardia refer to Table 3.4.

[Further related reading includes 104, 105, 115, 116, 146]

Cardiac Rhythm Disturbance

Table 3.3 – ASSESSMENT and MANAGEMENT of:

Bradycardia and Risk of Asystole

Bradycardia: A ventricular rate <60 bpm, but it is important to recognise patients with a relative bradycardia in whom the rate is inappropriately slow for their haemodynamic state.

ASSESSMENT	MANAGEMENT
Assess to determine if one or more adverse signs are present: – Systolic blood pressure <90 mmHg. – Ventricular rate <40 bpm. – Ventricular arrhythmias compromising BP requiring treatment. – Heart failure.	**If one or more signs are present:** ● Follow oxygen guidelines – aim for target saturation within the range 94–98%. ● Gain IV access. ● Administer atropine[a] (refer to atropine guideline) and repeat after 3–5 minutes if necessary, or transcutaneous pacing. ● Undertake a 12-lead ECG. ● Transfer to further care.

Risk of asystole: If the patient is initially stable (i.e. no adverse signs are present) or a satisfactory response is achieved with atropine, next determine the risk of asystole.

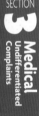

Assess for risk of asystole – this is indicated by:	

Assess for risk of asystole – this is indicated by:
– Previous episode of asystole.
– Möbitz II AV block.
– Complete (third degree) AV block, especially with a broad QRS complex or an initial ventricular rate <40 bpm.
– Ventricular standstill >3 seconds.
	If there is a risk of asytole (i.e. one or more signs are present) or the patient shows adverse signs and has not responded satisfactorily to atropine, transvenous pacing is likely to be required. One or more of the following interventions may improve the patient's condition during transport:
	● Transcutaneous pacing should be undertaken if available.
	If transcutaneous pacing is not available:
	● Fist pacing may produce ventricular contraction – give serial rhythmic blows with the closed fist over the lower left sternal edge to pace the heart at a rate of 50–70 bpm.
	NOTES:
	  a. **Do not** give atropine to patients with cardiac transplants; their hearts will not respond to vagal blocking by atropine and paradoxical high degree AV block or sinus arrest may result.
	  b. Complete heart block with a narrow QRS complex escape rhythm may not require pacing. The ectopic pacemaker (which is situated in the atrioventricular junction) may provide a stable rhythm at an adequate rate.
	  c. Initiate transcutaneous pacing (if equipment is available):
	    – if there is no response to atropine
	    – if patient is severely symptomatic, particularly when high degree block (Möbitz type II or third degree AV block) is present.
	NB Transcutaneous pacing may be painful; use analgesia. Verify mechanical capture. Monitor the patient carefully; try to identify the cause of the bradycardia.

[a] Caution – Doses of atropine lower than 500 mcg may paradoxically cause further slowing of ventricular rate. Use atropine cautiously in acute myocardial ischaemia or infarction; an increased rate may worsen ischaemia.

KEY POINTS

Cardiac Rhythm Disturbance
● **Gain venous access.**
● **Always take a defibrillator to any patient with suspected cardiac rhythm disturbance.**
● **Establish cardiac rhythm monitoring as soon as possible, preferably with a 12-lead ECG.**
● **Record the ECG rhythm during any intervention and archive. Ensure all ECGs are safely handed over to receiving staff and archive so further copies can be retrieved if necessary.**

Cardiac Rhythm Disturbance

Table 3.4 – ASSESSMENT and MANAGEMENT of:

Tachycardia, Broad Complex Tachycardia and Narrow Complex Tachycardia

ASSESSMENT	MANAGEMENT
Tachycardia ● These guidelines are intended for the treatment of patients who maintain a cardiac output in the presence of the tachycardia. ● **Pulseless ventricular tachycardia** is treated with immediate attempts at defibrillation following the algorithm for the treatment of pulseless VT/VF.	1. Support the ABCs. 2. Administer high levels of supplemental oxygen – aim for a target saturation 94–98%. 3. Gain IV access. 4. Establish cardiac rhythm monitoring. 5. Record and monitor BP and SpO$_2$. 6. Record a 12-lead ECG if possible, if not, record a rhythm strip. 7. If the rhythm changes at any time, make a further recording. 8. Make a continuous record of the rhythm during any therapeutic intervention (whether a drug or physical manoeuvre like carotid sinus massage). 9. The response to treatment can provide important additional information about the arrhythmia. 10. Identify and treat reversible causes; give analgesia if indicated. 11. Try to define the cardiac rhythm from the ECG. Determine the QRS duration and determine whether the rhythm is regular or irregular. If the QRS duration is 120 msec or more, the rhythm is a broad complex tachycardia. If less than 120 msec, the rhythm is a narrow complex tachycardia.
Broad complex tachycardia	● The rhythm is likely to be ventricular tachycardia, particularly in the context of ischaemic heart disease, patients showing adverse signs (reduced consciousness, SBP <90 mmHg, chest pain or heart failure), or in the peri-arrest situation. ● In all cases, maintain the supportive measures above and monitor the patient during transport. ● Provide an alert/information call according to local guidelines. ● Atrial fibrillation with aberrant conduction may produce an irregular broad complex tachycardia, but the diagnosis is difficult to make with certainty and often requires expert examination of the ECG. This emphasises the importance of recording the ECG when the arrhythmia is present. Ambulance personnel may greatly assist the subsequent diagnosis and management of patients by obtaining good quality ECG recordings. It is advantageous if these can also be archived electronically so that additional copies are available in the future.

Narrow complex tachycardia	If the rhythm is narrow complex (QRS <120 msec) **AND REGULAR,** it is likely to be either:
	  – sinus tachycardia. This is a physiological response, for example to pain, fever, blood loss or heart failure. Treatment is directed towards the cause. Trying to slow the rate is likely to make the situation worse
	  – supraventricular tachycardia (SVT). This is often seen in patients without other forms of heart disease. There may be a history of previous attacks
	  – atrial flutter with regular AV conduction (often 2:1 and a rate of 150 bpm).
	● In cases of SVT, start with vagal manoeuvres. In some cases the patient may be aware of techniques that have terminated previous episodes. The Valsalva manoeuvre (forced expiration against a closed glottis) may be effective and is conveniently achieved (especially in supine patients) by asking the patient to blow into a 20 ml syringe with sufficient force to push back the plunger. If this fails, perform carotid sinus massage provided no carotid bruit is heard on auscultation. A bruit may indicate the presence of atheromatous plaque, rupture of which may cause cerebral embolism and stroke.
	● Record the ECG (preferably multi-lead) during each manoeuvre. If the arrhythmia is successfully terminated by vagal procedures, it is very likely to have been SVT. If the rhythm is atrial flutter, slowing of ventricular rate may occur and allow the identification of flutter waves on the ECG.
	● Maintain the supportive measures above and monitor the patient during transport.
	● **AN IRREGULAR** narrow complex rhythm is most commonly atrial fibrillation, less commonly atrial flutter with variable block. Maintain the supportive measures above and monitor the patient during transport.
	● In all cases, ensure the patient is received into a suitable emergency department maintaining cardiac monitoring throughout. Ensure detailed hand-over to appropriate staff and that ECGs are safely handed over.

1. Introduction

- Patients presenting in pre-hospital care with an altered level of consciousness (ALoC) provide a major challenge.

- In patients with ALoC it is important to undertake a rapid assessment for **TIME CRITICAL** conditions.

- It is important to understand, where possible, the cause of altered consciousness which can range from diabetic collapse, to factitious illness (refer to Table 3.5 and Table 3.6).

- The patient history may provide valuable insight into the cause of the current condition. Consider the following in formulating your diagnosis; ask relatives or bystanders:

  - is there any history of recent illness or pre-existing chronic illness (e.g. diabetes, epilepsy)?
  - any past history of mental health problems?
  - any preceding symptoms such as headache, fits, confusion?
  - any history of trauma?

NOTE: Remember, an acute condition may be an exacerbation of a chronic condition or a 'new' illness superimposed on top of a pre-existing problem.

However, often there is little available information – in these circumstances the scene may provide clues to assist in formulating a diagnosis:

- Environmental factors (e.g. extreme cold, possible carbon monoxide sources)?

- Evidence of tablets, ampoules, pill boxes, syringes, including domiciliary oxygen (O_2), or administration devices (e.g. nebuliser machines)?

- Evidence of alcohol, or medication abuse?

Table 3.5 – RED FLAG CONDITIONS

Condition

Stroke/TIA (**refer to stroke/TIA guideline**).

Head injury (**refer to head trauma guideline**).

Epilepsy (**refer to convulsion guideline**).

Hypoglycaemia (**refer to glycaemic emergencies**).

Hyperglycaemia (**refer to glycaemic emergencies**).

Subarachnoid haemorrhage (**refer to headache**).

Overdose (**refer to overdose and poisoning**).

Table 3.6 – SOME CONDITIONS THAT MAY RESULT IN DLoC (Decreased level of consciousness)

Alterations in pO_2 (hypoxia) and/or pCO_2 (hyper/hypocapnoea)

Inadequate airway.

Inadequate ventilation or depressed respiratory drive.

Persistent hyperventilation.

Table 3.6 – SOME CONDITIONS THAT MAY RESULT IN DLoC continued

Inadequate perfusion

Hypovolaemia.

Cardiac arrhythmias.

Distributive shock.

Neurogenic shock.

Raised intracranial pressure.

Altered metabolic states

Hypoglycaemia and hyperglycaemia.

Intoxication or poisoning

Drug overdose.

Alcohol intoxication.

Carbon monoxide poisoning.

Medical conditions

Stroke.

Subarachnoid haemorrhage.

Epilepsy.

Meningitis.

Hypo/hyperthermia.

Head injury

This guideline contains guidance for managing patients with transient loss of consciousness (section 1) and coma (section 2).

2. SECTION 1 – Transient Loss of Consciousness (TLoC)

- Transient loss of consciousness (TLoC) may be defined as spontaneous loss of consciousness with complete recovery, that is full recovery of consciousness without any residual neurological deficit.

- An episode of TLoC is often described as a 'blackout' or a 'collapse'. There are various causes of TLoC, including:

  - cardiovascular disorders (which are the most common)
  - neurological conditions such as epilepsy, and psychogenic attacks.

- The diagnosis of the underlying cause of TLoC is often inaccurate and delayed.

Assessment and management

For the assessment and management of transient loss of consciousness refer to Table 3.7.

3. SECTION 2 – Coma

Introduction

- Coma is defined as U on the AVPU scale or a Glasgow Coma Score (GCS) (refer to **Appendix**) of 8 or less; however, any patient presenting with a decreased level of consciousness (GCS<15) mandates further assessment and, possibly, treatment.

Altered Level of Consciousness

Table 3.7 – ASSESSMENT and MANAGEMENT of:

Transient Loss of Consciousness

ASSESSMENT (ADULTS)	MANAGEMENT (ADULTS)

● Assess ABCD	● If any of the following **TIME CRITICAL** features are present:
	  – major **ABCD** problems
	  – unexpected OR persistent loss of consciousness, then:
	● Start correcting any **ABCD** problems.
	● Undertake a **TIME CRITICAL** transfer to nearest appropriate receiving hospital.
	● Continue patient management en-route.
	● Provide an alert/information call.

● Assess for TIME CRITICAL features	
● Ascertain from the patient or witnesses what happened before, during and after the event	**Record details about:** ● Circumstances of the event. ● The patient's posture immediately before loss of consciousness. ● Prodromal symptoms (such as sweating or feeling warm/hot). ● Appearance (whether eyes were open or shut) and colour of the patient during the event. ● Presence or absence of movement during the event (limb-jerking and its duration). ● Any tongue-biting (record whether the side or the tip of the tongue was bitten). ● Injury occurring during the event (record site and severity). ● Duration of the event (onset to regaining consciousness). ● Presence or absence of confusion during the recovery period. ● Weakness down one side during the recovery period.
● If TLoC is confirmed:	Assess and record: ● Details of any previous TLoC, including number and frequency. ● The patient medical history and any family history of cardiac disease (personal history of heart disease or family history of sudden cardiac death). ● Current medication that may have contributed to TLoC (diuretics). ● Routine observations (pulse rate, respiratory rate and temperature) – repeat if clinically indicated. ● Lying and standing blood pressure if clinically appropriate. ● Other cardiovascular and neurological signs.
● Assess for concomitant injuries	● Refer to relevant guideline.
● Assess heart rhythm	● Undertake a 12-lead ECG using automated interpretation (refer to local guidelines).
● If an underlying cause is suspected	● Undertake relevant examinations and investigations, for example, check blood glucose levels if hypoglycaemia is suspected – refer to relevant guideline.

● Assess for uncomplicated faint and situational syncope	Diagnose uncomplicated faint (uncomplicated vasovagal syncope) on the basis of the initial assessment when:
	● There are no features that suggest an alternative diagnosis (NOTE: that brief seizure activity can occur during uncomplicated faints and is not necessarily diagnostic of epilepsy).
	AND
	● There are features suggestive of uncomplicated faint (the 3 'P's) such as:
	  – **posture** – prolonged standing, or similar episodes that have been prevented by lying down.
	  – **provoking** factors (such as pain or a medical procedure).
	  – **prodromal** symptoms (such as sweating or feeling warm/hot before TLoC).
	Diagnose situational syncope on the basis of the initial assessment when:
	● There are no features from the initial assessment that suggest an alternative diagnosis.
	AND
	● Syncope is clearly and consistently provoked by straining during micturition (usually while standing) or by coughing or swallowing.

● Care pathway	● Only patients with a GCS 15, with normal blood sugar and responsible adult supervision present may be left at scene, for example if a diagnosis of uncomplicated faint or situational syncope is made, and there is nothing in the initial assessment to raise clinical or social concern. ● **Advise the patient to take a copy of the patient report form and the ECG record to their GP and follow local protocols to safely hand over clinical responsibility.**

- There are a number of causes of coma; refer to Tables 3.5 and 3.6.

Assessment and management

For the assessment and management of coma refer to Table 3.8.

Table 3.8 – ASSESSMENT and MANAGEMENT of:

Coma (GCS <8)

ASSESSMENT (ADULTS)	MANAGEMENT (ADULTS) NOTE: TAKE A DEFRIBILLATOR TO THE INCIDENT – many calls to unconscious patients are cardiac arrests.
● Assess **ABCD**	● Start correcting any **ABCD** problems. ● Undertake a **TIME CRITICAL** transfer to the nearest appropriate receiving hospital. ● Continue patient management en-route. ● Provide an alert/information call.
● Oxygen	● Administer high levels of supplementary oxygen and aim for a target saturation within the range of 94–98% (refer to oxygen guideline).
● Assess for hypoxia	● Apply pulse oximetry. ● Obtain IV access if appropriate.
● Assess heart rhythm for arrhythmias	● Undertake a 12-lead ECG.
● Assess level of consciousness	● Assess using the AVPU scale or Glasgow Coma Scale (GCS) (refer to Appendix): A – Alert V – Response to voice P – Responds to painful stimulus U – Unresponsive. ● Assess and note pupil size, equality and response to light. ● Check for purposeful movement in all four limbs and note sensory function.
● Assess blood glucose level	● If hypoglycaemic (<4.0 mmol/l) or suspected, **refer to glycaemic emergencies.**.
● Blood pressure	● Measure blood pressure.
● Assess for significant injury especially to the head	● If trauma detected or suspected, immobilise spine and **refer to neck and back trauma**.
● Assess for other causes	● Breath for ketones, alcohol and solvents. ● Evidence of needle tracks/marks. ● MedicAlert® type jewellery (bracelets or necklets) which detail the patient's primary health risk (e.g. diabetes, anaphylaxis, Addison's disease etc) – also list a 24-hour telephone number to obtain a more detailed patient history. ● Warning stickers, often placed by the front door or the telephone, directing the health professional to a source of detailed information (one current scheme involves storing the patient details in a container in the fridge, as this is relatively easy to find in the house). ● Patient-held warning cards, for example, those taking monoamine oxidase inhibitor (MAOI) medication. **For management refer to relevant guideline(s).**
● Assess for respiratory depression	● In cases of severe respiratory depressions, refer to airway and breathing management guideline. ● If the level of consciousness deteriorates or respiratory depression develops in cases where an overdose with opiate-type drugs may be a possibility, consider naloxone (refer to naloxone guideline). ● In a patient with fixed pinpoint pupils suspect opiate use/overdose. NOTE: any patient with a decreased level of consciousness may have a compromised airway.

● Re-assess ABCD	● Document any changes/note trends in:
	  – GCS
	  – altered neurological function
	  – base line observations.

Appendix

GLASGOW COMA SCALE

Category	Element	Score
Eyes opening	Spontaneously	4
	To speech	3
	To pain	2
	None	1
Motor response	Obeys commands	6
	Localises pain	5
	Withdraws from pain	4
	Abnormal flexion	3
	Extensor response	2
	No response to pain	1
Verbal response	Orientated	5
	Confused	4
	Inappropriate words	3
	Incomprehensible sounds	2
	No verbal response	1

KEY POINTS

Decreased Level of Consciousness
- Maintain patent airway.
- Support ventilation if required.
- Address treatable causes.
- History – obtain as much information as possible.
- Consider an alert/information call.

1. Introduction

- Dyspnoea is defined as *'a subjective experience of breathing discomfort that consists of qualitatively distinct sensations that vary in intensity'*.

- Dyspnoea is an important clinical symptom that may indicate underlying pathology for a large range of conditions (refer to Table 3.9), particularly those affecting the respiratory and cardiac systems.

- Acute episodes of dyspnoea often have a pulmonary or cardiac cause. Asthma, cardiogenic pulmonary oedema, chronic obstructive pulmonary disease (COPD), pneumonia, cardiac ischaemia, and interstitial lung disease are common causes and account for approximately 85% of all ED cases of dyspnoea. In 15% of cases dyspnoea is unexplained.

2. Incidence

- Dyspnoea is the most common reason for emergency department (ED) attendance. Approximately 25–50% of dyspnoea patients presenting to the ED are admitted to hospital.

3. Severity and Outcome

- Dyspnoea is an important clinical symptom which in some circumstances can be severe or life-threatening. Dyspnoea varies in intensity and can be a distressing symptom, especially for patients at the end of life. **For details of the severity and outcome for specific conditions refer to individual guidelines.**

4. Pathophysiology

- Dyspnoea is multi-dimensional process involving physiological and psychological systems.

- The respiratory system is designed to match alveolar ventilation with metabolic demand. Disruption of this process may lead to the conscious awareness of breathing and dyspnoea. Dyspnoea is an uncomfortable sensation and may include chest tightness, air hunger, effortful breathing, the urge to cough and a sense of suffocation.

5. Assessment and Management

- Diagnosis of the underlying cause of the patient's presenting illness can be difficult, and may require in-hospital investigations. Assessment must include a detailed history and a thorough physical examination. For the assessment and management of patients with dyspnoea refer to Table 3.11.

Table 3.9 – CAUSES OF DYSPNOEA

Pulmonary causes	Cardiac causes	Other causes
Acute exacerbation of asthma.	Cardiac arrhythmia.	Anaphylaxis.
Acute heart failure.	Cardiac tamponade.	Chemicals/poisons.
Bronchiectasis.	Ischaemic heart disease.	Diabetic ketoacidosis.
Acute exacerbation of COPD.	Myocardial infarction.	Diaphragmatic splinting.
Flail chest.	Valvular dysfunction.	Hyperventilation.
Interstitial lung disease.	Pericarditis.	Panic attack/anxiety.
Lung/lobar collapse.		Severe hypovolaemia.
Massive haemothorax.		Metabolic causes.
Pleural effusion.		Obesity.
Pneumonia.		Pain.
Pneumothorax.		Severe anaemia.
Pulmonary embolism.		
Upper airway obstruction.		

Table 3.10 – DIFFERENTIAL DIAGNOSIS FOR COMMON CONDITIONS

Condition	Symptoms	Signs	Auscultation sounds	History
Acute Asthma (**refer to asthma guideline**)	Dyspnoea Cough Unable to complete sentences	Wheeze Tachypnoea Tachycardia Pulsus paradoxus Hyperresonant chest Accessory muscle use	Decreased or absent breath sounds if severe	Previous asthma Recent increase in inhaler use Allergen exposure
Acute Coronary Syndrome (**refer to acute coronary syndrome guideline**)	Central chest pain for >15 minutes constricting or crushing that radiates to left arm/neck	Wheeze Tachycardia Arrhythmia	Crackles	Symptoms suggestive of ischaemic heart disease and previous investigations for chest pain
Acute Heart Failure (**refer to heart failure guideline**)	Dyspnoea especially on exertion Orthopnoea/paroxysmal nocturnal dyspnoea Cough producing frothy, white or pink phlegm	Peripheral oedema Tachycardia	Rales Heart murmur Crepitations	IHD Hypertension History of heart failure
Anaphylaxis (**refer to allergic reactions including anaphylaxis guideline**)	Dyspnoea Dysphagia Chest tightness	Tachycardia Tachypnoea Wheeze Erythema Urticaria Angioedema	Decreased breath sounds	Allergen exposure
Chronic Obstructive Pulmonary Disease (COPD) (**refer to COPD guideline**)	Progressive dyspnoea Wheezing Chest tightness Cough – purulent sputum	Wheeze Cyanosis	Rales	Smoking >35 years of age
Foreign Body Airway Obstruction (FBAO) (refer to FBAO guideline)	Dyspnoea	Wheeze Clutching at neck Silent cough	Audible stridor	Eating – especially fish, meat, or poultry
Pneumonia (**refer to medical emergencies guideline**)	Dyspnoea Fever Cough	Tachycardia	Rhonchi	Smoking IHD
Pneumothorax (**refer to thoracic trauma guideline**)	Dyspnoea Sudden onset pleuritic chest pain	Dyspnoea Sudden onset pleuritic chest pain	Decreased breath sounds	Trauma Previous pneumothorax COPD Asthma Smoking
Pulmonary Embolism (**refer to pulmonary embolism guideline**)	Dyspnoea Pleuritic chest pain Cough Possible DVT Leg oedema	Tachycardia Tachypnoea Fever ECG: Non-specific ST wave changes	Focal rales	Prolonged immobilisation Recent surgery Thrombotic disease

3 SECTION **Medical** Undifferentiated Complaints

Dyspnoea

Table 3.11 – ASSESSMENT and MANAGEMENT of:

Dyspnoea

NB Take a defibrillator at the earliest opportunity and keep with the patient until hand-over

ASSESSMENT	MANAGEMENT

● Assess **ABCD**	● If any of the following **TIME CRITICAL** features present:
	  – major **ABCD** problems
	  – extreme breathing difficulty (**refer to medical emergencies guideline**)
	  – cyanosis (**refer to medical emergencies guideline**)
	  – hypoxia – SpO$_2$ <94% or not responding to oxygen therapy (refer to oxygen guideline)
	  – features of life-threatening asthma (**refer to asthma guideline**)
	  – features of tension pneumothorax or major chest trauma (**refer to thoracic trauma guideline**)
	  – acute myocardial infarction (**refer to acute coronary syndrome guideline**)
	  – anaphylaxis (**refer to allergic reactions including anaphylaxis guideline**)
	  – loss of consciousness (**refer to altered level of consciousness guideline**), then:
	● Start correcting **A** and **B** and undertake a **TIME CRITICAL** transfer to nearest receiving hospital.
	● Continue patient management en-route.
	● Provide an alert/information call.

● Ask the patient if they have an individualised treatment plan	● Follow the treatment plan if available. ● The patient will often be able to guide their care.

● If non-**TIME CRITICAL** – obtain a thorough history to help identify cause of dyspnoea	**Specifically assess:**
	● Respiratory rate.
	● Effort and effectiveness of ventilation – rate and depth.
	● Degree of dyspnoea.
	● Length of difficulty breathing – sudden or gradual onset?
	● Pain associated with breathing – any pattern of breathing/depth of respiration?
	● Do certain positions exacerbate breathing (e.g. unable to lie down, must sit upright)?
	● Does the patient have a cough?
	● If yes, is the cough productive:
	  – **sputum or bubbling:** consider infection or heart failure
	  – **frothy white/pink sputum:** consider acute heart failure
	  – **yellow/green sputum:** consider chest infection
	  – **haemoptysis:** consider PE, chest infection or carcinoma of the lung.
	● Has the patient increased their medication recently?
	● Signs of anaphylaxis:
	  – itchy rash
	  – facial swelling
	  – circulatory collapse.

● Percuss the chest	● To determine if there are collections of fluid in the lungs.

● Auscultate the chest	● To determine adequacy of air entry on both sides of the chest.
	● To determine chest sounds:
	  – audible wheeze on expiration – consider asthma, ACS, anaphylaxis, COPD or heart failure (especially in older patients with no history of asthma)
	  – audible stridor (upper airway narrowing) consider anaphylaxis, or FBAO
	  – crepitations (fine crackling in lung bases) – ACS, heart failure
	  – rhonchi (harsher, rattling sound) indicating collections of fluid in larger airways – pneumonia.

Consider possible causes (refer to Table 3.9 and Table 3.10) if there is a history of:

Consider specific respiratory problems	● Asthma – consider acute exacerbation (**refer to asthma guideline**). ● COPD – consider acute exacerbation (**refer to COPD guideline**). ● Pulmonary embolism (**refer to PE guideline**). ● Heart failure (e.g. left ventricular failure, right ventricular failure, congestive heart failure, cor pulmonale, hypertension) – consider acute exacerbation (**refer to heart failure guideline**). ● Other respiratory disorder? ● Smoking.

Table 3.11 – ASSESSMENT and MANAGEMENT of:

Dyspnoea continued

Consider specific cardiovascular problems	Acute coronary syndrome (e.g. STEMI, NSTEMI)? NB Some patients with acute myocardial infarction may have breathlessness as their only symptom (**refer to ACS guideline**). <ul><li>Constricting pain (**refer to ACS guideline**).</li><li>Angina (**refer to ACS guideline**).</li><li>Ischaemic heart disease.</li><li>Valvular dysfunction/congenital heart problems.</li></ul>
Consider other conditions	<ul><li>Recent trauma (**refer to thoracic trauma guideline**).</li><li>Recent surgery or immobilisation (**refer to PE guideline**).</li><li>Hyperventilation – often accompanied by numbness and tingling in the limbs and around the mouth (**refer to hyperventilation syndrome guideline**). NB Ensure other more serious conditions are excluded before considering this diagnosis.</li></ul>
● Known cause	● If cause of dyspnoea known follow relevant guideline.
● Unknown cause	● If cause of dyspnoea unknown **refer to medical emergencies guideline** and follow management below.
● ECG	● Undertake a 12-lead ECG.
● Oxygen	● Administer supplemental oxygen if indicated (refer to oxygen guideline).
● Ventilation	Consider assisted ventilation at a rate of 12–20 breaths per minute if (refer to airway and breathing management guideline): <ul><li>SpO_2 is <90% on high concentration O_2.</li><li>Respiratory rate is <10 or >30.</li><li>Expansion is inadequate.</li></ul>
● Fluid	● Administer fluid as required (refer to intravascular fluid therapy guideline).
● Pain management	● Administer pain relief if indicated (refer to pain management guideline).
● Position	● Position for comfort – usually sitting upright.
● Degree of dyspnoea	● Re-assess the response to using the visual analogue scale or other locally agreed scale.
● Transfer to further care	<ul><li>All patients with an unexplained cause of dyspnoea.</li><li>Where the cause is known refer to the relevant guideline for care pathway.</li></ul>

3 **Medical** Undifferentiated Complaints SECTION

KEY POINTS

Dyspnoea
- **Is breathlessness a result of respiratory, cardiac, both or other causes?**
- **Consider time critical causes.**
- **Assess degree of dyspnoea and response to treatment using a visual analogue score.**
- **Consider possible causes and refer to relevant guidelines for assessment and management.**

Headache [160–163]

1. Introduction

- Headache is a common condition presenting in pre-hospital care.
- Most headaches are simple and not serious, but care must be taken to ensure that **TIME CRITICAL** conditions are not missed. A **detailed history is vital** when dealing with headache, as aetiology may go back hours, days, months (or even years in relation to family history or childhood illness; e.g. tumours).

2. History

- Exclude the following or refer to the specific guidelines for:
  - **stroke**
  - **head injury**
  - **glycaemic episode.**
- Assess the **SOCRATES** of the pain:
  - **S**ite – where exactly is the pain.
  - **O**nset – what was the patient doing when the pain came on.
  - **C**haracter – what does the pain feel like.
  - **R**adiates – where does the pain spread to.
  - **A**ssociated symptoms – e.g. nausea, dizziness.
  - **T**iming – how long has the patient had pain.
  - **E**xacerbating/relieving factors – what makes it better or worse.
  - **S**everity – obtain an initial pain score.
- Key questions for patients with headache:
  - Is this the worst headache ever?
  - Is it different from your usual headache?
  - Is this a new headache?

Headaches can be broadly defined as primary or secondary.

Primary headaches are those which occur spontaneously (simple headache); in response to a lifelong condition (e.g. migraine); 'tension type' headaches (various aetiologies[a]) or cluster headache (severe short lasting headache). These should not considered as being pathophysiological; that being normal for the patient.

Secondary headaches are secondary to illness or injury and are pathological in origin, for instance head trauma (skull fracture), infective origin (i.e. meningitis); intracranial haemorrhage (i.e. spontaneous subarachnoid bleed or sub dural bleed following trauma) or vascular (i.e. temporal arteritis).

- It is difficult to accurately differentiate between a simple headache, which requires no treatment, and a potentially more serious condition. Table 3.12 lists '**red flag**' symptoms that require the patient to undergo hospital assessment. NB This does not mean that any patient presenting without these symptoms is automatically safe to be left at home.

Consideration should be given to transferring all first presentations of severe headache to the emergency department for further investigation.

Table 3.12 – RED FLAG SIGNS AND SYMPTOMS

Signs and symptoms
Headache of severe, sudden (thunderclap) onset.
Headache localised to the vertex (top of head).
Escalating headache of unusual nature.
Changed visual acuity.
Meningeal irritation.
Changed mental state and inappropriate behaviour.
Newly presenting ataxia.
Cranial nerve palsy.
Posture-related headache.
Headache triggered by cough/valsava manoeuvre.

NB Multiple red flags increase significantly the risk of serious pathology.

3. Incidence

Refer to Table 3.13 for details of the incidence of different types of primary headache.

Table 3.13 – INCIDENCE BY TYPE FOR PRIMARY HEADACHES

Type	Incidence
Migraine	6–8% in men 15–18% in women
(Episodic) Tension Type Headache	Up to 70% of whole population during life Most prevalent up to age of 30
Cluster Headache	Less than 1 in every 1000 people

- Secondary headache data are not meaningful in the emergency setting as the intention is not to exclude these potentially more serious presentations in the pre-hospital environment.

4. Severity and Outcome

- The severity of headaches varies from patient to patient in terms of the pain the patient experiences. Although the pain may be the primary concern of the patient, it may belie the true severity of the underlying cause.
- The outcome for patients presenting through the 999 system for headache will be varied as the cause of the headache, the clinical significance of the headache and the progression are all dependent on the presenting factors.
- Patients may deteriorate rapidly if they have a space occupying condition (e.g. haemorrhage resulting in mass effect).
- Clinicians must ensure that the patient receives the safest pathway of care and it is always better to be cautious, especially in children and those patients who are on their own.

[a] Tension type or chronic daily headaches can be caused by medication overuse or withdrawal. These should be considered to be secondary headache.

Headache

- It is preferable to be cautious when dealing with patients with headaches, as diagnosis can be challenging.
- Where patients are not conveyed, follow-up care MUST be arranged. Always liaise with the patient's GP (or out-of-hours doctor) to discuss onward care.

Ensure that, where practicable, the patient is not left alone whilst awaiting follow-up.

5. Assessment and Management

- For the assessment and management of headache refer to Table 3.14.

KEY POINTS

Headache

- **Crescendo headaches are significant.**
- **Headaches with different or unusual characteristics are significant.**
- **Migraineurs are at risk of serious intracranial events.**
- **In headache, blood pressure must be checked.**
- **Any persistent headache or any headache associated with altered conscious levels or unusual behaviour is significant.**
- **Sinister headaches may or may not be accompanied by neurology. Do not exclude simply based on physical examination – HISTORY IS KEY.**

Table 3.14 – ASSESSMENT and MANAGEMENT of:

Headache

ASSESSMENT	MANAGEMENT
● Assess ABCD	● Start correcting any ABCD problems – **refer to medical emergencies guideline..**
● Specifically assess: Levels of consciousness	● Assess AVPU: NB The only normal GCS is 15. A – Alert V – Responds to voice P – Responds to painful stimulus U – Unresponsive.
Temperature	
Pulse rate	● Do not administer supplemental oxygen unless the patient is hypoxaemic (SpO$_2$ <94%) (refer to oxygen guideline).
Respiratory rate	
Blood pressure	● Measure systolic/diastolic.
Blood glucose level	
Record pain score	● Consider symptomatic pain relief for clinically benign headaches using appropriate drug. ● **Avoid morphine** due to potential side effects which could worsen the patient's condition and/or hinder further assessment: – Respiratory depression – Nausea and vomiting – Drowsiness – Pupillary constriction.
Assess for: ● Any evidence of a rash. ● Neck stiffness and photophobia (light sensitivity of eyes). ● Loss of function or altered sensation. ● Flushed face but cool, pale trunk and extremities.	
● Assess for red flag symptoms (refer to Table 3.12)	● Undertake a **TIME CRITICAL** transfer to nearest suitable receiving hospital. ● Provide an alert/information call.

Mental Disorder

1. Introduction

DEFINITIONS

WHO has defined mental health as a state of well-being in which every individual realises his or her own potential, can cope with the normal stresses of life, can work productively and fruitfully, and is able to make a contribution to her or his community. Problems and disorders that affect people's mental health are often referred to colloquially as 'mental health problems'. Such broad use of this term gives little indication of the severity of their conditions or of the likely courses of events in particular patients' circumstances. Sometimes, people who have a severe mental disorder are described as having a mental illness.

This guideline uses the term 'mental disorder' to distinguish those conditions that are primarily related to people's mental ill health from the very common and understandable anxieties and emotional reactions of people who are casualties or who require ambulance services for any other reason. These more general and frequent psychosocial responses to accidents, injuries and illness are better referred to as 'distress' rather than calling them mental health problems or disorders. People who are distressed should be managed according to principles of psychological first aid.

This guideline provides general advice about matters related to people who have mental disorders. There have been rapid developments in recent years of knowledge and agreement about the most effective ways to care for people who are distressed. Therefore the future intention is to develop several additional guidelines relating to distress, public mental health, and mental disorders.

THE PREVALENCE OF MENTAL DISORDERS

The prevalence of common mental health disorders varies greatly across all populations

Although mental disorders are widespread, serious cases are concentrated among a relatively small proportion of people who experience more than one mental health problem [164]. The World Health Organization estimates that up to 450 million people worldwide have a mental health problem [165]. In the UK, 1 in 4 British adults experience at least one diagnosable mental health problem in any one year, and 1 in 6 experiences this at any given time (The Office for National Statistics Psychiatric Morbidity report, 2001). More than half of people aged 16 to 64 years who meet the diagnostic criteria for at least one common mental health disorder experience comorbid anxiety and depressive disorders.

Mental disorders vary from mild anxiety, phobic states and mild to severe depression, to severe and enduring mental illnesses, unipolar and bipolar affective disorders (otherwise termed depression, hypomania and mania), serious problems from misuse of alcohol and drugs, and schizophrenia. Comorbidity (having more than one disorder) is common. The causes of mental disorders are often unclear, with mental health being influenced not only by individual attributes, but also by the social circumstances in which individuals find themselves and the environment in which they live. These determinants interact with each other dynamically, and are known as protective or risk factors. Risk factors include genetic inheritance, where a family history of mental illness plays a part; life experiences such as childhood abuse or stress;

experience of traumatic events such as in war torn countries; biological factors have also been identified as potential causes. Other factors such as a traumatic brain injury or a pregnant woman's exposure to viruses or toxic chemicals can lead to a mental disorder. Many disorders, for example, are provoked by, maintained by or associated with consumption of alcohol and illicit substances. Not uncommonly, people who develop mental disorders may present first to the emergency and ambulance services. Commonly, ambulance services meet people who have had a mental disorder previously, but who develop a new episode or an exacerbation of a chronic problem. Ambulance services may also be called to people who are already under the care of mental health services.

VULNERABILITY

Certain groups in society may be particularly susceptible to the development of mental disorders depending on the local context, including households living in poverty, people with chronic health conditions, ethnic minority groups, and persons exposed to and/or displaced by war or conflict.

People with a mental disorder have their own set of vulnerabilities and risks, including an increased likelihood of experiencing disability and premature mortality, stigma and discrimination, social exclusion and impoverishment. They may also be vulnerable to exploitation and abuse from other members of society.

PSYCHOTROPIC DRUGS THAT ARE USED TO TREAT PEOPLE WHO HAVE MENTAL DISORDERS

Table 3.15 provides a very brief overview of three categories of drugs that are used to treat people who

---

TABLE 3.15 – DRUGS USED IN MENTAL HEALTH

ANXIOLYTICS

- Benzodiazepines are among the most frequently used drugs in this category. They can be used to induce sleep and also to reduce anxiety. In excess, they are principally sedative. Examples of anxiolytics include lorazepam, clonazepam and diazepam

ANTIDEPRESSANTS

- Antidepressants are a class of drugs that reduce symptoms of depressive disorders by correcting chemical imbalances of neurotransmitters in the brain. They include a number of different groups of drugs that are used over weeks and months rather than days, and some types may take up to three weeks to begin to show an effect. They are grouped into four main types:
  - SSRIs (selective serotonin reuptake inhibitors) These are a widely used group of antidepressants. In general, SSRIs are better tolerated than most other types of antidepressants although some people will experience a few mild side effects when taking them. Examples include fluoxetine, fluvoxamine, sertraline and paroxetine
  - SNRIs (serotonin and noradrenaline reuptake inhibitors) Third generation of antidepressants which are commonly prescribed. The common side effects of serotonin-noradrenaline reuptake inhibitors (SNRIs) are the same as those that are associated with SSRIs. Examples include duloxetine, venlafaxine,

TABLE 3.15 – DRUGS USED IN MENTAL HEALTH continued

TRICYCLICS

- These are a group of the older antidepressants which are very dangerous in excess. Agitations followed by sedation and cardiac arrhythmias are the most significant effects in poisoning. They too can cause significant side effects. Examples include amitriptyline, clomipramine, trimipramine

  - MAOIs (monoamine oxidase inhibitors)
    These are now used rarely and only then by people who are resistant to more recently developed drugs. However, this group of antidepressants is raised here because it has an important range of severe drug interactions and, in the ambulance context, morphine must be avoided. When they interact with other drugs, they can cause a dangerous increase in blood pressure. Examples include phenelzine and tranylcypromine.

ANTIPSYCHOTICS

- They are a range of medications that are used in the medium- to long-term management of people who have disorders such as schizophrenia and other psychotic illnesses. They can also be used in the setting to sedate. Some people refer to them as neuroleptics. They can be taken orally or given by injection as depot antipsychotic medication and are powerful tranquillizers.

- There are two basic types of antipsychotics:

  - *Typical antipsychotics:* Older or first-generation antipsychotics These are the original antipsychotic medications. Examples include chlorpromazine, haloperidol, fluphenazine
  - *Atypical antipsychotics:* Newer or second-generation antipsychotics. They have largely replaced the first generation antipsychotics, due to the lower risk of side effects (particularly extrapyramidal side effects). Examples include risperidone, olanzapine, aripiprazole

have mental disorders. Some of the more modern drugs may require close supervision of certain parameters of the physical health of people who take them. The brevity of this table and the possible side effects of psychotropic medications are two reasons why ambulance clinicians are strongly advised to consult the British National Formulary or another source of information that is approved by their employers when they assess people who are taking psychotropic medications.

2. Who is who in the Mental Health Services

APPROVED MENTAL HEALTH PROFESSIONALS (AMHP)

An AMHP is responsible for organising and coordinating assessments under the Mental Health Act (1983) as amended 2007. The role is often held by specially trained social workers, but can also be carried out by occupational therapists, community mental health nurses and psychologists.

PSYCHIATRIST

A medically trained doctor who specialises in mental health problems and is trained to deal with prevention, diagnosis and treatment and can prescribe medication.

PSYCHOLOGIST

A professional who is interested in how people think, act, react, interact and behave. Psychologists who have undergone specialist training in the treatment of people with mental health problems are called clinical psychologists.

CARE COORDINATOR/KEY WORKER

Mental health teams often use these terms interchangeably to refer to the named individual who is designated as the main point of contact and support for a person who has a need for on-going care. This can be a nurse, social worker or other mental health worker; whomever is deemed appropriate for the person's situation. They keep in close contact with service users who are receiving mental health care and monitor how that care is delivered in the community. They usually work as part of a community mental health team (CMHT).

COMMUNITY PSYCHIATRIC NURSE (CPN)

A CPN is a qualified mental health nurse who supports people with mental health problems who are living in the community. This is most often in the person's own home but it can also be in clinics based, for example, in a GP's surgery.

SUPPORT WORKERS

Support workers work in the community as part of the mental health team. They supplement the work of CPNs, (e.g. by helping a patient to socialise more by taking them out or helping them with their shopping). They are supervised by qualified members of the mental health team.

POLICE OFFICERS

Although police officers are not mental health professionals, they have a crucial role in working with and supporting people with mental health problems. They may be the first to respond to urgent situations involving people with mental health problems, and have to make quick decisions to assess the situation as well as the needs of the individuals involved, ensuring their safety and that of the general public. They can also use their powers under the MHA (1983) to detain mentally unwell people found in a public place.

3. Specialities

ADULT MENTAL HEALTH SERVICES (AMH)

AMH services offer a wide range of interventions for adults aged 18–65 in a community.

CHILD AND ADOLESCENT MENTAL HEALTH SERVICES (CAMHS)

NHS-provided specialist mental health services for children and young adults, up to school-leaving age.

MENTAL HEALTH SERVICES FOR OLDER PEOPLE (MHSOP)

Mental Health Services for Older People provide specialist diagnosis and care to people of all ages with probable dementia and people over 65 years of age with depression, anxiety and psychotic illnesses. A range of services offer different levels of support dependent on the severity of the illness at that time.

4. Other disorders

LEARNING DISABILITY

A person with a learning disability is someone who, from childhood, has had difficulty in learning and processing information so that it significantly reduces his or her ability to carry out the full range of everyday tasks. It is normally recognised as an IQ below 70. It is diagnosed as moderate, profound or severe. This guide does not cover learning disability as it is not a mental illness but effective communication is important when dealing with people with learning disability.

DEMENTIA

The term dementia is used to describe a range of conditions which affect the brain and result in an overall impairment of the person's function. The person may experience memory loss, problems with communication, impaired reasoning and difficulties with daily living skills. This can result in changes in behaviour, which can disrupt their ability to live independently and may affect social relationships.

Some people with dementia will have dementia passports – This is a simple communication tool that articulates a person's normal everyday needs and thus helps services including ambulance clinicians deliver person-centred care.

ASPERGER'S SYNDROME /DISORDER

Asperger's syndrome is a form of autism which is a lifelong disability that affects how a person makes sense of the world, processes information and relates to other people.

It is a type of development disorder which involves delays in the development of many basic skills, most notably the ability to socialise with others, to communicate and to use imagination. Autism is often described as a 'spectrum disorder' because the condition affects people in many different ways and to varying degrees

Generally it is not possible to tell that someone has the condition from their outward appearance. People with the condition have difficulties in three main areas:

  – social communication
  – social interaction
  – social imagination.

Some people with Asperger's syndrome will have a 'Hospital Passport'.

The passport is designed to help people with autism to communicate their needs to doctors, nurses and other healthcare professionals.

5. IPAP Suicide Risk Assessment

Risk assessment – in mental health terms – is about identifying and considering a range of factors that may suggest an increased probability of an event or incident happening (i.e. self harm and/or suicide). Assessment should include examination of past incidents (both the context and detail) in the light of the current circumstances, which will inform and influence the subsequent management plan. Suicide is the main cause of premature death in people with mental illness.

IPAP is a basic suicide risk assessment process which can be used by non-mental health professionals to identify and assess the presence of suicidal risk.

Intent	thoughts.
Plans	access to the means.
Actions	current and/or past.
Protection	family, social network, services.

It is important to note that each additional element, relevant to the patient, represents increased risk.

IPAP uses key elements of various evidence based suicide risk assessment tools used throughout the UK. It is a simple process, ideal for use in the pre-hospital emergency care environment, and will assist in identifying risk factors required to formulate a safe and effective care plan for patients who have expressed suicidal ideation. This will include the key issues required at handover to other health/social care agencies and/or professionals.

Summary:

● No risk – no thoughts of killing self.

● Mild risk – some thoughts of killing self, no plan.

● Moderate risk – thoughts of killing self, vague plan, low on lethality, would not do it.

● Severe risk – thoughts of killing self, specific plan and lethal, would not do it now.

● Extreme risk – thoughts of killing self, specific plan and lethal, will do it/has done it.

Remember:

● Seriously expressed intent is the best indicator of intended behaviour.

● Asking someone about suicide isn't going to put the idea into their head. People appreciate openness, honesty and being treated with respect.

● Risk is dynamic and the level of risk can change rapidly depending on the patient's circumstances (e.g. social, interpersonal relationships, and stability of mental health).

Rationale for use of IPAP:

● A lot of suicide risk assessment tools are quite specialised and if not used by MH professionals are subject to inaccurate results and interpretation.

● NICE Guidelines don't recommend use of assessment tools because most of them are not accurate enough when used in isolation.

● Impractical to use an existing tool because there isn't one single tool that would be recognised across the country.

Figure 3.1 outlines a clinical decision outcome pathway which could be used in conjunction with IPAP.

6. Management

Ambulance clinicians should be aware that successfully managing the acute distress from mental health problems can involve many different aspects, subtleties and intervention strategies. Ambulance clinicians may well be the first contact that a person with a mental health problem has with health services, and as such need to recognise the importance of their role. A person may contact ambulance services due to a physical health problem but which their mental health may have bearing on the outcome or the onward treatment provided.

Mental Disorder

Alternatively ambulance clinicians may be called to attend to a person who appears to have a mental health problem but also has significant physical care needs, for example when a person has self-harmed.

The value of the assessment should not be underestimated, a person suffering with a mental health problem may appreciate the time and care taken to establish what, why and how something has happened, and this may help alleviate some of their distress. The practical management of the situation therefore starts with the assessment. This will then indicate the direction and help with the formulation for where a person's needs may best be met. Fundamental to the management of any mental health problem is the approach taken by a health professional; they must try and engage the person in meaningful dialogue. Management of acute distress thus involves the use of effective communication skills.

Communication

Effective communication is fundamental to successfully working with someone who presents in crisis with a mental health problem. For ambulance clinicians managing dynamic situations that deal with both physical and mental health components these can be stressful and challenging. Engaging a person using effective communication skills can be challenging when there are multiple unknown aspects. What is described below may help with this.

De-escalation of acute distress

Mental health problems can be highly distressing times and ambulance clinicians may be faced with highly distressed people for many different reasons. De-escalation is often taught within mental health settings as the distress and challenging nature of care can lead to more distress. The basis for de-escalation includes using highly developed communication skills, empathy, non-confrontation, threat minimisation, compromise and distraction. The literature indicates that there is a lack of consensus and consistency within training. However, overarching themes from de-escalation literature recognise the importance of understanding the individual in their social and cultural context. Alongside this are effective communication skills, with an emphasis on using empathy, genuineness, transparency and non-verbal awareness to help de-escalate.

Gaining an understanding of the person's situation is vital, and as such the assessment of the situation will assist with this. Doing so using exploratory questions such as 'what, when, where, how' type questions and giving the person time to speak can be a foundation for this. Being able to reflect your understanding of the situation by explaining back to the person what you have learnt from them will demonstrate that you have listened and understood, which will relieve anxieties. Including the person as much as possible is vital, remembering to explain and check with the person so they feel that they have control helps reduce anxiety where they feel that they have lost control.

MANAGING ACUTE BEHAVIOURS FOR PARTICULAR MENTAL HEALTH PROBLEMS.

Anxiety

Anxiety is a normal and usually transitory experience related to a threat or perceived danger. The nature and degree of the anxiety can lead to more prolonged or disabling anxiety which is treated by specialist services. It is highly likely that ambulance clinicians will be responding to people who exhibit a degree of anxiety related to their situation.

There can be many different responses that a person can have to their anxiety. This can include physical symptoms such as shortness of breath, dizziness, trembling and so on, but also behaviours that can be a way of coping for the person. These can include impulsive acting out behaviours such as shouting or self-harm.

During an episode of heightened anxiety simple strategies include:

- Staying with the person
- Encouraging them to sit
- Calming your own breathing rate and speaking in short sentences
- Reassuring the person
- Demonstrating control of the situation, being firm but caring
- Encouraging the person to breathe in and out slowly
- Considering the environment, how much is noise and external stimulation influencing the anxiety? Can this be reduced?

Self-harm

Self-harm can be and should be distinguished from suicide attempts, although a person can exhibit both behaviours. Self-harm is considered by NICE as 'self-poisoning or self-injury, irrespective of the apparent purpose of the act'. However, a history of self-harm can be a strong predictor for repeated self-harm and completion of suicide.

Self-harm is often viewed negatively by healthcare clinicians, often as attention seeking and manipulative. This can perhaps be attributed to the difficulty and anxieties of working with someone who self-harms. Instead it should be recognised that self-harm is a way of coping that the person uses. This coping can be for various reasons, such as coping with negative thoughts and feelings. These may be associated with a person's depression or if the person has a diagnosis of personality disorder. Self-harm is also highly associated with past traumas and abuse. Self-harm can often be viewed as a problem largely for young people, and it is thought that up to 1 in 10 young people have self-harmed. As a coping strategy it could be related to the self-harm as way of:

- Release or catharsis
- Making an emotional pain a 'real' physical pain
- Having control when feeling out of control
- As a punishment for oneself
- When in a dissociative state, that is an out of body experience

Self-harm can be a complex and difficult behaviour to respond to and to try and understand. It is recognised that when a person feels worthless, they might adopt ways of being that help maintain that perception. This might involve or maintain self-harm behaviours and the feelings of worthlessness might also be compounded if they are received negatively by health professionals. Self-harm is thought to also be maintained by its power to bring relief, although the act is then strongly associated with feelings of shame that perpetuate negative feelings and further punishing behaviour, increasing the risk of self-harm.

A large part of the work for the ambulance clinician is likely to be centred on the physical nature of the self-harm. However, talking about the self-harm is vital as part of the assessment, it acknowledges what has happened and with this it communicates to the person that you are not rejecting them. This helps reduce feelings of shame and stigma which can help maintain self-harm. When working with someone who has self-harmed it is important that these factors are addressed:

- What led up to it? That is the triggers – interpersonal stressors and situational triggers.
- The intent of the act?
- What was the motivation?
- Was it planned? Impulsive?
- Protective factors?

These questions may overlap those if the person was also suicidal, but ambulance clinicians should be aware to separate these two aspects and to treat accordingly.

Acute psychosis

The term psychosis is often used to indicate the presence of behaviours such as hallucinations, delusions, behavioural changes (e.g. over-activity or excitement) and thought disorder. Psychosis is often associated with a diagnosis of schizophrenia but is also associated with severe depression and bipolar disorder.

Because presentations can be very varied, specific management can be difficult. Establishing rapport with the person is vital. This can be challenging if the person is experiencing hallucinations of distressing voices which make it difficult to concentrate or hold a conversation. The person may well find it difficult to follow the flow of a conversation due to problems with thought, for example, inability to articulate thoughts clearly and words become jumbled up or words get loosely associated with other words but lead to a different topic. This requires

the ambulance clinician to be patient and understanding and go at the pace of the person in distress.

As an acute psychotic episode could be attributed to a variety of mental health issues and physical conditions, being able to establish this may be very difficult in the pre-hospital environment. Preferably the person is assessed and seen as soon as possible by specialist mental health services in the community or in a hospital setting. Treatment through specialist services for an episode of psychosis usually involves a combination of medication and therapeutic interventions such as CBT (cognitive behavioural therapy) and family therapy.

Pathways for referral

It is recommended that providers of pre-hospital care have clear policies and procedures that set out the routes for onward referral to other agencies.

The routes open to decision making as to conveyance to hospital or otherwise may be as follows:

Contacting local Mental Health Services – this could be a Crisis Team or a team which specialises in the rapid assessment of people who present with mental health problems (RAID). This could be for advice or to wait for specialist services to attend and assess. This may lead to further assessment such as a specific Mental Health Act Assessment which may involve the person being subject to detention under the Mental Health Act (1983, as amended 2007).

Ambulance clinicians may have options to convey the person to an Accident and Emergency Department for further physical or mental health care.

If felt necessary the police may assist ambulance clinicians where there is potential for a variety of risks. This may involve the person being conveyed to a Place of Safety under s136 or s135 of the Mental Health Act (1983 as amended 2007). Depending on local services this may be to a specific Place of Safety unit within a mental health hospital, an Accident & Emergency Department, a police station if the situational risk dictates this, or to any place designated as a place of safety.

KEY POINTS

It is not vital that ambulance clinicians are able to fully assess and diagnose patients with mental health issues. However it is important that clinicians are able to recognise common mental health signs, symptoms and behaviours when attempting to decide upon the need for transportation or referral of a patient. Below is a guide that should help clinicians in the decision making process.

It is not exhaustive and similarly it is not necessary for all signs and symptoms to be present. In fact it will usually be the case that only some will be evident.

It is important that clinicians gain as much information as possible and should not be afraid to ask questions when done so politely and professionally.

Remember, if in doubt ask for help.

Behaviour Observe both verbal and non-verbal signs.	• Eye contact yes or no? • Calm and relaxed or anxious, upset, aggressive, suspicious or pre-occupied? • Is the patient's body language appropriate or are they hyperactive or hypoactive? • Is the patient's conduct appropriate to the situation or are they overly intrusive or maybe very withdrawn?
Appearance Again assessed through observation	• Is the patient dressed properly, are they unkempt or have poor hygiene or other evidence or poor self-care? • Are there signs of self-harm, for instance cutting marks, drug and alcohol misuse, overdose?

Mental Disorder

KEY POINTS

Speech and rapport	● Is the volume of speech normal or very loud or quiet? ● Is the rate of speech normal for the situation or is it pressured or especially slow? ● Is the conversation spontaneous? Does the patient talk far too much or only minimally and is it in response to questions? ● Is the patient friendly and cooperative or is speech forced or monotone?
Mood/affect	● Does the patient present in a way that fits with their current mood for instance, are they flat, restricted or blunted, or alternatively does their mood appear to vary quickly and seem inappropriate to the situation? ● Bearing this in mind , does the patient describe or appear, elated, anxious, angry, agitated or even disinterested and lacking any motivation ● At this point it is worth considering potential risks to the patient or others (for instance suicidal ideas or violent thoughts). Don't be afraid to ask as the vast majority of people will be relieved to disclose such feelings especially to clinicians who appear interested and empathetic. There is no evidence to suggest that enquiring about this will implant any new ideas.
Cognition	● GCS ● Orientated to time, person and place? ● Short-term memory, is the patient able to retain and recall information and use it appropriately? ● Is the patient able to concentrate and pay attention as would be expected for the situation? ● Does the patient express a normal level of general knowledge and ability to identify familiar items, objects, people and places? ● Can the patient easily follow simple instructions?

Thoughts:
The Nature and Content
The Process and form
Perception
	● Does the patient have any thoughts of self-harm, suicide or thoughts of harming others?
	● Do they appear pre-occupied or to have obsessive thoughts?
	● Do they display any unusual beliefs or delusional, unrealistic ideas about themselves, others or the world in general?
	● Are they very anxious or very low or depressed,
	● Do they describe feeling hopeless or appear unmotivated, even to complete small tasks like eating, drinking or appropriate levels of self-care?
	● Does the thought process of the patient flow logically and naturally within the conversation or when taking the history or do they:
	  – Change subject often and quickly to unrelated topics or to whatever changes in front of them?
	  – Do their thoughts seem overly fast or unusually slow?
	  – Is their speech very fast or unusually slow?
	  – Are they very vague with answers questions, rarely addressing or coming to a point or conclusion?
	  – Are they using nonsense words or very mixed up sentences, sometimes described as a "word salad"?
	
	The following symptoms and traits are often associated with psychosis type illness and can feel very real and very disturbing for the patient. They are less likely to be found in the very young (under 18 years old)
	Hallucinations
	● Visual disturbances and visions not apparent to others, these can be described as people, animals or objects and are individual to the patient
	● Auditory hallucinations, often hearing voices not belonging to the patient and outside of their head. These can be derogatory, commanding or abusive. Similarly auditory hallucinations may not be voices at all and again vary from patient to patient.
	Delusions: These can include:
	● The belief of a patient that their thoughts can be read, changed or removed from their minds.
	● The patient may feel that they themselves are not real or that the situation they are in is not real.
	● A patient may describe feeling detached or removed from themselves akin to watching themselves or their situation from afar with little control.

Insight	● Does the patient acknowledge that they have a current mental health problem? ● Do they acknowledge the need for help or further input and are they willing to comply with this? ● Are they able to evaluate different treatment options and choices? ● Are they able to weigh up and identify any risks to themselves or others?

Table 3.16 – IPAP Suicide Risk Assessment Tool

Risk Factor	Context/Explanation	Examples of some questions which may be used. Questions should be clear, unambiguous, single and relevant to the circumstances.
I Intent	• Explore what thoughts the patient is having. Concrete, intrusive and upsetting thoughts over a prolonged period could indicate that the patient is very vulnerable. • So: Is the patient experiencing suicidal thoughts now? – How intrusive are the thoughts? Are they fleeting and unspecific or are they intrusive and troubling? – How frequent are the thoughts and for how long have they been there? – How often are they occurring, where, when, with whom? – If a patient is psychotic and is hallucinating or has delusional beliefs, this presents an increased risk. **Explore the content of these beliefs and experiences and accept that they are real for the patient concerned.**	• Are you feeling so bad that you have thought of suicide? • Are you feeling so bad that you are thinking of suicide? • Are you feeling so bad that you have considered killing yourself? • Do you feel like killing yourself now? • Are you feeling so bad at the moment that you feel unable to go on living?
P Plan	• Plans are a powerful indication of risk. A formulated, realistic and practical plan is an indication of vulnerability. Specifically, access to the means is a key indicator of risk. • So: Does the patient have any plans to take their own life? If so: – What are they? – Are they practical? – Have they been rehearsed? – Does he/she have access to the means and are the means readily available?	• Have you thought about how you would kill yourself? • Have you thought about when you would do it? • Do you have a plan? If the answer is 'yes'...... • Tell me about your plan?/What is your plan?/What have you planned to do? • Do you have access to the means to do this now? • Have you rehearsed this at all? • Do you have what you need to do it?
A Action	• *PAST.* Previous behaviours are a good gauge for future behaviours. • So: Has the patient attempted to take his or her own life before? If so: – How many attempts have they made? – When was the last attempt? – How harmful were the previous attempts? – What methods were used? – How do they/did they feel about surviving?	• Have you ever felt like this before? • Have you ever attempted suicide before? • Have you ever felt suicidal before? • Tell me about what happened • How did you feel about that? • How do feel now compared to how you felt then?
	Does the patient have a history of self-harm or substance misuse?	*Be aware that people with a history of self-harm and/or substance misuse have a higher risk of completing suicide than those without.*
	PRESENT. If there have been no previous attempts, establish if they have carried out any part of their 'action' this time and, if so, what have they done?	Questions will need to relate to whatever plan the person has outlined so might include things like. • Have you bought a rope? • What tablets/medication have you been storing?/Have you taken any tablets/medication now? • Have you been to the bridge?
P Protective measures	• Support – family and friends can be a powerful restraining factor for those at risk of taking their own life. If the patient, or you, are able to mobilise support it can help to reduce the immediate risk (with the patient's consent). • So: – What support does the patient have? For example involvement with a specialist mental health team, access to a 'crisis' service (or equivalent)? – Is the patient alone or with others? – Who can the patient call upon for support? (As above or others). – What restraints are there to stop the patient taking their own life (e.g. family, children, friends, religious beliefs, pets, work, hobbies)?	• What would prevent you from doing this? • What support have you got access to? • What would help stop you feeling like this? • Do you feel lonely? • Do you feel that you are a burden to others? • Do you feel that you have let other people down?

Table 3.17 – IPAP Suicide Risk Levels

No risk	No thoughts of killing self.	• If "No" to all the 'Intent' questions and the patient has immediate support available (from family, friends, mental health team), then the patient is safe for "self care". • Advice should include: – Make a routine appointment to see GP to discuss feelings. – Ring Samaritans if they want to talk to someone (08457 909090 available 24hrs/day). Please note that if there is any worsening in symptoms the patient must seek emergency care, e.g. GP, Urgent Care Centre, Emergency Dept (ED), OOH service, or a repeat call to the ambulance service.
Mild risk	Some thoughts of killing self, no plan.	• The patient must be seen by a specialist mental health practitioner. You should consider: – Mental Health Alternative Care Pathway. – GP. – GP triage scheme (or similar). If these are not available, take the patient to ED.
Moderate risk	Thoughts of killing self, vague plan, low on lethality, would not do it at this moment.	
Severe risk	Repeated thoughts of killing self, specific plan and lethal, would not do it at this moment.	• The patient must be seen by a specialist mental health practitioner as soon as possible. • If the patient is known to local mental health (MH) services and has NOT yet acted on the persistent and intrusive thoughts/disordered thinking, and has no medical need/injury, contact the appropriate Team/Care Coordinator/GP. Consult local Alternative Care Pathways. • If the patient is not known to local MH services and/or HAS attempted suicide; the patient must be transported to hospital (ED). Consider: – IV access / ECG monitoring. – Use of Mental Capacity Act 2005 if necessary.
Extreme risk	Persistent thoughts of killing self, specific plan and lethal, will do it/has done it.	

SECTION 3 Medical – Undifferentiated Complaints

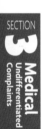

Is the patient expressing active suicidal ideation? (E.g. Persistent and intrusive thoughts of suicide; or responding to disordered thoughts such as delusions/hallucinations?).

Has the patient attempted suicide?

Has the patient taken a deliberate overdose (prescribed/over the counter/illicit medicines)?

Has there been any deterioration in their cognitive functioning or physical condition?

Is the result 'severe' or 'extreme' on the IPAP Suicide Risk Assessment tool?

Does the patient feel that they have no future? (E.g. Hopelessness, feeling that nothing will ever get better).

Is the patient under 16 years of age?

If "YES" to any question the patient must be seen be a specialist mental health practitioner as soon as possible.

If the patient is known to local mental health (MH) services and has NOT yet acted on the persistent and intrusive thoughts/disordered thinking, and has no medical need/injury, contact the appropriate Team/Care Co-ordinator/GP. Consult local Alternative Care Pathways.

If the patient is not known to local MH services and/or HAS attempted suicide; the patient must be transported to hospital (ED).

Consider:
- IV access / ECG monitoring.
- Use of Mental Capacity Act 2005 if necessary.

Does the patient have any definite plans to take their own life?

What are they? (Are they practical? Have they been rehearsed?).

Does the patient have access to the means, and are the means readily available?

Has the patient attempted to take his or her own life before? If so:
- How many attempts have they made?
- When was the last attempt?
- How harmful were the previous attempts?
- What methods were used?
- How do they/did they feel about surviving?

Does the patient have a history of self harm?

Is the result 'mild' or 'moderate' on the IPAP Suicide Risk Assessment tool?

If "YES" to these questions the patient must be seen by a specialist mental health practitioner. You should consider:
- Mental Health Alternative Care Pathway
- GP
- GP triage scheme

If these are not available, take the patient to ED.

If "NO" to all the above questions and the patient has immediate support available (from family, friends, mental health team) then the patient is safe for "self care".

Advice should include:
- Make a routine appointment to see GP to discuss feelings.
- Ring Samaritans if they want to talk to someone (08457 909090 available 24hrs/day).

Please note that if there are any worsening in symptoms the patient must seek emergency care, e.g. GP, Walk in centre, ED, OOH service or a repeat call to the ambulance service.

If "NO" to any of these questions then refer to the green box.

Recommended minimum observations include:
- Respiratory Rate
- Pulse
- Blood Pressure
- GCS
- Temperature
- Blood Glucose

Figure 3.1 – Suicidal Ideation (adults aged 18 years and over).

This flow chart is designed to assist in your decision making when caring for a patient with suicidal ideation. It does not replace your clinical judgement.

1. Introduction

The Mental Capacity Act 2005 (MCA) was implemented in England and Wales to provide protection and powers to individuals aged 16 years and over who may lack capacity to make some (or all) decisions for themselves. It is also for people working with, or caring for them. It applies to public and private locations.

2. What is the MCA?

The MCA empowers individuals to make their own decisions where possible and protects the rights of those who lack capacity. Where an individual lacks capacity to make a specific decision at a particular time, the MCA provides a legal framework for others to act and make that decision on their behalf, in their best interest. This include decisions about their care and/or treatment.

3. What is mental capacity?

'Capacity' is "the ability of an individual to make decisions regarding specific elements of their life" (MCA, 2005) and it is crucial within the pre-hospital emergency care environment since everything done to/for a conscious patient requires their consent. Patients must have mental capacity in order to give (or withhold) consent and, apart from situations where the Mental Health Act 1983 (MHA) applies, mental capacity is central to determining whether treatment and care can be given to someone who refuses.

For the person's wishes to be overridden there must be evidence that some impairment or disturbance of mental functioning exists, rendering the person unable to make an informed decision at the time it needs to be made. In simple terms 'capacity' is the ability to a make a decision *at the time it needs to be made*. In order to demonstrate capacity a person must be able to:

- Understand information relevant to the decision.
- Retain the information relevant to the decision.
- Consider all the factors involved i.e. weigh up the pros and cons.
- Communicate their decision.

4. Responsibilities under the Act

Ambulance staff have a formal duty of regard to the Act and the Code of Practice; and every Ambulance Trust should as best practice have a formal process (i.e. a policy/protocol) for establishing the capacity of patients to give, or withhold, consent for assessment, treatment and/or being transported for further care, when required.

There must always be a presumption of capacity. In every situation, staff must assume that a person can make their own decision(s) unless it is found - beyond reasonable doubt - that they are unable to do so.

Doubts about mental capacity may arise for many reasons including the person's behaviour, circumstances, or concerns raised by someone else. Approximately two million people in England and Wales may lack capacity to make decisions for themselves because of:

- Dementia.
- Learning disabilities.
- Mental health problems.
- Stroke and brain injuries.
- Temporary impairment due to medication, intoxication, injury or illness.

Staff must always act in the best interests of any person who lacks capacity; but if the impairment is temporary you should consider if it is safe to wait until the patient regains capacity before acting on their behalf.

5. Legal context

The MCA has five Key Principles which emphasise the fundamental concepts and core values of the Act. These must be considered and applied when you are working with, or providing care or treatment for, people who lack capacity.

They are:

1. Every adult has the right to make decisions and must be assumed to have capacity to do so unless it is proved otherwise.

   - This means that you cannot assume that someone is unable to make a decision for themselves just because they have a particular medical/neurological condition, disability or because of their age.

2. People must be supported as much as possible to make a decision before anyone concludes that they cannot make their own decision.

   - This means that you should make every effort to encourage and support the person to make the decision for themselves. If a lack of capacity is established, it is still important that you involve the person as much as possible in making decisions.

3. People have the right to make what others might regard as an unwise or eccentric decision.

   - This means that capacity should not be confused with an assessment of the reasonableness of the person's decision. A person is entitled to make a decision which others might perceive to be unwise, eccentric or irrational, *as long as they have the capacity to do so.*
   - However, it is important to note that when an apparently irrational decision is based on a misperception of reality (e.g. someone experiencing hallucinations/delusions/disordered thinking), rather than a different *value system* to that held by the assessor, then the patient may not truly be able to understand. This would lead to doubts about their ability to make a decision and an assessment should be completed.

4. Apply best interest principles.

   - This means that anything done for, or on behalf of, a person who lacks mental capacity must be done in their best interests.

5. Anything done for, or on behalf of, people without capacity should be the least restrictive of their basic rights and freedoms.

   - This means that you must choose the option that interferes least with their rights and freedom of action. Make sure that whatever you do, you do not limit their freedom of movement any more than is absolutely necessary. Always use the least restrictive intervention.

6. Helping people to make decisions for themselves

When a person in your care needs to make a decision you must start from the assumption that the person *has* capacity to make the decision in question (Principle 1). You should make every effort to encourage and support the person to make the decision themselves (Principle 2) and you will have to consider a number of factors to assist in the decision making process.

These could include:

- Does the person have all the relevant information needed to make the decision? If there is a choice, has all the information been given on the alternatives?

- Could the information be explained or presented in a way that is easier for the person to understand? Help should be given to communicate information wherever necessary. For example, a person with a learning disability might find it easier to communicate using pictures, photographs, or sign language.

- Are there particular times of the day when a person's understanding is better, or is there a particular place where they feel more at ease and able to make a decision? For example, if a person becomes drowsy soon after they have taken their medication this would not be a good time for them to make a decision.

- Can anyone else help or support the person to understand information or make a choice? For example, a relative, carer, friend or advocate.

When there is reason to believe that a person lacks capacity to make a decision you should consider the following:

- Has everything been done to help and support the person make the decision?

- Does the decision need to be made without delay?

- If not, is it possible to wait until the person does have the capacity to make the decision for him/herself?

7. Assessing capacity

There are two questions to consider when you are assessing a person's capacity:

- Is there an impairment of, or disturbance in the functioning of, the person's mind or brain (this can be temporary or permanent)?

And, if so.

- Is the impairment or disturbance sufficient to cause the person to be unable to make that particular decision at the relevant time?

Is the impairment or disturbance sufficient to cause the person to be unable to make that particular decision at the relevant time? A person may be mentally incapable of making the decision in question either because of a long-term mental disability or because of temporary factors such as unconsciousness, confusion or the effects of fatigue, shock, pain, anxiety, anger, alcohol or drugs (or drug withdrawal). When possible, attempts should be made to enhance capacity by, for example, pain management.

Assessments of capacity are 'functional', and are related to the individual decision that needs to be made – at the time it needs to be made (i.e. can the person complete the functions required to make the decision, thus demonstrating they have capacity?). The more serious or complex the decision, the greater the level of capacity required. If an adult is mentally capable of making the decision, then his or her decision about whether to receive treatment or care must be respected; even if a refusal may risk permanent injury to that person's health or even lead to premature death (unless he or she is mentally disordered and can be treated under the MHA). Refusals of treatment can vary in importance. Some may involve a risk to life or of irreparable damage to health; others may not. What matters is whether, at the time in question, the patient *has* capacity to make that decision.

When consent is refused by a competent adult the least you should do is:

- Respect the patient's refusal as much as you would their consent.

- Make sure that the patient is *fully* informed of the implications of refusal.

- Involve other members of the health care team (as appropriate).

- Ensure this is clearly and fully documented in the patient's records.

Local policy may require additional elements. **If there is uncertainty as to the consequences of the act of self-harm, then it should be assumed that the consequences will be serious.**

When an individual is reasonably believed to lack capacity to make the decision required, ambulance staff have a legal duty to act in that person's best interests – unless a valid and applicable Advance Decision to Refuse Treatment (ADRT) is in place.

The following flowchart outlines the assessment process. Assessors must be able to show how their assessment was completed if required later on and details must be included in the patient's clinical record.

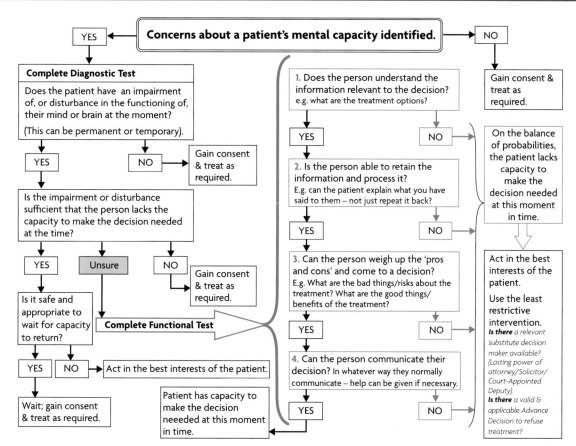

Figure 3.2 – Flow chart outlining MCA assessment for ambulance staff.
Reproduced with permission of S Putman.

Remember that an unwise decision made by a person does not itself indicate a lack of capacity. Most people will be able to make most decisions, even when they have a diagnosis that may seem to imply that they cannot. This is a general principle that cannot be over-emphasised. The more complex the decision is, the greater the level of capacity required to make it.

ALCOHOL

When determining if there is an impairment of the mind or brain, the consumption of alcohol is often a complicating factor. This does not necessarily mean that the patient is not aware of their behaviour, or aware of the decisions they make, but it may mean that they are less aware/ concerned about the consequences than they would otherwise be. Judging capacity in such circumstances is difficult and subjective, but the patient's safety is paramount, so consideration should be given to balancing the risk of getting the determination of capacity wrong against the clinical risk of non-intervention.

SELF HARM

The NICE Clinical Guideline 16 'Factors that can affect capacity' states:

"If the mental capacity of a person who has self-harmed has been impaired by the effects of alcohol or drugs, or by that person's emotional distress, staff must be satisfied that these temporary factors are operating to such a degree that the assumption of mental capacity is overridden. In such a case, where incapacity is temporary, staff should decide whether it is safe to defer treatment decisions until capacity is regained.

If a person appears to be calm but refuses potentially life-saving treatment, or expresses the wish to die by suicide, the assumption of capacity could be rebutted by evidence that the person does not truly comprehend the consequences of his or her decision, that the person is acting under the undue influence of another, that the person's emotional distress associated with the stated reason for wishing to be dead is impairing his or her judgement, or that the person's behaviour shows that he or she is deeply ambivalent about the decision (for example if the person initially sought help for the effects of the self-harm)" [175].

Once again, careful consideration should be given to balancing the risk of getting the determination of capacity wrong against the clinical risk of non-intervention.

Section 5 of the MCA Code of Practice (CoP) outlines specific actions taken by ambulance staff (and others) which will be protected from liability and includes the following:

● Carrying out diagnostic examinations and tests (to identify an illness, condition or other problem).

● Providing professional medical, dental and similar treatment.

● Giving medication.

● Taking someone to hospital for assessment or treatment.

● Providing nursing care (whether in hospital or the community).

● Carrying out any other necessary medical procedures (e.g. taking a blood sample) or therapies (e.g. physiotherapy or chiropody).

● Providing care in an emergency.

8. Best interests

If a person has been assessed as lacking capacity then any action taken, or any decision made for – or on behalf of – that person, must be made in their best interests (Principle 4).

'Best Interest Assessors' (BIA) are appointed to assist making complex decisions for those who are unable to do so for themselves (e.g. when deciding on long term treatment for a medical condition, or on where to live).

There is a significant difference between making a "best interest" decision involving a BIA and making a decision which is in the best interest of the patient in an emergency. BIAs are required to consider a wide range of elements when making such a decision on someone else's behalf. In emergencies, where there is limited or no information available, it will often be in a patient's best interests for urgent treatment to be provided without delay.

Key factors which you must consider when working out what is in the best interests of a person who lacks capacity (whenever possible) include:

Identify all relevant circumstances.
Try to identify all the things that the person would take into account if they were making the decision or acting for themselves.

Find out the person's views.
Try to find out the views of the person who lacks capacity, including:

- Their past and present wishes and feelings – these may have been expressed verbally, in writing or through behaviour or habits (e.g. an ADRT).

- Any beliefs and values (e.g. religious, cultural, moral or political) that would be likely to influence the decision in question.

- Any other factors the person themselves would be likely to consider if they were making the decision or acting for themselves.

  Relatives/friends/carers may be able to assist with this.

Avoid discrimination.
- Do not make assumptions about someone's best interests simply on the basis of the person's age, appearance, condition or behaviour.

Assess whether the person might regain capacity.
- Consider whether the person is likely to regain capacity. (If so, can the decision wait until then? It may be that the person lacks capacity to make a decision to accept *initial* treatment but, having received that treatment, regains capacity to refuse further treatment/intervention (including transport to hospital).

If the decision concerns life-sustaining treatment.
- This should not be motivated in any way by a desire to bring about the person's death.

- Always check for an advanced decision to refuse treatment – if the person has previously made arrangements for withholding life sustaining treatment (when they had capacity to do so) this should be recorded in an ADRT. If a **valid and applicable** ADRT is found, it must be respected and treatment withheld.

Consult others.
- As far as possible the decision maker must consult other people (e.g. family, friends, carers, Lasting Power of Attorney) if it is appropriate to do so, and take into account their views as to what would be in the best interests of the patient lacking capacity.

Avoid restricting the person's rights.
- Use the least restrictive intervention.

Take all of this into account.
- Whenever possible, weigh up all of these factors in order to work out what is in the person's best interests.

9. Record keeping

Decision-makers should ensure that where a capacity assessment is undertaken, this is recorded in the individual's care and treatment record in line with local policy. If the person was restrained the following should also be recorded:

- Why restraint was required.

- How the person was restrained.

- Who was involved?

- How long was restraint required?

It is recognised that it may not be possible to complete full details in an emergency situation but do remember that it is not sufficient to say a patient does not have capacity, without detailing how that decision was reached. A written record of the ambulance crew assessment and outcome must be made at the earliest opportunity.

10. Deprivation of Liberty/Restraint

Deprivation of Liberty Safeguards (DoLS) exist to protect the human rights of people who lack capacity to consent to arrangements for their care or treatment, and who might need to be deprived of their liberty. E.g. a person who has dementia may need to have doors locked to prevent them walking away from where they live and getting lost, or coming to harm, as a result.

Deprivation of liberty without lawful justification is prohibited under Article 5 of the European Convention on Human Rights. There is a distinction between restraining or *restricting* an individual's movements, and depriving that individual of their liberty.

Restraint is defined in Section 6 of the MCA as:

- The use or threat of force to secure the doing of an act that the individual resists; or

- the restriction of the individual's liberty, whether that individual resists or not.

Restraint, or restrictions, on an incapacitate individual's liberty can be justified under the MCA provided:

- The person lacks capacity and restraint is in their best interest.

- Restraint is used to prevent harm to the person.

- It is proportionate to the seriousness of the harm.

The least restrictive method must be used for the shortest amount of time.

SECTION **3** Medical Undifferentiated Complaints

Any power to restrain a person as a result of the MCA does not interfere with any other existing powers of arrest for criminal offences or powers under the Mental Health Act 1983.

However, the distinctions between restraining or restricting an individual, and depriving them of their liberty, are not always easy to identify. For example, it is possible to 'deprive' someone of their liberty not just by physical confinement, but also by virtue of the level of control exercised over an individual's movements. It is important to note however, that DoLS are highly unlikely to be a required for conveying patients.

The concepts of restraint, restriction, and deprivation of liberty are best understood as existing on the same continuum; with deprivation of liberty involving a higher degree or intensity, of restrictions over that individual. Ultimately, the concept is one to be interpreted in view of the specific circumstances of that individual at the time.

In simple terms - any person who is subject to regular and recurrent restrictions of their liberty should be considered for DoLS. Under this process safeguards are put in place to keep the person safe, this includes regular review of the need for restriction. DoLS only apply to an individual at a stated location (address). If the person moves to another address (e.g. goes into hospital) then a new DoLS application will be required by the agency caring for them; DoLS authority will not be required during transit from one place to another.

11. Use of restraint by ambulance staff

Ambulance staff are obliged under the MCA to act in the best interests of/for patients who lack capacity, even when the patient refuses treatment or is abusive, threatening or violent.

The MCA also protects carers from liability when "reasonable force" is required to ensure that patients lacking capacity receive care that is in their best interests; or to protect them from further harm. As stated previously, Section 6 of the Act defines restraint as the use or threat of force where an incapacitated person resists, and any restriction of liberty or movement, whether or not the person resists.

Ambulance staff have limited training in this aspect. Minimal restraint (i.e. reasonable force) can be used in cases where patients lack capacity, and there is no perceived risk of harm to the ambulance crew. If the behaviour of the patient exceeds what the crew can safely manage then assistance must be requested in line with local policy (this does not necessarily have to be police).

A Dynamic Risk Assessment should always be completed prior to the use of any form of restraint; recording decisions and actions in the Patient Clinical Record.

Ambulance staff should always monitor the physical well-being of the patient and should be familiar with the information elsewhere in this guidance pertaining to Acute Behavioural Disturbance, which may result after prolonged forcible restraint.

12. Transfer and continuing care of the patient

Ambulance staff must complete a clinical record (in line with local policy) with the normal clinical information including, full details of the capacity assessment, risk factors, and - where relevant – actions agreed with others such as the transport method and a description of any restraint applied by either ambulance staff or others.

Consider if a pre-alert to the receiving hospital/unit is required, and complete if necessary.

Ambulance staff must provide a full clinical handover at hospital and a copy of the completed patient clinical record. Emergency Department (ED) staff must be informed that the patient has been brought to ED using the provisions of the MCA. ED staff may need to re-assess the patient's capacity to make a decision regarding staying for further care, assessment and/or treatment.

13. Other Mental Capacity Act Safeguards

The MCA includes other safeguards to protect vulnerable people who have reduced capacity, and those using the Act to care for them.

Briefly, these include (amongst others):

- **Lasting Power of Attorney (LPA)** – An individual can give another person the authority to make a decision on their behalf if/when they become unable to do so. This is achieved by establishing a Lasting Power of Attorney. Once activated, the LPA can make decisions that are as valid as one made by the person. There are two types – Health and Wellbeing and Property and Financial Affairs. The LPA should always act in the best interest of the person.

- **Advance Decisions to Refuse Treatment.**

  Allow people to refuse treatment, providing that the decision to do so was made when the person had capacity.
  To make a valid ADRT the person must:
  – Be at least 18 years of age
  – Have capacity to make the decision.
  – Make a decision that is specific and able to be complied with (i.e. outline in detail what they want to refuse and the circumstances in which it can be refused).

  The ADRT doesn't need to be in writing, unless it relates to life sustaining treatment – in which case it must be in writing and witnessed.
  An ADRT is only valid and applicable when all of the conditions described are met, and the person lacks capacity to make the decision themselves.

  If ambulance staff are not aware of an ADRTs existence, when caring for someone who lacks capacity, then they should continue to act in the best interest of the patient.

- **Court of Protection.**

  Makes decisions on financial or welfare matters for people who can't make decisions at the time they need to be made, and have no one appropriate to do this for them. Most cases are heard by district judges and a senior judge but can sometimes be heard by High Court judges.

- **Court Deputies.**

  People who are appointed by the Court of Protection to act on behalf a person with reduced capacity when there is no LPA. Court Deputies have similar powers to that of an LPA.

- **Independent Mental Capacity Advocates (IMCAs).**

  IMCAs are a legal right for people over 16 who lack capacity and do not have an appropriate family member or friend to represent their views. An IMCA can be used to assist with decisions regarding serious medical treatment or a change of accommodation.

The position taken in this guideline is that staff of the ambulance services should refer to their employers any questions or concerns that they might have as regards gaining lawful consent from their patients, application of the relevant legislation (and associated codes of practice) that apply in the jurisdiction in which they work for assessing, caring for and treating apparently incapacitous persons.

Readers should be aware that there are different laws relating to capacity and consent, and different mental health primary and secondary legislation in England and Wales, Northern Ireland, and Scotland. This guideline cannot cover in detail any of that legislation, the associated codes of practice and governmental guidance. Therefore, this guideline provides a very brief overview of some facets of the process in England and Wales.

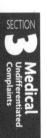

SECTION

3

Medical
Undifferentiated
Complaints

1. Introduction

Although the care of a wide range of medical conditions will be quite specific to the presenting condition, there are general principles of care that apply to most medical cases, regardless of underlying condition(s).

2. Patient Assessment

In order to gather as much relevant information as possible, without delaying care, the accepted format of history taking is as follows:

- Presenting complaint – why the patient or carer called for help at this time.

- The history of presenting complaint – details of when the problem started, exacerbating factors and previous similar episodes.

- Direct questioning about associated symptoms, by system. Ask about all appropriate systems.

- Past medical history, including current medication.

- Family history.

- Social history.

Combined with a good physical examination (primary and secondary survey), this format of history taking should ensure that you correctly identify those patients who are time critical, urgent or routine. The history taken must be fully documented. In many cases, a well-taken history will point to the diagnosis.

The presence of 'MedicAlert®' type jewellery (bracelets or necklets) can provide information on the patient's pre-existing health risk that may be relevant to the current medical emergency.

1. A primary survey should be undertaken for **ALL** patients as this will rapidly identify patients with actual or potential **TIME CRITICAL** conditions.

2. A secondary survey is a more thorough 'head-to-toe' assessment of the patient. It should be undertaken following completion of the primary survey, where time permits. The secondary survey will usually be undertaken during transfer to further care; however, in some patients with time critical conditions, it may not be possible to undertake the secondary survey before arrival at further care.

I. Primary survey

- The primary survey should take 60–90 seconds for assessment and follow **ABCD** approach (Table 3.19). Document the vital signs and the time the observations were taken.

- Assessment and management should proceed in a 'stepwise' manner and abnormalities should be managed as they are encountered, that is do not move onto breathing and circulation until the airway is managed (refer to airway and breathing management guideline). Every time an intervention has been carried out, re-assess the patient.

- If any of the features/conditions listed in Table 3.18 are identified during the primary survey or immediately un-correctable ABCD problems, then the patient should be considered **TIME CRITICAL. CORRECT A AND B PROBLEMS ON SCENE, THEN UNDERTAKE A TIME CRITICAL** transfer **TO NEAREST SUITABLE RECEIVING HOSPITAL.**

- If airway and breathing cannot be corrected, or haemorrhage cannot be controlled, evacuate immediately, continuing resuscitation as appropriate en-route.

- Provide an alert/information call.

- Continue patient assessment and management en-route.

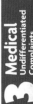

Table 3.18 – TIME CRITICAL FEATURES/CONDITIONS

- **Adrenal crisis (including Addisonian crisis)** – is a life-threatening condition resulting from adrenal insufficiency – refer to hydrocortisone guidelines.

- **Airway impairment.**

- **Anaphylaxis** – is a life-threatening condition resulting from an immune response to an allergen – **refer to allergic reactions including anaphylaxis guideline**.

- Any patient with **GCS <15** – check the airway and blood glucose levels in all patients with a decreased GCS.

- **Cardiac chest pain.**

- **Cardiogenic shock.**

- **Sepsis** – is a life-threatening condition resulting from infection. Suspect sepsis in patients who have signs and symptoms of infection, a systolic blood pressure below 90 mmHg and tachypnoea – refer to intravascular fluid guidelines.

- **Failing ventilation.**

- **Severe breathlessness** – unable to complete a sentence.

- **Severe haemorrhage** – **refer to trauma emergencies in adults overview guideline** and gastrointestinal bleeding.

- **Severe hypotension** – due to bradycardia or extreme tachycardia.

- **Status epilepticus** – is a life-threatening condition defined as a convulsion lasting >30 minutes – **refer to convulsion guidelines**.

NB This list is not inclusive; patients with other signs may also be time critical; this is where the clinical judgement of the paramedic is important.

Table 3.19 – ASSESSMENT and MANAGEMENT of:

Medical Emergencies

- All stages should be considered but some may be omitted if not considered appropriate and only if capnography is available.

At each stage consider the need for:
- **TIME CRITICAL** transfer to further care.
- Early senior clinical support.

STAGE	ASSESSMENT	MANAGEMENT
A	**AIRWAY** – assess the airway (refer to airway and breathing guideline). **Look for** obvious obstructions, e.g. teeth/dentures, foreign bodies, vomit, blood. **Listen for** noisy airflow, e.g. snoring, gurgling or no airflow. **Feel for** air movement.	Correct any airway problems immediately by: - Positioning – head tilt, chin lift, jaw thrust. - Suction (if available and appropriate). - Oropharyngeal airway. - Nasopharyngeal airway. - Laryngeal mask airway (if appropriate). - Endotracheal intubation (if appropriate and only if capnography is available). - Needle cricothyroidotomy.

BREATHING – expose the chest and assess (refer to airway and breathing guideline).

Look for:
- Respiratory rate (<10 or >30).
- Respiratory depth.
- Breaths per minute.
- Adequacy and depth of chest movements.
- Symmetry of chest movement.
- Equality of air entry.
- Effectiveness of ventilation.
- Cyanosis or pallor peripherally and centrally.
- Position of trachea in suprasternal notch.

Feel for:
- Any instability of chest wall and note any areas of tenderness and note depth and equality of chest movement.

Note any:
- Wheezing, noisy respiration on inspiration or expiration.
- Stridor (higher pitched noise on inspiration), suggestive of upper respiratory obstruction.

Listen for:
- Altered breathing patterns with a stethoscope – ask the patient to take deep breaths in and out briskly through their mouth if possible – listen on both sides of the chest:
  - above the nipples in the mid-clavicular line
  - laterally in the mid-axillary line
  - below the shoulder blade (front and back).
- Auscultate to assess air entry and compare sides.
- Wheezing on expiration.
- Crepitations at the rear of the chest (crackles, heard low down in the lung fields at the rear – may indicate fluid in the lung in heart failure).
- Additional crackles and wheeze on inspiration may be associated with inhalation of blood or vomit.

Percuss for:
- Dullness or hyperresonance.

B

Correct any breathing problems immediately.
- If breathing is absent refer to appropriate resuscitation guidelines. If the breathing is inadequate refer to airway and breathing guideline.
- Treat underlying cause of unilateral chest movement if tension pneumothorax.
- Administer supplemental oxygen if the patient is hypoxaemic – aim for target saturation (SpO_2) within the range of 94–98% except for patients with COPD or other risk factors for hypercapnia (refer to oxygen guideline).
- In patients with a decreased level of consciousness (Glasgow Coma Scale (GCS) <15) administer the initial supplemental oxygen dose until the vital signs are normal, then reduce the oxygen dose and aim for a target saturation (SpO_2) within the range of 94–98%.
- In patients with sickle cell crisis administer supplemental oxygen via an appropriate nasal mask/cannula until a reliable SpO_2 measurement is available; then adjust the oxygen flow to aim for target saturation within the range of 94–98%.

Consider assisted ventilation at a rate of 12–20 respirations per minute if any of the following are present:
- Oxygen saturation (SpO_2) <90% on levels of supplemental oxygen.
- Respiratory rate <10 or >30 bpm.
- Inadequate chest expansion.

NB **Restraint (positional) asphyxia** – If the patient is required to be physically restrained (e.g. by police officers) in order to prevent them injuring themselves or others, or for the purpose of being detained under the Mental Health Act, then it is paramount that the method of restraint allows both for a patent airway and adequate respiratory volume.

Under these circumstances it is essential to ensure that the patient's airway and breathing are adequate at all times.

Table 3.19 – ASSESSMENT and MANAGEMENT of:

Medical Emergencies *continued*

STAGE	ASSESMENT	MANAGEMENT
	● Assess for evidence of external haemorrhage (e.g. epistaxis, haemoptysis, haematemesis, melaena).	● Arrest external haemorrhage. ● In cases of internal or uncontrolled haemorrhage undertake a **TIME CRITICAL** transfer to further care; provide an alert/information call. ● Patients with sepsis will benefit from early fluid therapy and an appropriate hospital alert/information call.

MANAGEMENT

Fluid therapy
- If fluid replacement is indicated refer to intravascular fluid therapy guideline.
- Rapid fluid replacement into the vascular compartment can overload the cardiovascular system particularly where there is pre-existing cardiovascular disease and in the elderly. Gradual rehydration over many hours rather than minutes is indicated. NB Monitor fluid replacement closely in these cases.

STAGE C

ASSESMENT
- Assess skin colour and temperature.
- Palpate for a radial pulse – if present this implies adequate perfusion of vital organs, but this is highly variable. If absent feel for a carotid pulse. NB The estimation of blood pressure by pulse is inaccurate and unreliable; however, the presence of a radial suggests adequate perfusion of major organs. The presence of a femoral pulse suggests perfusion of the kidneys, while a carotid pulse and coherent mentation suggests adequate perfusion of the brain.
- Assess pulse rate, volume and rhythm.
- Check capillary refill time centrally (forehead or sternum – normal <2 seconds).

Consider hypovolaemic shock and be aware of its early signs:
- Pallor.
- Cool peripheries.
- Anxiety, abnormal behaviour.
- Increased respiratory rate.
- Tachycardia.

Recognition of shock
Shock is difficult to diagnose. In certain groups of patients the signs of shock appear late (e.g. pregnant women, patients on medication such as beta-blockers, and the physically fit).
Blood loss of 750–1000 ml will produce little evidence of shock; blood loss of 1000–1500 ml is required before more classical signs of shock appear. NB This loss is from the circulation **NOT** necessarily visible externally.

STAGE D

DISABILITY (mini neurological examination)
Note the initial level of responsiveness on AVPU scale, and time of assessment.
- **A** – Alert
- **V** – Responds to voice
- **P** – Responds to painful stimulus
- **U** – Unresponsive

Assess and note pupil size, equality and response to light.

- Check for purposeful movement in all four limbs.
- Check sensory function.

- Assess blood glucose levels in all patients with a history of diabetes, impaired consciousness, convulsions, collapse or alcohol consumption.

Check blood glucose level to rule out hypo or hyperglycaemia as the cause – **refer to glycaemic emergencies guideline in adults**.

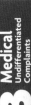

II. Secondary survey

- A secondary survey should only commence after the primary survey has been completed and an assessment of the patient's critical status has been made.

- The secondary survey is a more thorough 'head-to-toe' assessment of the patient including their past medical history (refer to Table 3.20). It is important to monitor the patient's vital signs during the survey.

- The secondary survey will usually be undertaken during transfer to hospital; however, in some patients with critical conditions, it may not be possible to undertake the secondary survey before arrival at further care.

Table 3.20 – SECONDARY SURVEY

Assessment

HEAD
- Re-assess airway, breathing, and circulation.
- Re-assess levels of consciousness (AVPU), pupil size and activity.
- Establish Glasgow Coma Scale (refer to Table 3.19).

CHEST
- Re-assess rate and depth of breathing.
- Re-listen for breath sounds in all lung fields, and record.
- Assess for pneumothorax – in small pneumothorax no clinical signs may be detected. A pneumothorax causes breathlessness, reduced air entry and chest movement on the affected side. If this is a tension pneumothorax, then the patient will have increasing respiratory distress, distended neck veins, and tracheal deviation (late sign) away from affected side may also be present.
- Assess skin colour, temperature, and record.
- Assess heart sounds and heart rate.
- Obtain a blood pressure reading using a sphygmomanometer.
- Document and record all results.
- Record pulse oximeter reading.
- Re-assess and continue management as appropriate en-route to further care.

ABDOMEN
- Feel for tenderness and guarding in all four quadrants.
- Check for bowel sounds.
- Listen and asculate.

LOWER/UPPER LIMBS
Check for MSC in **ALL** four limbs:
- **MOTOR** – Test for movement and power.
- **SENSATION** – Apply light touch to evaluate sensation.
- **CIRCULATION** – Assess pulse and skin temperature.

MANAGEMENT

Correcting:
- Airway.
- Breathing.
- Circulation.
- Disability (mini neurological examination).

- Ensure adequate oxygen therapy and support ventilation if required.

- Apply ECG and pulse oximetry monitoring, as required. Consider ECG monitoring for patients on dialysis to check for the presence of hyperkalaemia.

- Consider patient positioning (e.g. sitting upright for respiratory problems).

- Check blood glucose levels in all patients with history of diabetes, impaired consciousness, seizures, collapse or alcohol/drug consumption. Provide drug therapy as required; refer to appropriate drug guidelines. In adrenal crisis refer to hydrocortisone guideline.

- If the level of consciousness deteriorates or respiratory depression develops in cases where an overdose with opiate type drugs may be a possibility, consider administering naloxone (refer to naloxone guideline).

- In patients with fixed pinpoint pupils suspect opiate use. Follow ADDITIONAL MEDICAL guidelines as indicated by the patient's condition (e.g. cardiac rhythm disturbance):
  - correct A and B problems on scene
  - undertake a **TIME CRITICAL** transfer to nearest suitable further care
  - provide an alert/information call required
  - provide a comprehensive verbal hand-over and a completed patient report form to the receiving staff.

ADDITIONAL INFORMATION

- The patient history can provide valuable insight into the cause of the current condition.

The following may assist in determining the diagnosis:

- Relatives, carers or friends with knowledge of the patient's history.

- Packets or containers of medication (including domiciliary oxygen) or evidence of administration devices (e.g. nebuliser machines).

- MedicAlert® type jewellery (bracelets or necklets) which detail the patient's primary health risk (e.g. diabetes, anaphylaxis, Addison's disease etc) but also list a 24-hour telephone number to obtain a more detailed patient history.

- Warning stickers, often placed by the front door or the telephone, directing the health professional to a source of detailed information (one current scheme involves storing the patient details in a container in the fridge, as this is relatively easy to find in the house).

- Patient-held warning cards denoting previous thrombolysis, at-risk COPD patients, or those taking monoamine oxidase inhibitor (MAOI) medication.

- Patients' individualised treatment plans.

- Patients on long-term steroids or who have adrenal insufficiency may deteriorate rapidly because of steroid insufficiency. If significantly unwell, the patient should be given hydrocortisone and fluids if required.

Appendix

Table 3.21 – GLASGOW COMA SCALE

Category	Element	Score
Eyes Opening	Spontaneously	4
	To speech	3
	To pain	2
	None	1
Motor Response	Obeys commands	6
	Localises pain	5
	Withdraws from pain	4
	Abnormal flexion	3
	Extensor response	2
	No response to pain	1
Verbal Response	Orientated	5
	Confused	4
	Inappropriate words	3
	Incomprehensible sounds	2
	No verbal response	1

KEY POINTS

Medical Emergencies in Adults (Overview)

- Detect TIME CRITICAL problems early.
- Minimise time on scene.
- Continuously re-assess ABCD, AVPU.
- Initiate treatments en-route if deterioration.
- Provide an alert/information call for TIME CRITICAL patients.

3 Medical Undifferentiated Complaints SECTION

1. Introduction

- Chest pain is one of the most common symptoms of acute coronary syndrome (ACS).

- It is also a common feature in many other conditions such as aortic dissection, chest infection with pleuritic pain, pulmonary embolus, reflux oesophagitis, indigestion, and simple musculoskeletal chest pain.

- There must be a high index of suspicion that any chest pain is cardiac in origin.

- **Taking and assessing a history** – there are a number of specific factors that may help in reaching a reasoned working diagnosis, and applying appropriate management measures to the patient. ACS cannot be excluded on clinical examination (**refer to ACS guideline**).

- Do not assess symptoms differently in women and men or patients from different ethnic groups.

2. Incidence

It is estimated that over 360,000 patients attend emergency departments with acute chest pain each year.

3. Severity and Outcome

Some cases of chest pain may be life-threatening (e.g. aortic dissection).

4. Assessment and Management

For the assessment and management of non-traumatic chest pain/discomfort refer to Table 3.23.

Table 3.22 – FEATURES OF DIFFERENT TYPES OF PAIN

Features which suggest a diagnosis of myocardial ischaemia include:

- Central chest pain.
- Crushing or constricting in nature.
- Persists for >15 minutes.
- Pain may also present in:
  - the shoulders
  - upper abdomen
  - referred to the neck, jaws and arms.

Features which suggest a diagnosis of stable angina include:

- Pain is typically related to exertion and tends to last minutes but should it persist for >15 minutes, or despite usual treatment, ACS is more likely.

Features of pleuritic type pain:

- Stabbing.
- Generally one-sided.
- Worse on breathing in.
- Usually have cough with sputum.
- Raised temperature (>37.5°C).

Features of indigestion type pain:

- Central.
- Related to food.
- May be associated with belching and burning.
  NB Some patients with ACS may also suffer indigestion type pain and belching.

Features of muscular type pain:

- Sharp/stabbing.
- Worse on movement.
- Often associated with tenderness.

KEY POINTS

Non-Traumatic Chest Pain/Discomfort

- **Most chest pain is not acute coronary syndrome – but this possibility needs to be excluded rapidly.**
- **Is there another life-threatening cause (e.g. aortic dissection)?**
- **Have a low threshold for recording a 12-lead ECG.**
- **A normal ECG cannot reliably exclude ACS.**

Non-Traumatic Chest Pain/Discomfort

Table 3.23 – ASSESSMENT and MANAGEMENT of:

Non-Traumatic Chest Pain/Discomfort

NB A defibrillator must always be taken at the earliest opportunity to patients with symptoms suggestive of a heart attack and remain with the patient until hand-over to hospital staff.

ASSESSMENT	MANAGEMENT
● Assess **ABCD**	If any of the following **TIME CRITICAL** features are present: ● Major ABC problems. ● Suspected acute coronary syndrome especially ST-segment-elevation myocardial infarction (STEMI) (**refer to acute coronary syndrome guideline**). ● Pulmonary embolism. ● Aortic dissection. ● Pneumonia. ● Respiratory rate <10 or >30 breaths per minute. ● Oxygen saturation (SpO$_2$) <94% on air. ● Start correcting any **ABC** problems. ● Undertake a **TIME CRITICAL TRANSFER.** Provide an alert/information call. ● Continue management en-route.
● Assess whether the chest pain may be cardiac	● For the features of specific types of pain refer to Table 3.22 ● Note time of onset, duration, characteristics (type including radiation and aggravating and alleviating factors). ● Ask the patient if they have a previous history of coronary heart disease.
● Assess for accompanying features	● Nausea. ● Vomiting. ● Sweating. ● Pallor. ● Cough. ● Radiation of pain to the arm(s). ● Breathlessness – NB If breathlessness is a predominant symptom/sign with tightness in the chest, then causes of breathlessness must also be considered.
● Undertake a clinical assessment specifically for:	● Haemodynamic problems. ● Heart failure. ● Cardiogenic shock. ● Other non-coronary causes (e.g. aortic dissection).
● Other conditions	● If clinical examination and a 12-lead ECG make a diagnosis of ACS less likely, assess for other acute conditions (pulmonary embolism, aortic dissection, pneumonia). **NB DO NOT exclude an acute coronary syndrome when patients have a normal resting 12-lead ECG – a normal ECG cannot reliably exclude ACS.**
● Measure and record	● Respiratory rate. ● Pulse. ● Blood pressure. ● Monitor with ECG for arrhythmias. ● Undertake and assess a 12-lead ECG. Where facilities exist for telemetry, transmit ECG to appropriate hospital department according to local protocols.
● Assess oxygen saturation	● Closely monitor the patient's SpO$_2$ but do not administer oxygen unless the patient is hypoxaemic on air (SpO$_2$ <94%) (refer to oxygen guidelines).
● Assess patient's pain	● Measure and record pain score (**refer to pain management guideline**). ● Consider analgesia (**refer to pain management guideline**).
● Documentation	● Complete documentation. [92]

3 SECTION

Medical Undifferentiated Complaints

1. Introduction

- Recognising (and acting upon) the signs and symptoms of serious illness in a child is much more important than reaching the correct diagnosis.

- Good patient assessment will allow potentially life-threatening illnesses or injuries to be recognised sooner, allowing treatments and interventions to be given at the earliest opportunity. (This includes the need for rapid hospital transfer when urgent assessment and further treatments are required.)

- Assessment priorities include the detection of respiratory distress, circulatory impairment or decreased consciousness.

Cardiac arrest

- Adults often suffer sudden cardiac arrest while well perfused and in a relatively normal metabolic state, because the heart suddenly stops with an arrhythmia.

- In contrast, cardiac arrest in children is much more likely to occur as a result of unrecognised or prolonged hypoxia. As a consequence of hypoxia and acidosis, the heart becomes bradycardic and can result in asystole. Hypoxia and acidosis decrease the likelihood of successful resuscitation and so it is essential that serious childhood illnesses are recognised long before this chain of events can occur if child deaths are to be avoided.

- Recognition of the seriously ill or injured child involves the identification of a number of key signs affecting the child's airway, breathing, circulatory and neurological systems.

- If any of these signs are present, the child must be regarded as time critical.

2. Assessment

Primary assessment

AIRWAY – assessment of the airway

Check the airway for obstruction, foreign material or vomit.

Position the head to open the airway

The younger the child the less neck extension will be required. A newborn's head should be placed in the neutral position whilst older children should be extended into a 'sniffing the morning air' position.

Abnormal upper airway sounds should be sought

- Inspiratory noises (stridor) suggest an airway obstruction near the larynx.

- A snoring noise (stertorous breathing) may be present when there is obstruction in the pharynx (e.g. massive tonsils).

3. Breathing – Assessment and Recognition of Potential Respiratory Impairment

Measure the respiratory rate

- A rapid respiratory rate (tachypnoea) at rest in a child indicates a need for increased ventilation and suggests:

  - an airway problem
  - a lung problem

  - a circulatory problem, or
  - a metabolic problem.

Table 3.24 – NORMAL RESPIRATORY RATES

Age	Respiratory Rate
<1 year	30–40 breaths per minute
1–2 years	25–35 breaths per minute
2–5 years	25–30 breaths per minute
5–11 years	20–25 breaths per minute
>12 years	15–20 breaths per minute

Recession (indrawing, retraction)

- Children have pliable rib cages so when respiratory effort is high, indrawing is seen between the ribs (intercostal recession) and along the costal margins where the diaphragm attaches (subcostal recession). The sternum itself may even be drawn in (sternal recession) in tiny babies but as children get older, the rib cage becomes less pliable and other signs of accessory muscle use (other than recession) will be seen (see below). If recession is seen in older children, it suggests severe respiratory difficulty.

Accessory muscle use

- As in adult life, when the work of breathing is increased, the sternocleidomastoid muscle may be used as an accessory respiratory muscle. In infants this may cause the head to bob up and down with each breath.

Flaring of the nostrils

- This is a subtle sign that is easily missed. It indicates significant respiratory distress.

Inspiratory or expiratory noises

- Wheezing indicates lower airway narrowing and is most commonly heard on expiration. The volume of wheeze is **NOT** an indicator of severity and may diminish with increasing distress because less air is being moved.

Inspiratory noises (stridor)

- Suggests an imminent danger to the airway due to reduction in airway circumference to approximately 10% of normal. Again, the volume of stridor does **NOT** reflect severity and may also diminish with increasing distress as less air is moved.

Grunting

- Is produced by exhalation against a partially closed laryngeal opening (glottis). This is more likely to be seen in infants and is a sign of severe respiratory distress.

Effectiveness of breathing – chest expansion and breath sounds

Note the degree of expansion on both sides of the chest and whether it is equal.

Auscultate the chest with a stethoscope

A silent chest is a pre-terminal sign, as it indicates that very little air is moving in or out of the chest.

Pulse oximetry

This can be used at all ages to measure oxygen saturation (readings are less reliable in the presence of shock, hypothermia and other conditions such as carbon monoxide poisoning and severe anaemia).

Table 3.25 – THE EFFECTS OF RESPIRATORY INADEQUACY ON OTHER SYSTEMS

Heart rate
- Tachycardia (or eventually bradycardia) may result from hypoxia and acidosis.
- Bradycardia in a sick child is a pre-terminal sign.

Skin colour
- Flushing of the skin (vasodilation) is seen in early respiratory distress due to elevated carbon dioxide levels.
- Hypoxia causes vasoconstriction and skin pallor.
- Cyanosis is a pre-terminal sign of hypoxia.

Mental status
- Hypoxia makes children agitated and drowsy.
- Agitation may be difficult to recognise due to the child's distress. Use parents to help make this assessment.
- Drowsiness gradually progresses leading to unconsciousness.

4. Circulation – Recognition of Potential Circulatory Failure (Shock)

- Circulatory assessments in children are difficult as each physical sign may have a number of confounding variables.
- When assessing whether a child is shocked, it is important to assess and evaluate each of the signs below.

Heart rate

- Tachycardia results from loss of circulatory volume. Heart rates, particularly in infants, can be very high (up to 220 bpm) (heart rates greater than 220 bpm are seen in supraventricular tachycardia).
- Bradycardia becomes apparent before cardiac arrest (see above).

Table 3.26 – NORMAL HEART RATES

Age	Heart Rate
<1 year	110–160 beats per minute
1–2 years	100–150 beats per minute
2–5 years	95–140 beats per minute
5–11 years	80–120 beats per minute
>12 years	60–100 beats per minute

Pulse volume

- Peripheral pulses become weak and then absent as shock advances.
- Children peripherally vasoconstrict their extremities as shock progresses, initially cooling skin distally and then more proximally as shock advances.
- There is no validated relationship between the presence of certain peripheral pulses and the systemic blood pressure in children.

Capillary refill

- This should be measured on the forehead or the sternum.
- A capillary refill time of >2 seconds indicates poor perfusion, although this is influenced by a number of factors, including cold and poor lighting conditions.

Blood pressure

- Varies with age.
- Is difficult to reliably measure, increasing on-scene times, and, as a result, is not routinely measured in pre-hospital practice.
- Hypotension is a very late (and pre-terminal) sign in shocked children and so other signs of circulatory inadequacy will manifest (and should have been recognised!) long before hypotension occurs.

Table 3.27 – THE EFFECTS OF CIRCULATORY INADEQUACY ON OTHER SYSTEMS

Respiratory rate
- The combination of both rapid respiratory rate and no recession may indicate circulatory insufficiency.
- Tachypnoea occurs as the body tries to correct metabolic derangements.

Skin
- Mottled, cold, pale skin reflects poor perfusion.

Mental status
- Agitation is seen in early shock, progressing to drowsiness as shock advances.
- Poor cerebral perfusion may ultimately result in loss of consciousness.

5. Disability – Recognition of Potential Central Neurological Failure

Level of consciousness/alertness/the 'AVPU' score:

A Alert
V Responds to voice
P Responds to painful stimulus
U Unresponsive

Response to a painful stimulus

Pinch a digit or pull frontal hair. A child who is unconscious or who only responds to pain has a significant degree of coma (refer to Glasgow Coma Scale – Appendix).

Posture: observe the child's posture

- Children may be:
- Floppy (hypotonia) – recent floppiness in a child suggests serious illness.
- Stiffness (hypertonia) or back arching (opisthotonus)
  - new onset stiffness suggests severe cerebral disturbance
  - decerebrate or decorticate postures suggest a serious underlying cerebral abnormality.

Pupils

- Test pupil size and reaction.
- Pupils should be equal, of normal size and react briskly to light.
- Any abnormality or change in pupil size or reaction may be significant.

Table 3.28 – THE EFFECTS OF NEUROLOGICAL IMPAIRMENT ON OTHER SYSTEMS

Respiratory system

Brain insults produce abnormal breathing patterns e.g. hyperventilation, Cheyne–Stokes breathing or apnoea.

Circulatory system

Bradycardia may be a result of dangerously raised intracranial pressure.

NOTE: the whole assessment should take less than 2 minutes unless intervention is required.

Frequent re-assessment of ABCDs is necessary to assess the response to treatment or to detect deterioration. (Blood glucose levels should be measured in any seriously ill child.)

6. Management

Any child believed to have a serious problem involving:

- Airway
- Breathing
- Circulation
- Disability

must be considered to have a **TIME CRITICAL** condition and receive immediate management of airway, breathing and circulation, and be rapidly transferred to an appropriate receiving hospital with a suitable pre-alert message.

Remember: **A** and **B** problems should be addressed on scene and **C** problems managed en-route to further care.

7. Airway Management

- The child's airway should be managed in a stepwise manner.
- If epiglottitis is possible, then extreme caution must be exercised (**refer to respiratory illness in children guideline**).

Manual extension manoeuvres, head tilt, chin lift or jaw thrust

- Do not place pressure on the soft tissues under the chin or in front of the neck as this can obstruct the airway.

Aspiration, foreign body removal

- Avoid blind finger sweeps as they may push material further down the airway or damage the soft palate.
- Use paediatric suction catheters where available.

Oropharyngeal airway (OPA)

- Ensure the OPA is of the appropriate size (refer to page-for-age) and inserted using the correct technique. Discontinue insertion or remove if the child gags (**refer to paediatric resuscitation guidelines**).

Nasopharyngeal airway

- Correct sizing is essential (refer to page-for-age).
- In small children, a smaller size may be required.
- Care should be taken not to damage tonsillar/adenoidal tissues.

Endotracheal intubation

- The hazards associated with intubation in children are considerable and usually outweigh the advantages. It should **ONLY** be attempted where other more basic methods of ventilation have failed and only when capnography is available (**refer to paediatric resuscitation charts** (or page-for-age) for ET sizes).

Needle cricothyroidotomy

- Surgical airways should not be performed in children under the age of 12 years.
- Needle cricothyroidotomy is a method of last resort.
- The initial oxygen (O_2) flow rate in litres per minute should be set equal to the child's age in years and gradually increased until adequate chest wall movements are seen (**refer to foreign body airway obstruction in children guideline**).

8. Breathing Management

- **Ensure adequate oxygenation (refer to oxygen guideline)**.
- All sick children require adequate oxygenation.
- Administer high levels of supplemental oxygen (O_2) via a non-rebreathing mask.
- In children with sickle cell disease or cardiac disease, high levels of O_2 should be administered routinely, whatever their oxygen saturation.
- If the child finds the facemask distressing, ask the parent to help by holding the mask as close to the child's face as possible. If this still produces distress, wafting O_2 across the face directly from the tubing (with the facemask detached from the tubing) is better than nothing.
- Consider assisted ventilation at a rate equivalent to the normal respiratory rate for the age of the child (refer to paediatric resuscitation charts for normal values) if:
  - the child is hypoxic (SpO_2 <90%) and remains so after 30–60 seconds on high concentration O_2

- respiratory rate is <50% normal or >3 times normal (see Table 3.24)
- expansion is inadequate.

- Use an appropriately sized mask to ensure a good seal.

- Try to avoid hyperventilation to minimise the risks of i) gastric insufflation or ii) barotrauma. The bag-valve-mask should have a pressure release valve as an added safety measure. If this is not available, extreme care must be taken not to overexpand the lungs. No bag smaller than 500 ml volume should be used for bag-valve-mask ventilation unless the child is <2.5 kg (pre-term baby size).

Wheezing

The management of asthma is discussed elsewhere (**refer to asthma in children guideline**).

9. Circulation Management

Arrest external haemorrhage

Do not waste time attempting to gain intravenous (IV) or intraosseous (IO) access at the scene. Obtain access en-route unless delay is unavoidable.

Cannulation

Attempt cannulation with the widest bore cannula that can be confidently placed. The vehicle can be stopped briefly to allow for venepuncture and disposal of the sharp with transport being recommended before applying the IV dressing.

The intraosseous route may be required where venous access has failed on two occasions or no suitable vein is apparent within a reasonable timeframe. The intraosseous route is the preferred route for vascular access in all cases of cardiac arrest in young children.

Blood glucose level should be measured in i) all children in whom vascular access is being obtained and ii) any child with decreased conscious level (**refer to altered level of consciousness guideline**).

Fluid administration

- Use sodium chloride 0.9% to treat shock.
- Fluids should be measured in millilitres and documented as volume administered – not the volume of fluid chosen.
- Fluids should be administered as boluses rather than 'run in'.

Hand-over at the receiving unit must include details of volume and type of fluid administered.

Fluid volumes

Children found to have shock (circulatory failure[a]) as a result of medical illness are usually resuscitated with 20 ml/kg boluses of sodium chloride 0.9%, to restore vital signs to normal.

No more than two boluses should be given except on medical advice (refer to intravascular fluid and sodium chloride 0.9% guidelines).

Exceptions

- In diabetic ketoacidosis, fluids are administered more cautiously to reduce the risk of cerebral oedema (**refer to glycaemic emergencies in childhood guideline**).

- In diabetic ketoacidosis, fluid should be withheld unless severe shock is present when 10 ml/kg should be administered over 10–15 minutes (**refer to glycaemic emergencies in childhood guideline**).

- If a child has heart failure or renal failure give a 10 ml/kg bolus but stop if the patient deteriorates. Transfer to hospital as a priority.

- Where exceptional circumstances are present (e.g. long transfer time), medical advice should be obtained.

10. Disability Management

The aim of management of any child with a cerebral insult is to minimise further insult by optimising their circumstances.

This usually concerns management strategies designed to:

- prevent hypoxia (see above).
- normalise circulation (without causing fluid overload).
- identify and treat hypoglycaemia (**refer to glycaemic emergencies in childhood guideline**).

Other conditions which can be treated before hospital and are discussed elsewhere include:

- convulsions (**refer to childhood convulsions guideline**).
- opiate poisoning (refer to naloxone guideline).
- meningococcal septicaemia (**refer to meningococcal septicaemia guideline**).

Summary

The primary assessment of the child should establish whether the child is **TIME CRITICAL or not**.

Immediate correction of **A** and **B** problems must be undertaken without delay at the scene.

C problems can be corrected en-route to hospital.

Children who are found to be seriously ill must be considered **TIME CRITICAL** and **MUST BE** taken to the nearest suitable receiving hospital without delay.

A hospital alert/information call should be made whenever a seriously ill child is transported.

NB Paediatric drug doses are expressed in 'mg/kg' (refer to specific drug guidelines for dosages and information).

Drug doses MUST be checked prior to ANY drug administration, no matter how confident the practitioner may be.

Additional Information

Remember that the child/parent's history provides invaluable insights into the cause of the current condition.

The following may be of great help in making an assessment:

- Relatives, carers or friends with knowledge of the child's history.

[a] The signs of circulatory failure (cold peripheries, delayed capillary refill time, mottled skin, a weak thready pulse) are detailed above.

- Packets or containers of medication or evidence of administration devices (e.g. inhalers, spacers etc).
- MedicAlert® type jewellery (e.g. bracelets), which detail the child's primary health risk (e.g. diabetes, anaphylaxis, drug allergy etc) as well as a 24-hour telephone number to obtain a more detailed patient history.
- Child protection concerns may become apparent during the initial medical assessment and should be appropriately dealt with (**refer to safeguarding children guideline**).

KEY POINTS

Medical Emergencies

- **The child/parent's history will provide a valuable insight into the cause of the child's current condition.**
- **Emergency airway management rarely requires intubation.**
- **Hypoxia and hypovolaemia need urgent correction.**
- **Check the blood glucose in all seriously ill children and those with a decreased level of consciousness.**
- **A and B should be corrected on scene and C problems managed en-route to further care.**

Appendix

Glasgow Coma Scale and modified Glasgow Coma Scale.

GLASGOW COMA SCALE

Item		Score
Eyes opening:		
	Spontaneously	4
	To speech	3
	To pain	2
	None	1
Motor response:		
	Obeys commands	6
	Localises pain	5
	Withdraws from pain	4
	Abnormal flexion	3
	Extensor response	2
	No response to pain	1
Verbal response:		
	Orientated	5
	Confused	4
	Inappropriate words	3
	Incomprehensible sounds	2
	No verbal response	1

MODIFICATION OF GLASGOW COMA SCALE FOR CHILDREN UNDER FOUR YEARS OLD

Item		Score
Eyes opening:		As per adult scale
Motor response:		As per adult scale
Best verbal response:		
	Appropriate words or social smiles, fixes on and follows objects	5
	Cries, but is consolable	4
	Persistently irritable	3
	Restless, agitated	2
	Silent	1

Minor Illness in Children
[For references, refer to individual medical guidelines]

1. Introduction

- Traditional ambulance priorities 'focused' on the recognition and management of both serious illness and major injury prior to hospital transfer (**refer to medical emergencies in children – overview guideline**).

- Recent changes in pre-hospital care mean that children with less serious illnesses are now increasingly managed either at home or in the community rather than in emergency departments or on 'children's units', as before.

- Fever is the commonest reason for parents to seek medical attention for their child and usually suggests an underlying infection.

- Thereafter, respiratory illnesses and episodes of gastroenteritis make up a large proportion of the remaining acute paediatric presentations.

Paediatric Considerations

i) The paediatric population

- Children should not simply be viewed as 'little adults'. They pose many pitfalls for the unwary and inexperienced and present healthcare providers with significant challenges wherever the setting.

- Children display important differences in their anatomy, their physiology, their immunity and the illnesses they encounter, as well as the ways in which these conditions present, develop and progress.

- Difficulties verbalising and communicating their condition further add to these challenges.

ii) 'Major' and 'minor' illnesses

- Before considering 'minor' illnesses in children, it is crucial to both appreciate and understand that 'major' childhood illnesses – including life-threatening conditions such as meningococcal disease – rarely present in extremis, but more commonly present with relatively innocent features that can easily be mistaken for minor illnesses.

- Children with advanced major illness (or significant injury) typically have deranged vital signs that are usually readily detected. Earlier in their illness, these children may well have had normal physiology and appeared relatively well – if assessed early in their illness, these children might be misdiagnosed as only having a minor illness.

- Using the febrile child as an example, children with '**RED**' traffic light features clearly require transfer to hospital. Disease progression is much harder to predict in those with '**GREEN**' or '**AMBER**' features. These children will most probably have a minor illness but (as described above) they may be within the early stages of a more significant infection, when their symptoms and signs have not progressed and fully developed, hiding the seriousness of the evolving, underlying condition.

- This scenario is not uncommon in early meningococcal disease which classically presents with non-specific signs (e.g. fever, sore throat, lethargy, vomiting, diarrhoea, decreased appetite etc), mimicking either an upper respiratory tract infection or gastroenteritis.

- Identifying a child with a serious infection early in their illness significantly improves their outcome and so it is essential that the very subtle, early signs of serious illness are sought (**refer to febrile illnesses in children guideline**).

2. Assessment and Management

- Refer to the following guidelines that facilitate the assessment and management of children with minor illnesses, offering i) clinical management strategies, and ii) guidance to help identify the group of children with relatively insignificant symptoms that are masking a more serious underlying illness, requiring further medical assessment and intervention.

See following guidelines on:
i) **febrile illness in children**
ii) respiratory illnesses in children
iii) gastroenteritis in children.

KEY POINTS

Minor Illness in Children

- **Pre-hospital practices are changing.**
- **Children should not be viewed simply as 'little adults'.**
- **Childhood febrile illnesses, respiratory illnesses and gastroenteritis are frequently encountered.**
- **Major illnesses (e.g. meningococcal septicaemia) will often mimic otherwise trivial conditions.**
- **See guidelines on febrile illness in children, respiratory illnesses in children, gastroenteritis in children, and meningococcal septicaemia.**

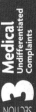

Febrile Illness in Children [142, 181–186]

1. Introduction

- Sick children are notoriously difficult to assess except for the times when they are obviously very ill or injured, with grossly deranged vital signs. (The younger the child the more difficult the assessment.)

- In critically ill children, temperature is not routinely recorded as part of the 'ABC' assessment as it delays treatment without altering management.

- Temperature should however be measured in the less ill child, where it forms part of the picture of their illness and is essential in informing decision making.

- Staff should be familiar with NICE's published guidance on this topic (on which this guideline is based).

Fever

- Normal body temperature is 37°C. A temperature of 38°C and above is likely to be significant.

- Fever is part of the immune system's response to infection and is not thought to be harmful (although lay people often assume that it is).

- It can herald a significant underlying infection hence the importance of identifying its cause.

- Throughout most of childhood, the height of the fever bears little relationship to the gravity of the illness, although in babies aged <6 months, a high temperature is much more likely to be significant.

- When facing serious infections, small babies often have unstable body temperatures and may paradoxically present with a low body temperature.

- Febrile illnesses in children aged between 6 months and 6 years can produce a seizure – a febrile convulsion – following a rapid rise in body temperature (**refer to convulsions in children guideline**).

2. Incidence

- Febrile illness is the commonest medical problem in childhood and suggests an underlying infection. Younger children are the most vulnerable due to the immaturity of their immune systems. By the age of 18 months, an otherwise healthy child would be expected to have had around eight acute febrile illnesses.

3. Severity and Outcome

- Infectious diseases are a major cause of childhood mortality and morbidity.

- Most febrile illnesses are due to self-limiting viral infections requiring little or no intervention. However, fever is a common presenting feature of serious bacterial infections (SBI) such as meningitis, septicaemia, urinary tract infections and pneumonia, and distinguishing between a simple viral infection and a more serious bacterial infection can be a real diagnostic challenge. 1% of the UK's under 5 population will have an SBI each year.

4. Assessment

a) TEMPERATURE MEASUREMENT

Do not take temperatures orally in the under 5s. Even in older children, it may be easier to avoid using the oral method.

The best method to measure a small baby's temperature (aged <1 month) is an electronic axillary thermometer.

Between 1 month and 5 years, both chemical 'dot' thermometers and aural tympanic thermometers are reliable and are equally effective.

The thermometer must be left in place for at least the minimum recommended time, otherwise it may well under-record.

Chemically sensitive strips placed on the forehead are inaccurate and should not be used.

Mercury-containing, glass thermometers are no longer used for safety reasons.

If a parent states that their child has been feverish this should be accepted as evidence of fever and taken seriously (even if they had not measured the temperature with a thermometer at the time).

b) FEBRILE CHILD ASSESSMENT

Carry out a primary survey immediately on any ill child to exclude any evidence of life-threatening illness.

Assuming this is negative, take and record a full history of the illness, including at a minimum:

1. Length of illness.
2. Other symptoms besides fever, specifically asking about:

   - Urinary symptoms.
   - Abdominal pain.
   - Headache, photophobia, neck stiffness.
   - Abnormal skin colour, cold hands and feet, muscle pains, or
   - Other complaints such as a painful joints, sore throat, ear pain etc.
3. Is fluid intake adequate? A febrile child needs extra fluids to prevent dehydration.

   If they are vomiting, they may:
   i) become dehydrated, and
   ii) be unable to absorb medication.
   Diarrhoea also increases fluid losses, increasing the risk of dehydration.
4. Underlying (chronic) medical problems, including advice that the parent may have been given by specialists regarding actions to be taken if their child develops a fever. (This should include whether the child is under current investigation or management by a doctor.)
5. Medications, antibiotics or steroids (or other drugs reducing immunity). To assess a child properly, you will need to be aware of the action of any drug that they are taking as this may be relevant. If in doubt, this must be checked.
6. Any other illness in the family, the nursery or school etc?
7. Recent foreign travel – consider malaria or other tropical illness.

Examination

Following the history, perform a detailed examination including:

1. Overall assessment/general impression – lively, miserable, disinterested, playful, floppy etc.

2. Physiological parameters – measure respiratory rate[a], heart rate[a], capillary refill time (CRT) and temperature. Oxygen saturations and an AVPU score may also be useful.

Important clinical points

As a general rule, **tachycardia** accompanies fever and raises the possibility of sepsis, whilst **tachypnoea** suggests an underlying respiratory illness.

A child's resting heart rate increases 10 bpm for every 1°C rise in body temperature.

A **disproportionate tachycardia** – i.e. above the accepted normal range (refer to Table 3.29) having taken account of the fever – is seen in early sepsis and meningococcal disease. Such children must receive further medical assessment.

Other features suggesting sepsis include cold hands and feet, abnormal skin colour and muscle pains in the legs.

Infants and small children with meningococcal disease rarely exhibit 'classical' textbook signs (**neck stiffness, photophobia** and **non-blanching rash**), but more commonly present with features that might suggest a non-specific viral illness such as an upper respiratory tract infection (URTI) or gastroenteritis.

In such circumstances, seek (and document) evidence to rule out the possibility of meningococcal disease.

1. Assessment of dehydration (**refer to gastroenteritis in children guideline**).
2. Examine all other systems (including skin) to determine the source of the fever and estimate the disease severity.

   A positive sign must be 'seen' rather than assumed – (e.g. otitis media cannot be diagnosed on a history of 'earache' alone. Direct visualisation of the tympanic membrane using an auroscope is required to make the diagnosis!)
   NB It is possible for a child to have a common infection as well as a more serious underlying one; a child with coryza and runny nose could still have meningitis.
3. Perform a 'Traffic Light' assessment (refer to Tables 3.30–3.32). This tool was developed by NICE to prioritise febrile children into three groups according to the presence of certain symptoms and signs:

   '**Green**' is low risk,
   '**Amber**' is intermediate risk and,
   '**Red**' is high risk.

Note: The traffic light system does not seek to make a specific diagnosis but simply identifies which symptoms and signs should receive the highest priority, guiding subsequent management.

c) SPECIFIC FEBRILE ILLNESSES

The following potential diagnoses must each be specifically considered:

- **Meningococcal septicaemia** – often the child may not present as acutely as tradition would have it.

- **Meningitis (under 1 year olds do not always have neck stiffness).**

- **Urinary tract infection (UTI)** – particularly common in babies and young children and can cause permanent kidney damage. UTIs can also progress to life-threatening septicaemia. Symptoms can again be very non-specific and include: poor feeding, lethargy and abdominal pains. In hospital practice, clean catch urine samples are collected on every febrile child to exclude UTIs.

- **Pneumonia** – typical chest signs may be absent.

- **Herpes simplex encephalitis** – classical pointers include focal neurological signs and focal seizures.

- **Septic arthritis/osteomyelitis** – fever plus very tender swollen joint(s)/bone(s), refusal to weight-bear.

- **Kawasaki's disease** – a collection of signs including: fever for >5 days; cervical lymphadenopathy; mucosal changes in the upper respiratory tract (e.g. redness and cracked lips); peripheral changes in the distal limbs (e.g. oedema, peeling skin); a non-specific, blanching 'measles-like' rash; bilateral conjunctival redness.

5. Management

Giving an **antipyretic** such as paracetamol or ibuprofen purely to treat the fever is not necessary, but parental sensitivities should be observed.

An analgesic/antipyretic may help relieve misery and other unpleasant symptoms that often accompany febrile illnesses (e.g. aches, pains and other symptoms which the child is often unable to fully describe).

Antipyretics do not protect against febrile convulsions. Giving antipyretics to a child who has either just had a seizure or who is thought to be at risk of having a seizure has not been shown to be beneficial.

Note: Antipyretics are effective, even in children with serious bacterial infections. It would therefore be wrong to assume that a clinical improvement seen following an antipyretic excludes a serious underlying infection.

Combinations of paracetamol and ibuprofen should not be given. Only consider alternating these agents if the distress persists or recurs before the next dose is due.

Antibiotics should not be given to a febrile child where the diagnosis is not known. This can delay the subsequent diagnosis of a serious infection such as meningitis.

6. Referral Pathway

Febrile children fulfilling the following criteria **must** be transported to hospital:

- Any child <5 years old fulfilling **RED** criteria, no matter how well they may otherwise appear.

- Any febrile baby <1 month old (irrespective of the absolute temperature).

- Any febrile child <3 months old without an obvious cause (as a minimum, an urgent urine sample will be required).

- Those aged <3 years without an obvious cause, if a urine sample cannot be arranged at the time through the GP.

- Those with any signs of serious illness (**refer to medical emergencies in children guideline**).

[a] These signs must be documented and interpreted using the age-specific, normal ranges for that child, listed in Table 3.29.

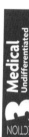

- Any child with a significant fever but no localising symptoms or signs, who has received antibiotics within the last 48 hours (signs of meningitis can be masked by antibiotic use; so called 'partially treated' meningitis).

- Any child on steroids or other medication known to suppress the immune system.

- Any child, regardless of age, where there is any doubt that they could be seriously ill.

- Any child where the social or psychological environment suggests that they may not receive adequate supervision or care if left at home.

- Those with a medical protocol saying that this is necessary.

Other categories (includes AMBER and **GREEN** groups).

Give serious consideration to transporting any child <5 years old that meets AMBER criteria to hospital, no matter how well they appear (see below).

Note: if a child fulfils AMBER criteria and a decision is made **not** to transport the child OR a child falls into the **GREEN** category but a cause for the fever has not been found, one of the following 'safety nets' **MUST** be put in place:

Safety netting

a. Provide written information on warning symptoms to the parent/carer with advice regarding further management and how further healthcare can be accessed. A parental information sheet detailing suitable advice is available in the NICE Feverish Child quick reference guide. (NICE suggest either 'verbal or written' advice, but an anxious parent/carer absorbs verbal information poorly so written instructions should be given.)

b. Make urgent follow-up arrangements for any child fulfilling AMBER criteria with a GP or other paediatric healthcare professional giving a specified time and place (e.g. for the child to be seen within the next 2–6 hours, exact timing to be decided by the attending staff).
Direct verbal hand-over to the doctor is important but may not always be possible.

The arrangements must be made by the attending ambulance staff.

It is not adequate to tell the parents to make their own arrangements to see the GP.

c. Liaison with other healthcare professionals such as the GP or out-of-hours service, to ensure the parent or carer has direct access to them if they are worried.

Finally, if in any doubt about your decision, consult the doctor responsible for the child (either their GP or out-of-hours doctor).

Febrile Illness in Children

- **Febrile illness is the commonest paediatric presentation and suggests underlying infection.**

- **Always seek the underlying cause of the fever.**

- **All febrile children must be assessed with a full history and examination.**

- **Physiological parameters must be measured, documented and compared against age-specific, 'normal' values.**

- **Significant tachycardia suggests sepsis.**

- **Use the NICE 'traffic light' system.**

- **Early non-specific features are common in serious infections (e.g. meningococcal disease often mimics URTIs and gastroenteritis).**

- **Small children rarely exhibit the 'classical' meningococcal signs – neck stiffness, photophobia or non-blanching rash; these features are more likely in older children and teenagers. In all age groups important early features include fever, cold hands and feet, abnormal skin colour and muscle pains or confusion.**

- **Improvement following antipyretics does not rule out a serious underlying infection.**

- **Do not blindly give antibiotics to a febrile child where the diagnosis is not known.**

- **Where a justifiable clinical reason not to transport a child to hospital has been found and a decision made to stay at home, these decisions must be carefully documented.**

- **Provide a 'safety net,' with written information, to any febrile child not transferred to hospital.**

- **If uncertain, seek advice from either their GP or out-of-hours doctor.**

- **The GP should be routinely informed of any consultation.**

Table 3.29 – 'NORMAL' PAEDIATRIC PHYSIOLOGICAL VALUES

Age	Respiratory rate (bpm)	Heart rate (bpm)
<1 year	30–40	110–160
1–2 yrs	25–35	100–150
2–5 yrs	25–30	95–140
5–12 yrs	20–25	80–120
Over 12 yrs	15–20	60–100

Table 3.30 – GREEN: NICE 'TRAFFIC LIGHTS' CLINICAL ASSESSMENT TOOL

Colour	Normal colour of skin, lips and tongue
Activity	Responds normally to social cues Content/smiles Stays awake or awakens quickly Strong/normal cry/not crying
Hydration	Normal skin and eyes Moist mucous membranes
Other	No amber or red symptoms or signs

Table 3.31 – AMBER: NICE 'TRAFFIC LIGHTS' CLINICAL ASSESSMENT TOOL

Colour	Pallor reported by parent/carer
Activity	Not responding normally to social cues Wakes only with prolonged stimulation Decreased activity No smile
Respiratory	Nasal flaring Tachypnoea: ● RR >50/min age 6–12 months ● RR >40/min age >12 months O₂ sat ≤95% in air Crackles
Hydration	Dry mucous membranes Poor feeding in infants Capillary Refill Time (CRT) ≥3 seconds ↓ Urinary output
Other	Fever for ≥5 days Swelling of a limb or joint Non-weight bearing/not using an extremity A new lump >2 cm

Table 3.32 – RED: NICE 'TRAFFIC LIGHTS' CLINICAL ASSESSMENT TOOL

Colour	Pale/mottled/ashen/blue
Activity	No response to social cues Appears ill to a healthcare professional Unable to rouse, or if roused, does not stay awake Weak/high pitched/continuous cry
Respiratory	Grunting Tachypnoea: RR >60/min Moderate or severe chest indrawing
Hydration	Reduced skin turgor
Other	0–3 months, temp ≥38°C 3–6 months, temp ≥39°C Non blanching rash Bulging fontanelle Neck stiffness Status epilepticus Focal seizures Focal neurological signs Bile-stained vomiting

3 SECTION Medical Undifferentiated Complaints

Introduction

Childhood respiratory illnesses include:

1. Asthma.
2. Bronchiolitis.
3. Croup.
4. URTIs (tonsillitis, otitis media).
5. Pneumonia.

1. Asthma

For the management of mild, moderate, severe and life-threatening asthma **refer to the asthma in children guideline**.

2. Bronchiolitis

2.1 Introduction

Bronchiolitis is an acute, self-limiting respiratory infection that is usually caused by respiratory syncytial virus (RSV) and occurs predominantly in the autumn and winter months. It is characterised by inflammation of the bronchioles.

2.2 Assessment

- Clinical presentation: a coryzal baby (peak age 2–5 months) with their first wheezy episode.

- Irregular breathing and apnoeas are frequently reported.

- During the first 72 hours, bronchiolitic infants may deteriorate clinically, before symptomatic improvements are seen.

- The baby's parents and siblings often have concurrent respiratory illnesses and may report sore throats or dry coughs.

- Examination may reveal:
    - ↓oxygen saturations
    - ↑respiratory rate
    - recession
    - fine, bilateral inspiratory crackles
    - high-pitched expiratory wheezes
    - low grade fever
    - high fevers (temp >38.5 °C) suggest bacterial pneumonia rather than bronchiolitis.

- Premature babies, those with chronic lung disease, children with congenital heart disease, cystic fibrosis, congenital or acquired immune deficiency (HIV), and those either aged <2 months or having apnoeas are at highest risk and **must** be transferred to further care.

- Previously well babies with diminished feeding, irregular breathing, hypoxia (O_2 saturations <95% on air), tachypnoea or tachycardia should also be transferred to further care where they will receive respiratory support and help with feeding/hydration.

2.3 Management

- Treatments aim to provide respiratory support and support feeding/hydration.

- Antivirals, antibiotics, steroids, nebulisers, physiotherapy, steam treatments, nasal decongestants, homeopathy and complementary therapies have not been shown to be effective.

- Acute bronchiolitis lasts approximately two weeks from its onset, but can last up to four weeks.

- Ongoing cough and persisting wheeze are not uncommonly seen after the initial illness has passed but should prompt further medical assessment.

3. Croup

3.1 Introduction

- Croup is a common, acute, respiratory illness of gradual onset, characterised by stridor that typically is mild and self-limiting.

3.2 Incidence

- Croup mostly affects children between the ages of six months and six years.

- It can occur all year round but peaks are seen in both spring and autumn.

3.3 Pathophysiology

- Croup results from viral infections, most commonly parainfluenza, but also RSV, influenza A and B, as well as *Mycoplasma pneumoniae*.

- Stridor, hoarseness and a barking 'seal-like' cough result from inflammation and narrowing around the subglottic region of larynx. (This is the narrowest point of the paediatric airway.)

NB Stridor may also be caused by epiglottitis, bacterial tracheitis, retropharyngeal abscesses, foreign bodies, anaphylaxis and angio-oedema, blunt trauma, glandular fever, inhalation of hot gases and diphtheria; all children with these conditions **must** be transferred to further care.

3.4 Assessment

- The child with croup may have mild clinical features in keeping with a simple, upper respiratory tract infection although they can present with more worrying features including respiratory distress, respiratory failure and respiratory arrest.

- The features of respiratory distress – increased respiration rate, increased work of breathing, recession, nasal flaring, grunting, use of accessory muscles and stridor – are described in the **medical emergencies in childhood guideline**.

- The Modified Taussig Score is a simple clinical assessment tool that can be used to determine the severity of croup and the need for medication by scoring i) stridor and ii) recession (refer to Table 3.33).

Table 3.33 – MODIFIED TAUSSIG CROUP SCORE

		Score*
Stridor	None	0
	Only on crying, exertion	1
	At rest	2
	Severe (biphasic)	3
Recession	None	0
	Only on crying, exertion	1
	At rest	2
	Severe (biphasic)	3

* Mild: 1–2; Moderate: 3–4; Severe: 5–6

- Hypoxia (O_2 saturations <95% on air), cyanosis, physical exhaustion (quietening stridor, reduced recession in a child that is becoming more unwell), restlessness, irritability and altered consciousness are ominous signs.

- Croup (and the differentials listed above) can cause: respiratory distress, but may also progress exceedingly rapidly to produce complete upper airway obstruction and respiratory arrest. Therefore **all children with stridor must be transferred** to further care for further medical assessment and observation.

- Keep the child in a position of comfort, sat upright and supported on a parent's lap – children often 'know' how to maintain their own airways in an optimal position (they often adopt a so-called 'tripod' posture).

- At all times, a calm approach is to be encouraged. Any intervention likely to upset the child – examining their ears, nose or throat, blood sugar measurement, cannulation, and even nebulisation (see below) – must be avoided, as distressing the child can precipitate an acute deterioration and complete airway obstruction. This is of increased importance in pre-hospital settings as skills for expert airway intervention will not be immediately available.

3.5 Severity and outcome

- Using the Modified Taussig Score, croup can be described as mild (1–2), moderate (3–4) or severe (5–6) (refer to Table 3.33).

3.6 Management

- **Steroids** are the mainstay of treatment – usually oral dexamethasone (nebulised budesonide may alternatively be used but may distress the child, adversely worsening their symptoms) – and work by relieving subglottic inflammation.

- Children with moderate or severe croup (Modified Taussig Score >3), may benefit from early steroid treatment but must still be transferred to further care for subsequent observation.

  - Oral dexamethasone (refer to dexamethasone guideline) is preferred to nebulised budesonide, as nebulisation frequently distresses small children, producing further airway narrowing.
  - NB The intravenous preparation of **dexamethasone** is administered **ORALLY** (refer to dexamethasone guideline).

3.7 Referral pathway

As above, irrespective of whether steroids are given, all children with stridor must still be transferred to further care for subsequent observation, even if clinical improvements are noted at home.

4. Upper Respiratory Tract Infections (URTIs) e.g. tonsillitis (sore throat, acute pharyngitis, acute exudative tonsillitis), otitis media, etc

4.1 Introduction

Upper respiratory tract infections (URTIs) are one of the commonest reasons for paediatric presentation, especially during the winter months.

4.2 Incidence

25% of all under five year olds see their GPs each year for tonsillitis.

4.3 Assessment

- Children with URTIs may complain of:

  - sore throat
  - cough
  - fever
  - headache
  - earache
  - systemic illness
  - anorexia and lethargy.

- Physical examination may reveal:

  - cervical lymphadenopathy
  - offensive breath
  - inflamed, purulent tonsils.

Breathing may also be compromised by either stridor or respiratory distress. In these circumstances, avoid attempts to examine the throat (see croup guidance above) and transfer urgently to further care.

Children with 'muffled' voices that sound as if they have something hot in their mouths must also be transferred to further care, to exclude quinsy (peritonsillar abscess).

Tenderness behind the ear (over their mastoid process) in a child with otitis media, whose ear may/may not be starting to 'stickout' suggests mastoiditis (a dangerous infection of the bone around the ear) and must be transferred to further care.

The child's hydration status should be estimated as fluid intake can be significantly decreased.

4.4 Management

URTIs are usually self-limiting. Parents should be offered advice about managing their child's symptoms (rest, extra fluids, analgesia, antipyretics etc) and informed about the likely duration of their child's illness (refer to Table 3.34).

Antibiotics are not prescribed routinely. Most URTIs are viral and so do not respond to antibiotics. Bacteria (e.g. Streptococci) also cause URTIs but even in these cases antibiotics are rarely needed; they don't improve the child's symptoms and they can often cause diarrhoea, vomiting and rashes.

Table 3.34 – TYPICAL DURATION OF ACUTE RESPIRATORY ILLNESSES

Condition	Duration
acute otitis media	4 days
acute sore throat/pharyngitis/tonsillitis	1 week
common cold	1½ weeks
acute rhinosinusitis	2½ weeks
acute cough/bronchitis	3 weeks

GPs tend to use one of three antibiotic strategies:

1. **no prescribing** – no antibiotics are needed where the URTI is thought likely to clear up on its own.
2. **delayed prescribing** – delayed antibiotics are useful when symptoms fail to improve or even worsen.

3. **immediate prescribing** – immediate antibiotic prescriptions are reserved for the most severe cases, including:

- Under twos with acute bilateral otitis media.
- Children with acute otitis media and otorrhoea (ear discharge).
- Children with acute streptococcal URTIs (no cough but fever, pustular tonsils and tender lymph nodes).

Antibiotics are also prescribed for children who are:

- Systemically very unwell.
- At high risk of serious complications because of pre-existing illnesses (heart, lung, renal, liver or neuromuscular disease, diabetes, cystic fibrosis, prematurity, immunosuppression or previous hospitalisations).

  Cough mixtures: over-the-counter cough and cold preparations often contain sedatives and antihistamines that are dangerous if taken accidentally by small children in overdose. As a result, these medicines are no longer available for children aged two years or under. Children in this age group with colds and fever should now only be offered paracetamol or ibuprofen to manage their temperature, if needed.
  Simple cough syrups containing glycerol, and honey and lemon may still be given, as well as vapour rubs and inhalant decongestants (see individual labelling).

4.5 Referral pathway

Hospital admission may also be indicated when:

- There is diminished fluid intake (e.g. young child with severe tonsillitis and teenagers with glandular fever), and
- Where concerns regarding the diagnosis persist (NB early **meningococcal disease** is frequently misdiagnosed as an URTI in small children – where this diagnosis cannot be excluded, arrangements for an urgent medical opinion should be made). (**Refer to febrile illness in children guideline**.)

4.6 Non-conveyance

As when managing the febrile child, if a decision not to transfer a child to further care has been reached, a clinically justifiable reason should be present and properly documented.

'Safety netting,' with written advice, should again be encouraged and follow-up arrangements should be provided.

Where doubts persist seek senior advice or review.

Again, remember that early **meningococcal disease** is frequently misdiagnosed in small children simply as an URTI.

5. Pneumonia (lower respiratory tract infections, 'chest infections')

Children with pneumonia are likely to have the following signs and symptoms:

- Fever.
- Cough.

- Tachypnoea.
  - RR > 60 breaths/min, age 0–5 months
  - RR > 50 breaths/min, age 6–12 months
  - RR > 40 breaths/min, age > 12 months
- Nasal flaring.
- Chest indrawing.
- Oxygen saturations <95%.
- Crackles in the chest.
- Cyanosis.

Such children are likely to require antibiotics and possibly additional oxygen and should be seen by either their GP or a paediatrician.

KEY POINTS

Respiratory Illness

- **Childhood respiratory illnesses are common and usually self-limiting.**
- **Antibiotics are rarely indicated.**
- **Children with underlying conditions (e.g. prematurity, chronic lung disease, congenital heart disease, cystic fibrosis, congenital or acquired immune deficiency (HIV), cerebral palsy), are especially vulnerable and must be seen either by their GP or in hospital.**
- **Tachypnoea is seen in all respiratory illnesses.**
- **Respiratory distress causes increased respiration rate, increased work of breathing, recession, nasal flaring, grunting, use of accessory muscles and stridor.**
- **Exhaustion suggests respiratory failure and respiratory arrest may rapidly follow.**
- **Stridor can progress rapidly to complete upper airway obstruction and respiratory arrest.**
- **Approach a child with stridor calmly and gently. Sit them upright, in a position of comfort and avoid painful/distressing procedures.**
- **Transfer all children with stridor for further medical assessment and observation.**
- **Steroids (dexamethasone) are used in moderate and severe croup.**
- **Children with pneumonia require antibiotics and possibly oxygen therapy. They should be seen by either their GP or a paediatrician.**
- **Whilst URTIs are very common, early meningococcal disease can easily be misdiagnosed as an URTI. (When unable to exclude this diagnosis, make arrangements for an urgent second opinion.)**
- **Provide a 'safety net' (with written information) for all children with respiratory illness not transferred to hospital.**
- **If uncertain, seek advice from either the child's GP or the out-of-hours doctor.**

Heat Related Illness [92, 103, 198–281]

1. Introduction

- Heat related illness is a relatively uncommon presenting condition to ambulance services but it can be life-threatening.
- Heat related illness can be **exogenous,** caused by environmental factors (e.g. the sun) or **endogenous** (e.g. drugs and exercise).
- Heat related illness is a continuum of heat related conditions (refer to Figure 3.3).

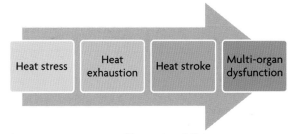

Figure 3.3 – Continuum of heat related illness.

The management of heat related illness is supportive: refer to Table 3.38.

Heat stress

- Heat stress is a mild form of heat illness, characterised by the features below (refer to Table 3.35). This level of heat disorder is often self-managed, but if left untreated can progress to more serious conditions.

Table 3.35 – FEATURES OF HEAT STRESS (EUROPEAN RESUSCITATION COUNCIL GUIDELINES)

Heat stress
- **Temperature:** normal or mildly elevated.
- **Heat oedema:** swelling of feet and ankles.
- **Heat syncope:** vasodilation and dehydration causing hypotension.
- **Heat cramps:** sodium depletion causing cramps.

Heat exhaustion

- A less severe heat illness than heat stroke, lacking the defining neurological symptoms of this condition. Symptoms are mainly due to excess fluid loss and electrolyte imbalance.

Table 3.36 – FEATURES OF HEAT EXHAUSTION (ERC)[60]

Heat exhaustion
- Systemic reaction to prolonged heat exposure (hours to days).
- Temperature >37°C and <40°C.
- Headache, dizziness, nausea, vomiting, tachycardia.
- Hypotension, sweating, muscle pain, weakness and cramps.
- Haemoconcentration.
- Hyponatraemia or hypernatraemia.
- May progress rapidly to heat stroke.

Heat stroke

- A 'systemic inflammatory response' to a core body temperature >40.6°C in addition to a change in mental status and organ dysfunction (European Resuscitation Council Guidelines)[60].

There are two types of heat stroke:

a. **Non-exertional heat stroke** due to very high external temperatures and/or high humidity; it tends to be more common in very hot climates. It tends to occur in the:
  – elderly
  – very young
  – chronically ill.

b. **Exertional heat stroke** is due to excess heat production. This tends to occur in:
  – athletes including marathon and fun-runners
  – manual workers
  – firefighters
  – military recruits.

Table 3.37 – FEATURES OF HEAT STROKE (ERC)[60]

Heat stroke
- Core temperature ≥40°C.
- Hot, dry skin (sweating is present in about 50% of cases of exertional heat stroke).
- Early signs and symptoms are extreme fatigue, headache, fainting, facial flushing, vomiting and diarrhoea.
- Cardiovascular dysfunction including arrhythmias and hypotension.
- Respiratory dysfunction including acute respiratory distress syndrome (ARDS).
- Central nervous system dysfunction including seizures and coma.
- Liver and renal failure.
- Coagulopathy.
- Rhabdomyolysis.

2. Incidence

The exact incidence of heat stroke is unknown, with many sufferers self-managing their condition. Mortality, in the absence of a heat wave is relatively low; in the United Kingdom it is estimated to be 40 deaths per million annually.

A variety of medications may predispose to the development of heat illness. In addition, individuals who take drugs of abuse (e.g. cocaine, ecstasy, amphetamines) and then engage in vigorous dancing in crowded 'rave' settings may also develop heat illness.

3. Severity and Outcome

- Heat stroke is a life-threatening emergency that requires prompt appropriate treatment, with estimates of mortality of 10–50%. Recovery from heat stroke even after appropriate treatment and rehabilitation may be incomplete and leave patients with persistent functional impairment.

- **Systemic effects** – heat stroke can lead to a variety of life-threatening systemic conditions including: disseminated intravascular coagulation, rhabdomyolysis, renal failure, hepatic necrosis, metabolic acidosis and decreased tissue perfusion, in addition to cerebral and cerebellar damage.

4. Pathophysiology

- In heat illnesses there is an imbalance in the metabolic production and subsequent loss of heat by the body. This increase in core body temperature has multiple undesirable effects on many body systems. Systemically this increased temperature leads to swelling and degeneration at both cellular and tissue levels.

- **Cellular changes** – at increased temperatures cellular organelles swell and stop functioning properly. Cell membranes become distorted, leading to unwanted increased permeability and inappropriate movement of ions into and out of cells. Red blood cells also change shape at elevated temperatures and their capacity to carry oxygen is decreased. At higher temperatures cells will also undergo inappropriate apoptosis and die.

5. Assessment and Management

- For the assessment and management of heat related illness refer to Table 3.38.

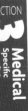

KEY POINTS

Heat Related Illness

- Heat exhaustion/heat stroke occurs in high external temperatures, as a result of excess heat production and with certain drugs. The higher the level of activity the lower the environmental temperature required to produce heat stroke.

- Do not assume that collapse in an athlete is due to heat – check for other causes.

- In heat exhaustion the patient may present with flu-like symptoms, such as headache, nausea, dizziness, vomiting, and cramps; the temperature may not be elevated.

- In heat stroke the patient will have neurological symptoms such as decreased level of consciousness, ataxia and convulsions, and the temperature will usually be elevated, typically >40°C.

- Remove the patient from the hot environment or remove cause, if possible, remove clothing and cool.

Table 3.38 – ASSESSMENT and MANAGEMENT of:

Heat Related Illness

ASSESSMENT	MANAGEMENT

● Assess ABCD	● If any of the following **TIME CRITICAL** features are present:
	  – major **ABC** problems
	  – haemodynamic compromise
	  – decreased level of consciousness, then:
	● Start correcting **A** and **B** problems.
	● Undertake a **TIME CRITICAL** transfer to nearest appropriate receiving hospital.
	● Provide an alert/information call.
	● Continue patient management en-route.

● Assess	Undertake physical examination and assess for the presence of features of heat related illness (refer to Tables 3.35–3.37) ● Remove the patient from the hot environment or remove cause if possible. ● Remove to an air-conditioned vehicle where available. ● Remove all clothing. ● Commence cooling with fanning, tepid sponging, water misting or with a wet sheet loosely over the patient's body. NB Consider other potential causes (e.g. diabetes or cardiac problems).
● Temperature	Measure and record: ● The patient's core temperature. ● If possible and time allows measure the environmental temperature. NB The core temperature may or may not be elevated, but patients may be tachycardic, hypotensive and/or sweating excessively.
● Heat stroke	Heat stroke is potentially fatal and the patient needs to be cooled as an emergency. ● If cold or iced water is used, massaging of the skin may be needed to overcome cold induced vasoconstriction and ensure effective heat loss. ● Apply ice packs, if available, wrapped in a thin cloth or towel to the patient's neck, axilla and groin. NB Ice packs applied directly to the skin can cause frostbite. ● Transfer the patient with air conditioning turned on or with windows open. NB Immersion in ice water is effective but usually not possible in the pre-hospital environment.
● GCS	● Check Glasgow Coma Score.
● Oxygen	● If the patient is hypoxaemic, administer high levels of supplemental oxygen and aim for a target saturation within the range of 94–98% – refer to oxygen guideline.
● Fluid therapy	● If fluid therapy is indicated refer to intravascular fluid therapy guidelines. ● **DO NOT** delay on scene for fluid replacement; administer en-route.
● Blood glucose	● Measure blood glucose – **refer to glycaemic emergencies guidelines**.
● Vital signs	● Monitor vital signs. ● Monitor ECG.
● Transfer	● Transfer patients to nearest appropriate receiving hospital. ● Continue management en-route. ● Complete documentation. [92]

1. Introduction

- Hyperventilation syndrome (HVS) is a common presentation in pre-hospital care.
- **It is defined as 'a rate of ventilation exceeding metabolic needs and higher than that required to maintain a normal level of plasma carbon dioxide (CO_2)'.**
- Hyperventilation can occur in a number of conditions, including life-threatening conditions such as:
  - pulmonary embolism
  - diabetic ketoacidosis
  - asthma
  - hypovolaemia.

The cause of hyperventilation cannot always be determined in the pre-hospital environment, especially in the early stages.

2. Incidence

- It is estimated that 6–11% of primary care patients may suffer from some form of HVS. The condition is more common in women.
- HVS most commonly occurs between 15 and 55 years of age, although it can occur at any age, but it is rare in children, where the most likely cause is physical illness.

3. Severity and Outcome

- Although death is rare, the condition can be debilitating with physical signs and symptoms and is distressing.

4. Pathophysiology

- The cause of HVS is unknown but it is hypothesised that stress may result in an exaggerated respiratory response. Stressors may include psychological distress, caffeine, isoprenaline, cholecystokinin and deficiencies in sodium lactate metabolism. Other causes include elevated level of CO_2, and some have argued that sufferers have a lower threshold trigger for the 'fight-flight response'.
- HVS presents in two forms, acute and chronic. Acute HVS accounts for 1% of cases.

- Over-breathing results in hypocapnia (decreased level of carbon dioxide in the blood) causing respiratory alkalosis and a decreased level of serum ionised calcium, resulting in a number of physical and psychological signs and symptoms. Patients may present with one or more of the signs and symptoms listed in Table 3.39.

Table 3.39 – PRESENTING FEATURES

Signs and symptoms

Breathing:
- Sudden dyspnoea.
- Hyperpnoea.
- Tachypnoea.

Electrolyte imbalance:
- Tetany due to calcium imbalance.
- Paraesthesia (numbness and tingling of the mouth and lips and extremities).
- Carpopedal spasm.

Psychological:
- Acute agitation and anxiety.

Other:
- Chest pain – may resemble angina pectoris.
- Palpitations.
- Tachycardia and electrocardiographic changes.
- Aching of the muscles of the chest.
- Feeling of light-headedness or dizziness.
- Weakness and fatigue.
- Frequent sighing.
- Non-diaphragmatic respiratory effort.

Assessment and Management

For the assessment and management of hyperventilation syndrome refer to Table 3.40 and Figure 3.4.

KEY POINTS

Hyperventilation Syndrome
- **HVS is a diagnosis of exclusion.**
- **Medical conditions can cause hyperventilation.**
- **In children a medical cause is more likely than stress.**
- **Administer supplemental oxygen if hypoxaemic (SpO_2 <94%)**
- **Tetany, paraesthesia and carpopedal spasm may occur.**

Hyperventilation Syndrome

Table 3.40 – ASSESSMENT and MANAGEMENT of:

Hyperventilation Syndrome

ASSESSMENT	MANAGEMENT

● Assess ABCD	● If any of the following **TIME CRITICAL** features present:
	  – major **ABCD** problems
	  – cyanosis
	  – reduced level of consciousness – **refer to altered level of consciousness guideline**.
	  – hypoxia – refer to oxygen guideline.
	● Start correcting **A** and **B** problems.
	● Undertake a **TIME CRITICAL** transfer to nearest receiving hospital.
	● Continue patient management en-route.
	● Provide an alert/information call.
	NB If any of the **TIME CRITICAL** features listed above are present, it is unlikely to be due to hyperventilation syndrome but is more likely to be physiological hyperventilation, secondary to an underlying pathological process.

Ask the patient if they have an individualised treatment plan	● Follow individualised treatment plan if available. ● The patient will often be able to guide their care.
Specifically assess: **History**	⚠️**Always presume hyperventilation is secondary to hypoxia or other underlying respiratory or metabolic disorder until proven otherwise and such is a diagnosis of exclusion.** ● Cause of hyperventilation. ● Previous episodes of hyperventilation. ● Previous medical history. ● Features of hyperventilation syndrome refer to Table 3.39.
Differential diagnosis	Consider differential diagnosis such as: ● Heart failure – **refer to heart failure guideline**. ● Acute asthma – **refer to asthma guidelines**. ● Chest infection – **refer to medical emergencies guideline**. ● Pulmonary embolism – **refer to pulmonary embolism guideline**. ● Diabetic ketoacidosis or other causes of metabolic acidosis – **refer to glycaemic emergencies guideline**. ● Pneumothorax – **refer to thoracic trauma guideline**. ● Drug overdose – **refer to overdose and poisoning guidelines**. ● Acute myocardial infarction – **refer to acute coronary syndrome guideline**.
Oxygen saturation	● Apply pulse oximeter. ● **DO NOT** administer supplemental oxygen unless hypoxaemic (SpO_2 <94%) – refer to oxygen guideline. NB Low SpO_2 is not a presenting feature of HVS and will indicate an underlying clinical condition.
Breathing	● Consider auscultation of breath sounds during assessment of breathing. ● Aim to restore a normal level of pCO_2 over a period of time by reassuring the patient and coaching them regarding their respirations. ● Try to remove the source of the patient's anxiety – this is particularly important in the management of children. ● **Refer to dyspnoea guideline**.
● Transfer	Transfer to further care: ● Patients experiencing their first episode. ● Known HVS sufferers whose symptoms have not settled, or re-occur within 10 minutes. ● Patients who have an individualised care plan and a responsible adult present may be considered for non conveyance and managing at home according to local protocols. Provide details of local care pathways if symptoms re-occur.

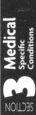

3 Medical
Specific Conditions

SECTION

Hyperventilation Syndrome

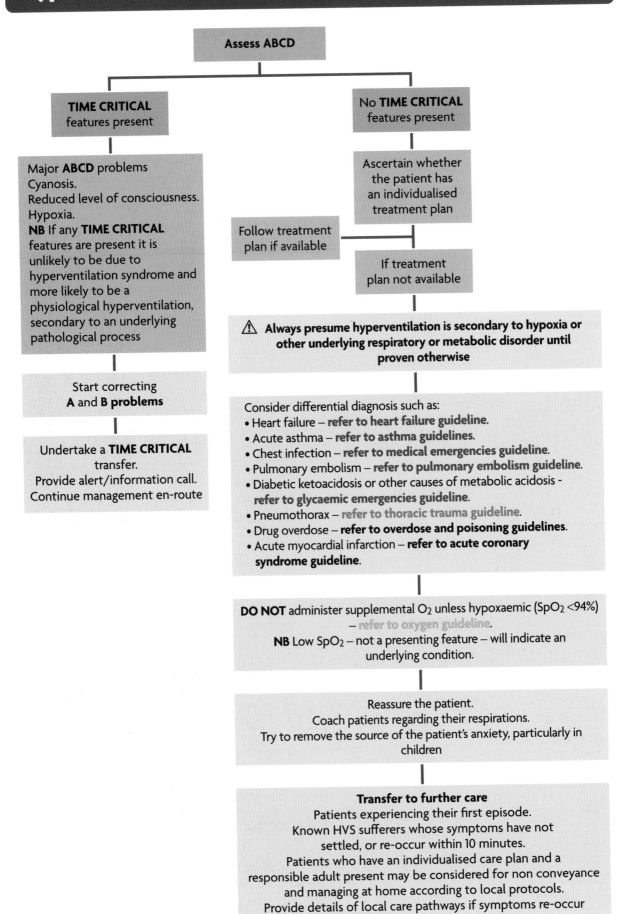

Assess ABCD

TIME CRITICAL features present

Major **ABCD** problems
Cyanosis.
Reduced level of consciousness.
Hypoxia.
NB If any **TIME CRITICAL** features are present it is unlikely to be due to hyperventilation syndrome and more likely to be a physiological hyperventilation, secondary to an underlying pathological process

Start correcting **A** and **B problems**

Undertake a **TIME CRITICAL** transfer.
Provide alert/information call.
Continue management en-route

No **TIME CRITICAL** features present

Ascertain whether the patient has an individualised treatment plan

Follow treatment plan if available

If treatment plan not available

⚠ **Always presume hyperventilation is secondary to hypoxia or other underlying respiratory or metabolic disorder until proven otherwise**

Consider differential diagnosis such as:
• Heart failure – **refer to heart failure guideline**.
• Acute asthma – **refer to asthma guidelines**.
• Chest infection – **refer to medical emergencies guideline**.
• Pulmonary embolism – **refer to pulmonary embolism guideline**.
• Diabetic ketoacidosis or other causes of metabolic acidosis - **refer to glycaemic emergencies guideline**.
• Pneumothorax – **refer to thoracic trauma guideline**.
• Drug overdose – **refer to overdose and poisoning guidelines**.
• Acute myocardial infarction – **refer to acute coronary syndrome guideline**.

DO NOT administer supplemental O_2 unless hypoxaemic (SpO_2 <94%) – refer to oxygen guideline.
NB Low SpO_2 – not a presenting feature – will indicate an underlying condition.

Reassure the patient.
Coach patients regarding their respirations.
Try to remove the source of the patient's anxiety, particularly in children

Transfer to further care
Patients experiencing their first episode.
Known HVS sufferers whose symptoms have not settled, or re-occur within 10 minutes.
Patients who have an individualised care plan and a responsible adult present may be considered for non conveyance and managing at home according to local protocols.
Provide details of local care pathways if symptoms re-occur

Figure 3.4 – Assessment and management of hyperventilation syndrome algorithm.

CTION
3
Medical
Specific

1. Introduction

- Hypothermia is defined as a core body temperature below 35°C (refer to Figure 3.5). It is a potentially life-threatening condition.

- There are three main types of hypothermia depending on the speed at which a person loses heat:

i. Acute hypothermia (immersion hypothermia)

- This occurs when a person loses heat very rapidly (e.g. by falling into cold water). It is associated with near-drowning. Acute hypothermia may also occur in a snow avalanche when it may be associated with asphyxia.

ii. Subacute hypothermia (exhaustion hypothermia)

- This typically occurs in a hill walker who is exercising in moderate cold who becomes exhausted and is unable to generate enough heat. Heat loss will occur more rapidly in windy conditions or if the patient is wet or inadequately clothed. It may be associated with injury or frostbite. Do not forget that if one person in a group of walkers is hypothermic, others in the party who are similarly dressed and who have been exposed to identical conditions may also be hypothermic.

iii. Chronic hypothermia

- In chronic hypothermia heat loss occurs slowly, often over days or longer. It most commonly occurs in the elderly person living in an inadequately heated house or the person who is sleeping rough. It can be associated with injury or illness (e.g. the patient who falls or has a stroke and who is on the floor overnight).

- Mixed forms of hypothermia may occur e.g. the exhausted walker who collapses and falls into a stream.

Diagnosis

- In order to measure core body temperature accurately and make a diagnosis, a low-reading thermometer is required. In the pre-hospital environment, measuring the patient's temperature using an oesophageal, bladder or rectal approach may not be practical. However, tympanic thermometry in cold environments may not be reliable (as the probe is not well insulated) and if the patient is in cardiac arrest, with no blood flow in the carotid artery.

- Because of the difficulty of diagnosing hypothermia in the pre-hospital environment, patients should be treated as having hypothermia if there is clinical suspicion of the diagnosis based on the risk factors in Table 3.41, the clinical history, examination, and the presence of concurrent injuries or illness which may suggest hypothermia.

Table 3.41 – RISK FACTORS FOR HYPOTHERMIA

Factors

- Older patients > 80 years due to impaired thermoregulation.
- Children due to their proportionately larger body surface area.
- Some medical conditions (e.g. hypothyroidism, stroke etc) due to impaired thermoregulation.
- Intoxicated patients (e.g. alcohol, recreational drugs).
- In association with near-drowning and in patients exposed to cold, wet and windy environments especially if inadequately dressed.
- Patients suffering from exhaustion.
- Injury and immobility.
- Decreased level of consciousness.

2. Incidence

- The true incidence is unknown but the ONS report fewer than 400 deaths per annum in England and Wales. However, it is suggested that hypothermia may be under-diagnosed in temperate climates such as the UK.

- Death from hypothermia is more common in women than men and in people over 80 years old.

3. Pathophysiology

As the core body temperature falls there may be:

- Progressive decrease in the level of consciousness **(refer to altered level of consciousness guideline)**.

- Other brain dysfunction (e.g. slurring of speech, muscular incoordination).

- Slowing heart rate.

- Slowing respiratory rate.

- Development of cardiac arrhythmias (sinus bradycardia → atrial fibrillation → ventricular fibrillation → asystole).

- Cooling the body decreases oxygen demand and is protective for the brain and vital organs; therefore **DO NOT STOP CARDIAC RESUSCITATION IN THE FIELD** as good outcomes have resulted from prolonged resuscitation of hypothermic patients.

4. Severity and Outcome

The severity of hypothermia can be classified into mild, moderate and severe depending on the patient's core body temperature (refer to Figure 3.5).

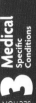

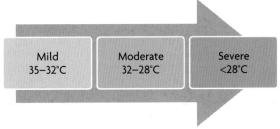

Mild	Moderate	Severe
35–32°C	32–28°C	<28°C

Figure 3.5 – Severity of hypothermia.

Hypothermia

- However, in the pre-hospital environment, core temperature is difficult to measure, and it may be better to define the severity clinically (refer to Table 3.42).

5. Assessment and Management

For the assessment and management of hypothermia refer to Table 3.43.

Table 3.42 – CLINICAL STAGES OF HYPOTHERMIA

Stage	Clinical signs
I	Clearly conscious and shivering.
II	Impaired consciousness without shivering.
III	Unconscious.
IV	No breathing.
V	Death due to irreversible hypothermia.

Table 3.43 – ASSESSMENT and MANAGEMENT of:

Hypothermia

ASSESSMENT	MANAGEMENT
Assess ABCD	**If any of the following TIME CRITICAL features are present:** ● Major ABC problems. ● Haemodynamic compromise. ● Decreased level of consciousness. ● Cardiac arrest, then: Start correcting **A** (with cervical spine protection if indicated) and **B** problems. Undertake a **TIME CRITICAL** transfer to nearest appropriate receiving hospital. Provide an alert/information call. Continue patient management en-route.
Assess	Undertake physical examination and assess for the presence of features of hypothermia (refer to Table 3.42): early symptoms are non-specific and include ataxia, slurred speech, apathy, irrational behaviour, and decrease in the level of consciousness (**refer to altered level of consciousness guideline**), heart rate and rhythm, and respiratory rate.
Temperature	Measure and record the patient's core temperature – temperature measurement in the field is difficult, therefore it is important to suspect and treat hypothermia from the history and circumstances of the situation. NB Shivering occurs early but will cease when the temperature falls further (refer to Table 3.42); the patient will feel cold to the touch.
Warming	**PREVENT FURTHER HEAT LOSS** as in the mildly hypothermic patient, preventing further heat loss will enable the patient to warm up by their own metabolism. ● Place in vehicle. ● **DO NOT** wrap cold patients in foil blankets directly next to skin. Wrap them in fabric blankets first and then place a foil blanket on top. ● If the patient is conscious provide a hot drink/food if available and appropriate. ● **DO NOT** rub the patient's skin as this causes vasodilatation and may increase heat loss. ● **DO NOT** give the patient alcohol as this causes vasodilatation and may increase heat loss. ● Manage co-existing trauma or medical conditions as they arise (refer to appropriate **trauma/medical** guidelines).
Resuscitation	**BEWARE:** Hypothermia may mimic death with very slow and weak or undetectable pulse, very slow and shallow respiration, fixed dilated pupils and increased muscle tone. ● Airway – clear the airway. ● Ventilation – if there are no signs of respiration, ventilate with high concentrations of oxygen (refer to appropriate resuscitation guidelines). ● Signs of life – look for signs of life (palpate central artery, ECG monitoring etc) for up to 1 minute. ● Cardiac arrest – refer to appropriate resuscitation guidelines and additional information below. ● Rough handling can invoke cardiac arrhythmias (including VF and pulseless VT) so handle patients carefully. ● Cardiac arrythmias (except VF) will usually revert spontaneously with re-warming and do not need treatment unless they persist after re-warming.
Oxygen	If the patient is hypoxaemic, administer high levels of supplemental oxygen and aim for a target saturation within the range 94–98% – refer to oxygen guideline.

Hypothermia

Table 3.43 – ASSESSMENT and MANAGEMENT of:

Hypothermia *continued*

Fluid therapy	● If fluid therapy is indicated, refer to **intravascular fluid therapy guidelines**. NB The use of cold fluids should be avoided if possible. ● **DO NOT** delay on scene for fluid replacement; administer en-route.
Blood glucose	● Measure blood glucose level, if <4.0 mmol/l treat for hypoglycaemia (**refer to glycaemic emergencies guidelines**).
Vital signs	● Monitor ECG. ● Respiratory rate may be very slow – measure for 10 seconds.
Transfer	● Transfer patients to nearest appropriate receiving hospital. ● In severe hypothermia, the fastest way to re-warm patients is by extracorporeal warming: – this may not be available in every hospital so follow any local care pathways. ● Continue management en-route. ● Complete documentation. [92]
	Additional information for cardiac arrest in hypothermia: Follow the usual procedure (refer to appropriate resuscitation guidelines) with the following minor changes: ● **Signs of life** – because the heart rate and respiratory rate may be slow and difficult to detect, look for signs of life (palpate central artery, ECG monitoring etc) for up to 1 minute. ● Hypothermia may cause chest wall stiffness, and ventilations and compressions may be more difficult. ● Drugs are less likely to be effective at low body temperatures: do not give drugs if the core temperature is below 30°C. ● Defibrillation is less likely to be effective at low body temperatures: if VF persists after 3 shocks, delay further defibrillation until the core temperature is above 30°C. ● **DO NOT STOP CARDIAC RESUSCITATION IN THE FIELD,** hypothermia is protective and good outcomes have resulted from prolonged resuscitation of hypothermic patients. **Trauma** (refer to appropriate trauma guidelines) – hypothermia worsens the prognosis of trauma patients, so it is important that patients who are initially normothermic, are not allowed to become hypothermic. This may occur for example during a prolonged extrication from a road traffic collision or from the cooling of burns.

3 Medical Specific Conditions — SECTION

KEY POINTS

Hypothermia

● Hypothermia is defined as a core body temperature below 35°C.

● There are three main classifications depending on the speed at which a person loses heat: acute, subacute, and chronic hypothermia.

● Prevent further heat loss; wrap the patient appropriately, do not rub the skin or give alcohol.

● Patients with decreased level of consciousness may develop VF or pulseless VT and should be immobilised and managed horizontally.

● Cardiac arrest is treated in the usual way, bearing in mind that drugs/defibrillation are less likely to be effective at low body temperatures.

1. Introduction

- Sickle cell disease is a hereditary condition affecting the haemoglobin contained within red blood cells.

- A previous history of sickle cell disease and sickle cell crisis will be present in most cases, with the patient almost always being aware of their condition.

- The signs and symptoms include (**any of those listed below may apply**):
  - severe pain, most commonly in the long bones and/or joints of the arms and legs, but also in the back and abdomen
  - stroke
  - high temperature
  - difficulty in breathing, reduced oxygen (O_2) saturation, cough and chest pain may indicate acute chest syndrome
  - pallor
  - tiredness/weakness
  - dehydration
  - headache
  - priapism.

2. Incidence

- There are different types of sickle cell disease found mainly in people of African or Afro-Caribbean origin, but these can also affect people of Mediterranean, Middle Eastern and Asian origin. In the United Kingdom it is estimated that 15,000 adults and children suffer from sickle cell disease with 1 in every 2,000 babies born with the condition.

3. Severity and Outcome

- These painful crises can result in damage to the patient's lungs, kidneys, liver, bones and other organs and tissues. The recurrent nature of these acute episodes is the most disabling feature of sickle cell disease, and many chronic problems can result, including leg ulcers, blindness and stroke. Acute chest syndrome[a] is the leading cause of death amongst sickle cell patients.

4. Pathophysiology

- The red cells of patients with sickle cell disease are prone to assuming a permanently sickled shape when exposed to a variety of factors including hypoxia, cold or dehydration. These cells are prone to mechanical damage, hence the haemolytic anaemia in this group of patients, and to occluding the microvasculature leading to tissue hypoxia and pain and end organ damage.

- A crisis may follow as a result of an infection, during pregnancy, following surgery or a variety of other causes including mental stress.

5. Assessment and Management

For the assessment and management of patients with sickle cell crisis refer to Table 3.44 or Figure 3.6.

KEY POINTS

Sickle Cell Crisis

- **Sickle cell disease is a hereditary condition affecting the haemoglobin contained within red blood cells; the cells are irregular in shape and occlude the microvasculature leading to tissue ischaemia.**

- **Sickle cell crises can result in damage to the lungs, kidneys, liver, bones and other organs and tissues.**

- **Sickle cell crises can be very painful and patients should be offered pain relief.**

- **In sickle cell crisis and acute chest syndrome, aim for an oxygen saturation of 94–98% or aim for the saturation level that is usual for the individual patient.**

- **Patients with sickle cell disease can be dangerously ill but in no pain (e.g. aplastic crisis, stroke, hepatic sequestration, PE, etc).**

- **Acute chest syndrome is a leading cause of death amongst sickle cell patients and is characterised by hypoxia and tachypnoea.**

---

[a] **Acute Chest Syndrome (also known as chest crisis).** This is a common and potentially life-threatening complication of painful crises, and is often precipitated by a chest infection. The patient becomes breathless, hypoxic and tachypnoeic/tachycardic over a short period of time. Chest pain is often present, and the hypoxia responds poorly to inhaled oxygen. Crackles are often present in the lung bases and will ascend rapidly to involve the whole lung fields in severe cases. Radiological changes follow late and patients may be critically ill with near normal radiology. If a chest crisis is suspected, treatment should be initiated with inhaled oxygen and intravenous fluids. In hospital, intravenous antibiotics and urgent exchange transfusion are likely to be instituted after discussion with the haematology team. Intensive care and mechanical ventilation may be required in some cases. Pulmonary embolus is an important differential diagnosis.

Sickle Cell Crisis

Table 3.44 – ASSESSMENT and MANAGEMENT of:

Sickle Cell Crisis

ASSESSMENT	MANAGEMENT

● Assess ABCD	● If any of the following **TIME CRITICAL** features present:
	  – major **ABCD** problems
	  – acute chest syndrome[a], then:
	● Start correcting **A** and **B** and undertake a **TIME CRITICAL** transfer to nearest receiving hospital.
	● Continue patient management en-route.
	● Provide an alert/information call.

● Ask the patient if they have an individualised treatment plan	● Follow the treatment plan if available. ● The patient will often be able to guide their care. ● Follow **medical emergencies guideline** in addition to the specific management detailed below.
● Oxygen	Administer supplemental oxygen to **ALL** patients including those with chronic sickle lung disease; oxygen helps to counter tissue hypoxia and reduce cell clumping. ● **Adults** – administer supplemental oxygen via an appropriate nasal mask/cannula until a reliable SpO_2 measurement is available; then adjust the oxygen flow to aim for target saturation within the range of 94–98%. ● **Children** – administer high levels of supplemental oxygen. ● Apply pulse oximeter. NB It is safer to over-oxygenate until a reliable SpO_2 measurement is available.
● ECG	● Undertake a 12-lead ECG in patients with chest pain to exclude obvious cardiac causes (**refer to acute coronary syndrome guideline**).
● Fluid	Patients with a sickle cell crisis will not have acute fluid loss, but may present with dehydration if they have been ill for an extended period of time. ● If fluid resuscitation is indicated (refer to intravascular fluid therapy guideline).
● Pain management	● Offer **ALL** patients pain relief. ● **Entonox** – administer initially but do not administer for extended periods (refer to Entonox guideline). ● **Opiate analgesia** – administer orally or subcutaneously rather than intravenously if possible (refer to morphine guidelines). The dose should be guided by the patient's hand-held record if available, otherwise refer to **pain management guidelines**.
● Transfer to further care	● Transfer to specialist unit where the patient is usually treated. ● Patients should not walk to the ambulance as this will exacerbate the effects of hypoxia in the tissues.

[a] **Acute Chest Syndrome (also known as chest crisis).** This is a common and potentially life-threatening complication of painful crises, and is often precipitated by a chest infection. The patient becomes breathless, hypoxic and tachypnoeic/tachycardic over a short period of time. Chest pain is often present, and the hypoxia responds poorly to inhaled oxygen. Crackles are often present in the lung bases and will ascend rapidly to involve the whole lung fields in severe cases. Radiological changes follow late and patients may be critically ill with near normal radiology. If a chest crisis is suspected, treatment should be initiated with inhaled oxygen and intravenous fluids. In hospital, intravenous antibiotics and urgent exchange transfusion are likely to be instituted after discussion with the haematology team. Intensive care and mechanical ventilation may be required in some cases. Pulmonary embolus is an important differential diagnosis.

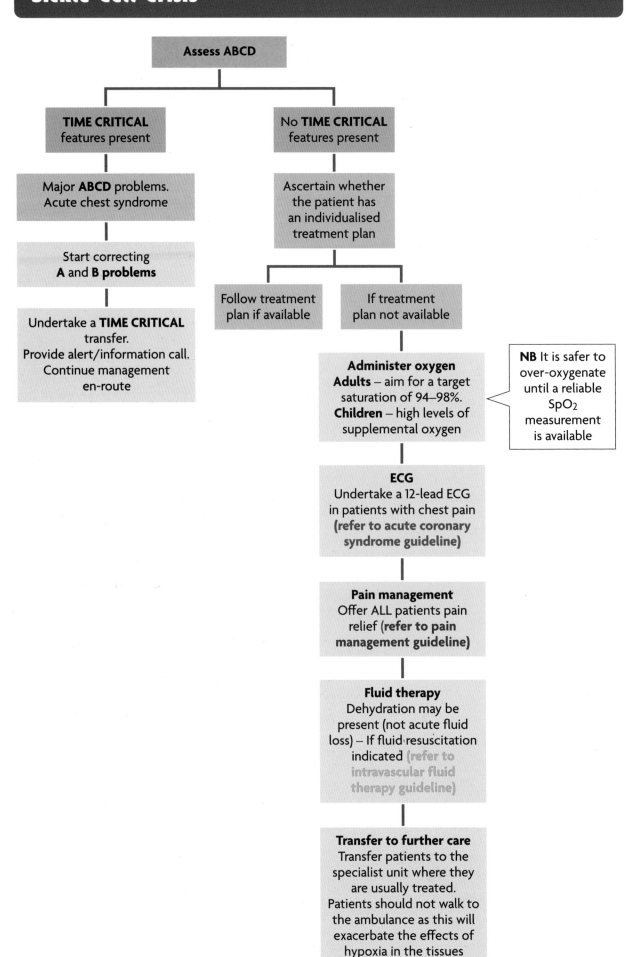

Assess ABCD

TIME CRITICAL features present

Major **ABCD** problems. Acute chest syndrome

Start correcting **A and B problems**

Undertake a **TIME CRITICAL** transfer. Provide alert/information call. Continue management en-route

No **TIME CRITICAL** features present

Ascertain whether the patient has an individualised treatment plan

Follow treatment plan if available

If treatment plan not available

Administer oxygen
Adults – aim for a target saturation of 94–98%.
Children – high levels of supplemental oxygen

NB It is safer to over-oxygenate until a reliable SpO2 measurement is available

ECG
Undertake a 12-lead ECG in patients with chest pain **(refer to acute coronary syndrome guideline)**

Pain management
Offer ALL patients pain relief **(refer to pain management guideline)**

Fluid therapy
Dehydration may be present (not acute fluid loss) – If fluid resuscitation indicated (refer to intravascular fluid therapy guideline)

Transfer to further care
Transfer patients to the specialist unit where they are usually treated. Patients should not walk to the ambulance as this will exacerbate the effects of hypoxia in the tissues

Figure 3.6 – Assessment and management algorithm for sickle cell crisis.

Meningococcal Meningitis and Septicaemia [183, 185, 324–337]

1. Introduction

- Meningococcal disease is the leading cause of death by infection in children and young adults and can kill a healthy person of any age within hours of their first symptoms.

2. Incidence

- There are 1,200 confirmed cases of meningococcal disease in England and Wales each year, although the true figure is probably twice this number.

3. Pathophysiology

- Two clinical categories are described, although they often overlap:
  i. meningitis.
  ii. septicaemia.

- In meningitis, the meninges covering the brain and spinal cord are infected by bacteria causing inflammation.

- In septicaemia, bacteria invade the bloodstream, releasing toxins and producing a clinical picture of shock and circulatory collapse. Deterioration can be rapid and may be irreversible, with treatment becoming less effective by the minute. Early recognition and prompt treatment improves clinical outcomes.

4. Severity and Outcome

- The mortality from septicaemia can be up to 40% but if recognised early, resuscitated aggressively and managed on ITU, mortalities of less than 5% can be achieved.

5. Assessment

- **Refer to medical emergencies in adults or children**.
- The 'classical features' – **neck stiffness, photophobia** and **haemorrhagic rash** – should be sought and are useful clinical discriminators when present, but less helpful and potentially falsely reassuring when absent.
- These features are more common in adults, older children and teenagers but quite rare in pre-school children. Small children often present with non-specific signs such as nausea, vomiting, loss of appetite, sore throat and coryzal symptoms – features that might otherwise suggest a diagnosis of viral illness.

Airway:
- Added sounds (e.g. grunting).
- Upper airway obstruction (e.g. coma, fitting).

Breathing:[a]
- Respiratory rate.
- Breathing effort.
- Oxygen saturations (SaO_2).

Circulation:[a]
- Pulse.
- Capillary refill time.

Disability:
- **A** Alert
- **V** Responds to voice
- **P** Responds to painful stimulus
- **U** Unresponsive

Expose:
- Examine for rashes (see below).
- Measure temperature if appropriate.

The patient may have been previously unwell with non-specific symptoms, for example

- Irritability.
- Pyrexia.
- 'Flu-like' symptoms.

THE RASH

Presentation – the classical, haemorrhagic, non-blanching rash (may be petechial or purpuric) is seen in approximately 40% of infected children.

In pigmented skin it can be helpful to look at the conjunctiva under the lower eyelid.

In an unwell patient, a non-blanching rash suggests meningococcal septicaemia.

The 'glass' or 'tumbler' test

A petechial or purpuric rash does **NOT** blanch/fade when pressed with a glass tumbler, **remaining visible through the glass.**

If the 'glass' test is negative, do not assume that meningococcal disease has been excluded; often there will be **NO** rash.

If meningococcal disease is suspected in any patient (irrespective of the presence or absence of a rash) undertake a TIME CRITICAL transfer (refer to Figure 3.7).

CLINICAL FINDINGS

The patient may be 'unwell' and deteriorate rapidly. Clinical features include:

- Fever (may be masked by peripheral shutdown or antipyretics).
- Cold, mottled skin (especially extremities) (the skin may rarely be warm and flushed; features of 'warm shock').
- Vomiting, abdominal pain and diarrhoea.
- Pain in joints, muscles and limbs.
- Rash – progressive petechial rash becoming purpuric – like a bruise or blood-blister. (NB These rashes are often **absent** at presentation.)
- Raised respiratory rate and effort.
- O_2 saturations – reduced or unrecordable (poor perfusion).
- Raised heart rate.
- Capillary refill time >2 seconds.
- Rigors.
- Seizures.

---

[a] For the 'normal' paediatric age-related respiratory and cardiovascular parameters **refer to medical emergencies in children – overview guideline**.

Level of consciousness:

- Alert/able to speak during early stages of shock.
- As shock advances:
  - **babies:** limp, floppy, drowsy, fitting
  - **older children and adults:** difficulty walking / standing, drowsiness, confusion, convulsions.

6. Management

- Open airway.

Oxygen:

- **Children:** administer high levels of supplemental oxygen (O_2).
- **Adults:** administer high levels of oxygen via a non rebreathing mask, ensuring oxygen saturations (SpO_2) of >94%.
- Consider assisted ventilation (rate: 12–20 breaths/min.) if:
  - SpO_2 is <90% on high concentration O_2
  - respiratory rate is <10 or >30
  - expansion is inadequate.
- Correct **A** and **B** problems at scene then **DO NOT DELAY TRANSFER** to nearest receiving hospital.
- When meningococcal septicaemia is suspected (e.g. a non-blanching rash is seen), administer **benzylpenicillin EN-ROUTE** to further care (**refer to Figure 3.7 and to benzylpenicillin guideline**). NB Meningococcal septicaemia can progress rapidly – the sooner antibiotics are administered the better.

Fluid therapy:

Hypovolaemia occurs in meningococcal septicaemia and requires fluid resuscitation (refer to intravascular fluid therapy guidelines).

- **DO NOT** delay at scene for fluid replacement; cannulate and give fluid **EN-ROUTE TO HOSPITAL** wherever possible.
- Measure blood glucose level and treat if necessary.
- Provide hospital alert message (include child's age if paediatric) en-route, repeat ABC assessments and manage as necessary.

7. Risk of Infection to Ambulance Personnel

- Meningococcal bacteria are very fragile and do not survive outside the nose and throat.
- Ambulance personnel directly exposed to large respiratory particles, droplets or secretions from patients with meningococcal disease should be offered preventative antibiotics. Such exposure is unlikely to occur unless working in very close proximity to the patient (e.g. inhaling droplets coughed or sneezed by the patient, or when undertaking airway management).
- If a case of meningococcal disease is confirmed, Public Health will provide antibiotics for exposed contacts who may otherwise be at increased risk of infection.

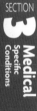

SECTION
3
Medical
Specific
Conditions

KEY POINTS

Meningococcal Meningitis and Septicaemia

- Meningococcal disease is the leading cause of death from infection in children and young adults. It can kill a healthy person of any age within hours of their first symptoms.
- Two clinical categories are described – meningitis and septicaemia – although they often overlap.
- Non-specific symptoms, such as pyrexia or a 'flu-like' illness may be the only clinical features at first presentation.
- Look for a rash; a non-blanching rash suggests meningococcal septicaemia (but is not universally present).
- Whenever meningococcal disease is suspected (irrespective of the presence or absence of a rash) undertake a TIME CRITICAL transfer.
- Administer benzylpenicillin if septicaemia is suspected. The illness progresses rapidly and early antibiotics improve outcomes.

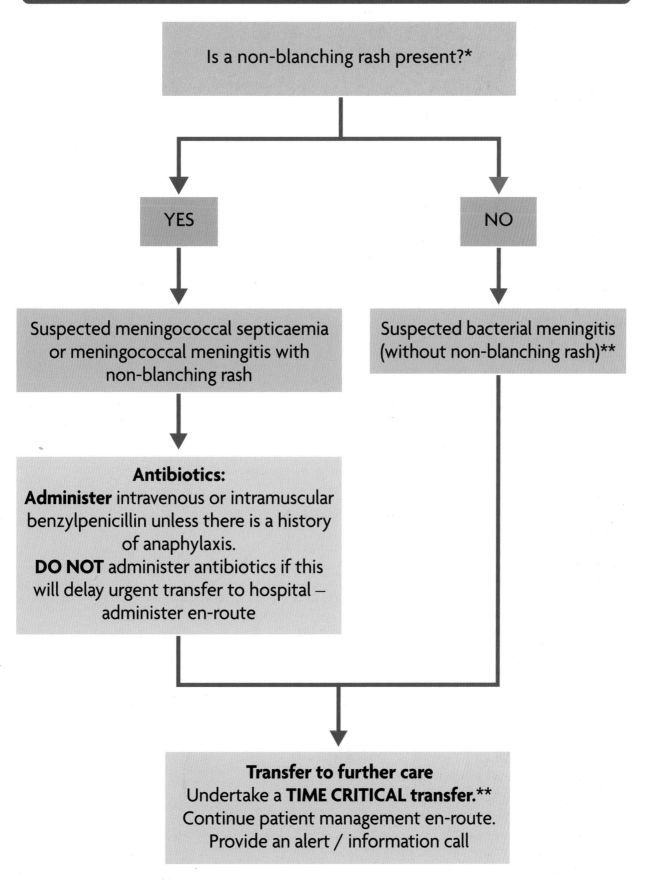

Figure 3.7 – Management algorithm for patients with suspected meningococcal disease.

* The term non-blanching rash is interchangeable with 'haemorrhagic rash', 'petechial rash' and 'purpuric rash'.

** If bacterial meningitis is suspected and urgent transfer is not possible, administer antibiotics even in the absence of a non-blanching rash.

Medical
Specific
Conditions

3
SECTION

1. Introduction

- Acute coronary syndrome (ACS) covers a range of conditions including:
  i. unstable angina
  ii. non-ST-segment-elevation myocardial infarction (NSTEMI)
  iii. ST-segment-elevation myocardial infarction (STEMI).

Chest pain is a cardinal, but not the only, symptom of ACS or 'heart attack' (refer to Table 3.45).

Table 3.45 – FEATURES OF DIFFERENT TYPES OF PAIN

Features which suggest a diagnosis of myocardial ischaemia include:

- Central chest pain.
- Crushing or constricting in nature.
- Persists for >15 minutes.
- Pain may also present in:
  - the shoulders
  - upper abdomen
  - referred to the neck, jaws and arm.

Features which suggest a diagnosis of stable angina include:

- Pain is typically related to exertion and tends to last minutes but should it persist for >15 minutes, or despite usual treatment, ACS is more likely.

- Coronary heart disease (CHD) is a major single cause of death in the UK.
- **Time is of the essence in restoring coronary blood flow in patients with ST-segment-elevation myocardial infarction (STEMI).**
- **The benefits of reperfusion with primary percutaneous coronary intervention (PPCI) or thrombolytic treatment are time-dependent.**
- **PPCI is now the most common form of reperfusion treatment.**
- Patients with STEMI who are ineligible for thrombolysis have a high mortality rate and should be referred for PPCI where facilities exist.

2. Incidence

- In 2010/11 the MINAP database recorded 79,863 heart attacks of which 40% were STEMI, but this is possibly an underestimation.

3. Severity and Outcome

- Approximately two-thirds of STEMI patients will die before they reach hospital.
- The risk of cardiac arrest from ventricular fibrillation (VF) or other arrhythmia is highest in the first few hours from symptom onset. VF can occur without warning.
- Survival from VF occurring in the presence of ambulance personnel with a defibrillator immediately available is as high as 40%. This falls rapidly to 2% or less if the defibrillator is not immediately available.
- Patients with NSTEMI and unstable angina manifestations of ACS are at significant risk of death and should be treated as medical emergencies.

4. Pathophysiology

- ACS occurs when there is an abrupt reduction in blood supply to the muscle of the heart; leading to myocardial ischaemia.
- Myocardial ischaemia is usually caused by a disruption of the internal artery wall, at the site of an atheroma plaque, causing a blood clot to form, occluding the coronary artery.

5. Assessment and Management

For assessment and management of ACS refer to Table 3.46 and Figure 3.8.

KEY POINTS

Acute Coronary Syndrome

- **Acute coronary syndrome refers to a spectrum of conditions.**
- **Always take defibrillator to the patient.**
- **Patients with ECG evidence of STEMI should be assessed for suitability for reperfusion with PPCI or thrombolysis according to local care pathways.**
- **Patients with NSTEMI remain at high risk and should be treated as a MEDICAL EMERGENCY.**

SECTION
3 Medical Specific Conditions

Table 3.46 – ASSESSMENT and MANAGEMENT of:

Acute Coronary Syndrome

NB A defibrillator must always be taken at the earliest opportunity to patients with symptoms suggestive of a heart attack and remain with the patient until hand-over to hospital staff.

ASSESSMENT	MANAGEMENT
● Assess ABCD	● If any of the following **TIME CRITICAL** features are present: 　– major ABC problems 　– 12-lead ECG shows STEMI or LBBB with other clinical features suggestive of ACS 　– suspected acute coronary syndrome with haemodynamic instability, then: ● Start correcting any **ABC** problems. ● Undertake a time **CRITICAL TRANSFER. NB For patients with STEMI undertake a direct admission to a 'cardiac facility'** (access to cardiological advice). ● Provide an alert/information call. ● Continue management en-route: 　– send a 12-lead ECG for expert review where possible 　– patients with ECG evidence of STEMI should be assessed for suitability for reperfusion treatment (refer to Figure 3.8) 　– administer aspirin as soon as possible (refer to the aspirin guideline) 　– administer **clopidogrel** (refer to the clopidogrel guideline) – follow local guidelines 　– administer **glyceryl trinitrate (GTN)** for patients with ongoing ischaemic discomfort (refer to the GTN guideline).
● Assess whether the chest pain may be cardiac	● Pain typically comes on over seconds and minutes rather than starting abruptly – 'classical presentation' is detailed in Table 3.45. NB Many patients do not have 'classical presentation' as described above and some people, especially the elderly, and those with diabetes, may not experience pain as their chief complaint. This group have a high mortality rate.
● Assess for accompanying features	● Nausea and vomiting. ● Marked sweating. ● Breathlessness. ● Pallor. ● Combination of chest pain associated with haemodynamic instability. ● Feelings of impending doom. ● Skin that is clammy and cold to the touch. **NB These may not always be present.**
● ECG	● **DO NOT exclude an ACS where patients have a normal resting 12-lead ECG.** ● Use clinical judgement as to whether a repeat 12-lead ECG is required after normal or equivocal ECG but history suggestive of ACS (continuing or worsening pain or heamodynamic instability).
● Assess oxygen saturation	● Closely monitor the patient's SpO_2 but do not administer oxygen unless the patient is hypoxaemic on air (SpO_2 <94%) (refer to oxygen guidelines).
● Undertake further assessment and management in the order appropriate to the circumstances	● Monitor ECG for arrhythmias. ● Obtain intravenous access if clinically indicated. ● Monitor vital signs. ● Repeat dose of GTN if chest discomfort persists. ● 12-lead ECG (as above).
● Assess patient's pain	● Measure and record pain score (**refer to pain management guideline**). ● Consider analgesia (**refer to pain management guideline**).
● Documentation	● Complete documentation. [92]
	Additional Information: ● The treatment of patients with ACS is a rapidly developing area of practice. ● National and international standards and guidelines for ACS care consistently emphasise the importance of rapid access to defibrillation and reperfusion and specialist cardiological care. ● Pre-alerting the hospital can speed up appropriate treatment of STEMI patients. ● Pre-hospital thrombolysis may be an option where PPCI is not available, but patients can subsequently be transferred to a PPCI capable hospital.

3 Medical
Specific Conditions
SECTION

Acute Coronary Syndrome

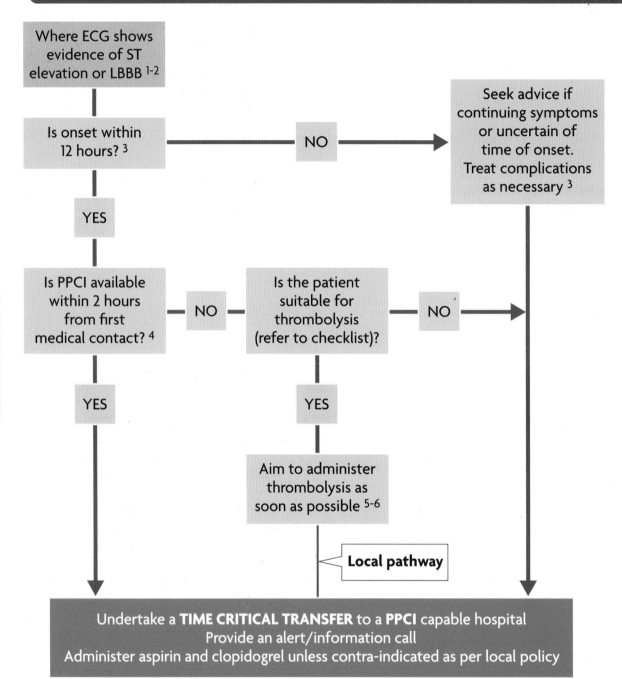

Where ECG shows evidence of ST elevation or LBBB [1-2]

Is onset within 12 hours? [3]

NO → Seek advice if continuing symptoms or uncertain of time of onset. Treat complications as necessary [3]

YES

Is PPCI available within 2 hours from first medical contact? [4]

NO → Is the patient suitable for thrombolysis (refer to checklist)?

NO →

YES

YES

Aim to administer thrombolysis as soon as possible [5-6]

Local pathway

Undertake a **TIME CRITICAL TRANSFER** to a **PPCI** capable hospital
Provide an alert/information call
Administer aspirin and clopidogrel unless contra-indicated as per local policy

1. Up to a third of patients with MI will have atypical presentations such as shortness of breath or collapse, without chest pain. This is particularly so in patients with diabetes or the elderly. **Have a low threshold for performing a 12-lead ECG in any patient presenting as 'unwell'.** Seek advice in 'atypical' patients who have ST elevation or LBBB (see below) as urgent reperfusion may still be indicated.

2. ECG criteria for reperfusion include ST segment elevation ($\geq$ 2mm in 2-standard or 2 adjacent precordial leads, not including V1) or **LBBB** in patients with other clinical features suggestive of ACS. Patients who have ST depression rather than elevation are a high risk group who need urgent specialist assessment. **Seek advice.**

3. If there is uncertainty about the time of symptom onset, or any ongoing chest pain/discomfort or haemodynamic upset beyond 12 hours, seek advice as urgent reperfusion may still be indicated.

4. Refer to local policies for target 'call to balloon' time.

5. Thrombolytic treatment should not be regarded as the end of the emergency care of a STEMI patient. Rapid transfer to an appropriate hospital for timely therapy to prevent re-infarction, and assessment of the need for rescue PPCI, is essential.

6. Refer to reteplase or tenecteplase guidelines for the checklist to identify eligibility for pre-hospital thrombolysis.

Figure 3.8 – The management of patients presenting with STEMI or LBBB.

1. Introduction

- The incidence of allergic reactions continues to rise.
- The symptoms range from mild to life-threatening and include:
  - urticaria (hives)
  - itching
  - angio-oedema (swelling of the face, eyelids, lips and tongue)
  - a petechial or purpuric rash
  - dyspnoea
  - wheeze
  - stridor
  - hypoxia
  - hypotension
  - abdominal pain
  - diarrhoea/vomiting.
- The most common triggers are food, drugs and venom (refer to Table 3.47) but in 30% of cases the trigger is unknown.
- Injected allergens commonly result in cardiovascular compromise, with hypotension and shock predominating.
- Slow release drugs prolong absorption and exposure to the allergen.

Table 3.47 – COMMON TRIGGERS OF ALLERGIC REACTIONS

1 – Foods

Nuts (e.g. peanuts, walnut, almond, brazil, and hazel), pulses, sesame seeds, milk, eggs, fish/shellfish.

2 – Venom – insect sting/bites

Insect stings and bites (e.g. wasps and bees).

NB Bees may leave a venom sac which should be scraped off (not squeezed).

3 – Drugs

Antibiotics (e.g. penicillin, cephalosporin, ciprofloxacin, and vancomycin), non-steroidal anti-inflammatory drugs, angiotensin converting enzyme inhibitor, gelatins, protamine, vitamin K, amphotericin, etoposide, acetazolamide, pethidine, local anaesthetic, diamorphine, streptokinase.

4 – Other causes

Latex[a], hair dye, semen and hydatid.

2. Incidence

- It is estimated that allergic reactions affect 30% of adults, with anaphylaxis estimated to affect up to 2% of the population.

3. Severity and Outcome

- The severity of symptoms varies from a localised urticaria to life-threatening pulmonary and/or cardiovascular compromise – anaphylaxis.
- Generally, the longer it takes for anaphylactic symptoms to develop, the less severe the overall reaction.

- Some patients relapse after an apparent recovery (biphasic response), therefore, patients who have experienced an anaphylactic reaction should be transferred to hospital for further evaluation.
- The mortality associated with anaphylaxis is estimated to be <1%. Death occurs quickly (venom: 10–15 minutes; food: 30–35 minutes) after contact with the trigger usually as a result of respiratory arrest from airway obstruction.

4. Assessment and Management

For the assessment and management of anaphylaxis and allergic reactions refer to Figure 3.9.

Patients with previous episodes:

- May wear 'MedicAlert®' bracelets/necklets.
- Carry an adrenaline pen.
- May experience panic attacks.

KEY POINTS

Allergic Reactions including Anaphylaxis (Adults)

- **Remove from trigger if possible.**
- **Anaphylaxis can occur despite a long history of previously safe exposure to a potential trigger.**
- **Consider anaphylaxis in the presence of acute cutaneous symptoms and airway or cardiovascular compromise.**
- **Anaphylaxis may be rapid, slow or biphasic.**
- **Adrenaline is key in managing anaphylaxis.**
- **The benefit of using appropriate doses of adrenaline far exceeds any risk.**
- **Half doses of adrenaline are no longer recommended for anaphylaxis in patients who are prescribed beta-blockers or tricyclic anti-depressants and a standard adult dose should be administered.**

[a] Latex allergy has implications for equipment use.

Allergic Reactions including Anaphylaxis (Adults)

Quickly remove from trigger if possible (e.g. environmental, infusion etc).
DO NOT delay definitive treatment if removing trigger not feasible

Assess ABCDE
If **TIME CRITICAL** features present - correct **A** and **B** and
transfer to nearest appropriate receiving hospital.
Provide an alert/information call

Consider mild/moderate allergic reaction if:
onset of illness is minutes to hours
AND
cutaneous findings (e.g. urticaria
and /or angio-oedema)

Consider chlorphenamine
(refer to chlorphenamine guideline)

Consider anaphylaxis if:
Sudden onset and rapid progression
Airway and/or **Breathing problems** (e.g.
dyspnoea, hoarseness, stridor, wheeze,
throat or chest tightness)
and/or **Circulation** (e.g. hypotension,
syncope, pronounced tachycardia)
and/or **Skin** (e.g. erythema, urticaria,
mucosal changes) problems

Administer high levels of supplementary
oxygen and aim for a target saturation
within the range of 94–98%
(refer to oxygen guideline)

Administer adrenaline (IM only)
(refer to adrenaline guideline)

If haemodynamically compromised
consider fluid therapy
(refer to fluid therapy guideline)

Consider chlorphenamine
(refer to chlorphenamine guideline)

Consider administering hydrocortisone
(refer to hydrocortisone guideline)

Consider nebulised salbutamol for
bronchospasm (refer to salbutamol
guideline)

Monitor and re-assess ABC
Monitor ECG, PEFR (if possible),
BP and pulse oximetry en-route

Figure 3.9 – Allergic reactions including anaphylaxis algorithm.

Asthma (Adults) [103, 293, 358–359]

1. Introduction

- Asthma is one of the commonest of all medical conditions. Asthma has varying levels of severity and patients usually present to pre-hospital care with one of four presentations: mild/moderate, severe, life-threatening, and near fatal (refer to Table 3.48).

- Typically in patients requiring hospital admission the symptoms will have developed gradually over a number of hours (>6 hours). Usually patients are known asthmatics and may be on regular inhaler therapy for this. Patients may have used their own treatment inhalers and in some cases will have used a home-based nebuliser.

- Patients may report a history of increased wheezy breathlessness, often worse at night or in the early morning, associated either with infection, allergy or exertion as a trigger.

2. Incidence

- Asthma is rare in the elderly population and practitioners should be aware that many people will describe a range of other respiratory conditions as 'asthma', and therefore other causes of breathlessness need to be considered.

- In adults, asthma may often be complicated and mixed in with a degree of bronchitis, especially in smokers. This can make the condition much more difficult to treat, both routinely and in emergencies. The majority of asthmatic patients take regular 'preventer' and 'reliever' inhalers.

3. Severity and Outcome

- The obstruction in its most severe form can be **TIME CRITICAL** and some 2,000 people a year die as a result of asthma. Patients with severe asthma and one or more risk factor(s) (refer to Table 3.49) are at risk of death.

- In patients ≤40 years, deaths from asthma peak in July/August in contrast to patients aged >40 years where deaths peak in December/January.

4. Pathophysiology

- Asthma is caused by a chronic inflammation of the bronchi, making them narrower. The muscles around the bronchi become irritated and contract, causing sudden worsening of the symptoms. The inflammation can also cause the mucus glands to produce excessive sputum which further blocks the air passages.

- The obstruction and subsequent wheezing are caused by three factors within the bronchial tree:
  i. increased production of bronchial mucus
  ii. swelling of the bronchial tube mucosal lining cells
  iii. spasm and constriction of bronchial muscles.

  These three factors combine to cause blockage and narrowing of the small airways in the lung. Because inspiration is an active process involving the muscles of respiration, the obstruction of the airways is overcome on breathing in. Expiration occurs with muscle relaxation, and is severely delayed by the narrowing of the airways in asthma. This generates the wheezing on expiration that is characteristic of this condition.

Table 3.48 – FEATURES OF SEVERITY

Near-fatal asthma

- Raised $PaCO_2$ and/or requiring mechanical ventilation with raised inflation pressures.

Life-threatening asthma

Any one of the following in a patient with severe asthma:
- Altered conscious level.
- Exhaustion.
- Arrhythmia.
- Hypotension.
- Cyanosis.
- Silent chest.
- Poor respiratory effort.
- PEF <33% best or predicted.
- SpO_2 <92%.
- PaO_2 <8 kPa.
- 'Normal' $PaCO_2$ (4.6–6.0 kPa).

Acute severe asthma

Any one of:
- PEF 33–50% best or predicted.
- Respiratory rate ≥25/minute.
- Heart rate >110/minute.
- Inability to complete sentences in one breath.

Moderate asthma exacerbation

- Increasing symptoms.
- PEF >50–75% best or predicted.
- No features of acute severe asthma.

Table 3.49 – RISK FACTORS FOR DEVELOPING NEAR-FATAL ASTHMA

Medical

- Previous near-fatal asthma (e.g. previous ventilation or respiratory acidosis).
- Previous hospital admission for asthma especially if in the last year requiring three or more classes of asthma medication.
- Heavy use of β2 agonist.
- Repeated emergency department attendance for asthma care especially if in the last year.
- Brittle asthma.

Psychological/behavioural

- Non-compliance with treatment or monitoring.
- Failure to attend appointments.
- Fewer GP contacts.
- Frequent home visits.
- Self-discharge from hospital.
- Psychosis, depression, other psychiatric illness or deliberate self-harm.
- Current or recent major tranquilliser use.
- Denial.
- Alcohol or drug abuse.
- Obesity.
- Learning difficulties.
- Employment problems.
- Income problems.
- Social isolation.
- Childhood abuse.
- Severe domestic, marital or legal stress.

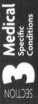

Section 3 Medical Specific Conditions

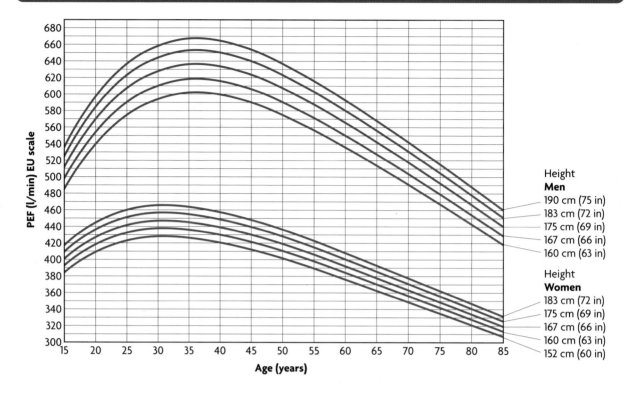

Figure 3.10 – Peak flow charts – Peak expiratory flow rate – normal values. For use with EU/EN13826 scale PEF meters only.[a]

[a] Adapted by Clement Clarke for use with EN13826 / EU scale peak flow meters from Nunn AJ Gregg I, Br Med J 1989:298;1068–70.

- Asthma is managed with a variety of inhaled and tablet medications. Inhalers are divided into two broad categories: preventer and reliever.

1. The preventer inhalers are normally anti-inflammatory drugs and these include steroids and other milder anti-inflammatories such as Tilade. The common steroid inhalers are beclomethasone (Becotide), budesonide (Pulmicort) and luticasone (Flixotide). These drugs act on the lung over a period of time to reduce the inflammatory reaction that causes the asthma. Regular use of these inhalers often eradicates all symptoms of asthma and allows for a normal lifestyle.

2. The reliever inhalers include salbutamol (Ventolin), terbutaline (Bricanyl), tiotropium (Spiriva) and ipratropium bromide (Atrovent). These inhalers work rapidly on the lung to relax the smooth muscle spasm when the patient feels wheezy or tight chested. They are used in conjunction with preventer inhalers. Inhalers are often used through large plastic spacer devices, such as the Volumatic. This allows the drug to spread into a larger volume and allows the patient to inhale it more effectively. In mild and moderate asthma attacks some patients may be treated with high doses of 'relievers' through a spacer device. This has been shown to be as effective as giving a salbutamol nebuliser.

5. Assessment

- Assess **ABCD** as per medical emergencies in adults overview, but specifically assess for the severity of the asthma attack (refer to asthma algorithm – Figure 3.11 and Table 3.48).

6. Management

- Refer to the asthma algorithm (Figure 3.11 and Table 3.50) for the management of mild/moderate, severe, life-threatening, and near-fatal.

For less severe attacks:

- Where possible the patient's own β2 agonist should be given (ideally using a spacer) as first line treatment. Increase the dose by two puffs every 2 minutes according to response up to ten puffs.

- If symptoms are not controlled by ten puffs, then start nebulised salbutamol whilst transferring to the emergency department.

- Patients (or friends/bystanders) who have previously experienced a severe asthma attack may be more likely to call for help early in the development of an attack, and the symptoms may appear mild on arrival of the ambulance.

- Some patients may be appropriate for alternative care pathways, for example, early referral to a general practitioner. However, apparently minor symptoms should not preclude onward referral especially where an alternative pathway is not readily accessible. Local care pathways should be followed where patients are considered for non conveyance. However, caution should be exercised in known severe asthmatics and robust safety netting of patients must be in place.

Peak expiratory flow rate (PEFR)

- Peak flow is a rapid measurement of the degree of obstruction in the patient's lungs. It measures the maximum flow on breathing out, or expiring and therefore can reflect the amount of airway obstruction. Whenever possible, peak flow should be performed before and after nebulised treatment. Many patients now have their own meter at home and know what their normal peak flow is. Clearly, when control is good, their peak flow will be equivalent to a normal patient's measurement, but during an attack it may drop markedly (refer to Figure 3.10).

KEY POINTS

Asthma in Adults
- Asthma is a common life-threatening condition.
- Its severity is often not recognised.
- Accurate documentation is essential.
- A silent chest is a pre-terminal sign.

Table 3.50 – ASSESSMENT and MANAGEMENT

Asthma

ASSESSMENT	MANAGEMENT

• Assess **ABCD**
 Specifically assess for the severity of the asthma attack (refer to Figure 3.11)
	• If any of the following **TIME CRITICAL** features present:
	   – major ABCD problems
	   – extreme difficulty in breathing or requirement for assisted ventilations
	   – exhaustion
	   – cyanosis
	   – silent chest
	   – SpO_2 <92%
	   – PEF <33% best or predicted.
	 • Start correcting A and B problems.
	 • Undertake a **TIME CRITICAL** transfer to nearest receiving hospital.
	 • Continue patient management en-route.
	 • Provide an alert/information call.

• Mild/moderate asthma
 Increasing symptoms, PEF >50–75% best or predicted, no features of acute severe asthma
	• Move to a calm quiet environment.
	 • Encourage use of own inhaler, using a spacer if available. Ensure correct technique is used (refer to Figure 3.11).
	 • If unresponsive:
	   – administer high levels of supplementary oxygen
	   – administer nebulised salbutamol (refer to salbutamol guideline).

• Severe asthma
 Any one of:
   – PEF 33–50% of best or predicted
   – Respiratory rate >25/minute
   – Heart rate >110/minute
   – Inability to complete sentences in one breath
	• Administer high levels of supplementary oxygen.
	 • Administer nebulised salbutamol (refer to salbutamol guideline).
	 • If no improvement administer ipratropium bromide (refer to ipratropium bromide guideline).
	 • Administer steroids (refer to relevant steroids guideline).
	 • Continuous salbutamol nebulisation may be administered unless clinically significant side effects occur (refer to salbutamol guideline).

• Life-threatening asthma
 Any one of:
   – Altered conscious level
   – Exhaustion
   – Arrhythmia
   – Hypotension
   – Cyanosis
   – Silent chest
   – Poor respiratory effort
   – PEF<33% best or predicted
   – SpO_2 <92%
	• Continuous salbutamol nebulisation may be administered unless clinically significant side effects occur (refer to salbutamol guideline).
	 • Administer adrenaline 1 in 1000 IM only (refer to adrenaline guideline).

• Near fatal asthma
   – Requiring bag-valve-mask ventilation with raised inflation pressures
   – Transfer
	• Positive pressure ventilation using a nebulising T piece. Assess for bilateral tension pneumothorax.
	 • Transfer rapidly to nearest receiving hospital.
	 • Provide an alert/information call.
	 • Continue patient management en-route.
	 • For cases of mild asthma that respond to treatment consider alternative care pathway where appropriate. Note: exercise caution in known severe asthmatics.

3 Medical Specific Conditions
SECTION

Asthma (Adults)

MILD/
MODERATE
ASTHMA

Move to a calm, quiet environment

Encourage use of own inhaler, preferably using a spacer.
Ensure correct technique is used; two puffs, followed by
two puffs every 2 minutes to a maximum of ten puffs

Administer high levels of
supplementary **oxygen**

Administer nebulised **salbutamol** using
an oxygen driven nebuliser
(refer to salbutamol guideline)

SEVERE
ASTHMA

If no improvement, administer
ipratropium bromide by nebuliser
(refer to ipratropium bromide guideline)

Administer steroids
(refer to relevant steroids guideline)

Continuous **salbutamol** nebulisation may be
administered unless clinically significant side
effects occur (refer to salbutamol guideline)

LIFE-
THREATENING
ASTHMA

Administer **adrenaline**
(refer to adrenaline guideline)

Positive pressure nebulise using a bag-valve-mask and 'T' piece.
Assess for bilateral tension pneumothorax and treat if present.
Provide an alert/information call

NEAR-FATAL
ASTHMA

As you progress through the treatment algorithm consider the
patient's overall response on the condition arrow and transfer
as indicated

IMPROVING

CONSIDER TRANSFER

DETERIORATING

TIME CRITICAL TRANSFER

Figure 3.11 – Asthma assessment and management algorithm.

Chronic Obstructive Pulmonary Disease [358, 360–369]

1. Introduction

- Chronic obstructive pulmonary disease (COPD) is a chronic progressive disorder characterised by airflow obstruction ('reduced post-bronchodilator FEV 1/FVC ratio (where FEV 1 is forced expiratory volume in 1 second and FVC is forced vital capacity), such that FEV 1/FVC is less than 0.7').

- A diagnosis of COPD is usually made in the presence of airflow obstruction in people >35 years of age, who are or were previously smokers and may have one or more risk factors (refer to Table 3.51).

Table 3.51 – SIGNS/SYMPTOMS OF COPD

Signs/symptoms
- Exertional breathlessness.
- Chronic cough.
- Regular sputum production.
- Frequent winter 'bronchitis'.
- Wheeze.
- No clinical features of asthma.

- Patients with COPD usually present to the ambulance service with an acute exacerbation of the underlying illness. COPD is a concomitant/secondary illness in many incidents with other chief complaints.

- Some patients with severe COPD may have an individualised treatment plan to assist in their care. This can be used to guide therapy.

2. Incidence

- It is estimated that approximately 3 million people have COPD affecting 2–4% of the population over 45 years of age. However, only 1.5% of the population are diagnosed with the condition.

- In the UK, COPD is the fifth leading cause of death and it is estimated that by 2020 it will be the third leading cause of death worldwide.

3. Severity and Outcome

- COPD results in disability and impaired quality of life leading to 30,000 deaths per annum in the UK.

- COPD is the second leading cause of emergency admission, with 130,000 cases per annum, in the UK and direct costs estimated at £800 million and indirect costs of £24 million.

4. Pathophysiology

- Airflow obstruction is the result of airway and parenchymal damage due to chronic inflammation.

- COPD increases the risk of co-morbidities such as lung cancer and cardiovascular disease.

- An acute exacerbation refers to a worsening of the patient's symptoms (refer to Table 3.52). There is no one feature that defines an exacerbation, although there are a number of known causes (refer to Table 3.54), however, in 30% of cases the cause is unknown.

- COPD patients generally have lower than normal SpO_2 levels and British Thoracic Society oxygen guidelines should be followed to maintain an SpO_2 of 88–92%.

- Some exacerbations are mild and self-limiting whilst others are more severe, potentially life-threatening, and require intervention – not all features will be present (refer to Table 3.52).

- Some conditions may present with symptoms similar to an exacerbation of COPD – consider these when diagnosing an exacerbation of COPD (refer to Table 3.53).

5. Assessment and Management

For assessment and management of chronic obstructive pulmonary disease refer to Table 3.55 and Figure 3.12.

Table 3.52 – FEATURES OF AN ACUTE EXACERBATION OF COPD

Features
- Increased dyspnoea – particularly on exertion.
- Increased sputum volume/purulence.
- Increased cough.
- Upper airway symptoms (e.g. colds and sore throats).
- Increased wheeze.
- Chest tightness.
- Reduced exercise tolerance.
- Fluid retention.
- Increased fatigue.
- Acute confusion.
- Worsening of a previously stable condition.

Severe features
- Marked dyspnoea.
- Tachypnoea.
- Purse lip breathing.
- Use of accessory respiratory muscles (sternomastoid and abdominal) at rest.
- Acute confusion.
- New-onset cyanosis.
- New-onset peripheral oedema.
- Marked reduction in activities of daily living.

Table 3.53 – CONDITIONS WITH SIMILAR FEATURES TO AN ACUTE EXACERBATION OF COPD

Features
- Asthma.
- Pneumonia.
- Pneumothorax.
- Left ventricular failure/pulmonary oedema.
- Pulmonary embolus.
- Lung cancer.
- Upper airway obstruction.
- Pleural effusion.
- Recurrent aspiration.

Table 3.54 – CAUSES OF EXACERBATION OF COPD

Infections

- Rhinoviruses (common cold).
- Influenza.
- Parainfluenza.
- Coronavirus.
- Adenovirus.
- Respiratory syncytial virus.
- *C. pneumoniae.*
- *H. influenzae.*
- *S. pneumoniae.*
- *M. catarrhalis.*
- *S. aureus.*
- *P. aeruginosa.*

Pollutants

- Nitrogen dioxide.
- Particulates.
- Sulphur dioxide.
- Ozone.

SECTION

3

Medical
Specific
Conditions

KEY POINTS

Chronic Obstructive Pulmonary Disease

- Early respiratory assessment (including oxygen saturation) is vital.
- If in doubt, provide oxygen therapy, titrating en-route, aiming for oxygen saturation of 88–92%.
- Provide nebulisation with salbutamol and assess response.

Chronic Obstructive Pulmonary Disease

Table 3.55 – ASSESSMENT and MANAGEMENT of:

Chronic Obstructive Pulmonary Disease

ASSESSMENT	MANAGEMENT

● Assess ABCD	● If any of the following **TIME CRITICAL** features present:
	  – major **ABCD** problems
	  – extreme breathing difficulty (by reference to patient's usual condition)
	  – cyanosis (although peripheral cyanosis may be 'normal' in some patients)
	  – exhaustion
	  – hypoxia (oxygen saturation <88%) unresponsive to oxygen (O_2) – COPD patients normally have a lower than normal oxygen saturation (SpO_2).
	● Start correcting **A** and **B** problems.
	● Undertake a **TIME CRITICAL** transfer to nearest receiving hospital.
	● Continue patient management en-route.
	● Provide an alert/information call.

● Ask the patient if they have an individualised treatment plan	● Follow the individualised treatment plan if available. ● The patient will often be able to guide their care.
Specifically assess: **Diagnosis**	● Assess whether this is an acute exacerbation of COPD – refer to Table 3.52 for the features of COPD. ● Or another condition – refer to Table 3.53 for conditions with similar features to an acute exacerbation of COPD. NB Chest pain and fever are uncommon symptoms of COPD – therefore consider other possible causes.
Airway	● Maintain airway patency. NB Noises (e.g. 'bubbling' or wheeze) associated with breathing indicating respiratory distress.
Breathing	● Note and monitor respiratory rate and effort.
● Bronchodilators	● Administer nebulised salbutamol (refer to salbutamol guideline) or, in severe cases, the initial nebulised salbutamol may be administered concurrently with ipratropium bromide (refer to ipratropium bromide guideline). ● If inadequate response after 5 minutes, a further dose of nebulised salbutamol may be administered. Ipratropium bromide may be given concurrently ONLY if not administered in initial nebulisation treatment (refer to ipratropium bromide guideline). ● Ipratropium can only be administered ONCE; salbutamol may be repeated at regular intervals unless the side effects of the drug become significant. NB Limit oxygen-driven nebulisation to 6 minutes. If journey time is significant, consider a further 6 minutes of nebulisation therapy ONLY if clinically indicated, but aim for a target saturation within the range of 88–92%.
● Position	● Position patient for comfort and ease of respiration – often sitting forwards – but be aware of potential hypotension.
● Oxygen[a]	● Measure oxygen saturation.[b] ● Administer supplemental oxygen; aim for a target saturation within the range of 88–92% or the prespecified range – refer to the patient's individualised treatment plan if available. NB The aim of oxygen therapy is to prevent life-threatening hypoxia – administer cautiously as a proportion of COPD sufferers are chronically hypoxic and when given oxygen may develop increasing drowsiness and loss of respiratory drive. If this occurs, reduce oxygen concentration and support ventilation if required.
● ECG	● Undertake a 12-lead ECG.
● Ventilation	● Consider non-invasive ventilation if not responding to treatment.
● Cardiorespiratory arrest	● Be prepared for cardiorespiratory arrest – refer to appropriate resuscitation guideline.
● Transfer	● Transfer rapidly to nearest receiving hospital. ● Provide an alert/information call. ● Continue patient mangement en-route. ● Consider alternative care pathway where appropriate.

[a] If the primary illness in a patient with COPD requires high concentration oxygen (refer to oxygen guideline) then this should **NOT BE WITHHELD.** The patient should be continually monitored closely for changes in respiratory rate and depth and the inspired concentration adjusted accordingly. In the short time that a patient is in ambulance care, hypoxia presents a much greater risk than hypercapnia in most cases.

[b] Pulse oximetry, whilst important in COPD patients, will not indicate carbon dioxide (CO_2) levels which are assessed by capnometry or more commonly, blood gas analysis in hospital.

Chronic Obstructive Pulmonary Disease

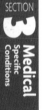

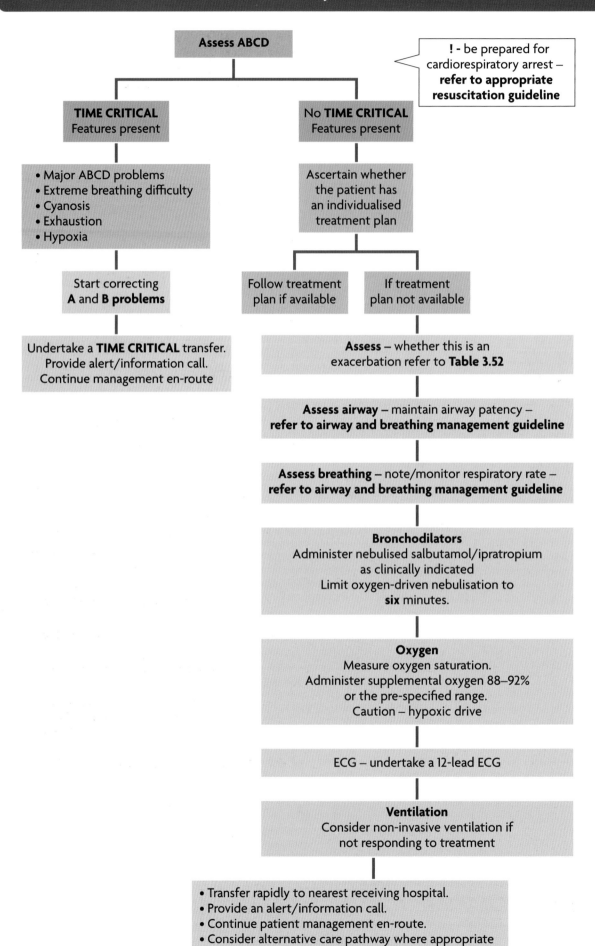

Assess ABCD

! - be prepared for cardiorespiratory arrest – **refer to appropriate resuscitation guideline**

TIME CRITICAL Features present

No **TIME CRITICAL** Features present

- Major ABCD problems
- Extreme breathing difficulty
- Cyanosis
- Exhaustion
- Hypoxia

Ascertain whether the patient has an individualised treatment plan

Start correcting **A** and **B problems**

Follow treatment plan if available

If treatment plan not available

Undertake a **TIME CRITICAL** transfer. Provide alert/information call. Continue management en-route

Assess – whether this is an exacerbation refer to **Table 3.52**

Assess airway – maintain airway patency – **refer to airway and breathing management guideline**

Assess breathing – note/monitor respiratory rate – **refer to airway and breathing management guideline**

Bronchodilators
Administer nebulised salbutamol/ipratropium as clinically indicated
Limit oxygen-driven nebulisation to **six** minutes.

Oxygen
Measure oxygen saturation.
Administer supplemental oxygen 88–92% or the pre-specified range.
Caution – hypoxic drive

ECG – undertake a 12-lead ECG

Ventilation
Consider non-invasive ventilation if not responding to treatment

- Transfer rapidly to nearest receiving hospital.
- Provide an alert/information call.
- Continue patient management en-route.
- Consider alternative care pathway where appropriate

Figure 3.12 – Assessment and management of chronic obstructive pulmonary disease algorithm.

1. Introduction

- Convulsion, seizure, and fit are all terms used to describe an 'an abnormal and excessive depolarisation of a set of neurons in the brain'.

- Clinical presentation depends on the area of the brain affected by the depolarisation, the cause and age. Often patients experience a period of involuntary muscular contraction, followed by a **post-ictal** recovery period, often characterised by lethargy and confusion and, in some cases, profound sleep. It is not uncommon for patients to act out of character when in the post-ictal state. This may include verbal or physical aggression. Oxygen therapy, in line with BTS guidelines, and a calm approach are important.

- There are a number of types of convulsion:

  - **epileptic** – neurological condition resulting in recurrent convulsions. Persistent and continual convulsions lasting >30 minutes are termed **status epilepticus and are potentially life-threatening**
  - **eclamptic** – occurs peri-natally and is often associated with pregnancy induced hypertension.

2. Incidence

2.1 Epilepsy

- Epilepsy affects 50 per 100,000 per annum in the UK. Convulsions affect 60% of patients, with two-thirds experiencing focal and one-third generalised tonic-clonic convulsions.

- Approximately 30% of sufferers develop chronic epilepsy; the remainder will experience a period of remission, being convulsion-free for five years.

  The number of convulsions experienced varies:
  - 33% – <1 per year
  - 33% – 1–12 per year
  - 33% – 1 per month.

- Patients with chronic epilepsy may present regularly to the Ambulance Service.

2.2 Eclamptic convulsion

- For information regarding the incidence of eclamptic convulsion **refer to pregnancy induced hypertension (including eclampsia)**.

3. Severity and Outcome

- In 80% of cases convulsions will have stopped after 10 minutes. However, seizures lasting 5 minutes or more and serial seizures of three or more in an hour are medical emergencies.

3.1 Epilepsy

- In a few cases, sudden death, termed 'sudden unexpected death in epilepsy (SUDEP)', can occur during a convulsion and results in 500 deaths per year in the UK. This is often due to non-compliance with medication.

- In patients recently diagnosed with epilepsy, death is generally a result of an underlying disease (e.g. vascular disease, tumour).

3.2 Fever

- A fever can reduce the threshold for a convulsion when there is underlying pathology. Investigation and treatment are indicated to prevent recurrence.

3.3 Eclamptic convulsion

- For information regarding the severity and outcome of eclamptic convulsion **refer to pregnancy induced hypertension (including eclampsia)**.

4. Pathophysiology

- The classification of convulsion is based on clinical presentation and underlying neurological disorder.

4.1 Epilepsy

- There are a number of causes of epilepsy (see above). However, in some cases the cause remains unknown. In newly diagnosed, or suspected epilepsy, in 60% of cases the cause is unknown.

- The commonest presentation to ambulance services is the tonic/clonic seizure, previously known as 'grand mal'.

4.2 Eclamptic convulsion

- See above.

5. Assessment and Management

- For the assessment and management of convulsion in adults refer to Table 3.56 and Figure 3.13.

KEY POINTS

Convulsions (Adults)

- **Most tonic/clonic convulsions are self-limiting and do not require drug treatment.**

- **Convulsions may be caused by other medical conditions (e.g. hypoxia, hypoglycaemia), which may be easily treated.**

- **Administer drugs if convulsion lasts longer than 5 minutes.**

- **Assume eclampsia as a cause of the convulsion in the peri-natal patient.**

- **Only consider leaving a patient at home who makes a full recovery following a convulsion if they are known to suffer from epilepsy, and can be supervised adequately.**

- **Consider referral to local epilepsy service for review/follow-up.**

Medical
Specific
Conditions

3
SECTION

Table 3.56 – ASSESSMENT and MANAGEMENT of:

Convulsions in Adults

NB Always take a defibrillator to a convulsing patient – this may be the presenting sign of circulatory arrest at the onset of sudden cardiac arrest.

ASSESSMENT	MANAGEMENT
● Assess **ABCD**	● If any of the following **TIME CRITICAL** features present: – major **ABCD** problems – **hypoxia may cause convulsions** – serious head injury – status epilepticus – following failed treatment – underlying infection (e.g. meningococcal septicaemia) (refer to benzylpenicillin guideline), then: – eclampsia – **refer to pregnancy induced hypertension (including eclampsia)**, then: ● Start correcting **A** and **B** problems. ● Check blood glucose to ensure hypoglycaemia is identified and treated. ● Undertake a **TIME CRITICAL** transfer to nearest receiving hospital if the patient can be moved despite convulsing – it is important to reach hospital for definitive care as rapidly as possible. ● Continue patient management en-route. ● Provide an alert/information call.
If not **TIME CRITICAL**	● Take a history from patient/eyewitness – if possible, to ascertain if a convulsion has occurred.
If the patient is known to suffer from epilepsy, check if they have an individualised treatment plan	● Follow the individualised treatment plan if available. ● Patients are usually on anti-epileptic medication such as phenytoin, sodium valproate (Epilim), carbamazepine (Tegretol), and lamotrigine (Lamictal).
Specifically assess: **Type of convulsion**	Ascertain type of convulsion if still convulsing: ● Epileptic. ● Eclamptic convulsion (**refer to pregnancy induced hypertension (including eclampsia) guideline**).
Blood glucose level	● Convulsion may be a presenting sign of **HYPOGLYCAEMIA** – consider in **ALL** cases. ● Check blood glucose level if <4.0 mmol/l or clinically suspected, administer glucose (**refer to glycaemic emergencies guideline;** glucose 10% guideline and glucagon guideline).
Heart rate and rhythm	● Monitor heart rate and rhythm for **ARRHYTHMIA (refer to cardiac rhythm disturbance guideline)**, for example a burst of rapid ventricular tachycardia may drop the blood pressure, and cause transient cerebral **HYPOXIA**, giving rise to a convulsion.
Temperature	● A raised temperature and any sign of a rash may indicate meningococcal septicaemia (**refer to meningococcal septicaemia guideline**). NB Patients often feel warm to touch following generalised convulsions due to the heat generated by excessive muscular activity.
Blood pressure	● Severe hypotension can trigger a convulsion (e.g. with syncope or a vasovagal attack where the patient remains propped up). ● In these instances there will usually be a clear precipitating event and no prior history of epilepsy. Once the patient lies flat and the blood pressure is restored the convulsion may stop.
Alcohol/drug usage	● Convulsions are more common in alcoholics, are associated with hypoglycaemia and can be triggered by a number of prescription or illegal drugs (e.g. tricyclic antidepressants) – **refer to glycaemic emergencies guideline**.
Injury	● Assess for mouth/tongue injury – often accompanies an epileptic convulsion. ● Is there any history of head injury? ● Dislocated shoulder. ● Road traffic collision may have resulted from a convulsion – **refer to appropriate trauma guideline**. NB Wherever possible, obtain contact details of any witnesses and pass this to the receiving hospital.
Incontinence	● Often accompanies a convulsion.

SECTION **3** Medical Specific Conditions

Table 3.56 – ASSESSMENT and MANAGEMENT of:

Convulsions in Adults *continued*

● Airway	**DO NOT** attempt to force an oropharyngeal airway into a convulsing patient. A nasopharyngeal airway is a useful adjunct in such patients – **NB Caution in patients with suspected basal skull fracture or facial injury.**
● Position	● Position patient for comfort and protect from dangers, especially the head.
● Oxygen	**ACTIVE CONVULSION** ● Administer 15 litres per minute until a reliable SpO_2 measurement can be obtained and then adjust oxygen flow to aim for a target saturation within the range of 94–98% – as a convulsion occurs the brain is acutely starved of oxygen. **POST-ICTAL** ● Apply pulse oximeter. ● Measure oxygen saturation. ● Administer supplemental oxygen if hypoxaemic (SpO_2 of <94%) (refer to oxygen guideline).

● Medication	Most tonic/clonic convulsions are self-limiting and do not require drug treatment. Establish if any treatment has already been administered.
	
	Midazolam – refer to patient's own midazolam guideline.
	● If a grand-mal convulsion is still continuing 10 minutes **after the first dose of midazolam:**
	  – the ambulance clinician can advise the carer to administer a second dose of midazolam
	  – ambulance paramedics and technicians can administer the patient's own prescribed midazolam – if they are competent to administer medication via the buccal or intranasal route and are familiar with the indications, actions and side effects of midazolam
	  – a paramedic can administer a single dose of diazepam intravenously (IV) or rectally (PR).
	NB Due to the time taken to cannulate and administer intravenous diazepam and the time it takes for rectal diazepam to act, a second dose of midazolam is preferable.
	
	If the patient does not have their own midazolam:
	
	Diazepam or midazolam
	● Administer diazemuls or midazolam IV. Rectal diazepam (stesolid or buccal midazolam) may be given when IV access cannot be obtained (refer to diazepam or midazolam guideline) for:
	  – fits lasting >5 minutes and **STILL FITTING**
	  – repeated fits in close succession – not secondary to an uncorrected hypoxia or hypoglycaemic episode
	  – status epilepticus
	  – eclamptic fits lasting >2–3 minutes or recurrent.
	If a grand-mal convulsion continues 10 minutes after the second dose, medical advice should be sought. **Refer to eclampsia guideline.**

● Transfer	Transfer to further care ● Patients suffering from serial convulsions (three or more in an hour). ● Patients suffering from an eclamptic convulsion (**refer to pregnancy induced hypertension (including eclampsia) guideline**). ● Patients suffering their first convulsion. ● Difficulties monitoring the patient's condition. NB Known epileptics who make a full recovery, are not at risk and can be supervised adequately, can be managed at home following local guidelines. For these patients: ● Measure and record vital signs with the explanation given to the patient. ● Advise the patients and carer to contact the general practitioner (GP) if the patient feels generally unwell or 999 if there are repeated convulsions. ● Document the reasons for the decision not to transfer to further care and this must be signed by the patient and/or carer. ● Ensure contact is made with the patient's GP particularly where the patient has made repeated calls. ● Provide an information sheet. NB It is important not to label a patient as epileptic unless there is a known diagnosis.

3 Medical Specific Conditions

SECTION

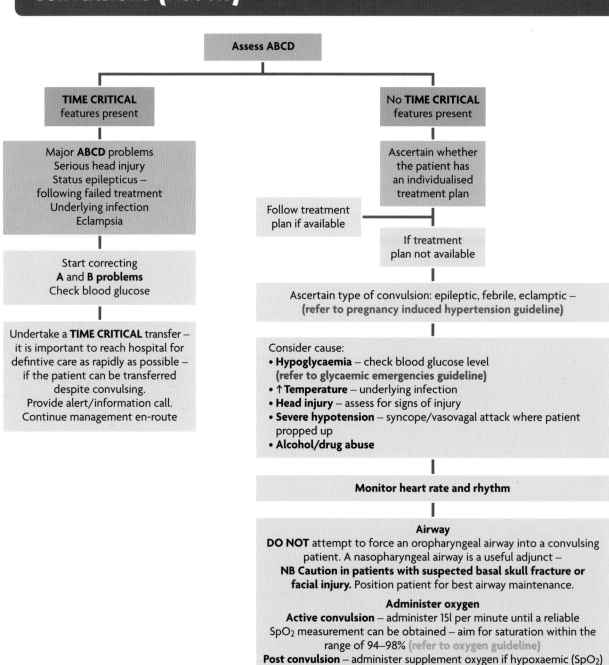

Assess ABCD

TIME CRITICAL
features present

Major **ABCD** problems
Serious head injury
Status epilepticus –
following failed treatment
Underlying infection
Eclampsia

Start correcting
A and **B** problems
Check blood glucose

Undertake a **TIME CRITICAL** transfer –
it is important to reach hospital for
defintive care as rapidly as possible –
if the patient can be transferred
despite convulsing.
Provide alert/information call.
Continue management en-route

No **TIME CRITICAL**
features present

Ascertain whether
the patient has
an individualised
treatment plan

Follow treatment
plan if available

If treatment
plan not available

Ascertain type of convulsion: epileptic, febrile, eclamptic –
(refer to pregnancy induced hypertension guideline)

Consider cause:
• **Hypoglycaemia** – check blood glucose level
(refer to glycaemic emergencies guideline)
• **↑ Temperature** – underlying infection
• **Head injury** – assess for signs of injury
• **Severe hypotension** – syncope/vasovagal attack where patient
propped up
• **Alcohol/drug abuse**

Monitor heart rate and rhythm

Airway
DO NOT attempt to force an oropharyngeal airway into a convulsing
patient. A nasopharyngeal airway is a useful adjunct –
**NB Caution in patients with suspected basal skull fracture or
facial injury.** Position patient for best airway maintenance.

Administer oxygen
Active convulsion – administer 15l per minute until a reliable
SpO$_2$ measurement can be obtained – aim for saturation within the
range of 94–98% (refer to oxygen guideline)
Post convulsion – administer supplement oxygen if hypoxaemic (SpO$_2$)
of <94% (refer to oxygen guideline)

Medication
Establish if any treatment has been given.
Patient's own buccal midazolam for a grand-mal convulsion still
continuing 10 minutes after the first dose of midazolam
recurrent **(refer to patient's own buccal midazolam guideline)**
Diazepam or midazolam for fits lasting >5 minutes and **STILL FITTING**;
repeated fits – not secondary to an uncorrected hypoxia or
hypoglycaemic episode; status epilepticus; eclamptic fits
lasting >2–3 minutes or recurrent
(refer to diazepam or midazolam guideline)

Transfer to further care
Patients suffering from: serial convulsions; an eclamptic convulsion
(refer to pregnancy induced hypertension
(including eclampsia) guideline); a first convulsion;
difficulties monitoring the patient's condition

Figure 3.13 – Assessment and management of convulsions in adults algorithm.

1. Introduction

Gastrointestinal (GI) bleeding is a common medical emergency accounting for 7,000 admissions per year in Scotland alone.

Gastrointestinal haemorrhage is commonly divided into:

- **Upper gastrointestinal bleeding.**
- **Lower gastrointestinal bleeding.**

2. Incidence

- Upper GI bleeding is more common than lower GI bleeding and is more prevalent in socioeconomically deprived areas.
- Upper GI bleeding accounts for up to 85% of gastrointestinal bleeding events.

3. Severity and Outcome

- The severity of gastrointestinal bleeding can range from clinically insignificant blood loss to significant life-threatening haemorrhage.
- Death is uncommon in patients less than 40 years of age, it is estimated that the overall mortality rate in the UK for patients admitted with acute GI bleeding is approximately 7%. The majority of deaths occur in the elderly, particularly those with comorbidities. There are many factors that are associated with a poor outcome including liver disease, acute haemodynamic disturbance, clotting abnormalities, continued bleeding, haematemesis, haematochezia, and elevated blood urea.
- Upper GI bleeding tends to be more severe and in extreme circumstances can rapidly lead to hypovolaemic shock.

4. Pathophysiology

- The upper gastrointestinal tract comprises the oesophagus, stomach and duodenum. For common causes of bleeding refer to Table 3.57.
- The lower gastrointestinal tract comprises the lower part of the small intestine, the colon, rectum and anus. Common causes of bleeding include diverticular disease, inflammatory bowel disease, haemorrhoids, and tumour.

ACUTE UPPER GI BLEEDING

- More than 50% of cases are due to peptic ulcers which, together with oesophagitis and gastritis, account for up to 90% of all upper GI bleeding in the elderly. 85% of deaths associated with upper GI bleeding occur in persons older than 65 years.
- Patients presenting with upper GI bleeding may have a history of aspirin or non-steroidal anti-inflammatory drug (NSAID) use.
  - Only 50% of patients present with haematemesis alone, 30% with melaena and 20% with haematemesis and melaena
  - Patients with haematemesis tend to have greater blood loss than those with melaena alone. Patients older than 60 years account for up to 45% of all cases (60% of these are women).

Table 3.57 – COMMON CAUSES OF UPPER GASTROINTESTINAL BLEEDING

Common causes

- Peptic ulcers:
  - Duodenal ulcers
  - Gastric ulcers
- Oesophageal varices
- Gastritis
- Oesophagitis
- Mallory–Weiss tears
- Caustic poison
- Tumour

Peptic ulcers

- Peptic ulcers are commonly associated with the use of aspirin, non-steroidal anti-inflammatory drugs, corticosteroids, anticoagulants, alcohol and cigarettes.

Oesophageal varices

- It is estimated that variceal bleeding is the cause of 10% of cases. These patients can bleed severely, with up to 8% dying within 48 hours from uncontrolled haemorrhage. It is commonly associated with alcoholic cirrhosis and increased portal pressure (causing progressive dilation of the veins and protrusion of the formed varices into the lumen of the oesophagus). Spontaneous rupture of the varices will cause the patient to become haemodynamically unstable within a very short period of time due to large volumes of blood loss.

Mallory–Weiss tears

- Approximately 10% are caused by oesophageal tears, which are more common in the young. Predisposing factors include hiatal hernia and alcoholism. Initiating factors are persistent coughing or severe retching and vomiting, often after an alcoholic binge; haematemesis presents after several episodes of non-bloody emesis. Bleeding can be mild to moderate.

Gastritis

- Drugs, infections, illnesses, and injuries can cause inflammation of the lining of the stomach and lead to bleeding.

Oesophagitis

- Gastroesophageal reflux disease or alcohol can lead to inflammation and ulcers in the lining of the oesophagus which may lead to bleeding.

Tumour

- In the oesophagus, stomach or duodenum can cause bleeding.

ACUTE LOWER GI BLEEDING

Patients with a lower GI bleed commonly present with bright red blood/dark blood with clots per rectum (PR); bright red blood PR in isolation excludes upper GI bleeding in over 98% of cases (unless the patient appears hypovolaemic). Lower GI bleeding is less likely to present with signs of haemodynamic compromise, is more prevalent in men and also has a common history of aspirin or NSAID use. The mean age for lower GI bleeding is 63–77 years, with mortality around 4% (even serious cases have rarely resulted in death). Common causes include:

Diverticular disease

- Diverticular bleeding accounts for up to 55% of cases. Patients commonly present with an abrupt but painless PR bleed. The incidence of diverticular bleeding increases with age.

Inflammatory bowel disease

- Major bleeding from ulcerative colitis and Crohn's disease is rare. Inflammatory bowel disease accounts for less than 10% of cases.

Haemorrhoids

- Haemorrhoids account for less than 10% of cases. Bleeding is bright red and usually noticed on wiping or in the toilet bowl. The incidence is high in pregnancy, a result of straining associated with constipation and hormonal changes. Further evaluation may be needed if the patient complains of an alteration of bowel habit and blood mixed with the stool.

Tumour

- Tumour in the large bowel can cause bleeding.

Differential diagnosis

- Post rectal bleeding can cause significant embarrassment for the patient and care must be taken when assessing female patients that PV bleeding is excluded.

5. Assessment and Management

For the assessment and management of gastrointestinal bleeding refer to Table 3.58.

KEY POINTS

Gastrointestinal Bleeding

- **Haematemesis or melaena indicates an upper GI source.**
- **Bright red or dark blood with clots per rectum indicates a lower GI source.**
- **Almost all deaths from GI bleeds occur in the elderly.**
- **Approximately 80% of all GI bleeds stop spontaneously or respond to conservative management.**

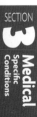

SECTION **3** Medical Specific Conditions

Gastrointestinal Bleeding

Table 3.58 – ASSESSMENT and MANAGEMENT of:

Gastrointestinal Bleeding

ASSESSMENT	MANAGEMENT

● Assess ABCD	● If any of the following **TIME CRITICAL** features are present:
	  – major **ABCD** problems
	  – haematemesis – large volume of bright red blood
	  – haemodynamic compromise
	  – decreased level of consciousness.
	● Start correcting **A** and **B** problems
	● Undertake a **TIME CRITICAL** transfer to nearest receiving hospital.
	● Provide an alert/information call.
	● Continue patient management en-route.

● Assess blood loss	Where does the bleeding originate – upper or lower GI tract? ● **Haematemesis** – vomited fresh/dark red/brown/black or 'coffee ground' blood (depending on how long it has been in the stomach). Did this occur after an increase in intra-abdominal pressure (e.g. retching or coughing)? ● Ascertain how many episodes of non-bloody emesis. ● **Melaena** – malodorous, liquid, black stool or bright red/dark blood with clots per rectum (PR). It can be difficult to estimate blood loss when mixed with faeces. ● Estimate blood loss – if not visible ask the patient or relatives/carers to estimate colour/volume – PR blood loss is difficult to estimate. (NB The blood acts as a laxative, but repeated blood-liquid stool, or just blood, is associated with more severe blood loss than maroon/black solid stool.) ● Has the patient suffered unexplained syncope – this may indicate concealed GI bleeding. Ensure PV bleeding is excluded in females.

● History	● **When did the bleeding begin?**
	● Is/has the patient:
	  – currently taking or recently taken aspirin or NSAID?
	  – currently taking iron tablets?
	  – consumed food or drink containing red dye(s)?
	  – currently taking beta-blockers or calcium-channel blockers – may mask tachycardia in the shocked patient?
	  – currently taking or recently taken anticoagulatory or antiplatelet therapy?
	
	● **Is there a history of:**
	  – bleeding disorders?
	  – liver disease?
	  – abdominal surgery in particular abdominal aortic surgery?
	  – alcohol abuse?
	  – syncope?

● Oxygen	● Administer supplemental oxygen if the patient is hypoxaemic (SpO$_2$ <94%).
● Vital signs	● Monitor vital signs. ● Monitor ECG.
● IV access	● Obtain if analgesia or fluid therapy are indicated.
● Pain management	● GI bleeding is not generally associated with pain. ● If pain relief is indicated **refer to pain management guidelines**.
● Fluid	● If fluid resuscitation indicated refer to intravascular fluid therapy guideline.
● Transfer to further care	● Continue patient management en-route. ● Provide an alert/information call.

1. Introduction

- A non-diabetic individual maintains their blood glucose level within a narrow range from 3.0 to 5.6 mmol per litre.

- This is achieved by a balance between glucose entering the blood stream (from the gastrointestinal tract or from the breakdown of stored energy sources) and glucose leaving the circulation through the action of insulin.

SECTION 1 – Hypoglycaemia

- A low blood glucose level is defined as <4.0 mmol/l, but the clinical features of hypoglycaemia may be present at higher levels and clinical judgement is as important as a blood glucose reading.

- Correction of hypoglycaemia is a medical emergency.

- If left untreated hypoglycaemia may lead to the patient suffering permanent brain damage and may even prove fatal.

- Hypoglycaemia occurs when glucose metabolism is disturbed – refer to Table 3.59 for risk factors.

- Any person whose level of consciousness is decreased, who is having a convulsion, is seriously ill or traumatised should have hypoglycaemia excluded.

- Signs and symptoms can vary from patient to patient (refer to Table 3.60) and the classical symptoms may not be present.

- Some patients are able to detect the early symptoms for themselves, but others may deteriorate rapidly and without apparent warning.

- Abnormal neurological features may occur, for example, one-sided weakness, identical to a stroke.

- Symptoms may be masked due to medication or other injuries, for example, with beta-blocking agents.

2. Assessment and Management

For the assessment and management of hypoglycaemia refer to Table 3.61 and or Figure 3.14.

SECTION 2 – Hyperglycaemia

- Hyperglycaemia is the term used to describe high blood glucose levels.

- Symptoms include unusual thirst (polydipsia), urinary frequency, and tiredness (refer to Table 3.62). They are usually of slow onset in comparison to those of hypoglycaemia.

Diabetic ketoacidosis (DKA)

- A relative lack of circulating insulin means that cells cannot take up glucose from the blood and use it to provide energy. This forces the cells to provide energy for metabolism from other sources such as fatty acids.

- This produces acidosis and ketones. The body tries to combat this metabolic acidosis by hyperventilation to blow off carbon dioxide. High blood glucose level means glucose spills over into the urine dragging water and electrolytes with it causing dehydration and glycosuria.

- New onset diabetes type 1 may present with DKA. More frequently it complicates intercurrent illness in

Table 3.59 – RISK FACTORS FOR HYPOGLYCAEMIA

Medical
- Insulin or other hypoglycaemic drug treatments.
- Tight glycaemic control.
- Previous history of severe hypoglycaemia.
- Undetected nocturnal hypoglycaemia.
- Long duration of diabetes.
- Poor injection technique.
- Impaired awareness of hypoglycaemia.
- Preceding hypoglycaemia (< 3.5 mmol/l).
- Severe hepatic dysfunction.
- Renal dialysis therapy.
- Impaired renal function.
- Inadequate treatment of previous hypoglycaemia.
- Terminal illness.
- Metabolic illness.
- Endocrine illness (including Addisonian crisis).
- Drug ingestion e.g. oral hypoglycaemic drugs, beta-blockers, alcohol.
- Sudden cessation of peritoneal dialysis.
- Hypothermia.
- Sudden cessation of tube or IV feeding.

Lifestyle
- Inadequate carbohydrate intake.
- Increased exercise (relative to usual)/excessive physical activity.
- Irregular lifestyle.
- Increasing age.
- Excessive or chronic alcohol intake.
- Early pregnancy.
- Breast feeding.
- Injection into areas of lipohypertrophy.
- Inadequate blood glucose monitoring.

Table 3.60 – SIGNS AND SYMPTOMS OF HYPOGLYCAEMIA

Autonomic	Neurological
Sweating	Confusion
Palpitations	Drowsiness
Shaking	Odd behaviour
Hunger	Speech difficulty
	In-coordination
	Aggression
General malaise	Fitting
Headache	Unconsciousness
Nausea	

a known diabetic. Infections, myocardial infarction (which may be silent) or a cerebrovascular accident (CVA) may precipitate the condition.

- Omissions or inadequate dosage of insulin or other hypoglycaemic therapy may also contribute or be responsible. Some medications, particularly steroids may greatly exacerbate the situation.

- Patients may present with one or more signs and symptoms (refer to Table 3.62) and this should alert the pre-hospital provider to the possibility of hyperglycaemia and DKA.

Glycaemic Emergencies (Adults)

MILD

Patient conscious, orientated and able to swallow.

Administer 15–20 grams of quick acting carbohydrate (sugary drink, chocolate bar/biscuit or glucose gel).

Test blood glucose level if <4 mmol/L, repeat up to 3 times.

Consider intravenous glucose 10% or 1 mg glucagon.

MODERATE

Patient conscious, but confused/ disorientated or aggressive and able to swallow.

If capable and cooperative, administer 15–20 grams of quick acting carbohydrate (sugary drink, chocolate bar/biscuit or glucose gel). Test blood glucose level.

Continue to test after 15 minutes and repeat up to 3 times consider intravenous glucose 10%. (Repeat up to 3 times until BGL above 4 mmol/L.)

Test blood glucose level, if <4 mmol/L administer 15–20 grams of quick acting carbohydrate.

Continue to test after 15 minutes and repeat up to 3 times, consider intravenous glucose 10% (Repeat up to 3 times until BGL above 4 mmol/L.)

SEVERE

Patient unconscious/ convulsing or very aggressive or nil by mouth or where there is an increased risk of aspiration/choking.

Assess ABCD Measure and record blood glucose level.

Administer IV glucose 10% by slow IV infusion (refer to glucose 10% guideline) – titrate to effect.

Re-assess blood glucose level after 10 minutes.

If <5 mmol/L administer a further dose of IV glucose – if IV not possible administer IM glucagon (onset of action 5–10 minutes).

Re-assess blood glucose level after a further 10 minutes.

If no improvement transfer immediately to nearest suitable receiving hospital. Provide alert/ information call.

Figure 3.14 – Hypoglycaemic emergencies algorithm.

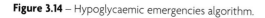

March 2016

Medical – specific conditions

175

1. Introduction

- Heart failure is not a specific disease entity, rather it is a clinical syndrome characterised by a number of clinical signs, symptoms and diagnostic findings. It occurs as a consequence of diastolic or systolic dysfunction resulting in the inability of the heart to provide adequate cardiac output for the body's metabolic needs.

- Acute heart failure (AHF) represents new or worsening signs or symptoms consistent with an underlying deterioration in ventricular function. It is characterised by dyspnoea resulting from acutely elevated cardiac filling pressures often, though not always, leading to rapid accumulation of fluid within the lung's interstitial and alveolar spaces (cardiogenic pulmonary oedema).

2. Incidence

- The overall prevalence of heart failure varies between 1% and 2%; it is the leading reason for hospital admission in patients over 65 years of age in westernised countries. Of heart failure cases, 80% are diagnosed following admission to hospital as an acute emergency.

3. Severity and Outcome

- The 60-day mortality following hospital admission because of an exacerbation of heart failure varies with estimates between 8% and 20%. Approximately 30% of heart failure patients will be re-admitted to hospital each year as a result of an acute exacerbation.

- The overall pre-hospital mortality rate for cases of acute cardiogenic pulmonary oedema has been reported at 8%.

4. Pathophysiology

- The pathophysiology underlying the worsening ventricular function is often coronary artery disease. Diseased coronary arteries become inelastic and intravascular pressures rise as a consequence – coronary artery perfusion will reduce unless mean arterial pressures are raised to ensure adequate coronary artery blood flow.

- As mean arterial pressures rise so too does cardiac afterload, which will lead to an increased end diastolic volume unless the force of ventricular contraction is raised. These combined processes initiate a spiral of increasing mean arterial pressures, increasing afterload and increasing preload.

Risk Factors
- Advancing age.
- History of CHF.
- Hypertension.

- Acute heart failure patients will often present with clinical signs of vascular congestion and the formation of oedema. The pathophysiology underlying the formation of oedema can vary depending on cause; however, in acute heart failure acute oedema occurs as a result of fluid shifts from the vascular compartment into the interstitial space.

- Left ventricular failure (LVF) may precipitate formation of pulmonary oedema as a result of reduced cardiac output and increasing pulmonary hypertension. As pulmonary vascular pressures rise, so increasing amounts of fluid will shift from the pulmonary vascular compartment into the lung interstitial spaces and alveoli. Pulmonary oedema occurs as a result of the accumulation of this fluid in the alveoli which decreases gas exchange across the alveoli, resulting in decreased oxygenation of the blood and, in some cases, accumulation of carbon dioxide (CO_2).

- The pathophysiology of pulmonary oedema can be thought of in terms of three factors (refer to Table 3.64):

  i.   flow
  ii. fluid
  iii. filter.

Table 3.64 – PULMONARY OEDEMA

i. Flow

The ability of the heart to eject the blood delivered to it depends on three factors:
1. the amount of blood returning to the heart (preload)
2. the coordinated contraction of the myocardium
3. the resistance against which it pumps (afterload).
Preload may also be increased by over-infusion of IV fluid or fluid retention. Coordinated contraction fails following heart muscle damage (myocardial infarction (MI), heart failure) or due to arrhythmias. Afterload increases with hypertension, atherosclerosis, aortic valve stenosis or peripheral vasoconstriction.

ii. Fluid

The blood passing through the lungs must have enough 'oncotic' pressure to 'hold on' to the fluid portion as it passes through the pulmonary capillaries. As albumin is a key determinant of oncotic pressure, low albumin states can also lead to the formation of pulmonary oedema (e.g. burns, liver failure, nephrotic syndrome).

iii. Filter

The capillaries through which the fluid passes may increase in permeability (e.g. acute lung injury (as in smoke inhalation), pneumonia or drowning).

- Right ventricular failure (RVF) may precipitate formation of peripheral oedema as a result of increasing right ventricular filling pressures, reduced right ventricular output and increasing systemic congestion. Peripheral oedema occurs as a result of the accumulation of fluid in the interstitial spaces and is most commonly noted in the lower legs and sacrum.

- The signs and symptoms of heart failure vary depending upon the extent of failure and underlying physiologic cause. However, three symptoms are common to nearly all forms: fatigue (including exercise intolerance), dyspnoea and congestion. It can be difficult to differentiate heart failure from other causes of breathlessness, such as exacerbation of chronic obstructive pulmonary disease (COPD), pulmonary embolism or pneumonia. Therefore, a thorough history and physical examination are required.

5. Assessment and Management

For the assessment and management of heart failure refer to Table 3.65.

Heart Failure

Table 3.65 – ASSESSMENT and MANAGEMENT

Heart Failure

ASSESSMENT	MANAGEMENT
Undertake ABCD assessment If the patient is **TIME CRITICAL** 1. Assess PERFUSION status Signs of **ADEQUATE** perfusion: ● Normal mentation ● Peripheral pulses present ● Systolic blood pressure >90 mmHg ● **NOT** pale ● Capillary Bed Refill Time <2 sec	● Start correcting ABC problems (**refer to medical emergencies overview**). ● Correct life-threatening conditions, airway and breathing on scene. ● Then commence transfer to nearest suitable receiving hospital. Refer to Figure 3.15.
Signs of **INADEQUATE** perfusion: ● Reduced consciousness ● Systolic blood pressure <90 mmHg ● Pallor ● Capillary Bed Refill Time >2 sec	Refer to Figure 3.15.
2. Assess CONGESTION status Signs of congestion: ● Pulmonary oedema ● Peripheral oedema ● Elevated jugular venous pulse	Refer to Figure 3.15. ● If pulmonary oedema is evident position the patient sitting upright if possible.
Record a 12-lead ECG	● It is uncommon for patients with heart failure to have a normal ECG. Where no ECG abnormalities are identified clinicians should consider the possibility of an alternative diagnosis. ● Where the ECG indicates that heart failure may be due to acute coronary syndrome manage as per the **ACS guideline.**

Table 3.66

Clinical Indicators of Potential Heart Failure

Pulmonary oedema
● Fine crackling sounds are suggestive of pulmonary oedema, commonly heard in the lung bases, but may be heard over other lung fields as well.
● Often accompanied by the coughing up of frothy sputum, white or pink (blood stained) in colour.

Peripheral oedema
● Although peripheral oedema is a common sign of chronic heart failure, it is not specific to heart failure and may be seen as a consequence of numerous pathologies. It usually only becomes apparent when the extracellular volume exceeds 5 litres.

Third heart sound
● An auscultated third heart sound (S3), or gallop rhythm, in an adult patient is usually a pathological indicator of reduced ventricular compliance.
● It is strongly associated with elevated atrial pressure; consequently it can be an important indicator of left ventricular failure and dilation.
Although a third heart sound is not sensitive (24%) for heart failure, it is highly specific (99%).

Jugular venous pressure
● Jugular venous pressure (JVP) provides an estimation of right atrial filling pressure as there are no valves between the right atrium and the internal jugular vein.
● Jugular venous pressure is assessed while the patient is supine with the upper body at a 30–45° angle from the horizontal plane.
● The vertical height of the crest of the internal jugular venous pulsation above the sternal angle determines the height of the venous pressure and provides the estimate of right atrial filling pressure.
● Any measurement greater than 3 cm suggests elevated right atrial filling pressure.
Elevated jugular venous pressure is a specific (90%) but not sensitive (30%) indicator of elevated left ventricular filling.

Table 3.67

Therapies in Heart Failure

GTN
- The use of nitrates in pulmonary oedema is associated with improved survival to hospital discharge.
- Buccal nitrates produce an immediate reduction in preload, comparable with IV GTN.
- Nitrates have some benefit as the first-line treatment in acute pulmonary oedema.

Furosemide
- There is little high-level evidence for or against the use of furosemide (**refer to furosemide protocol for dosage and information**) in the treatment of acute pulmonary oedema, but it has been standard treatment for many years.
- There is some evidence that furosemide can have a transient adverse vasoconstrictor effect; it is unclear whether this is beneficial or harmful.
- The acute vasodilator effect of furosemide is inhibited by aspirin.
- Pre-hospital trials comparing repeated furosemide vs. repeated nitrates favour the use of nitrates.

Furosemide should only be given after nitrates (which act on both preload and afterload).

Salbutamol
- The effectiveness of salbutamol in the treatment of pulmonary oedema presenting in the acute setting is unclear.
- Studies addressing the use of bronchodilators in chronic heart failure suggest worse outcomes following their use; however, a number of pre-hospital trials of combination drug therapies (including salbutamol) indicate improved outcomes.

Owing to the diagnostic uncertainty and possibility for misdiagnosis, salbutamol may still be considered in the management of heart failure where wheeze is present; this may avoid depriving COPD/asthma patients of vital bronchodilators.

Morphine
- Morphine and diamorphine are commonly used in the in-hospital emergency management of pulmonary oedema. The drugs act by reducing preload (venodilation) and also serve to decrease anxiety.

- Despite their widespread use, there is no conclusive trial evidence showing symptomatic improvement or mortality benefit.

Analysis of large heart failure registries suggest that the use of opiates in heart failure increases mortality; therefore they should not routinely be used unless they are being used to manage ACS and the patient is complaining of chest pain.

CPAP
- Non-invasive positive pressure ventilation (NiPPV) comprises two main treatment modalities – continuous positive airway pressure (CPAP) and bilevel positive airways pressure (BiPAP). The fundamental difference between these two modalities is the level of pressure maintained throughout the patient's respiratory cycle. In CPAP therapy pressure remains constant through the inspiratory and expiratory phases; in BiPAP therapy pressure is reduced during the expiratory phase and increases during the inspiratory phase.
- The objective of non-invasive positive pressure ventilation (NiPPV) is two-fold. First is to 'splint' open collapsing alveoli and increase intra-alveolar pressure. The increase in pressure helps shift fluid present in the alveoli back into the pulmonary capillaries thereby reducing pulmonary oedema. Second is to raise intrathoracic pressure throughout the respiratory cycle. This increase in intrathoracic pressure increases pressure in the vena cavae, and consequently serves to reduce filling pressures. Combined, these two actions serve to reduce congestion.
- Prospective randomised controlled trials have demonstrated that CPAP improves survival to hospital discharge, decreases intubation rates and has fewer complications.
- Pre-hospital studies exist suggesting CPAP is feasible in this setting, and may reduce severity of acute LVF, increase SpO_2 levels and improve survival to hospital discharge.

Expert opinion has recommended CPAP for use in the pre-hospital environment.

KEY POINTS

Heart Failure
- **Pulmonary oedema can be difficult to differentiate from other causes of breathlessness, such as exacerbation of COPD, pulmonary embolism or pneumonia; therefore, a thorough history and physical examination are needed.**

- **Symptoms include dyspnoea, worsening cough, pink frothy sputum, waking at night gasping for breath, breathlessness on lying down (sleeping on more pillows recently?), and anxiousness/restlessness.**

- **Sit the patient upright where possible.**

- **Early nitrate administration is the cornerstone of early treatment.**

- **Furosemide administration MUST be secondary to nitrate administration and should only be considered in cases with adequate perfusion and evidence of oedema.**

- **Morphine should be avoided unless there are signs of ACS.**

- **CPAP should be utilised where equipment and suitably trained personnel are available.**

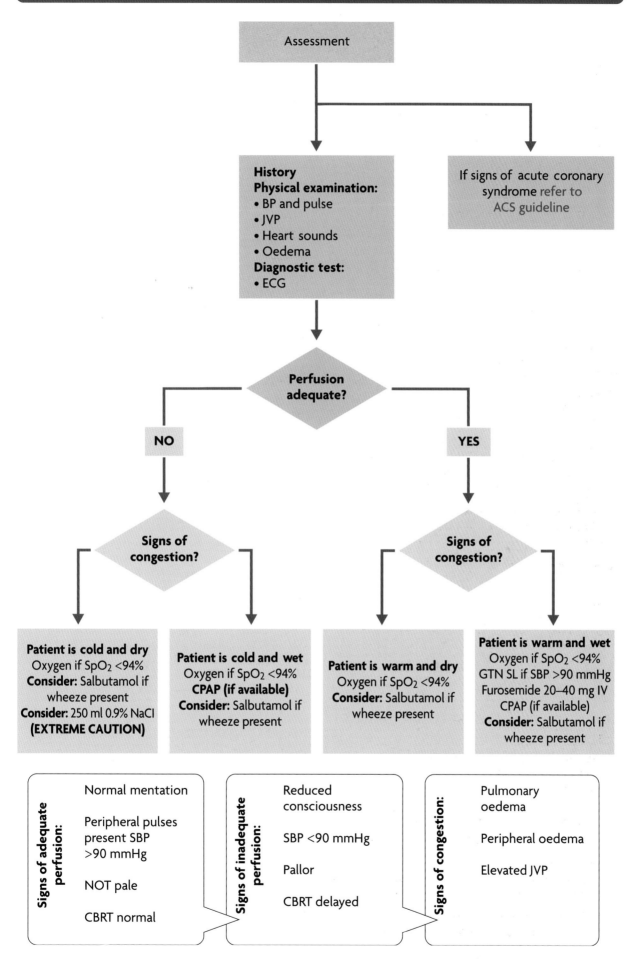

Figure 3.15 – Assessment and management algorithm of acute heart failure.

1. Introduction

The implantable cardioverter defibrillator (ICD) has revolutionised the management of patients at risk of developing a life-threatening ventricular arrhythmia. Several clinical trials have testified to their effectiveness in reducing deaths from sudden cardiac arrest in selected patients, and the devices are implanted with increasing frequency.

ICDs are used in both children and adults.

ICD systems consist of a generator connected to electrodes placed transvenously into cardiac chambers (the ventricle, and sometimes the right atrium and/or the coronary sinus) (refer to Figure 3.16). The electrodes serve a dual function allowing the monitoring of cardiac rhythm and the administration of electrical pacing, defibrillation and cardioversion therapy. Modern ICDs are slightly larger than a pacemaker and are usually implanted in the left subclavicular area (refer to Figure 3.16). The ICD generator contains the battery and sophisticated electronic circuitry that monitors the cardiac rhythm, determines the need for electrical therapy, delivers treatment, monitors the response and determines the need for further therapy.

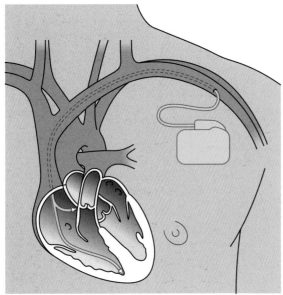

Figure 3.16 – Usual location of an ICD.

The available therapies include:

- Conventional programmable pacing for the treatment of bradycardia.

- Anti-tachycardia pacing (ATP) for ventricular tachycardia (VT).

- Delivery of biphasic shocks for the treatment of ventricular tachycardia and ventricular fibrillation (VF).

- Cardiac resynchronisation therapy (CRT) (biventricular pacing) for the treatment of heart failure.

These treatment modalities and specifications are programmable and capable of considerable sophistication to suit the requirements of individual patients. The implantation and programming of devices is carried out in specialised centres. The patient should carry a card or documentation which identifies their ICD centre and may also have been given emergency instructions.

The personnel caring for such patients in emergency situations are not usually experts in arrhythmia management or familiar with the details of the sophisticated treatment regimes offered by modern ICDs. Moreover, the technology is complex and evolving rapidly. In an emergency patients will often present to the ambulance service or emergency department (ED) and the purpose of this guidance is to help those responsible for the initial management of these patients.

2. General Principles

Some important points should be made at the outset.

On detecting VF/VT the ICD will usually discharge a maximum of eight times before shutting down. However, a new episode of VF/VT will result in the recommencing of its discharge sequence. A patient with a fractured ICD lead may suffer repeated internal defibrillation as the electrical noise is misinterpreted as a shockable rhythm.

These patients are likely to be conscious with a relatively normal ECG rate.

When confronted with a patient fitted with an ICD who has a persistent or recurring arrhythmia, or where the ICD is firing, expert help should be summoned at the outset. Outside hospital this will normally be from the ambulance service, who should be summoned immediately by dialling 999.

When confronted with a patient in cardiac arrest the usual management guidelines are still appropriate (**refer to cardiac arrest and arrhythmia guidelines**). If the ICD is not responding to VF or VT, or if shocks are ineffective, external defibrillation/cardioversion should be carried out. Avoid placing the defibrillator electrodes/pads/paddles close to or on top of the ICD; ensure a minimum distance of 8 cm between the edge of the defibrillator paddle pad/electrode and the ICD site. Most ICDs are implanted in the left sub-clavicular position (refer to Figure 3.16) and are usually readily apparent on examination; the conventional (apical/right subclavicular) electrode position will then be appropriate. The anterior/posterior position may also be used, particularly if the ICD is right sided.

Whenever possible, record a 12-lead electrocardiogram (ECG) and record the patient's rhythm (with any shocks). Make sure this is printed out and stored electronically (where available) for future reference. Where an external defibrillator with an electronic memory is used (whether for monitoring or for therapy) ensure that the ECG report is printed and handed to appropriate staff. Again, whenever possible, ensure that the record is archived for future reference. Record the rhythm during any therapeutic measure (whether by drugs or electricity). All these records may provide vital information for the ICD centre that may greatly influence the patient's subsequent management.

The energy levels of the shocks administered by ICDs (up to 40 Joules) are much lower than those delivered with external defibrillators (120–360 J). **Personnel in contact with the patient when an ICD discharges are unlikely to be harmed, but it is prudent to minimise contact with the patient while the ICD is firing.** Chest compression and ventilation can be carried out as normal and protective examination gloves should be worn as usual.

Placing a ring magnet over the ICD generator can temporarily disable the shock capability of an ICD. The magnet does not disable the pacing capability for treating bradycardia. The magnet may be kept in position with adhesive tape if required. Removing the magnet returns the ICD to the status present before application. The ECG rhythm should be monitored at all times when the device is disabled. An ICD should only be disabled when the rhythm for which shocks are being delivered has been recorded. If that rhythm is VT or VF, external cardioversion/defibrillation must be available. With some models it is possible to programme the ICD so that a magnet does not disable the shock capabilities of the device. This is usually done only in exceptional circumstances, and consequently, such patients are rare.

The manufacturers of the ICDs also supply the ring magnets. Many implantation centres provide each patient with a ring magnet and stress that it should be readily available in case of emergency. With the increasing prevalence of ICDs in the community it becomes increasingly important that emergency workers have this magnet available to them when attending these patients.

Decisions to apply a Do Not Attempt Resuscitation (DNAR) order will not be made in the emergency situation by the personnel to whom this guidance is directed. Where such an order does exist it should not be necessary to disable an ICD to enable the implementation of such an order.

Many problems with ICDs can only be dealt with permanently by using the programmer available at the ICD centre.

The guidelines should be read from the perspective of your position and role in the management of such patients. For example, the recommendation to 'arrange further assessment' will mean that the ambulance clinician should transport the patient to hospital. For ED staff, however, this might mean referral to the medical admitting team or local ICD centre.

Coincident conditions that may contribute to the development of arrhythmia (e.g. acute ischaemia worsening heart failure) should be managed as appropriate according to usual practice.

Maintain oxygen saturations at 94–98%.

Receiving ICD therapy may be unpleasant 'like a firm kick in the chest', and psychological consequences may also arise. It is important to be aware of these, and help should be available from implantation centres. An emergency telephone helpline may be available.

3. Management

The following should be read in conjunction with the treatment table (refer to Table 3.68) and algorithm (refer to Figure 3.17). Approach and assess the patient and perform basic life support according to current BLS guidelines.

Monitor the ECG

3.1. If the patient is in cardiac arrest.

3.1.1 Perform basic life support in accordance with current BLS guidelines. Standard airway management techniques and methods for gaining IV/IO access (as appropriate) should be established.

3.1.2 If a shockable rhythm is present (VF or pulseless VT) but the ICD is not detecting it, perform external defibrillation and other resuscitation procedures according to current resuscitation guidelines.

3.1.3 If the ICD is delivering therapy (whether by anti-tachycardia pacing or shocks) but is failing to convert the arrhythmia, then external defibrillation should be provided, as per current guidelines.

3.1.4 If a non-shockable rhythm is present manage the patient according to current guidelines. If the rhythm is converted to a shockable one, assess the response of the ICD, as in 3.1.2 above, performing external defibrillation as required.

3.1.5 If a shockable rhythm is converted to one associated with effective cardiac output (whether by the ICD or by external defibrillation), manage the patient as usual and arrange further treatment and assessment.

3.2. If the patient is not in cardiac arrest.

3.2.1 Determine whether an arrhythmia is present.

3.2.2 If no arrhythmia is present:
If therapy from the ICD has been effective and the patient is in sinus rhythm or is paced, monitor the patient, give O_2 and arrange further assessment to investigate possibility of new myocardial infarction (MI), heart failure, other acute illness or drug toxicity/electrolyte imbalance etc.
An ICD may deliver inappropriate shocks (i.e. in the absence of arrhythmia) if there are problems with sensing the cardiac rhythm or there are problems with the leads. Record the rhythm (while shocks are delivered, if possible), disable the ICD with a magnet, monitor the patient and arrange further assessment with help from the ICD centre. Provide supportive treatment as required.

3.2.3 If an arrhythmia is present:
If an arrhythmia is present and shocks are being delivered, record the arrhythmia (while ICD shocks are delivered if possible) on the ECG. Determine the nature of the arrhythmia. Transport rapidly to hospital in all cases.

TACHYCARDIA

3.2.3.1 If the rhythm is a **supraventricular tachycardia** (i.e. sinus tachycardia, atrial flutter, atrial fibrillation, junctional tachycardia, etc) and the patient is haemodynamically stable, and the patient is continuing to receive shocks, disable the ICD with a magnet. Consider possible causes, treat appropriately and arrange further assessment in hospital.

3.2.3.2 If the rhythm is **ventricular tachycardia:**

- Pulseless VT should be treated as cardiac arrest (3.1.2 above).
- If the patient is haemodynamically stable, monitor the patient and convey to the emergency department.
- If the patient is haemodynamically unstable, and ICD shocks are ineffective treat as per VT guideline.
- An ICD will not deliver antitachycardia pacing (ATP) or shocks if the rate of the VT is below the programmed detection rate of the device (generally 150 beats/min). Conventional management may be undertaken according to the patient's haemodynamic status.

● Recurring VT with appropriate shocks. Manage any underlying cause (acute ischaemia, heart failure etc). Sedation may be of benefit.

INAPPROPRIATE/INEFFECTIVE ICD FIRING

3.2.3.3 A ring magnet placed over the ICD box will stop the ICD from firing and may be considered in conscious patients where the ICD shocks are ineffective and the patient is distressed. In ICDs that have a dual pacing function, the magnet will also usually change the pacing function to deliver a paced output of 50 beats/min.

[Further related reading includes references 105, 116]

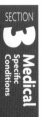

KEY POINTS

Implantable Cardioverter Defibrillators (ICDs)

● **ICDs deliver therapy with bradycardia pacing, ATP and shocks for VT not responding to ATP or VF.**

● **ECG records, especially at the time that shocks are given, can be vital in subsequent patient management. A recording should always be made if circumstances allow.**

● **Cardiac arrest should be managed according to normal guidelines.**

● **Avoid placing the defibrillator electrode over or within 8 cm of the ICD box.**

● **A discharging ICD is unlikely to harm a rescuer touching the patient or performing CPR.**

● **An inappropriately discharging ICD can be temporarily disabled by placing a ring magnet directly over the ICD box.**

Implantable Cardioverter Defibrillator

Table 3.68 – ASSESSMENT and MANAGEMENT of:

Patients Fitted with an ICD

ASSESSMENT	MANAGEMENT
If the patient is in cardiac arrest: ● Assess the patient ● Monitor the ECG	● Perform basic life support in accordance with current BLS guidelines. ● Standard airway management techniques. ● IV access (if required) should be used.
Assess rhythm: Shockable rhythm is present (VF or pulseless VT)	● **BUT** the ICD is not detecting it, perform external defibrillation and other resuscitation procedures according to current resuscitation guidelines. ● If the ICD is delivering therapy (whether by antitachycardia pacing or shocks) but is failing to convert the arrhythmia, then external defibrillation should be provided, as per current guidelines.
Non-shockable rhythm	● Manage the patient according to current guidelines. If the rhythm is converted to a shockable one, assess the response of the ICD, as in 3.1.2 above, performing external defibrillation as required.
If a shockable rhythm is converted to one associated with effective cardiac output (whether by the ICD or by external defibrillation)	● Manage the patient as usual and arrange further treatment and assessment.
If the patient is not in cardiac arrest	● Determine whether an arrhythmia is present.
If no arrhythmia is present	If therapy from the ICD has been effective, the patient is in sinus rhythm or is paced: ● Monitor the patient. ● Administer oxygen and aim for a saturation of 94–98% (refer to oxygen guideline). ● Arrange further assessment to investigate possibility of new myocardial infarction (MI), heart failure, other acute illness or drug toxicity/electrolyte imbalance etc. An ICD may deliver inappropriate shocks (i.e. in the absence of arrhythmia) if there are problems with sensing the cardiac rhythm or problems with the leads: ● Record the rhythm (while ICD shocks are delivered, if possible). ● Disable the ICD with a magnet. ● Monitor the patient. ● Arrange further assessment with help from the ICD centre. Provide supportive treatment as required.
If an arrhythmia is present	If an arrhythmia is present and shocks are being delivered: ● Record the arrhythmia (while ICD shocks are delivered, if possible) on the ECG. ● Determine the nature of the arrhythmia. ● Transport rapidly to hospital in all cases.
If the rhythm is **supraventricular** (i.e. sinus tachycardia, atrial flutter, atrial fibrillation, junctional tachycardia, etc)	If the patient is haemodynamically stable, and the patient is continuing to receive shocks, disable the ICD with a magnet: ● Consider possible causes, treat appropriately. Arrange further assessment in hospital.
If the rhythm is **ventricular tachycardia**	● Pulseless VT should be treated as cardiac arrest (3.1.2 above).
	If the patient is haemodynamically stable: ● Monitor the patient. ● Convey to the emergency department. **If the patient is haemodynamically unstable, and ICD shocks are ineffective, treat as per VT guideline.** ● An ICD will not deliver antitachycardia pacing (ATP) or shocks if the rate of the VT is below the programmed detection rate of the device. Conventional management may be undertaken according to the patient's haemodynamic status. ● For recurring VT with appropriate shocks, manage any underlying cause (acute ischaemia, heart failure etc). Sedation may be of benefit.

Implantable Cardioverter Defibrillator

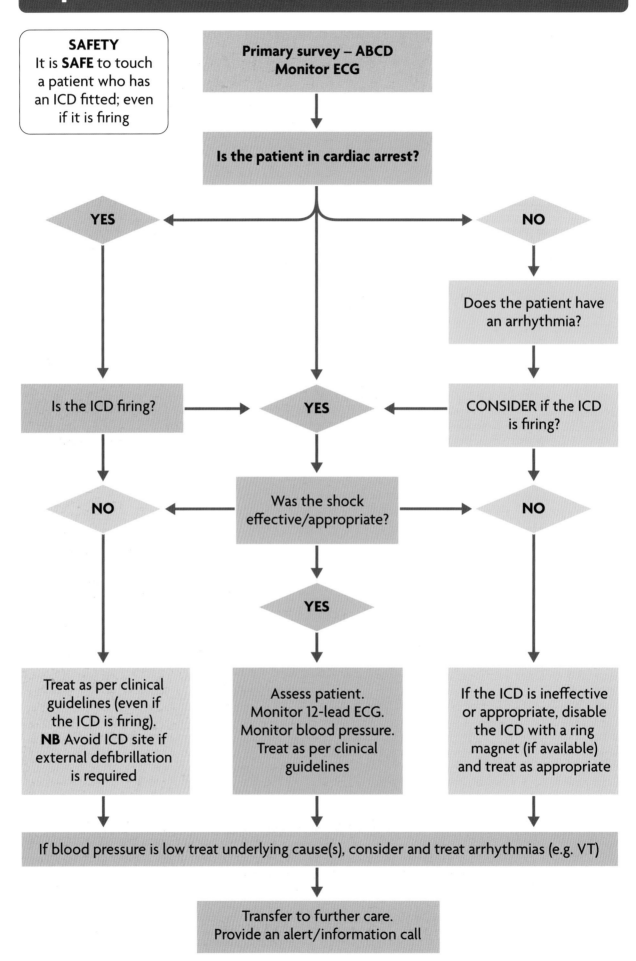

SAFETY
It is **SAFE** to touch a patient who has an ICD fitted; even if it is firing

Primary survey – ABCD
Monitor ECG

Is the patient in cardiac arrest?

YES — NO

Does the patient have an arrhythmia?

Is the ICD firing? → YES ← CONSIDER if the ICD is firing?

Was the shock effective/appropriate?

NO ← → NO

YES

Treat as per clinical guidelines (even if the ICD is firing). **NB** Avoid ICD site if external defibrillation is required

Assess patient. Monitor 12-lead ECG. Monitor blood pressure. Treat as per clinical guidelines

If the ICD is ineffective or appropriate, disable the ICD with a ring magnet (if available) and treat as appropriate

If blood pressure is low treat underlying cause(s), consider and treat arrhythmias (e.g. VT)

Transfer to further care. Provide an alert/information call

Figure 3.17 – Implantable cardioverter defibrillator algorithm.

Overdose and Poisoning (Adults) [103, 175, 467–478]

1. Introduction

Overdose and poisoning is a common cause of calls to the ambulance service accounting for 140,000 hospital admissions per year.

Poisoning

Exposure by ingestion, inhalation, absorption, or injection of a quantity of a substance(s) that may result in mortality or morbidity.

Common agents include:

- **Household products**, for example washing powders, washing-up liquids and fabric cleaning liquid/tablets, bleaches, hand gels and screen-washes, anti-freeze and de-icers, silica gel, batteries, petroleum distillates, white spirit (e.g. paints and varnishes), descalers and glues.

- **Pharmaceutical/recreational substances**, for example paracetamol, ibuprofen, co-codamol, aspirin, tricyclic antidepressants, selective serotonin uptake inhibitors (SSRIs), beta-blockers (atenolol, sotalol, propranolol), calcium channel blockers, benzodiazepines, opioids, iron tablets, cocaine and amphetamines.

- **Plants/fungi**, for example foxglove, laburnum, laurel, iris, castor oil plant, amanita palloides, etc. For further details of poisonous plants refer to: http://www.toxbase.org.

- **Alcohol**

- **Chemicals** – for details **refer to the Chemical, Biological, Radiological and Nuclear and Explosive Incidents guideline.**

- **Cosmetics.**

Poisoning may be:

1. accidental.
2. intentional (self-harm), mal-intent.
3. non-accidental.

Overdose

Exposure by ingestion, inhalation, absorption or injection of a quantity of a substance(s) above the prescribed/known safe dose; this is a common form of poisoning, involving prescribed or illicit drugs and may be accidental or intentional.

2. Incidence

- It is difficult to estimate the exact number of overdose and poisoning incidents, as not all cases are reported. In 2009/2010 there were 49,690 poison-related queries involving patients to the National Poisons Information Service.

3. Severity and Outcome

- There are a number of factors which will affect severity and outcome following exposure, including, age, toxicity of the agent, quantity and route of exposure.

- In 2009 there were 2,878 deaths related to drug overdose and poisoning in England and Wales. In patients that self-harm death commonly results from airway obstruction and respiratory arrest, secondary to a decreased level of consciousness.

4. Pathophysiology

- The mode of action following exposure will depend primarily on the nature of the toxin. For details of the actions of specific toxins refer to: http://www.toxbase.org.

5. Assessment and Management

For the assessment and management of overdose and poisoning in adults refer to Tables 3.69 and 3.70.

Duty of Care

It is not uncommon to find patients who have or claim to have taken an overdose and subsequently refuse treatment or admission to hospital. An assessment of their mental health state, capacity and suicide risk should be made; **refer to mental disorder guideline**. If, despite reasonable persuasion, the patient refuses treatment, it is not acceptable to leave them in a potentially dangerous situation without any access to care.

Assistance may be obtained from the medical/clinical director or a member of the clinical team and a judgement must be made to seek appropriate advice. Attendance of the police or local mental health team may be required, particularly if the patient is at risk.

KEY POINTS

Overdose and Poisoning
- **Establish: the event, drug or substance involved, the quantity, mode of poisoning, any alcohol consumed.**
- **NEVER induce vomiting.**
- **If caustics and petroleum products have been swallowed, dilute by giving milk at the scene wherever possible.**
- **If the patient vomits, retain a sample, if possible, for inspection at hospital.**
- **Bring the substance or substances and any containers for inspection at hospital.**

Overdose and Poisoning (Adults)

Table 3.69 – ASSESSMENT and MANAGEMENT

Overdose and Poisoning

⚠ **Safety First – DO NOT put yourself in danger – carry out a dynamic risk assessment and undertake measures to preserve your own safety.**

⚠ **Avoid mouth-to-mouth ventilation in cases of poisoning or suspected poisoning by cyanide, hydrogen sulphide, corrosives and organophosphates.**

SECTION **3** Medical Specific Conditions

ASSESSMENT	MANAGEMENT
● Assess ABCD	● If any of the following **TIME CRITICAL** features present: – major **ABCD** problems – cardiac and respiratory arrest – refer to resuscitation guidelines – decreased level of consciousness – NB Most poisons that impair consciousness also depress respiration – **refer to altered level of consciousness guideline** – respiratory depression – refer to airway management guideline – arrhythmias – **refer to cardiac rhythm disturbance guideline** – hypotension <70 mmHg – cardiac arrhythmias – **refer to cardiac rhythm disturbance guideline** – convulsions – **refer to convulsion guideline** – hypothermia – **refer to hypothermia guideline** – swallowed crack cocaine, then: ● Start correcting **A** and **B** problems. ● Undertake a **TIME CRITICAL** transfer to nearest appropriate receiving hospital. ● Continue patient management en-route. ● Provide an alert message/information call.
● Substance	● Ascertain what has been ingested/inhaled/absorbed/injected – ask relatives, friends, work colleagues etc. ● Examine the patient for odours, needle marks, pupil abnormalities, signs of corrosion in the mouth. ● Estimate the quantity. ● Ascertain what, if any, treatment has been given. ● Document the time the incident occurred. ● **NEVER** induce vomiting. ● In the case of caustic irritant (e.g. petroleum ingestion) encourage the patient to drink a glass of milk, if possible. Refer to Table 3.70 for specific management of certain toxins. ● If possible take and hand-over to staff at the hospital: – a sample of the ingested substance – all substances found at the scene whether thought to be involved or not – medicine containers – a sample of vomit – if present. Important information can be gained by contacting toxbase and local protocols should be followed to enable this
● Chemical exposure ● Oxygen	● If exposure to chemical substance is suspected – refer to CBRNE guideline chemical section for management ● If indicated, administer high levels of supplemental oxygen, particularly in cases of carbon monoxide poisoning or inhalation of irritant gases – refer to oxygen guideline ● Apply pulse oximeter. In poisoning by paraquat and bleomycin, give oxygen only if the saturation falls below 85% and reduce or stop oxygen therapy if the saturation rises above 88%.
● ECG	● Undertake a 12-lead ECG.
● Respirations	● Monitor respirations. ● Consider assisted ventilation if: – SpO_2 is <90% after administering high levels of oxygen for 30–60 seconds – respiratory rate is **<half normal rate** OR **>three times normal rate** – expansion is inadequate.
● Naloxone	● Opiates such as morphine, heroin etc, can cause respiratory depression; in cases of respiratory depression consider naloxone; monitor vital signs closely. NB Repeated doses of naloxone may be required – refer to naloxone guideline.
● Blood pressure	● Hypotension is common in severe cases of poisoning. ● Monitor blood pressure.
● Intravascular fluid	● In cases of drug induced symptomatic hypotension consider intravascular fluid – refer to intravascular fluid guideline.

Table 3.69 – ASSESSMENT and MANAGEMENT *continued*

Overdose and Poisoning *continued*

● Blood glucose level	● Measure blood glucose level – especially in cases of alcohol intoxication which is a common cause of hypoglycaemia (<4.0 mmol/l). ● Correct blood glucose level – **refer to glycaemic emergencies**; other relevant guidance: **glucose 10% guideline** and **glucagon guideline** – NB Glucagon is often not effective in overdoses.
● Thermoregulation	● Hypo- or hyperthermia can occur.
● Mental health assessment	● In cases of self-harm assess the patient's emotional and mental state – undertake a rapid mental health assessment – **refer to mental disorder guideline**. Do not delay treatment, but if possible, document the following information: ● The patient's home environment. ● The patient's social and family support network. ● The patient's emotional state and level of distress. ● The events leading to the incident.

● Transfer to further care	● All patients suffering an opioid overdose whether or not they have responded to naloxone – the effects of respiratory depression opioid overdose can last 4–5 hours.
	● All patients who have suffered an intentional overdose even if the substance is found to be harmless. If the patient does not require emergency treatment, but a mental health assessment may be required, consider alternative pathways (e.g. specialist mental health service) – as per local protocol. NB This decision should take into account the patient's preferences, and the views of the receiving service.
	Patients may be considered to be left at home if:
	    – The substance is verified by **TOXBASE/NPIS** as harmless.
	    – The incident is/was accidental.
	    – There is a responsible adult present.
	    – Advice given to seek medical advice if the patient becomes unwell.
	    – Arrangements have been made to inform the health visitor or GP.
	In patients that refuse transfer:
	● Assess mental capacity.
	● Explain the potential consequences of not receiving treatment.
	● If necessary seek medical advice – follow local protocol.

3 Medical
Specific Conditions

SECTION

Overdose and Poisoning (Adults)

Table 3.70 – SPECIFIC SUBSTANCES MANAGEMENT

SUBSTANCE	MANAGEMENT ⚠ Safety First – DO NOT put yourself in danger – carry out a dynamic risk assessment and undertake measures to preserve your own safety.
Alcohol (ethanol) Nausea, vomiting, slurred speech, confusion, convulsions, unconsciousness.	• Alcohol intoxication is a common emergency, especially in young adults, and is usually a transient problem. • Alcohol intoxication may cause alcohol-induced hypoglycaemia – Correct blood glucose level – **refer to glycaemic emergencies**; other relevant guidance: **glucose 10% guideline** and **glucagon guideline** – NB Glucagon is often not effective in overdoses. • When alcohol is combined with drugs in overdose, it may pose a major problem. For example, when combined with opiate drugs or sedatives, it will further decrease the level of consciousness with increased risk of respiratory depression and aspiration of vomit. In combination with paracetamol increases the risk of liver damage.
Carbon monoxide poisoning Disorientation, decreased consciousness. Unconscious. NB The supposed cherry red skin colouration in carbon monoxide poisoning is rarely seen in practice.	• Any patient found unconscious or disorientated in an enclosed space, for example, a patient involved in a fire in a confined space, where ventilation is impaired, or where a heating boiler may be defective, **MUST** be considered at risk of carbon monoxide poisoning. • The immediate requirement is to remove the patient from the source (and administer continuous supplemental oxygen in as high a concentration as possible) as carbon monoxide is displaced from haemoglobin more rapidly the higher the concentration of oxygen. SpO_2 monitoring is of no value in carbon monoxide poisoning as it measures bound haemoglobin and makes no distinction as to whether it is bound to O_2 or CO.
Orthochlorobenzalmalononitrile (CS gas) Lacrimation, burning sensation of the eyes, excessive mucus production, nausea and vomiting.	• Carried by police forces for defensive purposes. CS spray irritates the eyes (tear gas) and respiratory tract. **AVOID** contact with the gas, which is given off from patient's clothing. Where possible keep two metres from the patient and give them self-care instructions. Symptoms normally resolve in 15 minutes but may however potentiate or exacerbate existing respiratory conditions. If symptoms are present: • Remove patient to a well ventilated area. • Remove contaminated clothes and place in a sealed bag. • If possible remove contact lenses. • **DO NOT** irrigate the eyes as CS gas particles may dissolve and exacerbate irritation. If irrigation is required use copious amounts of saline. • Patients with severe respiratory problems should be immediately transported to hospital – **refer to airway management guideline** • Ensure good ventilation of the vehicle during transfer to further care.
Calcium-channel blockers diltiazem, verapamil, dihydrocodeine	• Overdose may lead to cardiac arrest. • Overdose of sustained release preparations can lead to delayed onset symptoms including: arrhythmias, shock, sudden cardiac collapse. • Refer to Table 3.69 for management. NB Immediate release preparations: problems are unlikely to develop in patients that are asymptomatic, and where the time interval is greater than 6 hours from time of ingestion.
Iron Nausea, vomiting blood, diarrhoea, black stools, metallic taste, convulsions, dizziness, flushed appearance, decreased level of consciousness, non-cardiac pulmonary oedema.	• Iron pills are regularly used by large numbers of the population including pregnant mothers. • They may cause extensive damage to the liver and gut and these patients will require hospital assessment and treatment. NB Charcoal is contra-indicated as it may interfere with subsequent treatment.
Cyanide Confusion, drowsiness, decreased level consciousness, dizziness, headache, convulsions.	• Cyanide poisoning requires specific treatment – seek medical advice. Provide full supportive therapy and transfer immediately to hospital. Provide an alert/information call. • Cyanide poisoning can occur in patients exposed to smoke in a confined space (e.g. house fire). Remove the patient from the source and administer continuous supplemental oxygen in as high a concentration as possible. If there are signs of decreased levels of consciousness transfer immediately to hospital. Provide an alert/information call. • In cases of CBRNE the HART/SORT team will provide guidance. • Poisoning may occur in certain industrial settings. Cyanide 'kits' should be available and the kit should be taken to hospital with the patient. The patient requires injection with dicobalt edetate **refer to dicobalt edetate guideline** or administration of the currently unlicensed drug hydroxycobalamin.

Table 3.70 – SPECIFIC SUBSTANCES MANAGEMENT *continued*

SUBSTANCE	MAGAGEMENT
Paracetamol and paracetamol containing compound drugs Nausea, vomiting, malaise, right upper quadrant abdominal pain, jaundice, confusion, drowsiness – unconsciousness may develop later. NB Presentation may be unreliable.	● There are a number of analgesic drugs that contain paracetamol and a combination of codeine or dextropropoxyphene. This, in overdose, creates two serious dangers: 1. Codeine and dextropropoxyphene are both derived from opioid drugs. This in overdose, especially if alcohol is involved, may well produce profound respiratory depression. This can be reversed with naloxone (refer to naloxone guideline). 2. Even modest doses of paracetamol may induce severe liver and kidney damage. It frequently takes 24–48 hours for the effects of paracetamol damage to become apparent and urgent blood paracetamol levels are required to assess the patient's level of risk.
Tricyclic antidepressants Central nervous system, excitability, confusion, blurred vision, dry mouth, fever, pupil dilation, convulsions, decreased level of consciousness, arrhythmias, hypotension, tachycardia, respiratory depression.	● Poisoning with tricyclic antidepressants may cause impaired consciousness, profound hypotension and cardiac arrhythmias. They are a common treatment for patients who are already depressed. Newer antidepressants such as fluoxetine (Prozac) and paroxetine (Seroxat) have different effects. ● Establish ECG monitoring. ● Arrhythmias – **refer to cardiac rhythm disturbance guideline**. ● The likelihood of convulsions is high – **refer to convulsion guidelines**. ● Monitor closely as the patient's physical condition can rapidly change.
Beta-blockers Bradycardia, hypotension, dizziness, confusion.	● Bradycardia – **refer to cardiac rhythm disturbance guideline**.
Opioids Drowsiness, nausea, vomiting, small pupils, respiratory depression, cyanosis, decreased level of consciousness, convulsions, non-cardiac pulmonary oedema.	● Ensure the airway is open – administer supplemental oxygen – refer to oxygen guideline. ● Profound respiratory depression can be reversed with naloxone – refer to naloxone guideline.
Benzodiazepines – diazepam, lorazepam, temazepam, flurazepam, loprazolam, etc Decreased level of consciousness, respiratory depression, hypotension.	Refer to Table 3.69 for management.

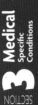

Table 3.71

Illegal Drugs

DRUG
Cocaine
(Powder cocaine, crack cocaine).

DESCRIPTION

Cocaine is a powerfully reinforcing psycho stimulant. Crack is made from cocaine in a process called freebasing.

OUTWARD SIGNS

Hyperexcitability, agitated, irritable and sometimes violent behaviour. Sweating. Dilated pupils.

EFFECTS

Induces a sense of exhilaration, euphoria, excitement and reduced hunger in the user primarily by blocking the re-uptake of the neurotransmitter dopamine in the midbrain, blocks noradrenaline uptake causing vasoconstriction and hypertension.

NB: Crack cocaine is pure and therefore more potent than street cocaine; it enters the bloodstream quicker and in higher concentrations. Because it is smoked, crack cocaine's effects are felt more quickly and they are more intense than those of powder cocaine. However, the effects of smoked crack are shorter lived than the effects of snorted powder cocaine. It is highly addictive even after only one use.

ADMINISTRATION

Cocaine comes in the form of a powder that is almost always 'cut' or mixed with other substances. It can be: snorted through the nose, rubbed into the gums, smoked or injected. Crack comes in the form of solid rocks, chips or chunks that are smoked.

SIDE EFFECTS

The symptoms of a cocaine overdose are intense and generally short lived. Although uncommon, people do die from cocaine or crack overdose, particularly following ingestion (often associated with swallowing 'evidence').

All forms of cocaine/crack use can cause coronary artery spasm, myocardial infarction and accelerated ischaemic heart disease, even in young people.

Various doses of cocaine can also produce other neurological and behavioural effects such as:
- dizziness.
- headache.
- movement problems.
- anxiety.
- insomnia.
- depression.
- hallucinations.

The unwanted effects of cocaine or crack overdose may include some or all of the following:
- tremors.
- dangerous or fatal rise in body temperature.
- delirium.
- myocardial infarction.
- cardiac arrest.
- seizures including status epilepticus.
- stroke.
- kidney failure.

TREATMENT

- Transfer patient rapidly to hospital.
- Administer supplemental oxygen – refer to oxygen guideline.
- Consider assisted ventilation at a rate of 12–20 breaths per minute if:
  - SpO$_2$ is <90% on high concentration O$_2$
  - respiratory rate is <10 or >30
  - expansion is inadequate.
- Undertake a 12-lead ECG – if the patient has a 12-lead ECG suggestive of myocardial infarction and a history of recent cocaine use then administer nitrates but do not administer thrombolysis.
- Administer aspirin and GTN if the patient complains of chest pain – refer to aspirin and GTN guidelines.
- **Chest pain** – administer diazepam if the patient has severe chest pain – refer to diazepam guideline.
- **Convulsions** – refer to convulsions guideline.
- **Hypertension** – if systolic BP > 220 and diastolic BP > 140 mmHg in the absence of longstanding hypertension – seek medical advice.
- **Hyperthermia** – administer paracetamol and cooling if the body temperature is elevated – refer to paracetamol guideline.

NB Swallowed crack cocaine represents a severe medical emergency and needs **URGENT** transportation to hospital **EVEN IF ASYMPTOMATIC**

Table 3.71

Illegal Drugs continued

DRUG
Amphetamines
(Amphetamines,
Methamphetamine)
Commonly known as:
Bennies, Billy Whizz,
Black Beauties,
Bumblebees, Clear Rocks,
Co-pilots, Crank, Croke,
Glass, LA Turnarounds,
Mollies, Oranges, Pep
Pills, Pink Champagne,
Pink Speed, Bombs,
Rippers, Rocks, Speed,
Splash, Sulph, Sulphate,
Wake Ups, Whizz.

DESCRIPTION
Amphetamines were developed in the 1930s and have been medically prescribed in the past for diet control and as a stimulant.

OUTWARD SIGNS
Mood swings, extreme hunger, sleeplessness, and hyperactivity.

EFFECTS
Increases energy levels, confidence and sociability.

ADMINISTRATION
They can be swallowed, sniffed or, rarely, injected. Onset approximately 30 minutes. Lasts for several hours. Used with other drugs or alcohol, the effects are magnified.

SIDE EFFECTS
Cardiovascular
- Tachycardia can lead to heart failure even in healthy individuals (**refer to cardiac rhythm disturbance guideline**).
- Hypertension can produce pinpoint haemorrhages in skin, especially on the face and even lead to stroke.

Central nervous system
- 'High' feelings, panic, paranoia can produce mental illness picture in long-term use, poor sleep, hyperpyrexia.

Gastrointestinal
- Liver failure.

TREATMENT
- **Vital signs** – monitor pulse, blood pressure, cardiac rhythm.
- **Agitation** – seek medical advice for consideration of diazepam use for severe agitation.
- **Convulsions – refer to convulsions guideline**.
- **Cardiac rhythm disturbance** – narrow-complex tachycardia with cardiac output is best left untreated.
- **Hypertension** – if systolic BP >220 and diastolic BP >140 mmHg in the absence of longstanding hypertension – seek medical advice.
- **Hypotension** – correct hypotension by raising the foot of the trolley and/or the administration of intravascular fluid – refer to intravascular fluid guideline.
- **Hyperthermia** – rapid transfer to hospital; cooling measures may be undertaken en-route – **refer to heat related illness guideline**.

DRUG
Opiates
(Heroin, Diamorphine,
Methadone-Amidone,
Dolophine, Methadose).

DESCRIPTION
Methadone is a synthetic opiate commonly used in the treatment of heroin addiction.

OUTWARD SIGNS
Withdrawal symptoms:
Sweating, shivering, muscle cramps, lacrimation.

EFFECTS
Reduce physical and psychological pain – relieving anxiety. The effects of methadone are less intense.

ADMINISTRATION
Injected, snorted or smoked.

SIDE EFFECTS
Cardiovascular system
Damage to veins and lungs. Infection. It is likely that babies are born underweight.

TREATMENT
Refer to Table 3.70 for management.

3 Medical Specific Conditions
SECTION

Table 3.71

Illegal Drugs *continued*

SECTION

3 Medical
Specific
Conditions

DRUG
3–4 methylene dioxymethamphetamine (MDMA) – Ecstacy 'E'
Commonly known as: doves, apples, strawberries, and diamonds.

DESCRIPTION
MDMA is a psychoactive drug with hallucinogenic effects.

OUTWARD SIGNS
Sweating, dilated pupils and elevated mood.

EFFECTS
Feeling warm, energetic, and friendly, rising to a state of euphoria.

ADMINISTRATION
'E' tablets may be white embossed 'headache' sized pills, or coloured capsules.
They take 40 minutes to work, lasting for 2–6 hours.
'E' may not be addictive but is illegal.

SIDE EFFECTS
Cardiovascular system
- Tachycardia (**refer to cardiac rhythm disturbance guideline**).
- Capillary rupture, causing red marking on the face in particular.

Central nervous system
- Some patients develop hyperpyrexia which can be life-threatening. These patients need urgent transfer to hospital for specialist care. Cooling measures (**refer to heat related illness guideline**) may be helpful but should not delay transfer to further care.
- Depression, panic and anxiety may also occur.

Liver and kidney damage
- Liver failure and severe kidney damage may occur.

Other
- Cystitis and heavy periods may occur in females who use 'E'.

TREATMENT
- Administer diazepam to control anxiety and agitation – refer to diazepam guideline.
- Treat convulsions with diazepam – refer to diazepam guideline.
- If the systolic BP > 220 and diastolic > 140 mmHg in the absence of longstanding hypertension give diazepam – refer to diazepam guideline.
- Correct hypotension by raising the foot of the bed and/or by giving fluids as per medical emergencies – refer to intravascular fluid guideline.
- Cooling measures (**refer to heat related illness guideline**) may be helpful but should not delay transfer to further care.
- Depression, panic and anxiety may also occur.

Table 3.71

Illegal Drugs *continued*

DRUG	
Lysergic Acid (Diethylamide (LSD) or 'acid')	**DESCRIPTION** It is a 'mind altering drug' that alters the brain's perception of things. It was discovered in 1943, and was used in the 1960s as a 'recreational drug'. **OUTWARD SIGNS** Agitated, unusual behaviour, clear mental disturbance. The patient may appear distant and display anxious behaviour. **DO NOT** interfere unduly as the 'trip' will self-limit, and communication is easier then. Keep the patient safe, and remember other drugs and alcohol will aggravate the effects of LSD. **EFFECTS** The alterations in perception may be pleasant or 'nightmarish', or a mix of both, and last for some 12 hours. **ADMINISTRATION** Produced on patches of blotting paper, called tabs or trips, often with printed motifs including cartoon characters. Once swallowed they take 30–60 minutes to work. The trip will last up to 12 hours and cannot be stopped. LSD is not addictive but is illegal. **SIDE EFFECTS** **Central nervous system** ● Visual hallucinations (distortion and delusions), which can cause dangerous behaviour. ● Nightmarish perceptions 'bad trips' may last for 12 hours. ● Nausea and vomiting. ● Personality changes and psychiatric illness. ● Nightmarish flashbacks that can last for years after drug use stops. ● Delusions – false sensations or visions – may affect taste, hearing and vision. ● Can trigger hidden mental illness in individuals. ● Permanent eye damage can occur. **TREATMENT** ● Usually self-limiting but sedate if necessary with intravenous diazepam – refer to diazepam guideline.

3 Medical
Specific
Conditions
SECTION

Pulmonary Embolism [103, 479–487]

1. Introduction

- Pulmonary embolism (PE) is an obstruction of the pulmonary vessels which usually presents as one of four types:

  1. **Multiple small pulmonary emboli** – characterised by progressive breathlessness more commonly identified at outpatients appointments than through emergency presentation due to the long-standing nature of the problem.

  2. **Segmental emboli with pulmonary infarction** – may present with pleuritic pain and/or haemoptysis but with little or no cardiovascular compromise.

  3. **Major pulmonary emboli obstruction of the larger branches of the pulmonary tree** – may present with sudden onset of shortness of breath with transient rise in pulse and/or fall in blood pressure. Often a precursor to a massive PE.

  4. **Massive pulmonary emboli** – often presenting with loss of consciousness, tachypnoea and intense jugular vein distension, and may prove immediately or rapidly (within 1 hour) fatal or unresponsive to cardiopulmonary resuscitation.

- Pulmonary embolism can present with a wide range of symptoms (refer to Table 3.72). The presence of predisposing factors (refer to Table 3.73) increases the index of suspicion of PE; which increases with the number of predisposing factors present. However, in approximately 30% of cases, the presentation is idiopathic.

- Symptoms such as dyspnoea, tachypnoea or chest pain have been found in >90% of cases of patients with PE; pleuritic chest pain is one of the most frequent symptoms of presentation.

- There may be sudden collapse with no obvious physical signs, other than cardiorespiratory arrest.

- Lesser risk factors include air, coach or other travel leading to periods of immobility, especially whilst sitting, oral oestrogen (some contraceptive pills) and central venous catheterisation.

- Over 70% of patients who suffer PE have peripheral vein thrombosis and vigilance is therefore of great importance – it may not initially appear logical to check the legs of a patient with chest pain but can be of great diagnostic value in such cases.

Table 3.72 – SIGNS AND SYMPTOMS OF PE

Symptoms

- Dyspnoea.
- Pleuritic chest pain.
- Substernal chest pain.
- Apprehension.
- Cough.
- Haemoptysis.
- Syncope.

Signs

- Respiratory rate >20 breaths per minute.
- Pulse rate >100 beats per minute.
- SpO$_2$ <92%.
- Signs of deep vein thrombosis (DVT).

Table 3.73 – PREDISPOSING FACTORS

Factor

Surgery especially recent

- Abdominal.
- Pelvic.
- Hip or knee surgery.
- Post operative intensive care.

Obstetrics

- Pregnancy.

Cardiac

- Recent acute myocardial infarction.

Limb problems

- Recent lower limb fractures.
- Varicose veins.
- Lower limb problems secondary to stroke or spinal cord injury.

Malignancy

- Abdominal and/or pelvic in particular advanced metastatic disease.
- Concurrent chemotherapy.

Other

- Risk increases with age.
- 65% ≥60 years of age.
- Previous proven PE/DVT.
- Immobility.
- Thrombotic disorder.
- Neurological disease with extremity paresis.
- Thrombophilia.
- Hormone replacement therapy and oral contraception.
- Prolonged bed rest >3 days.
- Other recent trauma.

2. Incidence

- Pulmonary embolism is a relatively common cardiovascular condition affecting approximately 21 per 10,000 per annum.

3. Severity and Outcome

- Pulmonary embolism can be life-threatening leading to death in approximately 7–11% of cases; however, treatment is effective if given early.

- Patients with a previous episode(s) of PE are three times more likely to experience a recurrence.

4. Pathophysiology

- The development of a pulmonary embolism occurs when a blood clot (thrombus), comprising red cells, platelets, and fibrin, forms in a vein, subsequently dislodges (embolism) and travels in the circulation. This is known as venous thromboembolism (VTE). If the embolism is small it may be filtered in the pulmonary capillary bed, but if the embolism is large it may occlude pulmonary blood vessels. The development of a VTE can also lead to deep vein thrombosis.

Pulmonary Embolism

- The haemodynamic problems occur when >30–50% of the pulmonary arterial bed is occluded.

- The probability of a PE can be assessed using a clinical predication tool such as the Wells Criteria (refer to Table 3.74). However a low probability cannot rule out PE.

5. Assessment and Management

For the assessment and management of pulmonary embolism refer to Table 3.75 and Figure 3.18.

Table 3.74 – WELLS CRITERIA FOR PE

Item	Score
Clinical signs and symptoms of DVT (leg swelling and pain with palpation of the deep veins).	3
An alternative diagnosis is less likely than pulmonary embolism.	3
Pulse rate >100 beats per minute.	1.5
Immobilisation or surgery in the previous 4 weeks.	1.5
Previous DVT/pulmonary embolism.	1.5
Haemoptysys.	1
Malignancy (treatment ongoing or within previous 6 months or palliative).	1
Clinical Probability of PE	**Total**
high >6 points	
moderate 2–6 points	
low <2 points	

KEY POINTS

Pulmonary Embolism

- **Common symptoms of PE are dyspnoea, tachypnoea, pleuritic pain, apprehension, tachycardia, cough, haemoptysis, leg pain/clinical DVT.**

- **Risk factors may be identifiable from the history.**

- **Ensure ABCD assessment and apply a pulse oximetry monitor early.**

- **Patients may present with unilateral swelling of the lower limbs; they may also be warm and red.**

- **Apply oxygen and if in respiratory distress, transfer to further care as a medical emergency.**

Table 3.75 – ASSESSMENT and MANAGEMENT of:

Pulmonary Embolism

ASSESSMENT	MANAGEMENT

● Assess ABCD	● If any of the following **TIME CRITICAL** features are present:
	   – major **ABCD** problems
	   – extreme breathing difficulty
	   – cyanosis
	   – severe hypoxia (SpO$_2$) <90% – unresponsive to oxygen.
	 ● Start correcting **A** and **B** problems.
	 ● Undertake a **TIME CRITICAL** transfer to nearest appropriate hospital.
	 ● Provide an alert/information call.
	 ● Continue patient management en-route.

● Specifically assess	● Respiratory rate and effort. ● Signs and symptoms combined with predisposing factors. ● Lower limbs for unilateral swelling; may also be warm and red. ● Calf tenderness/pain may be present – extensive leg clots may also lead to femoral tenderness. ● Differential diagnoses include pleurisy, pneumothorax or cardiac chest pain. ● High index of suspicion.
● Position	● Position patient for comfort and ease of respiration – often sitting forwards – but be aware of potential hypotension.
● Cardiorespiratory arrest	● Be prepared for cardiorespiratory arrest – refer to appropriate resuscitation guideline.
● Oxygen	● Administer supplemental oxygen, aim for a target saturation within the range of 94–98%.
● ECG	● Undertake a 12-lead ECG – be aware that the classic S1 Q3 T3 12-lead ECG presentation is often **NOT** present, even during massive PE. The commonest finding is a sinus tachycardia.
● Ventilation	● Consider assisted ventilation if indicated – refer to airway and breathing management guideline.
● Fluid	● If fluid therapy indicated – refer to intravascular fluid therapy guideline.
● Transfer to further care	● Transfer rapidly to nearest appropriate hospital. ● Provide an alert/information call. ● Continue patient management en-route.

ADDITIONAL INFORMATION

Whilst there is no specific pre-hospital treatment available, there may be a window of opportunity to manage massive PE before the patient progresses to cardiac arrest. Other in-hospital treatments may be effective including: haemodynamic and respiratory support, thrombolysis, surgical pulmonary embolectomy, percutaneous catheter embolectomy and fragmentation, and anticoagulation.

SECTION

3 Medical
Specific Conditions

Pulmonary Embolism

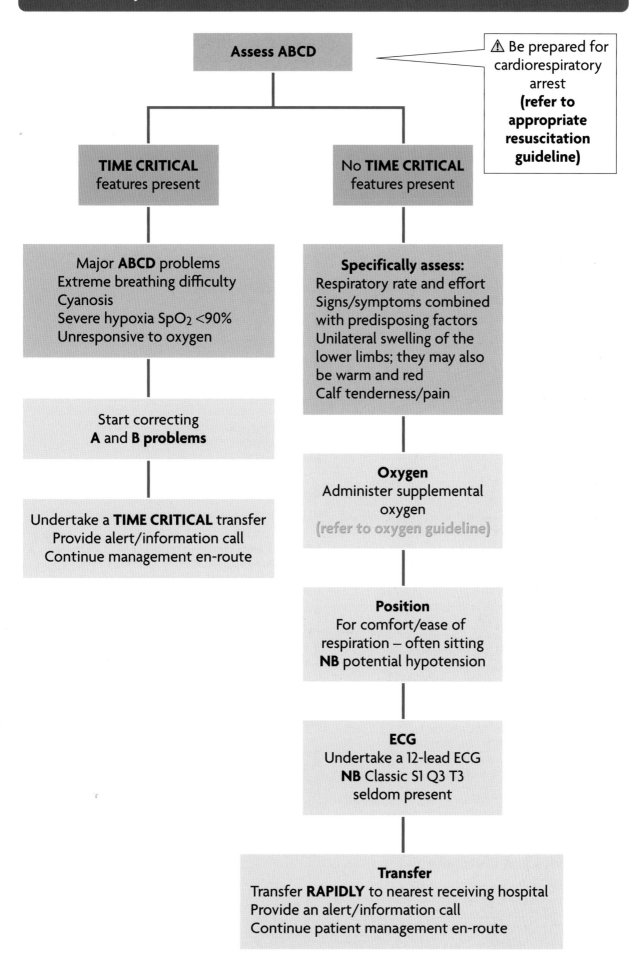

Assess ABCD

⚠ Be prepared for cardiorespiratory arrest **(refer to appropriate resuscitation guideline)**

TIME CRITICAL features present

No **TIME CRITICAL** features present

Major **ABCD** problems
Extreme breathing difficulty
Cyanosis
Severe hypoxia SpO$_2$ <90%
Unresponsive to oxygen

Specifically assess:
Respiratory rate and effort
Signs/symptoms combined with predisposing factors
Unilateral swelling of the lower limbs; they may also be warm and red
Calf tenderness/pain

Start correcting
A and **B problems**

Oxygen
Administer supplemental oxygen
(refer to oxygen guideline)

Undertake a **TIME CRITICAL** transfer
Provide alert/information call
Continue management en-route

Position
For comfort/ease of respiration – often sitting
NB potential hypotension

ECG
Undertake a 12-lead ECG
NB Classic S1 Q3 T3 seldom present

Transfer
Transfer **RAPIDLY** to nearest receiving hospital
Provide an alert/information call
Continue patient management en-route

Figure 3.18 – Assessment and management algorithm of pulmonary embolism.

Medical
Specific
Conditions

3
SECTION

Stroke/Transient Ischaemic Attack (TIA) [148, 488–493]

1. Introduction

Stroke is a major health problem in the UK. Improving care for patients with stroke and transient ischaemic attack (TIA) is a key national priority, with a National Stroke Strategy published by the Department of Health in 2007, and guidelines published by the National Institute for Health and Clinical Excellence (NICE) in 2008.

1.1 Acute stroke

Acute stroke is a medical emergency. For patients with thrombotic stroke, treatment with thrombolytic therapy (alteplase) is highly time-dependent. In order to determine suitability for treatment, patients must undergo a brain scan; therefore, patients need to be transferred to an appropriate hospital as rapidly as possible once the diagnosis is suspected.

It is important to remember that thrombolysis is not the only management proven to benefit stroke patients. Admission to a stroke unit for early specialist care is known to be life saving and to reduce disability, even if thrombolysis is not indicated.

Symptoms of stroke include:

- Numbness.
- Weakness or paralysis.
- Slurred speech.
- Blurred vision.
- Confusion.
- Severe headache.

The most sensitive features associated with diagnosing stroke in the pre-hospital setting are facial weakness, arm and leg weakness, and speech disturbance.

1.2 Transient ischaemic attack (TIA)

Transient ischaemic attack (TIA) is defined as stroke symptoms and signs that resolve within 24 hours. However, there are limitations to these definitions. For example, they do not include retinal symptoms (sudden onset of monocular visual loss), which should be considered as part of the definition of stroke and TIA. The symptoms of a TIA usually resolve within minutes or a few hours at most, and **anyone with continuing neurological signs when first assessed should be assumed to have had a stroke.**

The risk of a patient with TIA developing a stroke is high and symptoms should always be taken seriously.

2. Incidence

Each year in England, approximately 110,000 people have a first or recurrent stroke and a further 20,000 people have a TIA.

3. Severity and Outcome

Stroke accounted for over 56,000 deaths in England and Wales in 1999, which represents 11% of all deaths. Most people survive a first stroke, but often have significant morbidity.

More than 900,000 people in England are living with the effects of stroke, with half of these being dependent on other people for help with everyday activities.

4. Pathophysiology

The majority (70%) of strokes are ischaemic. Distinguishing between ischaemic and haemorrhagic strokes is not currently feasible in the pre-hospital setting.

A TIA occurs when blood supply to part of the brain is temporarily interrupted.

5. Assessment

Assess ABCDs

- Record time of onset if known.
- May have airway and breathing problems (**refer to dyspnoea guideline**).
- Level of consciousness may vary (**refer to altered level of consciousness guideline**).

Evaluate if the patient has any TIME CRITICAL features – these may include:

- Any major ABC problem.
- Positive FAST test.
- Altered level of consciousness.

If any of these features are present, start **correcting A and B problems then transport to the nearest suitable receiving hospital. Local arrangements will determine pathways (e.g. bypassing a local hospital for the nearest 'hyperacute' stroke centre).**

- Provide an alert/information call stating clearly that the patient is FAST positive/suspected acute stroke.
- En-route – continue patient **management** (see below).
- Assess blood glucose level, as **hypoglycaemia** may mimic a stroke.

Suspected acute stroke – a positive FAST test should be considered a TIME CRITICAL condition. Perform a brief secondary survey but do not allow this to delay transport to hospital:

- Assess blood pressure to provide a baseline for hospital assessment.
- Assess Glasgow Coma Scale (GCS) on **unaffected side** – eye and motor assessments may be more readily assessed if speech is badly affected.

Table 3.76 – FAST TEST

Facial weakness	Ask the patient to smile or show teeth. Look for NEW lack of symmetry.
Arm weakness	Ask the patient to lift their arms together and hold for 5 seconds. Does one arm drift or fall down? The arm with motor weakness will drift downwards compared to the unaffected limb.
Speech	Ask the patient to repeat a phrase. Assess for slurring or difficulty with the words or sentence.

These components make up the **FAST** (face, arms, speech test) assessment that should be carried out on **ALL** patients with suspected stroke/TIA. A deficit in any one of the three domains is sufficient for the patient to be identified as 'FAST positive'.

6. Management

Follow **medical emergencies guideline,** remembering to: Start correcting:

- **A**irway
- **B**reathing
- **C**irculation
- **D**isability (mini neurological examination)
- oxygen therapy is not recommended unless the patient is hypoxic (refer to oxygen guideline).

Consider recording 12-lead ECG en-route to hospital, but **do not delay transport** for this test.

Intravenous access is not essential unless the patient requires specific interventions, and may delay transport to hospital.

Specifically:

- Check blood glucose level (**refer to glycaemic emergencies guideline**).
- Conscious patients should be conveyed in the semi-recumbent position.
- Patients should be nil by mouth.

NOTE: Local policies will determine whether paramedics should use a risk score for suspected TIA patients and/or administer aspirin. In the absence of clear evidence relating to pre-hospital use of these interventions, JRCALC are unable to make a firm recommendation.

7. Referral Pathway

This will depend on locally commissioning arrangements. For example, bypassing local hospitals for a 'hyperacute' centre may require patients in some networks to meet specific criteria based on a positive FAST test and onset within the preceding 2 hours, so that the patient is within the 'time window' for thrombolysis.

Where possible, a witness should be asked to accompany the patient to hospital.

It is important to remember that thrombolysis is not the only management proven to benefit stroke patients. Admission to a stroke unit for early specialist care is known to be life saving and to reduce disability, even if thrombolysis is not indicated.

8. Audit Information

Ambulance services are required to monitor the use of the FAST test in patients with suspected stroke, and agree local pathways for patients with suspected stroke. Careful documentation of your assessment and management, including accurate timings, is essential to improving care for this group of patients.

KEY POINTS

Stroke/Transient Ischaemic Attack (TIA)

- **Time is of the essence in suspected acute stroke.**
- **Record time of onset if known.**
- **Stroke is common and may be due to either cerebral infarction or haemorrhage.**
- **The most sensitive features associated with diagnosing stroke in the pre-hospital setting are facial weakness, arm and leg weakness, and speech disturbance – the FAST test.**
- **FAST test should be carried out on ALL patients with suspected stroke/TIA.**
- **Patients with TIA may be at high risk of stroke and should be taken to hospital for further assessment.**

Further Reading

Comprehensive, high-quality information on stroke is available at:

- NHS Evidence – stroke
  http://www.evidence.nhs.uk/topic/stroke
- The Stroke Association
  http://www.stroke.org.uk

1. Introduction

- The incidence of allergic reactions continues to rise.
- The symptoms range from mild to life-threatening and include:
  - urticaria (hives)
  - angio-oedema (swelling of the face, eyelids, lips and tongue)
  - itching
  - dyspnoea
  - wheeze
  - stridor
  - hypoxia
  - abdominal pain
  - diarrhoea/vomiting
  - hypotension
  - pulmonary and/or cardiovascular compromise.
- The most common triggers are food, drugs and venom (refer to Table 3.77) but in 30% of cases the trigger is unknown.
- Injected allergens commonly result in cardiovascular compromise, with hypotension and shock predominating.
- Inhaled and ingested allergens typically cause rashes, vomiting, facial swelling, upper airway swelling and wheeze.
- Slow release drugs prolong absorption and exposure to the allergen.

Table 3.77 – COMMON TRIGGERS OF ALLERGIC REACTIONS

1 – Foods

Nuts (e.g. peanuts, walnut, almond, brazil and hazel), pulses, sesame seeds, milk, eggs, fish/shellfish.

2 – Venom – insect sting/bites

Insect stings and bites (e.g. wasps and bees).

NB Bees may leave a venom sac which should be scraped off (not squeezed).

3 – Drugs

Antibiotics (e.g. penicillin, cephalosporin, ciprofloxacin, and vancomycin), non-steroidal anti-inflammatory drugs, angiotensin converting enzyme inhibitor, gelatins, protamine, vitamin K, amphotericin, etoposide, acetazolamide, pethidine, local anaesthetic, diamorphine, streptokinase and other drugs.

4 – Other causes

e.g. Latex[a], hair dye.

[a] Latex allergy has implications for equipment use.

2. Incidence

- It is estimated that allergic reactions affect 40% of children, with anaphylaxis estimated to affect up to 2% of the population.

3. Severity and Outcome

- The severity of symptoms varies from a localised urticaria to life-threatening pulmonary and/or cardiovascular compromise, that is anaphylaxis.
- Generally, the longer it takes for anaphylactic symptoms to develop, the less severe the overall reaction.
- The mortality associated with anaphylaxis is estimated to be <1%. Death occurs quickly (venom: 10–15 minutes; food: 30–35 minutes) after contact with the trigger usually as a result of respiratory arrest from airway obstruction.

4. Assessment and Management

- For the assessment and management of anaphylaxis and allergic reactions refer to Figure 3.19.

Children with previous episodes:

- may wear 'MedicAlert®' bracelets/necklets
- they or their carers may carry an adrenaline pen (e.g. Anapen®, EpiPen®).

KEY POINTS

Allergic Reactions including Anaphylaxis (Children)

- **Remove from trigger if possible.**
- **Anaphylaxis can occur despite a long history of previously safe exposure to a potential trigger.**
- **Consider anaphylaxis in the presence of acute cutaneous symptoms and/or airway or cardiovascular compromise.**
- **Anaphylaxis may be rapid, slow or biphasic.**
- **Adrenaline is key in managing anaphylaxis.**
- **In anaphylactic reactions, the benefits of adminstering adrenaline, even at an inappropriate dose, far exceed the risk of giving no medication at all.**

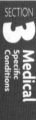

SECTION **3** Medical Specific Conditions

Allergic Reactions including Anaphylaxis (Children)

Quickly remove from trigger
if possible (e.g. environmental,
infusion etc)
DO NOT delay definitive treatment
if removing trigger not feasible

Assess ABCDE
If TIME CRITICAL features present –
correct A and B and transfer to nearest
suitable receiving hospital
Provide an alert/information call

**Consider mild/moderate allergic
reaction if:**
Onset of illness is minutes to hours
AND
Cutaneous findings (e.g. urticaria
and/or angio-oedema)

Consider chlorphenamine
(refer to chlorphenamine guideline)

Consider anaphylaxis if:
Sudden onset and rapid progression
Airway and/or **Breathing** problems (e.g.
dyspnoea, hoarseness, stridor, wheeze,
throat or chest tightness) and/or
Circulation (e.g. hypotension, syncope,
pronounced tachycardia) and/or **Skin** (e.g.
erythema, urticaria, mucosal changes) problems

Administer high levels of
supplementary oxygen
(refer to oxygen guideline)

Administer adrenaline 1 in 1000 IM only
(refer to adrenaline guideline)

If haemodynamically compromised
(refer to fluid therapy guideline)

Consider chlorphenamine
(refer to chlorphenamine guideline)

Consider administering hydrocortisone
(refer to hydrocortisone guideline)

Consider nebulised salbutamol
for bronchospasm
(refer to salbutamol guideline)

Monitor and re-assess ABC
Monitor ECG, PEFR (if possible),
BP and pulse oximetry en-route

Figure 3.19 – Allergic reactions including anaphylaxis algorithm.

1. Introduction

- Asthma is one of the commonest medical conditions requiring hospitalisation.

- The severity of asthma may be subdivided into mild/moderate, severe, or life-threatening (refer to Table 3.79).

- There may be a history of increasing wheeze or breathlessness (often worse at night or early in the morning). Respiratory infections, allergy and physical exertion are common triggers.

- Known asthmatics will be on regular medication, taking inhalers ('preventers' and/or 'relievers') and sometimes oral medications such as Montelukast (Singulair®) and theophyllines.

- Some children with asthma will have an individualised treatment plan with detailed information regarding their daily symptom control as well as what to do in an acute exacerbation.

- **Inhaled foreign body:** Consider an inhaled foreign body in a child experiencing their first wheezy episode, especially if there is a history of playing with small toys and the wheeze was of sudden onset and is unilateral. These children must be transferred for medical assessment. If they are unwell during transport, bronchodilators may provide some clinical benefit.

2. Severity and Outcome

- Children with previous hospital admissions (particularly intensive care admissions), are at risk of future severe or life-threatening episodes (and even death) – so this information should be sought.

Table 3.78 – RISK FACTORS FOR SEVERE ASTHMA

Risk Factors

- Previous severe or life-threatening episodes.
- Previous hospital admission for asthma especially if in the last year.
- Previous admission requiring intensive care.
- Back to back nebulisers with poor or no response.

3. Pathophysiology

- Asthma causes chronic bronchial inflammation which results in narrowing of the airways. In acute attacks, airway irritation causes smooth muscle contraction producing respiratory compromise. Inflammatory processes also cause i) excessive sputum production and ii) swelling of the bronchial mucosal which blocks the small airways.

  - Inspiration (an active process) generates sufficient pressures to overcome airway narrowing, but during expiration (a passive process) relaxation of the respiratory muscles causes airway narrowing, producing the characteristic wheeze.

  - Various medications are used to treat asthma. In children, these are typically delivered using a spacer device (e.g. a Volumatic® or Aerochamber®). Some children may also have a home nebuliser.

4. Assessment

Following an ABC assessment, the severity of the asthma attack should be established (refer to Table 3.79 and Asthma Algorithm – Figure 3.20).

Table 3.79 – FEATURES OF SEVERITY

Life-threatening asthma

- Silent chest.
- SpO_2 <92%.
- Cyanosis PEFR <33% best or predicted.
- Poor respiratory effort.
- Hypotension.
- Exhaustion.
- Confusion.

Severe asthma

- Can't complete sentences in one breath or too breathless to talk or feed.
- SpO_2 <92%.
- PEFR 33–50% best or predicted.
- Pulse:
  - >140 in children aged 2–5 years
  - >125 in children aged >5 years.
- Respiration:
  - >40 breaths/min aged 2–5 years
  - >30 breaths/min aged >5 years.

Moderate asthma exacerbation

- Able to talk in sentences.
- SpO_2 ≥92%.
- PEFR ≥50% best or predicted.
- Heart rate:
  - ≤140/min in children aged 2–5 years
  - ≤125/min in children >5 years.
- Respiratory rate:
  - ≤40/min in children aged 2–5 years
  - ≤30/min in children >5 years.

5. Management

The Asthma Algorithm (Figure 3.20) describes the management of mild/moderate, severe and life-threatening asthma. Adrenaline and hydrocortisone are now included in the management of severe/life threatening asthma in children.

Always ask if the child has an individualised asthma treatment plan and follow it, unless clinical circumstances dictate otherwise.

For some children alternative care pathways will already have been created (e.g. early referral to their GP). It is well recognised, however, that children with apparently minor symptoms can subsequently deteriorate and practitioners should therefore have a low threshold for onward referral (especially where an alternative pathway has not already been established).

Peak expiratory flow rate measurements (PEFR):
PEFR should be attempted where possible in children before and after nebulised therapy in mild to moderate

Asthma (Children)

asthma. However, care should be taken in severe life-threatening attacks as it could exacerbate the attack and the patient may deteriorate. Predicted PEFR are listed in Table 3.80.

Table 3.80 – PEAK EXPIRATORY FLOW CHART

Height (m)	Height (ft)	Predicted EU PEFR (L/min)
0.85	2'9'	87
0.90	2'11'	95
0.95	3'1'	104
1.00	3'3'	115
1.05	3'5'	127
1.10	3'7'	141
1.15	3'9'	157
1.20	3'11'	174
1.25	4'1'	192
1.30	4'3'	212
1.35	4'5'	233
1.40	4'7'	254
1.45	4'9'	276
1.50	4'11'	299
1.55	5'1'	323
1.60	5'3'	346
1.65	5'5'	370
1.70	5'7'	393

KEY POINTS

Asthma (Children)
- Clinical assessment should determine the severity of the attack.
- Bronchodilators (e.g. salbutamol) are the mainstay of treatment.
- High levels of oxygen may be required during an asthma attack.
- Mild/moderate attacks should be managed with inhaled bronchodilators via a spacer device.
- Nebulised treatments should be reserved for moderate/severe attacks where oxygen is required.
- In addition to β2 agonists, ipratropium is used in severe cases.

Section 3 Medical Specific

Table 3.81 – ASSESSMENT and MANAGEMENT

Asthma

ASSESSMENT	MANAGEMENT

● Assess **ABCD**
● Specifically assess for the severity of the asthma attack (refer to Figure 3.20)
	● If any of the following **TIME CRITICAL** features present:
	  – major ABCD problems
	  – extreme difficulty in breathing or requirement for assisted ventilations
	  – exhaustion
	  – cyanosis
	  – silent chest
	  – SpO_2 <92%
	  – PEF <33% best or predicted.
	● Start correcting A and B problems.
	● Undertake a **TIME CRITICAL** transfer to nearest receiving hospital.
	● Continue patient management en-route.
	● Provide an alert/information call.

● Mild/moderate asthma
  – Able to talk in sentences
  – SpO_2 >92%
  – PEFR >50% best or predicted
  – Pulse <140 in child ages 2–5, <125 in child >5
  – Respiration <40 in child ages 2–5
  – <30 in child ages >5
	● Move to a calm quiet environment.
	● Encourage use of own inhaler, using a spacer if available. Ensure correct technique is used (refer to Figure 3.20).
	● If unresponsive:
	  – administer high levels of supplementary oxygen
	  – administer nebulised salbutamol (refer to salbutamol guideline).

● Severe asthma
  – Can't complete sentences in one breath or too breathless to talk or feed
  – SpO_2 <92%
  – PEFR 33–50% best or predicted
  – Pulse >140 in child aged 2–5 years
  – >125 in child >5 years
  – Respiration >40 in child ages 2–5 years
  – >30 in child aged >5 years.
	● Administer high levels of supplementary oxygen.
	● Administer nebulised salbutamol (refer to salbutamol guideline).
	● If no improvement administer ipratropium bromide (refer to ipratropium bromide guideline).
	● Administer steroids (refer to relevant steroids guideline).
	● Continuous salbutamol nebulisation may be administered unless clinically significant side effects occur (refer to salbutamol guideline).

● Life-threatening asthma
  – Silent chest
  – SpO_2 <92%
  – Cyanosis
  – PEFR <33% best or predicted (exercise caution with PEFR in this patient group)
  – Poor respiratory effort
  – Hypotension
  – Exhaustion
  – Confusion
	● Continuous salbutamol nebulisation may be administered unless clinically significant side effects occur (refer to salbutamol guideline).
	● Administer adrenaline 1 in 1000 IM only (refer to adrenaline guideline).
	● Positive pressure ventilation using a nebulising T piece. Assess for bilateral tension pneumothorax.

● Transfer	● Transfer rapidly to nearest receiving hospital. ● Provide an alert/information call. ● Continue patient management en-route.
	● For cases of mild asthma that respond to treatment consider alternative care pathway where appropriate. ● **Note:** exercise caution in known severe asthmatics.

Asthma (Children)

MILD/ MODERATE ASTHMA

Move to a calm, quiet environment

Encourage use of own inhaler, preferably using a spacer. Ensure correct technique is used; two puffs, followed by two puffs every 2 minutes to a maximum of ten puffs

Administer high levels of supplementary **oxygen**

Administer nebulised **salbutamol** using an oxygen driven nebuliser *(refer to salbutamol guideline)*

SEVERE ASTHMA

If no improvement, administer **ipratropium bromide** by nebuliser *(refer to ipratropium bromide guideline)*

Administer steroids *(refer to relevant steroids guideline)*

Continuous **salbutamol** nebulisation may be administered unless clinically significant side effects occur *(refer to salbutamol guideline)*

LIFE-THREATENING ASTHMA

Administer **adrenaline** *(refer to adrenaline guideline)* NB Check the child is still receiving high levels of oxygen before administering

Positive pressure nebulise using a bag-valve-mask and 'T' piece. Provide an alert / information call

NEAR FATAL ASTHMA

As you progress through the treatment algorithm consider the child's overall response on the condition arrow and transfer as indicated

IMPROVING

CONSIDER TRANSFER

DETERIORATING

TIME CRITICAL TRANSFER

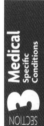

3 Medical Specific Conditions SECTION

Figure 3.20 – Asthma assessment and management algorithm.

1. Introduction

- Convulsions (also called 'tonic-clonic seizure' or 'fit') arise from abnormal electrical activity in the brain. They are usually **generalised** (affecting both sides of the body), but may also be **focal**, affecting just one side of the body. Fever is the commonest cause for convulsions (febrile convulsions) but they can also be caused by epilepsy, CNS infections (meningitis or encephalitis), hypoglycaemia, hypoxia, electrolyte imbalances, head injuries or (rarely) hypertension. Occasionally, cardiac arrest can be the presenting feature of an initial convulsion.

- Most convulsions stop within 4 minutes (>90%). After 5 minutes, a convulsion is unlikely to stop spontaneously. Prolonged fits become harder to stop with anticonvulsants. As a consequence, if a convulsion has not stopped within 5 minutes of its start, emergency (rescue) medication should be given.

- During febrile illnesses, small children (aged 6 months to 5 years) may develop febrile convulsions. These are not epilepsy. They can be seen in up to 1 in 20 children.

- A child having convulsions that are not triggered by fever requires further investigation.

2. Incidence

- 1 in 200 people have active epilepsy.

- It is twice as common in children as in adults.

- It can be related to another underlying condition such as cerebral palsy or a genetic disorder.

- Both meningitis and encephalitis cause fever and may cause convulsions (although these would not normally be classed as febrile convulsions).

3. Severity and Outcome

Febrile convulsions

- 66% of children only ever have the one febrile convulsion; the remainder may have further episodes during subsequent infections.

- 5% of children with febrile convulsions go on to develop epilepsy.

Convulsive Status Epilepticus (CSE)

- Convulsive status epilepticus is the most common neurological emergency in children.

- 1 in 20 febrile convulsions presents with CSE.

- 1 in 20 epileptic children have CSE (more common in children with Dravet syndrome and Lennox-Gastaut syndrome).

- CSE is defined as a convulsive seizure lasting 30 minutes or longer, or repeated tonic-clonic convulsions occurring over a 30 minute period without recovery of consciousness between each seizure.

- Prolonged convulsions (45–60 minutes or more) can result in death (observed mortality rate: 4%). They can also cause serious and irreversible consequences such as stroke, learning difficulties, visual impairment, behavioral problems and epilepsy. Adverse outcomes are more common in young children (<5 years of age).

4. Assessment

(refer to Table 3.82)

- Correct hypoxia and seek an underlying cause for the seizure. Ensure the child is not hypoglycaemic.

- Document if the child was unwell or feverish before the convulsion, any serious past medical history and any important events immediately preceding the convulsion (e.g. head injury).

- When managing a febrile convulsion, it is not sufficient to simply manage the convulsion. It is vitally important to seek and identify the underlying infection producing the child's fever, especially if managing in the community (although this should not delay immediate treatment priorities or hospital transport).

- Seizures are a feature of meningitis – if the fit has stopped and the child's condition permits, look for clinical signs (e.g. the typical rash of meningococcal septicaemia (and treat when present)).

- Establishing that a convulsion has fully stopped can be difficult. Following a tonic-clonic convulsion, the repeated, regular, rhythmic jerks of the limbs (the clonic phase of the seizure) become less frequent and eventually stop. In the following minutes, the child may show some or all of the following post-ictal ('post-convulsion') features:

  - brief and irregular jerks of one or more limbs
  - eye deviation
  - nystagmus (jerky eye movements to one side and then back to the midline)
  - noisy breathing.

- Since these features do not **necessarily** mean the child is still convulsing, additional emergency (rescue) medication (benzodiazepines) should not be given.

- Even when the above features are found to be part of an ongoing seizure, they are not thought to be harmful.

- Conversely, further doses of benzodiazepines can cause significant respiratory depression and respiratory arrest. When uncertain, do not give further benzodiazepines but transfer the child rapidly to hospital, for further assessment and ongoing treatment.

5. Management

(refer to Table 3.82 and Figures 3.21 and 3.22)

- This follows ABCDE priorities, treating the convulsion once ABC issues have been addressed.

- Manage airway, breathing and circulation as usual (also remember to measure the blood glucose as hypoglycaemia can cause seizures). An oropharyngeal airway may be helpful to maintain airway patency (alternatively, if the jaw is clenched a nasopharyngeal airway may prove useful). Administer oxygen and treat shock in the usual way. Oxygen saturation monitoring and nasal capnography (if available) should be applied.

- Epileptic children in the UK now carry individualised "Epilepsy Passports," containing essential information about their epilepsy, their emergency care plan and key professional contacts. These should be located, where possible, without delaying treatment.

Convulsions (Children)

- Most convulsions stop spontaneously (within 4 minutes).

- Anticonvulsant treatment should be given if the convulsion **has lasted 5 minutes or more or if the child has had three or more focal or generalised convulsions in an hour**. Pre-hospital treatments include buccal **midazolam** and **diazepam** (both rectal and intravenous preparations). Buccal midazolam is more effective than rectal diazepam but often diazepam is the only drug available. Both drugs may cause respiratory depression although this is uncommon.

- Do not delay the first dose of anticonvulsant medication whilst attempting venous access, for example use buccal or rectal routes.

- Before administration, ensure that the appropriate anticonvulsant dose for the child's weight and age is chosen, giving the **full** dose at the appropriate times. It is **not** appropriate to either i) gradually 'titrate the dose upwards' or ii) to only give a partial dose if the convulsion stops (even if the seizure has stopped, that full dose must be given). If this approach is followed, seizure recurrence is much less likely.

- A focal convulsion lasting longer than 5 minutes should be managed and treated in the same way as a generalised convulsion.

- If the convulsion is continuing 10 minutes after the first dose of medication has been given, a second dose of anticonvulsant can be given. Ideally, this should be given intravenously or intra-osseously e.g. **diazepam IV/IO** (refer to diazepam guideline) but if this is not possible a second dose can be given buccally or rectally. (This also applies if a carer has given the first dose of medication before the clinician arrives on scene.)

- Further doses of benzodiazepine should not be given even when there is uncertainty about whether the convulsion has stopped or not (see 'Assessment' above).

- Children may sometimes experience brief (i.e. <5 minute) repeated or 'serial' convulsions. Such children should be given an anticonvulsant if they have experienced three convulsions in an hour.

Hospital transfer

- Often it is safest to treat the convulsion before moving the child, although if the seizure has not stopped after one dose of anticonvulsant the child will have to be transferred while still convulsing.

- Pre-alert the hospital if the child continues to fit during the journey or appears to be otherwise very unwell.

- All children having their first convulsion should be transported to hospital for investigation.

- If the child has fully recovered and is a known epileptic it may not be necessary to take them to hospital.

KEY POINTS

Convulsions (Children)

- **Prolonged convulsions, called convulsive status epilepticus (CSE), is a medical emergency and may result in death or serious neurological impairments.**

- **Febrile convulsions are a very common cause for a childhood convulsion and occur between the ages of 6 months and 5 years.**

- **Most convulsions stop spontaneously within 4 minutes.**

- **A convulsion lasting 5 minutes (or more) should be treated with anticonvulsants.**

- **Buccal midazolam is the most widely available rescue medication used in childhood epilepsy.**

- **First choice anticonvulsants are usually given buccally or rectally, with buccal midazolam being the preferred treatment option.**

- **Wherever possible, the second dose of anticonvulsant should always be given intravenously (e.g. diazepam).**

- **The full dose for the child's age must be given when treating a convulsion.**

- **A child should not usually receive more than two doses of pre-hospital anticonvulsant.**

- **Always consider (and actively seek) the underlying cause for the convulsion.**

- **All first convulsions must be transported to hospital.**

Convulsions (Children)

Table 3.82 – ASSESSMENT and MANAGEMENT

Convulsions

ASSESSMENT	MANAGEMENT
Assess ABCD	Treat problems as they are found. ● The airway must be cleared. – Oropharyngeal or nasopharyngeal airways may be helpful. ● Administer high levels of supplemental oxygen – refer to oxygen guideline. ● Assist ventilations with a BVM if necessary. ● Check blood glucose level and manage if low – **refer to hypoglycaemia emergencies in children guideline**. ● Monitor vital signs. ● Manage the convulsion (see below).
Medication	● Administer an anticonvulsant. The first choice anticonvulsant is usually given buccally (midazolam) or rectally (diazepam): 　i. if the first convulsion lasts ≥5 minutes or 　ii. if the child has another convulsion that lasts ≥5 minutes within 10 minutes of the end of the first convulsion or 　iii. if the child continues to have brief (<5 minute) convulsions and has had three of these in a hour or has not regained consciousness between each convulsion. Ask whether the child has their own supply of medication. ● If the child **has** their own supply of medication: 　– if the child has their own buccal midazolam this should be used. 　– ask whether they have already received a dose, if not then administer the patient's own buccal midazolam*. ● If the child does **not** have their own buccal midazolam medication: 　– (and they have not yet received an anticonvulsant) give **buccal midazolam** (if carried) or (if midazolam is not available) **rectal diazepam** (refer to midazolam / diazepam guideline)*. ● If the child **has already received an anticonvulsant** (e.g. rectal **diazepam** or buccal **midazolam**): 　– If the convulsion is continuing **10 minutes** after this first anticonvulsant, one dose of an intravenous or intra-osseous anticonvulsant should be given e.g. **diazepam** IV/IO (refer to diazepam guideline). ● If it is not possible to gain intravenous or intra-osseous access for the second dose of medication, the child **should** be given another full dose of buccal or rectal medication; as continuing convulsive activity is more dangerous than the risk of side effects e.g. respiratory depression. ● In very rare cases a child may continue in convulsive status epilepticus 10 minutes after a second full dose of benzodiazepine. If at that point in time the hospital is still over 15 minutes away (total 25 minutes after the second dose) then a third dose of anticonvulsant may be considered. This must **only** be intravenous or intra-osseous.* *** Be ready to support ventilation as respiratory depression may occur.**
Other care	● Record the child's temperature. ● If transporting to hospital, ongoing assessments of ABCDEs and continuous ECG and oxygen saturation monitoring (and ETCO₂ if available) should be undertaken, continuing **oxygen** therapy as needed. ● If meningococcal septicaemia is diagnosed, treat with **benzylpenicillin** en-route to hospital (refer to benzylpenicillin guideline). ● Paracetamol may be given for fever (refer to paracetamol guideline). ● A febrile child should wear light clothing only. If the child begins to shiver (e.g. after stripping off all layers down to a nappy) this will potentially raise core temperature and will be counter productive.
Transfer to further care	The following should all be transported to hospital: ● Any child who is still convulsing or in status epilepticus must be transferred to further care as soon as possible, preferably after the first dose of anticonvulsant – undertake a **TIME CRITICAL** transfer, provide an alert/information call. ● Any child with suspected meningococcal septicaemia or meningitis – undertake a **TIME CRITICAL** transfer, provide an alert/information call. ● All first febrile convulsions even if the child has recovered. ● All children with seizures who have required more than one dose of anticonvulsant. ● Any child ≤ 2 years old who has had a seizure (even if totally recovered). ● Any child who has not fully recovered from their seizure. The following children may not require transport to hospital: ● Children following a febrile convulsion: 　– that is **not their first** and 　– **who have completely recovered** and 　– **where the carer is happy for the child not to be transported** may be left at home, providing that urgent review by the general practitioner (GP) or out of hours (OOH) GP is arranged to establish the cause of the fever. If this cannot be arranged by the attending crew, the child must be transported to hospital. ● Children who have recovered from a convulsion and **who are known to have epilepsy (and have followed their normal pattern) and have not required more than one dose of medication need not be transported** if they are otherwise well.

Section 3 Medical Specific Conditions

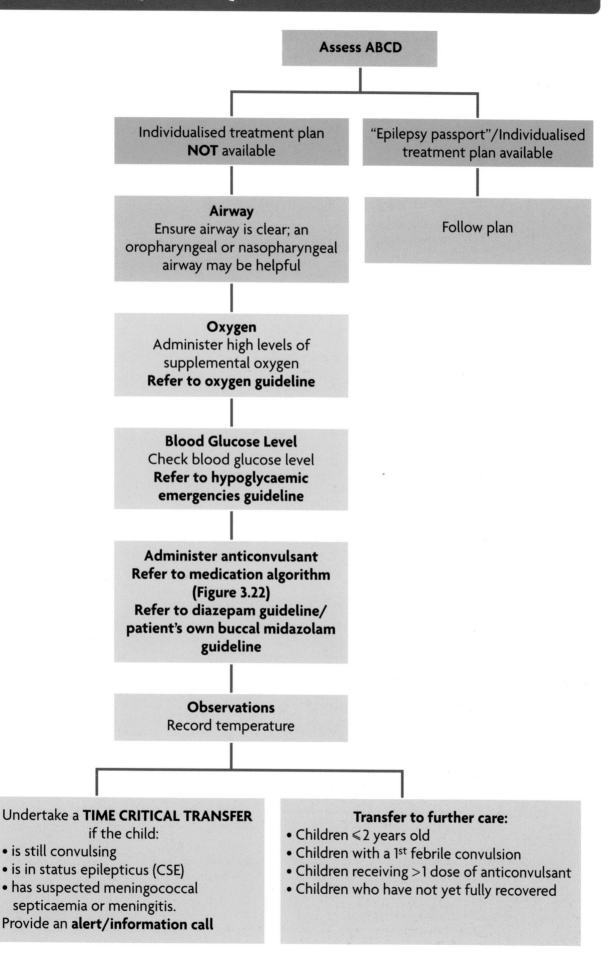

Figure 3.21 – Assessment and management algorithm of convulsions in children.

Section 3 — Medical Specific Conditions

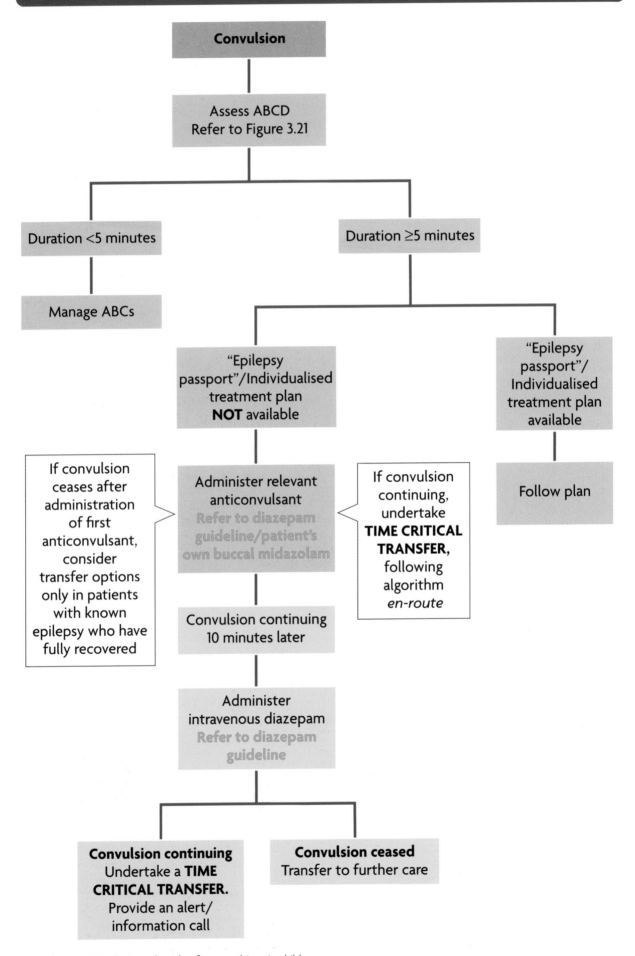

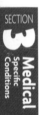

Figure 3.22 – Medication algorithm for convulsions in children.

1. Introduction

- Every year 10% of the UK's under-5s will have an episode of infective gastroenteritis.
- Characteristically they present with sudden onset of diarrhoea (with or without vomiting), which usually resolves without any specific treatment.
- When severe, dehydration can occur, which can be life-threatening. Younger children are most at risk of dehydration.

2. Severity and Outcome

In children with gastroenteritis:

1. vomiting usually lasts 1–2 days, and stops within 3 days.
2. diarrhoea usually lasts 5–7 days, and stops within 2 weeks.

3. Pathophysiology

Escherichia coli 0157:H7 infection

- *E. coli* 0157:H7 is a bacterium found in the intestines of healthy cattle that can cause serious human infections especially in the young and the elderly.
- It often leads to bloody diarrhoea and occasionally kidney failure (referred to as haemolytic uraemic syndrome or HUS). Outbreaks have occurred following school farm visits or following consumption of undercooked, contaminated beef. (Beef burgers are notorious as the meat comes from many animals.)
- When *Escherichia coli* 0157:H7 infection is suspected (e.g. contact with a confirmed case), urgent specialist advice must be sought.

4. Assessment

- Gastroenteritis is diagnosed on clinical findings and should be suspected where there is a sudden change in stool consistency to loose or watery stools and/or a sudden onset of vomiting.

History: consider the diagnosis when the child has had:

- recent contact with someone with acute diarrhoea and/or vomiting
- exposure to a known source of enteric infection (farm visits, contaminated water or food – see *Escherichia coli* 0157 infection above)
- recent overseas travel.

Differential diagnosis

Apart from gastroenteritis, alternative diagnoses must be considered when the following features are found and a more experienced paediatric assessment should be sought:

- Fever:
  - temp ≥38°C in child <3 months old
  - temp ≥39°C in child ≥3 months old.
- Shortness of breath or tachypnoea.
- Altered consciousness.
- Neck stiffness.
- Bulging fontanelle in infants.
- Non-blanching rash.

- Blood and/or mucus in stool.
- Bilious (green) vomit.
- Severe or localised abdominal pain.
- Abdominal distension or rebound tenderness.

Examination: clinical assessment for dehydration and shock

- Establish whether the child:
  - appears unwell
  - has altered responsiveness (e.g. irritability, lethargy)
  - has decreased urine output
  - has pale or mottled skin
  - has cold extremities.

  Use Table 3.83 to establish whether the child is clinically dehydrated or shocked.

Children most at risk of dehydration include:

- Infants of low birth weight (i.e. <2.5 kg).
- Children <1 year, especially those aged <6 months.
- >5 diarrhoeal stools in the previous 24 hours.
- >2 vomits in the previous 24 hours.
- Those who have not been offered/not been able to tolerate oral fluids.
- Breastfed infants who have stopped feeding.
- Malnourished children.

At the end of the clinical assessment three groups of children should have been identified:

1. Those that are **not dehydrated.**
2. Those that are **clinically dehydrated.**
3. Those that are **clinically shocked,** and their management is detailed below.

Stool samples are not normally required but should be obtained in certain situations:

- Diarrhoea ≥7 days.
- Recent overseas travel.
- Possible septicaemia.
- Blood/mucus in stool.
- Immunocompromise.
- Persisting diagnostic uncertainty.

Contact the GP or out-of-hours service where this is thought to be necessary.

5. Management

Most children with gastroenteritis can be managed at home with oral fluids, although dehydrated children require NG or IV fluid replacement and those in shock may require urgent intravenous fluid resuscitation. Fluid losses can be replaced either via the oral route, via a nasogastric tube or intravenously:

a) Oral (and nasogastric) fluids:

  - oral rehydration salt solutions (ORS) are given orally or via a nasogastric (NG) tube.
  - they should be given as small, frequent volumes.
  - response to oral rehydration must be monitored by regular clinical assessment.
  - commercially available ORS solutions include Dioralyte, Dioralyte Relief, Electrolade and Rapolyte.

b) Intravenous interventions (IV):

– IV fluids are required when shock is suspected or confirmed and requires urgent hospital transfer.
– when intravenous access cannot be established, intraosseous fluids may be required.

c) Other treatments:

– antibiotics, antidiarrhoeals and anti-emetics are not routinely used in the management of gastroenteritis.

Considering the three distinct groups of children identified by clinical assessment:

1. In those children **not clinically dehydrated:**

– fluid intake should be actively encouraged (e.g. milk, water, squash) – under fives need approximately 10 ml of fluid every 10 minutes.
– in infants, breastfeeding and other milk feeds should be continued.
– in older children, fruit juices and fizzy drinks must be stopped.
– oral rehydration salt (ORS) solutions should be offered to those at increased risk of dehydration as supplemental fluids, although toddlers and small children frequently refuse ORS because of the taste!
– if oral intake is insufficient or if the child is persistently vomiting, they should be transferred to secondary care for NG or IV fluid replacement. (Inpatient management often includes a trial of ORS or NG fluids prior to IV fluid replacement.)

2. Any child found to be **clinically dehydrated** must be taken to hospital (refer to red flag system, ⚑ see Table 3.83). They will need additional fluids to not just **maintain** their normal body water but also to replace their fluid losses.

3. **Clinically shocked** children require intravenous fluid resuscitation and urgent hospital transfer:

– a rapid 20 ml/kg IV of infusion **sodium chloride 0.9%** may be given but should not delay hospital transfer.
– clinical response to fluid boluses must be monitored.
– if shock persists, this infusion should be repeated and other causes of shock considered – refer to 0.9% sodium chloride guideline.

Information and advice for parents and carers

Advise parents, carers and children that:

● good handwashing is essential to prevent the spread of gastroenteritis to themselves and other family members; use soap (liquid if possible) in warm, running water followed by careful drying.

● wash hands after going to the toilet (children) or changing nappies (parents/carers) and before preparing, serving or eating food.

● infected children should not share towels.

● children should not go to school or other childcare facility while they have diarrhoea or vomiting caused by gastroenteritis and must stay away for at least 48 hours after the last episode of diarrhoea or vomiting.

● children should not swim in swimming pools for 2 weeks after the last episode of diarrhoea.

6. Referral Pathway

Children with gastroenteritis that are not dehydrated or shocked can initially be managed at home; if their

condition progresses seek an additional medical opinion (GP, OOH, emergency department, Paediatrician) (see 'Safety netting' below).

Hospital transfer is required if:

● Oral intake is insufficient.

● The child is persistently vomiting.

● A child is found to be clinically dehydrated.

● A child is found to be clinically shocked (Emergency Transfer).

● A child requires intravenous therapy.

● Suspicion of an alternative cause for the child's symptoms (e.g. UTI, meningococcal disease).

● Additionally some children's social circumstances will dictate additional/continued involvement of healthcare professionals.

Give the following advice for non-dehydrated children managed at home.

Nutritional considerations

During rehydration:

● Continue breastfeeding.

● Give full-strength milk straight away.

● Continue the child's usual solid food.

● Avoid fruit juices and fizzy drinks until the diarrhoea has stopped.

● Consider giving an extra 5 ml/kg of ORS solution after each large watery stool in children at increased risk of dehydration.

● If dehydration recurs after rehydration, restart oral rehydration therapy.

'**Safety netting**' should be provided for children who do not require referral, giving written information to parents and carers on how to:

● Recognise developing red flag symptoms (⚑ refer to Table 3.83), and get immediate help from an appropriate healthcare professional if red flag symptoms develop and

● (if necessary) make arrangements for follow-up at a specified time and place, that is face-to-face assessment.

Consider dehydration risk factors when interpreting symptoms and signs (refer to Table 3.83).

Within the category of 'clinical dehydration' there is a spectrum of severity indicated by increasingly numerous and more pronounced symptoms and signs.

Within the category of 'clinical shock' one or more of the symptoms and/or signs listed would be expected to be present.

Dashes (–) indicate that these clinical features do not specifically indicate shock but may still be present. Symptoms and signs with red flags (⚑) may help to identify children at increased risk of progression to shock.

If uncertain, manage as if the child has those red flag symptoms and/or signs.

Childhood Gastroenteritis

Table 3.83

Symptoms and signs of clinical dehydration and shock

Increasing severity of dehydration ⟶

Symptoms No clinically detectable dehydration	Clinically dehydrated	Clinically shocked
Appears well	⚑ Appears to be unwell or deteriorating	–
Alert and responsive	⚑ Altered responsiveness (e.g. irritable, lethargic)	Decreased level of consciousness
Normal urine output	Decreased urine output. Output often decreased in those with normal hydration as a compensatory mechanism Unreliable in those in nappies with diarrhoea	–
Skin colour unchanged	Skin colour unchanged	Pale or mottled skin
Warm extremities	Warm extremities	Cold extremities

Signs No clinically detectable dehydration	Clinically dehydrated	Clinically shocked
Alert and responsive	⚑ Altered responsiveness (e.g. irritable, lethargic)	Decreased level of consciousness
Skin colour unchanged	Skin colour unchanged	Pale or mottled skin
Warm extremities	Warm extremities	Cold extremities
Eyes not sunken	⚑ Sunken eyes	–
Moist mucous membranes (except after a drink)	Dry mucous membranes (except for 'mouth breather')	–
Normal heart rate	⚑ Tachycardia	Tachycardia
Normal breathing pattern	⚑ Tachypnoea	Tachypnoea
Normal peripheral pulses	Normal peripheral pulses	Weak peripheral pulses
Normal capillary refill time	Normal capillary refill time	Prolonged capillary refill time
Normal skin turgor	⚑ Reduced skin turgor	–
Normal blood pressure	Normal blood pressure	Hypotension (decompensated shock)

NB Rectal examinations should never be performed in the pre-hospital assessment of the paediatric acute abdomen.

KEY POINTS

Gastroenteritis

- Gastroenteritis is common, frequently viral and usually self-limiting.
- When severe, shock and life-threatening dehydration can occur.
- Clinical assessment determines whether dehydration or shock is present (seek Red Flag (🚩) symptoms and signs).
- Non-dehydrated children can frequently be managed at home with oral fluids or ORS.
- Failed oral rehydration requires either NG or IV fluid replacement in secondary care.
- Shocked children need urgent hospital treatment.
- Early meningococcal disease is known to mimic gastroenteritis in small children. An urgent second opinion should be sought if meningococcal disease cannot be excluded.
- Provide a 'safety net,' with written information, for all children with gastroenteritis not transferred to hospital.
- If uncertain, seek advice from either the child's GP or an out-of-hours doctor.

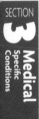

SECTION

3 Medical
Specific
Conditions

1. Introduction

- A non-diabetic individual maintains their blood glucose level within a narrow range from 3.0 to 5.6 mmol per litre.

- This is achieved by a balance between glucose entering the blood stream (from the gastrointestinal tract or from the breakdown of stored energy sources) and glucose leaving the circulation through the action of insulin.

- This guideline is for the assessment and management of children with glycaemic emergencies <18 years.

Section 1 – Hypoglycaemia

- Hypoglycaemia is the term used to describe low blood glucose levels.

- A low blood glucose level is defined as <4.0 mmol/l in children with diabetes and <3.0 mmol/l in non-diabetic children, but the clinical features of hypoglycaemia may be present at higher levels.

- Clinical judgement is as important as a blood glucose reading.

- Correction of hypoglycaemia is a medical emergency.

- If left untreated, hypoglycaemia may lead to the patient suffering permanent brain damage and may even prove fatal.

- Hypoglycaemia occurs when glucose metabolism is disturbed – refer to Table 3.84 for risk factors.

- Any child whose level of consciousness is reduced, who is having a convulsion or who is seriously ill or traumatised should have hypoglycaemia excluded.

- Signs and symptoms can vary from child to child (refer to Table 3.85).

Table 3.84 – RISK FACTORS FOR HYPOGLYCAEMIA

Medical – diabetic

- Insulin or other hypoglycaemic drug treatments.
- Tight glycaemic control.
- Previous history of severe hypoglycaemia.
- Undetected nocturnal hypoglycaemia.
- Preceding hypoglycaemia (< 3.5 mmol/l).
- Impaired awareness of hypoglycaemia.
- Increased exercise (relative to usual).
- Irregular lifestyle/supervision.
- Inadequate carbohydrate intake.
- Inadequate blood glucose monitoring.

Medical – non-diabetic

- Very sick or traumatised children.
- Metabolic illness.
- Endocrine illness (including Addisonian crisis).
- Ketotic hypoglycaemia of infancy.
- Sudden cessation of tube or IV feeding.
- Sudden cessation of peritoneal dialysis.
- Very young babies (especially pre-term).
- Hypothermia (especially in very young babies).
- Drug ingestion (e.g. oral hypoglycaemic drugs, beta-blockers, alcohol)

- Some children are able to detect early symptoms for themselves, but others may be too young, or deteriorate rapidly and without apparent warning.

- Abnormal neurological features may occur, for example, one-sided weakness, identical to a stroke.

- Symptoms may be masked due to medication or other injuries.

- The classical symptoms of hypoglycaemia may **NOT** be present and children may have a variety of unusual symptoms with low blood glucose.

- In **DIABETES MELLITUS** (DM) hypoglycaemia is due to a relative excess of exogenously administered insulin over available glucose.

Table 3.85 – SIGN AND SYMPTOMS

Autonomic

- Sweating.
- Palpitations.
- Shaking.
- Hunger.

General malaise

- Headache.
- Nausea.

Neurological

- Confusion.
- Drowsiness.
- Unusual behaviour.
- Speech difficulty.
- In-coordination.
- Aggression.
- Fitting.
- Unconsciousness.

2. Assessment and Management

For the assessment and management of hypoglycaemia refer to Table 3.86. The principles of assessment and management are essentially the same in diabetic and non-diabetic children and babies.

Section 2 – Hyperglycaemia

- Hyperglycaemia is the term used to describe high blood glucose levels.

- Symptoms include unusual thirst (polydipsia), passing large volumes of urine (polyuria) and tiredness and are usually of slow onset in comparison to those of hypoglycaemia.

- Children with diabetes mellitus are very likely to develop a raised blood glucose in response to infection and will have instructions as to how to deal with this – so called 'sick day rules'.

- Hyperglycaemia may also occur transiently in children who are severely physically stressed (e.g. during a convulsion).

- It is important to distinguish a simple raised blood sugar from the condition of diabetic ketoacidosis which is much more serious (see below). A raised blood glucose is not a pre-hospital emergency unless diabetic ketoacidosis is present. (However, the underlying reason for the raised blood sugar may, of course, be an emergency in its own right.)

Table 3.86 – ASSESSMENT and MANAGEMENT of:

Hypoglycaemia in Children

ASSESSMENT	MANAGEMENT
● Undertake ABCD assessment. ● Measure blood glucose level.[a]	● Start correcting ABC problems (**refer to medical emergencies in children**). ● Measure and record blood glucose level (pre-treatment).
SEVERE: patient unconscious (GCS ≤8), convulsing, very aggressive	● Keep nil by mouth, increased risk of choking/aspiration. ● Administer IV glucose 10% by slow IV infusion (refer to glucose 10% guideline). ● Titrate to effect – an improvement in clinical state and glucose level should be observed rapidly. Do not exceed 2 ml/kg. If IV route not possible administer IM glucagon[b] (onset of action 5–10 minutes) (refer to glucagon guideline). ● Re-assess blood glucose level after 10 minutes. ● If <5.0 mmol/l administer a further dose of IV glucose. ● Re-assess blood glucose level after a further 10 minutes. ● Transfer immediately to the nearest suitable receiving hospital. ● Monitor vital signs and conscious level en-route. Check glucose if deteriorates, or half hourly. ● Provide an alert/information call if necessary. NB **DO NOT** administer glucose 50% as there is a risk of brain damage.
MODERATE: Patient with impaired consciousness, uncooperative	● If capable and cooperative, administer quick acting carbohydrate (sugary drink, glucose tablets (2–3), or glucose gel). Do not give chocolate as it is slower acting. ● If **NOT** capable and cooperative, but able to swallow, administer 1–2 tubes of dextrose gel 40% to the buccal mucosa, or give intra-muscular glucagon[b] (refer to glucagon guideline). ● Re-assess blood glucose level after a further 10 minutes. ● Ensure blood glucose level has improved to at least 5.0 mmol/l in addition to an improvement in level of consciousness. ● If blood glucose not improved to 5 mmol/l, repeat treatment up to three times. Note: IM glucagon to be given ONCE ONLY. ● If no improvement after three treatments, consider intravenous glucose 10%. ● Transfer to the nearest suitable receiving hospital if requiring further treatment, otherwise can usually be safely left at home if with a responsible adult. ● Notify GP or out-of-hours provider if left at home. NB **DO NOT** administer glucose 50% as there is a risk of brain damage.
MILD: Patient conscious, orientated, able to swallow	● Administer quick acting carbohydrate (sugary drink, glucose tablets or glucose gel). Do not use chocolate (see above). ● Re-assess blood glucose level after a further 10 minutes. ● Ensure blood glucose level has improved to at least 5.0 mmol/l. ● If no improvement, repeat treatment up to three times. ● If no improvement after three treatments consider intravenous glucose 10% (refer to glucose 10% guideline). ● Transfer to the nearest suitable receiving hospital only if not responding to treatment. ● Notify GP or out-of-hours if left at home.

a Clean fingers prior to testing blood glucose levels as the child may have been in contact with sugary substances (e.g. sweets).
b Glucagon may take 5–10 minutes to take effect and requires the child to have adequate glycogen stores – thus, it may be ineffective if glycogen stores have been exhausted. This is likely in any children who have any NON diabetic causes of hypoglycaemia, although it is worth trying.

DIABETES MELLITUS

● Diabetes mellitus can even occur in infants. These children may have blood glucose levels that are particularly difficult to control and may be very difficult to manage.

● Known diabetic children will have protocols to follow if they become unwell – if available and appropriate, always follow them.

● Type 1 (insulin dependent) DM is nearly universal in children, although occasionally Type 2 (non-insulin dependent) DM is now seen, usually in association with severe obesity.

Diabetic ketoacidosis (DKA)

For the pathophysiology of this illness refer to glycaemic emergencies in adults.

● Patients may present with one or more signs as in Table 3.87.

Diabetic ketoacidosis (DKA) may occur relatively rapidly in children, sometimes without a long history of the classical symptoms. The absolute blood glucose level is not a good indicator of the presence of DKA – some children with blood glucose levels in the >20 range may appear quite well and not have DKA.

Glycaemic Emergencies (Children)

Table 3.87 – SIGN AND SYMPTOMS OF DKA

Symptoms
- Polyuria.
- Polydipsia.
- Abdominal pain.
- Vomiting.

Signs
- Weight loss.
- Lethargy, drowsiness confusion and ultimately coma and death.
- Dehydration, and occasionally circulatory failure due to hypovolaemia.
- Hyperventilation (Kussmaul breathing).
- Presence of ketones (measured) in the urine and/or blood.

- Children with DKA may present with significant dehydration – however, if IV fluid is given too fast this can lead to cerebral oedema and death. **Refer to intravascular fluid therapy guideline.** Do not give children DKA IV fluids unless they have good evidence of hypovolaemic shock.

- True shock (circulatory failure), as opposed to dehydration, is relatively uncommon in children with DKA, but does not require IV fluid resuscitation. Volumes must not exceed 10 ml/kg.

- Do not try to give oral fluids to children with DKA – they have a very high risk of aspiration.

- Ketone measurement (blood or urine) is useful in the diagnosis of DKA.

3. Assessment and Management

If a known diabetic child is well, not vomiting, fully conscious, has a blood glucose level >16 mmol/l but a blood ketone level <3 mmol/l, the family should contact their diabetes team or GP. Do not attempt to manage the patient yourself.

Once a blood ketone level is above 3 mmol/l (or urine ketones are high) and the child is unwell with vomiting then they should be managed as having DKA.

For the assessment and management of diabetic ketoacidosis refer to Table 3.88.

Table 3.88 – ASSESSMENT and MANAGEMENT of:

Diabetic Ketoacidisis in Children

ASSESSMENT	MANAGEMENT
- Undertake ABCD assessment	- Start correcting ABC problems (**refer to medical emergencies in children**). - Do not give IV fluids unless there is clear evidence of circulatory failure and no more than 10 ml/kg sodium chloride (refer to intravascular fluids/0.9% saline guideline).
- If the child is **TIME CRITICAL**	- Correct life-threatening conditions (airway and breathing on scene). - Then commence transfer to nearest suitable receiving hospital. NB DKA is a life-threatening condition requiring urgent hospital treatment.
- Measure blood glucose level	- Measure and record blood glucose level.
- Assess for signs of dehydration	- Do not give IV fluids to treat dehydration unless shocked (see above).
- Measure oxygen saturation (SpO$_2$)	- Administer high-flow oxygen as part of shock management. - Provide an alert/information call if necessary. - If the child has records of their blood or urine glucose levels, bring them with the patient.

KEY POINTS

Glycaemic Emergencies (Children)
- **Hypoglycaemia is a medical emergency.**
- **Treat hypoglycaemia with a suitable form of glucose (this will depend on the patient's condition).**
- **Glucagon may be used intramuscularly to treat hypoglycaemia if treatment with glucose is not possible.**
- **Children, whose hypoglycaemia is not due to diabetes, may not respond well to glucagon.**
- **DKA usually requires no emergency pre-hospital treatment except rapid transport to hospital.**
- **IV fluids can cause cerebral oedema in children with DKA.**
- **Do not give IV fluids to children with DKA unless significant shock is present and then only limited amounts.**

1. Introduction

Overdose and poisoning is a common cause of calls to the ambulance service accounting for 140,000 hospital admissions per year.

Poisoning

Exposure by ingestion, inhalation, absorption or injection of a quality of a substance(s) that results in mortality or morbidity.

Common agents include:

- **Household products**, for example washing powders, washing-up liquids and fabric cleaning liquid/tablets; bleaches, hand gels and screen-washes; anti-freeze and de-icers, silica gel, batteries, petroleum distillates, white spirit (e.g. paints and varnishes), descalers and glues. Exposure generally occurs as a result of ingestion but can arise from eye and skin contact; exposure can arise from multiple routes of exposure.

- **Pharmaceutical agents**, for example paracetamol, ibuprofen, co-codamol, aspirin, tricyclic antidepressants, selective serotonin uptake inhibitors (SSRIs), beta-blockers, calcium-channel blockers, cocaine, benzodiazepines, opioids, iron tablets.

- **Plants/fungi**, for example foxglove, laburnum, laurel, iris, castor oil plant, amanita palloides, etc. For further details of poisonous plants refer to: http://www.toxbase.org.

- **Alcohol**.
- **Chemicals**.
- **Cosmetics**.

Poisoning in children

1. **Accidental** exposure to a poisonous substance or medicine by an inquisitive child. This usually occurs in young children and ingestion of tablets is common, although, almost anything, however unpalatable to the adult palate, may be ingested. The event may not be obvious and may only be found on detailed questioning, if old enough to give a history.
2. **Intentional** poisoning (usually a medicine), as an act of deliberate self-harm. Over-the-counter medicine (e.g. paracetamol), or prescribed drugs are commonly used.
3. **Non-accidental** poisoning of children is extremely unlikely to be detected by the Ambulance Service, but if it is suspected it must be reported. **Refer to the safeguarding children guideline**.

Overdose

Exposure by ingestion, inhalation, absorption or injection of a quality of a substance(s) above the prescribed dose; this is a common form of poisoning, involving prescribed or illicit drugs and may be accidental or intentional.

2. Incidence

- It is difficult to estimate the exact number of overdose and poisoning incidents, as not all cases are reported. In 2009/2010 there were 49,690 poison-related queries involving patients to the National Poisons Information Service. Over one-third concerned children under the age of five. The majority of incidents were accidental and occurred in the home.

3. Severity and Outcome

- There are a number of factors which will affect severity and outcome following exposure, for example, age, toxicity of the agent, quantity and route of exposure.
- In 2009 there were 2,878 deaths related to drug overdose and poisoning in England and Wales.

4. Pathophysiology

- The mode of action following exposure will depend primarily on the nature of the toxin. For details of the actions of specific toxins refer to: http://www.toxbase.org

5. Assessment and Management

For the assessment and management of overdose and poisoning in children refer to Table 3.90.

Methodology

For details of the methodology used in the development of this guideline refer to the guideline webpage. Important information can be gained from toxbase and local protocols should be followed to obtain this information.

KEY POINTS

Overdose and Poisoning (Children)

- **Children and adolescents with serious poisoning and deliberate overdoses must be transferred to hospital.**
- **After an accidental poisoning that was found to be non-toxic, some children (refer to Table 3.90) may be considered for home management.**
- **Alcohol often causes hypoglycaemia even in adolescents.**
- **NEVER induce vomiting.**
- **If the child vomits, retain a sample, if possible, for inspection at hospital.**
- **Bring the substance or substances and any containers found to the hospital for inspection.**
- **Estimate the quantity of substance ingested.**

Table 3.89

Specific Substance Management

SUBSTANCE/SIGNS AND SYMPTOMS	MANAGEMENT
Alcohol (ethanol) • Nausea, vomiting, slurred speech, confusion, convulsions, unconsciousness.	• Alcohol poisoning follows the consumption of excessive amounts of alcohol. • It can be fatal so should be taken seriously. • It is not uncommon in teenagers. • Can cause severe hypoglycaemia even in teenagers. • **ALWAYS** check the blood glucose levels in any child or young person with a decreased conscious level, especially in children and young adults who are 'drunk', as hypoglycaemia (blood glucose <4.0 mmol/l) is common and requires treatment with oral glucose or glucose 10% IV (**refer to glycaemic emergencies in children**). NOTE: Glucagon is not effective in alcohol-induced hypoglycaemia.
Tricyclic Antidepressants • Central nervous system excitability, confusion, blurred vision, dry mouth, fever, pupil dilation, convulsions, coma, arrhythmias, hypotension, tachycardia, respiratory depression; physical condition can rapidly change.	• ECG monitoring and IV access should be established early in the treatment of tricyclic overdose. • The likelihood of fitting is high; this should be treated following the **convulsions in children guidelines**.
Iron • Nausea, vomiting blood, diarrhoea (black stools), metallic taste, convulsions, dizziness, flushed appearance, unconsciousness, non-cardiac pulmonary oedema.	• Iron pills are regularly used by large numbers of the population including pregnant mothers. In overdose, especially in children, they are exceedingly dangerous. They may cause extensive damage to the liver and gut and these children will require hospital assessment and treatment. NB Charcoal is contra-indicated as it may interfere with subsequent treatment.

Paracetamol
• Nausea, vomiting, malaise, right upper quadrant abdominal pain, jaundice, confusion, drowsiness – coma may develop later.
NB Frequently asymptomatic, symptoms are unreliable.
	• There are a number of analgesic preparations that contain paracetamol and a combination of codeine or dextropropoxyphene. This, in overdose, creates two serious dangers for the child:
	  1. The codeine and dextropropoxyphene are both derived from opioid drugs. This in overdose, especially if alcohol is involved, may well produce profound respiratory depression. This can be reversed with naloxone (refer to naloxone guideline).
	  2. Paracetamol, even in modest doses, is **dangerous** and can induce severe liver and kidney damage in susceptible children. Initially there are no clinical features to suggest this, which may lull the child's carers, the child, and ambulance clinicians into a false sense of security. It frequently takes 24–48 hours for the effects of paracetamol damage to become apparent and urgent blood paracetamol levels are required to assess the child's level of risk.

Opioids • Drowsiness, nausea, vomiting, small pupils, respiratory depression, cyanosis, coma, convulsions, non-cardiac pulmonary oedema.	• May produce profound respiratory depression. This can be reversed with naloxone (refer to naloxone guideline).

Section 3 Medical Specific

Overdose and Poisoning (Children)

Table 3.90 – ASSESSMENT and MANAGEMENT of:

Overdose and Poisoning

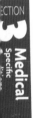

ASSESSMENT	MANAGEMENT

● Assess ABCD	● If any of the following **TIME CRITICAL** features present:
	  – major **ABCD** problems
	  – decreased level of consciousness – NB Most poisons that impair consciousness also depress respiration – **refer to altered level of consciousness guideline**
	  – respiratory depression
	  – hypotension <70 mmHg
	  – cardiac arrhythmias – **refer to cardiac rhythm disturbance guideline**
	  – convulsions – **refer to convulsion guideline**
	  – hypothermia – **refer to hypothermia guideline**, then:
	● Start correcting **A** and **B** problems.
	● Undertake a **TIME CRITICAL** transfer to nearest receiving hospital.
	● Continue patient management en-route.
	● Provide an alert/information call.

● Substance	● Ascertain what has been ingested.
	● The time the incident occurred.
	● Estimate the quantity of substance ingested/inhaled/absorbed/injected.
	● What if any treatment has been administered.
	● Refer to Table 3.89 for specific management.
	● **NEVER** induce vomiting.
	● In the case of caustic/petroleum ingestion encourage the child to drink a glass of milk, if possible.
	● If possible take to hospital:
	  – a sample of the ingested substance
	  – medicine containers
	  – a sample of vomit – if present.
	● Consider non-accidental injury – **refer to safeguarding children guideline**.

● Chemical exposure	● If exposure to chemical substance is suspected – **refer to CBRNE guideline chemical section** for management.
● Oxygen	● Administer high levels of supplemental oxygen, particularly in cases of carbon monoxide poisoning or inhalation of irritant gases – **refer to oxygen guideline**. ● Apply pulse oximeter. NB Supplemental oxygen maybe harmful in cases of paraquat poisoning.
● ECG	● Undertake a 12-lead ECG.

● Respirations	● Monitor respirations.
	● Consider assisted ventilation if:
	  – SpO$_2$ is <90% after administering high levels of oxygen for 30–60 seconds
	  – respiratory rate is **<$\frac{1}{2}$ normal rate** OR **>3 times normal rate**
	  – expansion is inadequate.
	● Opiates such as morphine or heroin can cause respiratory depression; consider naloxone – **refer to naloxone guideline**.

● Blood pressure	● Hypotension is common in cases of severe poisoning. ● Monitor blood pressure.
● Intravascular fluid	● If fluid is indicated **refer to intravascular fluid guideline**.
● Blood glucose level	● Measure blood glucose level. ● Blood glucose levels <4.0 mmol/l need correcting – **refer to glucose 10% guideline**. NB Glucagon is often not effective in overdoses.
● Mental health assessment	● In cases of attempted suicide undertake a rapid mental health assessment – **refer to mental disorder guideline**.

● Transfer to further care	● All children who have encountered a serious poisoning.
	● All children who have taken a deliberate overdose. (Even if the substance was harmless, they need to be transferred for a hospital-based assessment of their mental health).
	Following an accidental poisoning, it is possible for some children to be managed at home. This option may be considered when:
	  – the substance is/verified on **TOXBASE** as harmless
	  – the incident is/was accidental
	  – the carers know to seek medical advice if the child becomes unwell
	  – arrangements have been made to inform the health visitor or GP.

4

Trauma

Trauma

Trauma Emergencies Overview (Adults)   223

Trauma Emergencies Overview
(Children)   230

Abdominal Trauma   236

Head Injury   238

Limb Trauma   242

Neck and Back Trauma   246

Major Pelvic Trauma   252

Thoracic Trauma   255

Trauma in Pregnancy   260

Burns and Scalds (Adults)   262

Burns and Scalds (Children)   265

Electrical Injuries   268

Immersion and Drowning   271

1. Introduction

- Trauma is a leading cause of death in the UK. The wide range of traumatic injuries encountered in pre-hospital care can present a complex challenge. Research suggests that assessing and managing patients in a systematic way can lead to improved outcomes.

- This overview will outline the process of assessment and management of trauma patients. This guideline supports the following related guidelines:
  - abdominal trauma
  - head trauma
  - limb trauma
  - neck and back trauma
  - pelvic trauma
  - thoracic trauma
  - trauma in pregnancy
  - traumatic cardiac arrest
  - airway management
  - burns and scalds
  - electrical injuries
  - fluid therapy
  - oxygen therapy
  - pain management.

This guideline uses mechanism of injury and primary survey as the basis of care for all trauma patients.

2. Incidence

- In England it is estimated that there are approximately 20,000 cases of major trauma annually. Road traffic collisions (RTC) are the most common cause.

3. Severity and Outcome

- In England major trauma accounts for approximately 5,400 deaths each year, with many more cases leading to significant short- and long-term morbidity. In Scotland (1992–2002) there were 5,847 deaths resulting from trauma. Major trauma is the leading cause of death in patients under 45 years of age.

4. Incident Management

Overall control of the incident allows paramedics to concentrate on patient assessment and management and it is recommended that a model, such as SCENE, is used to assess the initial trauma scene so that it can be managed effectively (refer to Table 4.1).

5. Patient Assessment

A primary survey should be undertaken for **ALL** patients as this will rapidly identify patients with actual or potential **TIME CRITICAL** injuries (refer to **Table 4.3**).

A secondary survey is a more thorough 'head-to-toe' assessment of the patient. It should be undertaken following completion of the primary survey, where time permits. The secondary survey will usually be undertaken during transfer to further care; however, in some patients with time critical trauma, it may not be possible to undertake the secondary survey before arrival at further care (refer to Table 4.4).

5.1 Primary survey

- The primary survey should take no more than 60–90 seconds and follow the **<C>ABCDE** approach. Document the vital signs and the time they were taken.

- Consider mechanism of injury and the possible injury patterns that may result; but be aware that mechanism alone cannot predict or exclude injury and physiological signs should be utilised as well.

- Assessment and management should proceed in a **'stepwise'** manner and life-threatening injuries should be managed as they are encountered, that is do not move onto breathing and circulation until the airway is secured. Every time an intervention has been carried out, re-assess the patient.

- As soon as a life-threatening injury is identified and managed, it is recommended that transport should be immediately instigated to the appropriate trauma facility according to local procedures.

- If immediate transfer is not possible, consider mobilising senior clinical support if not already done during the SCENE assessment.

Table 4.1 – SCENE

S — Safety
Perform a dynamic risk assessment, are there any dangers now or will there be any that become apparent during the incident? This needs to be continually re-assessed throughout the incident. Appropriate personal protective equipment should be utilised according to local guidelines.

C — Cause including MOI
Establish the events leading up to the incident. Is this consistent with your findings?

E — Environment
Are there any environmental factors that need to be taken into consideration? These can include problems with access or egress, weather conditions or time of day.

N — Number of patients
Establish exactly how many patients there are during the initial assessment of the scene.

E — Extra resources needed
Additional resources should be mobilised now. These can include additional ambulances, helicopter or senior medical support. Liaise with the major trauma advisor according to local protocols.

MANAGEMENT OVERVIEW

If the patient has a life-threatening condition start immediate transfer to an appropriate trauma facility according to local procedures with treatment undertaken en-route to hospital.

- Provide an alert/information call.

- Continue patient re-assessment and management.

- If a patient requires IV fluids and fulfils the criteria in steps 1 or 2 of the Pre-Hospital Major Trauma Triage Tool (Appendix) then they should receive a bolus of tranexamic acid if available (refer to tranexamic acid guideline).

- **Pain management** – if analgesia is indicated **refer to pain management guideline**.

- Hand-over – it is recommended that the patient is handed over to receiving clinicians using the ATMIST format (refer to Table 4.2).

If the patient is **NON-TIME CRITICAL** undertake a secondary survey (refer to Table 4.4).

5.2 Secondary survey

- A secondary survey should only commence after the primary survey has been completed and in critical patients only during transport.

Table 4.2 – ATMIST

A	Age
T	Time of incident
M	Mechanism
I	Injuries
S	Signs and symptoms
T	Treatment given/immediate needs

Table 4.3 – ASSESSMENT and MANAGEMENT of:

Trauma Emergencies

- **All stages should be considered but some may be omitted if not considered appropriate.**
- **To reduce clot disruption avoid unnecessary movements.**
- **When available administer tranexamic acid to all patients who require TIME CRITICAL transfer, except isolated head injuries.**

At each stage consider the need for:
- **TIME CRITICAL – transfer to nearest appropriate hospital as per local trauma care pathway.**
- **Early senior clinical support.**

STAGE	ASSESSMENT	MANAGEMENT
<C>	**CATASTROPHIC HAEMORRHAGE** – assess for the presence of **LIFE-THREATENING EXTERNAL BLEEDING**	Follow the management in Figure 4.1.
A	**AIRWAY** – assess the airway and **AT ALL TIMES** consider C-spine injury and the need to immobilise (**refer to neck and back trauma guideline**). **Look for** obvious obstructions (e.g. teeth/dentures, foreign bodies, vomit, blood, trauma, soot/burns/oedema in burn patients). **Listen for** noisy airflow (e.g. snoring, gurgling or no airflow). **Feel for** air movement).	Correct any airway problems immediately by: ● Jaw thrust, chin lift (no neck extension). ● Suction (if appropriate). ● Nasopharyngeal airway. ● Oropharyngeal airway. ● Laryngeal mask airway (if appropriate). ● Endotracheal intubation (only if capnography available). ● Needle cricothyroidotomy.
B	Assess rate, depth and quality of respiration Grade breathing 1–5 1. patient not breathing 2. slow <12 per min 3. normal 12–20 but check depth 4. fast 20–30 observe very closely 5. very fast >30 Feel for depth and equality of chest movement, any instability of chest wall. Look for obvious chest injuries, wounds, bruising or flail segment. Auscultate lung fields assessing air entry on each side. Percuss the chest wall checking the pitch of the percussion note. In addition assess the chest and neck for the following using the mnemonic **TWELVE**: ● **T**racheal deviation ● **W**ounds, bruising or swelling ● **E**mphysema (surgical) ● **L**aryngeal crepitus ● **V**enous engorgement ● **E**xcluding open/tension pneumothorax, flail segment, massive haemothorax.	Administer 100% O_2 in all patients with critical trauma to target O_2 sats of 94–98%, even if there are risk factors such as COPD. ● Breathing graded at 1,2 should receive O_2 via BVM as should grade 5 if clinically appropriate. ● Breathing graded at 3,4 should receive supplemental 100% O_2 but be monitored very closely. ● Apply non-occlusive dressing to sucking chest wounds (**refer to thoracic trauma guideline**). ● Decompress a tension pneumothorax (**refer to thoracic trauma guideline**). ● Flail segments should not be splinted (**refer to thoracic trauma guideline**). NB **Restraint (POSITIONAL) asphyxia** – If the patient is required to be physically restrained (e.g. by police officers) in order to prevent them injuring themselves or others, or for the purpose of being detained under the Mental Health Act, then it is paramount that the method of restraint allows both for a patent airway and adequate respiratory volume. **Under these circumstances it is essential to ensure that the patient's airway and breathing are adequate at all times.**

Table 4.3 – ASSESSMENT and MANAGEMENT of:

Trauma Emergencies *continued*

STAGE	ASSESSMENT	MANAGEMENT
C	If massive external haemorrhage was controlled at start of assessment re-assess this now. Assess for radial and carotid pulses noting rate, rhythm and volume, assess central and peripheral capillary refill time, note skin colour, texture and temperature. Remain alert to the possibility of internal bleeding and assess for signs of blood loss in five places (blood on the floor and four more): 1. External 2. Chest (already done during breathing assessment) 3. Abdomen by palpation and observation of bruising or external marks 4. Pelvis – do not manipulate the pelvis – MOI may suggest a fracture 5. Long bones – assess for but do not be distracted by limb trauma. Consider hypovolaemic shock but be aware that blood loss of 1000–1500 ml is required before classical signs start to appear. Signs of hypovolaemic shock include pallor, cool peripheries, anxiety and abnormal behaviour, increased respiratory rate and tachycardia. Signs of shock also appear much later in certain patient groups (e.g. pregnant women, patients on beta-blockers and the physically fit). There may well be little evidence of shock; blood loss of 1000–1500 ml is required before more classic signs of shock appear.	Follow the management for haemorrhage control in Figures 4.1 and 4.2. Consider splinting: ● In the critical patient, **long bone fractures** should be splinted en-route to the trauma facility. ● **Pelvic fractures** should be stabilised at the earliest possible opportunity, preferably before the patient is moved – **refer to pelvic trauma guideline**. **Fluid therapy** If fluid replacement is indicated refer to intravascular fluid therapy guideline. **TRANEXAMIC ACID** If a patient requires IV fluids and fulfils the criteria in steps 1 or 2 of the Pre-Hospital Major Trauma Triage Tool (Appendix) then they should receive a bolus of tranexamic acid (refer to tranexamic acid guideline). In cases of internal or uncontrolled haemorrhage undertake a **TIME CRITICAL** transfer to appropriate hospital according to local procedures. To minimise clot disruption avoid unnecessary movement in victims of blunt trauma: ● Log roll should be avoided wherever possible. ● Patients should be lifted from the ground using a scoop (bivalve) stretcher. ● Once on a scoop (bivalve) stretcher patients should be transported on it. ● A long spinal board is an extrication device and should not be used unless required. Once on a long spinal board the patient should be transported on it – **refer to neck and back trauma guideline**. ● A patient with penetrating trauma who has no neurology and no possibility of direct trauma to the spinal column should NOT be immobilised.
D	**Disability** Obtain a full GCS (refer to Table 4.5) for the patient as this is required for the Pre-Hospital Major Trauma Triage Tool (Appendix)	
	Assess and note pupil size, equality and response to light.	
	Altered mental status.	Check blood glucose level to rule out hypo- or hyperglycaemia as the cause – **refer to glycaemic emergencies guideline in adults**.
E	**EXPOSURE and ENVIRONMENT** At this stage further monitoring may be applied.	
	Exposure.	Ensure patient does not suffer from exposure to cold/wet conditions.
	Trapped patient.	Consider mobilising early senior clinical support.

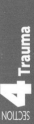

● A secondary survey should only commence after the primary survey has been completed, and in critical patients only during transport.

● The secondary survey is a more thorough "head-to-toe" survey of the patient; however, it is important to monitor the patient's vital signs during the survey.

● In some patients with critical trauma it may not be possible to undertake a secondary survey before arriving at a trauma facility. However, in patients with altered mental status it is recommended that a BM reading should be taken during transport.

Table 4.4 – SECONDARY SURVEY

ASSESSMENT

Head

- Re-assess airway.
- Check skin colour and temperature.
- Palpate for bruising/fractures.
- Check pupil size and reactivity.
- Examine for loss of cerebrospinal fluid.
- Establish Glasgow Coma Scale (refer to Table 4.5).
- Assess for other signs of basal skull fracture.

NB For further information **refer to the head trauma guideline**.

Neck

- The collar will need to be loosened for proper examination of the neck.
- Re-assess for signs of life-threatening injury using the mnemonic '**TWELVE**':
    - **T**racheal deviation
    - **W**ounds, bruising, swelling
    - **E**mphysema (surgical)
    - **L**aryngeal crepitus
    - **V**enous engorgement (jugular).
    - **E**xcluding open/tension pneumothorax, flail segment, massive haemothorax.
- Assess and palpate for spinal tenderness, particularly note any bony tenderness.

NB For further information **refer to the neck and back trauma guideline**.

Chest

- Assess rate, depth and quality of respiration and grade breathing 1–5:
1. patient not breathing
2. slow <12 per min
3. normal 12–20 but check depth
4. fast 20–30 observe very closely
5. very fast >30
- Breathing graded at 1,2 should receive O$_2$ via BVM as should grade 5 if clinically appropriate.
- Breathing graded at 3,4 should receive supplemental 100% O$_2$ but should be monitored very closely.
- Feel for rib fractures, instability and surgical emphysema.
- Look for contusions, seat belt marks and flail segments.
- Auscultate lung fields for signs of:
    - Pneumothorax
    - Tension pneumothorax
    - Haemothorax
    - Cardiac tamponade
    - Assess for signs of pulmonary contusion
    - Assess the front and as much of the back as is possible.

NB for further information **refer to the thoracic trauma guideline**.

Abdomen

- Examine for open wounds, contusions and seatbelt marks.
- Palpate the entire abdomen for tenderness and guarding.
- Examine the front and as much of the back as is possible.

NB For further information **refer to the abdominal trauma guideline**.

Table 4.4 – SECONDARY SURVEY continued

ASSESSMENT

Pelvis

- Blood loss may be visible either from the urethra or PV.
- The patient may have the urge to urinate.

NB For further information **refer to the pelvic trauma guideline**.

Lower/upper limbs

- Examine lower limbs then upper limbs.
- Look for wounds and evidence of fractures.
- Check for MSC in **ALL** four limbs:
    - **MOTOR** – Test for movement
    - **SENSATION** – Apply light touch to evaluate sensation
    - **CIRCULATION** – Assess pulse and skin temperature.

NB For further information **refer to the limb trauma guideline**.

6. Special Circumstances in Trauma

6.1 The trapped patient

Entrapment can be:

- **Relative:** trapped by difficulty in access/egress from the wreckage, including the physical injury stopping normal exit.
- **Absolute:** firmly trapped by the vehicle and its deformity necessitating specialised cutting techniques to free the patient.

All patients that have an **absolute** entrapment are at high risk of having suffered significant transfer of energy and therefore are at increased risk of severe injury.

6.2 Management

- Conduct a thorough assessment of the incident using SCENE or similar model.
- Consider mobilising senior clinical support at the earliest opportunity.
- Mobilise and liaise with other emergency services.
- Perform primary survey and manage as per trauma guideline.
- Form a rescue plan.
- Provide analgesia (**refer to pain management guidelines**).

Table 4.5 – GLASGOW COMA SCALE

Item		Score
Eyes opening:		
	Spontaneously	4
	To speech	3
	To pain	2
	None	1
Motor response:		
	Obeys commands	6
	Localises pain	5
	Withdraws from pain	4
	Abnormal flexion	3
	Extensor response	2
	No response to pain	1

Table 4.5 – GLASGOW COMA SCALE
continued

Item	Score
Verbal response:	
Orientated	5
Confused	4
Inappropriate words	3
Incomprehensible sounds	2
No verbal response	1

KEY POINTS

Trauma Emergencies Overview (Adults)

- **Overall assessment of safety: self, scene, casualties is of prime importance.**
- **The primary survey forms the basis of patient assessment, with due consideration for C-spine immobilisation.**
- **Arrest of external haemorrhage can be life saving.**
- **Consider mobilising senior clinical support at the earliest opportunity.**

Appendix – The NHS Clinical Advisory Group on Trauma

Pre-Hospital Major Trauma Triage Tool >12 years

Pre-Hospital Major Trauma Triage Tool

The Major Trauma Triage Tool presented below is based on the American College of Surgeons Guidelines for Field Triage 2006 with minor modifications. In Step 2 'Flail chest' has been changed to 'Chest injury with altered physiology' and 'Paralysis' has been changed to 'Sensory or motor deficit (new onset following trauma)'. In Step 3 'feet' have been changed to 'metres' for distance fallen. 'Entrapment' has been added. In Step 4 Burns are considered special if they are facial, circumferential or 20% body surface area (BSA).

Entry criteria for use of triage is a judgement that the patient may have suffered significant trauma.

Step 1

Physiological:

- GCS < 14 (refer to Table 4.5)
- SBP < 90 mmHg.

If any of the above factors are present, activate Major Trauma Alert and definitive care to be from Major Trauma Centre; otherwise proceed to Step 2.

Step 2

Anatomical:

- Penetrating to head/neck/torso/limbs proximal to elbow/knee.
- Chest injury with altered physiology.
- Two proximal long bone fractures.
- Crushed/degloved/mangled extremity.
- Amputation proximal to wrist/ankle.
- Pelvic fractures.
- Open or depressed skull fracture.
- Sensory or motor deficit (new onset following trauma).

If any of the above factors are present activate a Major Trauma Alert and definitive care to be from Major Trauma Centre; otherwise proceed to Step 3.

Step 3

Mechanism:

- Falls:
  - Fall > 6 m/2 storeys in adult
  - Fall > 3 m/2 times height in child.
- Motor vehicles:
  - Intrusion > 30 cm occupant site
  - Ejection partial/complete
  - Death in same passenger compartment
  - Vehicle telemetry data consistent with high risk of injury.
- Pedestrian/cyclist versus motor vehicle thrown/run over/with significant (> 20 mph) impact.
- Motorcycle crash > 20 mph.
- Entrapment.

If any of the above factors present consider a Major Trauma Alert with further assessment by either Trauma Unit or Major Trauma Centre; otherwise proceed to Step 4.

Step 4

- Special considerations that should lower the threshold for a Trauma Alert:
  - Older adults (age > 55)
  - Children (to Paediatric Trauma Centre)
  - Anticoagulation/bleeding disorders
  - Burns: full thickness facial, circumferential or 20% body surface area (BSA)
  - Time-sensitive extremity injury
  - Dialysis-dependent renal disease
  - Pregnancy > 20 weeks
  - EMS provider judgement.

If any of the above factors are present consider Major Trauma Alert with further assessment by either Trauma Unit or Major Trauma Centre.

SECTION **4** Trauma

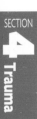

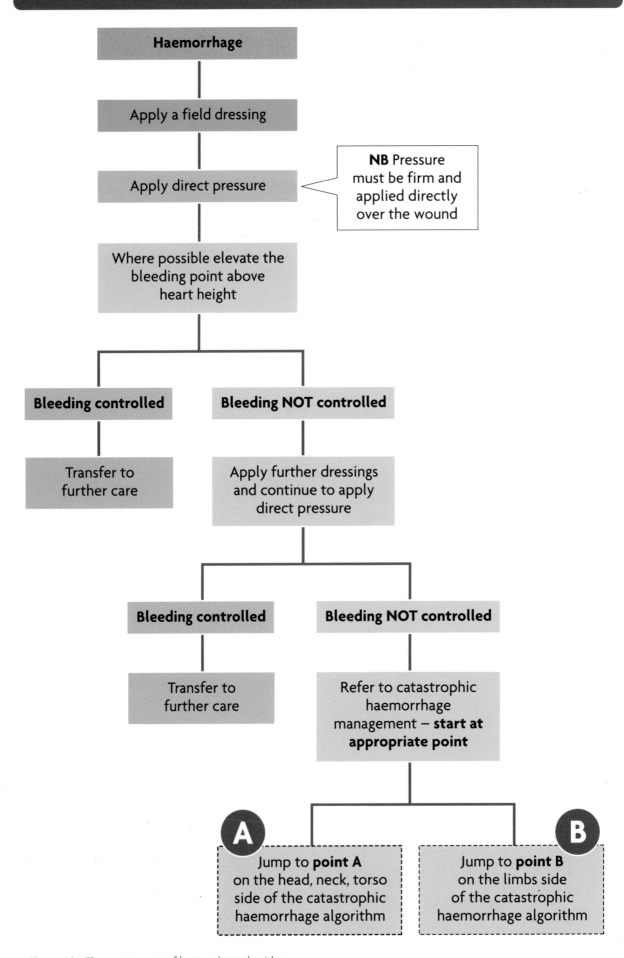

Haemorrhage

Apply a field dressing

Apply direct pressure

NB Pressure must be firm and applied directly over the wound

Where possible elevate the bleeding point above heart height

Bleeding controlled

Transfer to further care

Bleeding NOT controlled

Apply further dressings and continue to apply direct pressure

Bleeding controlled

Transfer to further care

Bleeding NOT controlled

Refer to catastrophic haemorrhage management – **start at appropriate point**

A

Jump to **point A** on the head, neck, torso side of the catastrophic haemorrhage algorithm

B

Jump to **point B** on the limbs side of the catastrophic haemorrhage algorithm

Figure 4.1 – The management of haemorrhage algorithm.

SECTION **4** Trauma

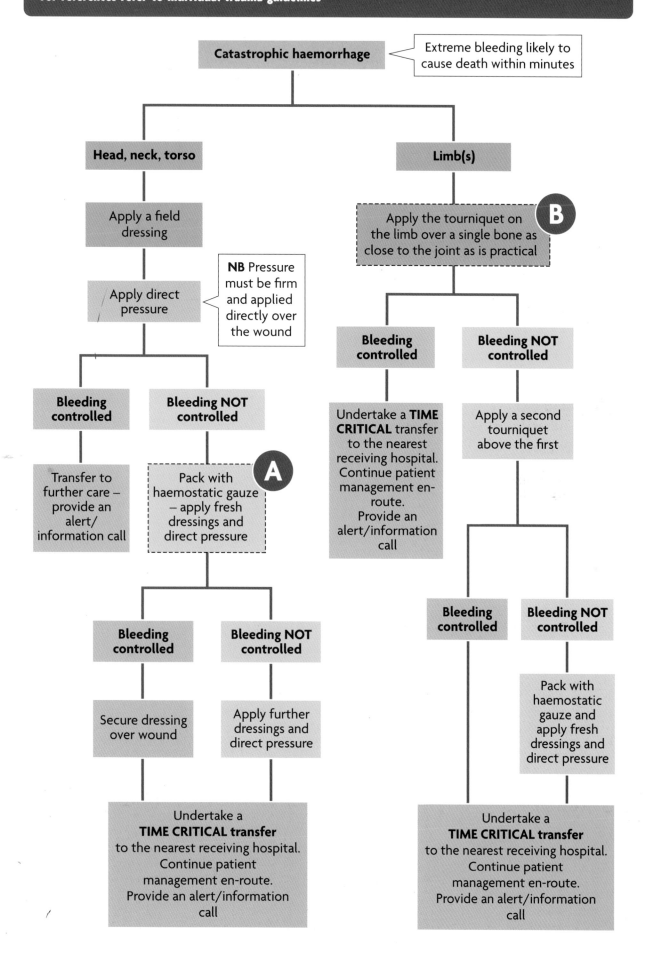

Figure 4.2 – The management of catastrophic haemorrhage algorithm.

1. Introduction

- Paediatric trauma is managed following the standard **<C>ABCDE** approach to trauma, taking into account differences in the child's anatomy, relative size and physiological response to injury. These differences are addressed below.

2. Incidence

- 700 children die as a result of accidents in England and Wales each year.

- 50% of child trauma deaths occur in motor vehicle incidents. Children travelling by car should legally be restrained but this law is not always followed and many deaths and serious injuries occur following vehicular ejection. Additionally, child deaths from cycle and pedestrian incidents are also very common.

- 30% of child trauma deaths occur at home with burns and falls being the leading causes.

- Child death reviews often identify circumstances that could potentially have been avoided had injury prevention methods been rigorously applied.

3. Assessment:
The Basic Trauma Approach

3.1 SCENE

Overall control of the incident allows paramedics to concentrate on patient assessment and management and it is recommended that a model, such as SCENE, is used to assess the initial trauma scene so that it can be managed effectively (see below).

S Safety

Risk assessment. Perform a dynamic risk assessment. Are there any dangers now or will there be any that become apparent during the incident? This needs to be continually re-assessed throughout the incident. Appropriate personal protective equipment should be utilised according to local protocols.

C Cause including MOI

Establish the events leading up to the incident. Is this consistent with your findings? Read the scene/wreckage looking for evidence that children were involved (e.g. toys or child seats). These may provide a clue that a child has been ejected from the vehicle or wandered off from the scene but may still require medical attention or other care. Ask if children were involved.

E Environment

Are there any environmental factors that need to be taken into consideration? These can include problems with access or egress, weather conditions or time of day.

N Number of patients

Establish exactly how many patients there are during the initial assessment of the scene

E Extra resources needed

Additional resources should be mobilised now. These can include additional ambulances, helicopter or senior medical support. Liaise with the major trauma advisor according to local protocols.

3.2 Primary survey

- Catastrophic haemorrhage (refer to Figure 4.4).

- Airway with cervical spine control (**refer to neck and back trauma guideline**).

- Breathing.

- Circulation.

- Disability.

- Exposure.

The management of a child suffering a traumatic injury requires a careful approach, with an emphasis on explanation, reassurance and honesty. Trust of the carer by the child makes management much easier.

If possible, it is helpful to keep the child's parents/carers close by for reassurance, although their distress can exacerbate that of the child.

3.3 Stepwise primary survey assessment

As for all trauma care, a systematic approach, managing problems as they are encountered before moving on is required.

4. Catastrophic Haemorrhage

Catastrophic blood loss must be arrested immediately (refer to catastrophic haemorrhage control, Figure 4.4).

5. Airway

In small children, the relatively large occiput tends to flex the head forward. In order to return the head to the neutral position it may be necessary to insert a small amount of padding under the shoulders.

Vomit, blood or foreign material may obstruct the airway. Apply gentle suctioning under direct vision. Blind finger sweeps are contra-indicated.

Head tilt should be avoided in trauma and a chin lift alone or a jaw thrust used to open the airway.

If an airway adjunct is needed, then an oropharyngeal airway should be inserted under direct vision. If it is necessary to insert a nasopharyngeal airway (e.g. because of trismus), care must be taken in all head injured children in case there is an underlying skull fracture, causing a risk of misplacement through the cribriform plate into the brain. It is also important to avoid damage to the adenoidal tissue. This can cause considerable bleeding making the airway even more difficult to manage.

High concentration oxygen (O_2) (**refer to oxygen guideline**) should be administered routinely, whatever the oxygen saturation, in children sustaining major trauma or long bone fractures.

Administer high concentration O_2 via a non-rebreathing mask, to maintain an oxygen saturation of at least 94%. If a high flow mask is not tolerated, the mask (or just the oxygen tubing) may be held near the child's nose or mouth.

Airway burns are considered as a 'special case' (**refer to burns and scalds in children guideline**). Examine for soot in the nostrils and mouth, erythema and blistering of the lips, and hoarseness of the voice. These suggest potential airway injury. These children require early endotracheal intubation and may deteriorate faster than adults due to the smaller diameter of their airway. Unless there is somebody at the scene who is trained in pre-hospital paediatric anaesthesia and difficult paediatric airway management who can electively intubate the child, it is best to transport the child rapidly (time critical transfer) and to pre-alert the hospital so they can have suitable experts standing by. If the airway swelling becomes life-threatening, and the airway cannot be controlled any other way, needle cricothyroidotomy may be required. Surgical airways should be avoided under the age of 12 years.

6. Cervical Spine

Cervical spinal immobilisation is essential when an injury to the neck has possibly occurred. Manual immobilisation is initially used although the subsequent use of a correctly sized cervical collar, head blocks and forehead/chin tapes and a scoop stretcher or a long board where the child has to be extricated is recommended. If the child is combative, this may not be possible and manual immobilisation may be the only possible method (**refer to neck and back trauma guideline**).

7. Breathing

A child's chest wall is readily deformable and may withstand significant force. As a result, significant intra-thoracic injuries can occur without any apparent external chest wall signs.

Auscultate the chest if practical.

Look at the chest for bruising and record the rate and adequacy of breathing. Chest wall movement and the presence of any wounds should be sought. Poor excursion may suggest an underlying pneumothorax.

Feel for rib fractures, or surgical emphysema.

This should reveal good, bilateral air entry and the absence of any added sounds. Listen specifically to the 3 areas:

1. above the nipples in the mid-clavicular line
2. in the mid-axilla under the armpits
3. at the rear of the chest, below the shoulder blades when it is possible to access this area.

Table 4.6 – NORMAL RESPIRATORY RATES

Age	Respiratory rate
<1 year	30–40 breaths per minute
1–2 years	25–35 breaths per minute
2–5 years	25–30 breaths per minute
5–11 years	20–25 breaths per minute
>12 years	15–20 breaths per minute

Assess for:

- Percuss the chest if possible assessing for hyporesonance or hyperresonance.
- Tension pneumothorax.

- Massive haemothorax.
- Sucking chest wounds (open pneumothorax).
- Flail chest.

NB **Refer to thoracic trauma guideline** for the management of these conditions.

NB Distended neck veins are very difficult to see in children and in shock may be absent.

Management

If ventilation is inadequate (see below) the child's respiratory effort may require support from bag-valve-mask ventilation and high flow oxygen. Assist ventilation at a rate equivalent to the normal respiratory rate for the age of the child (refer to Table 4.6) if:

- The child is hypoxic (SpO$_2$ <90%) and remains so after 30–60 seconds on high concentration O$_2$.
- Respiratory rate is <50% normal or >3 times normal.

Treat life-threatening chest injuries as per appropriate guideline (see above).

8. Circulation

Refer to Medical Emergencies – recognition of Circulatory Failure

Look firstly for evidence of significant external haemorrhage and treat as per haemorrhage guideline (refer to Figures 4.3 and 4.4).

Assess the:

- Brachial or carotid pulses; record rate and volume (refer to Table 4.7):
  - tachycardia (with a poor pulse volume) suggests shock
  - bradycardia also occurs in the shocked child but is a **PRE-TERMINAL SIGN**.
- Respiratory rate: elevated due to compensatory mechanisms in shock.
- Capillary refill time: measure on the forehead or sternum.
- Colour.
- Conscious level.
- Examine the abdomen for signs of intra-abdominal bleeding (if present assume a pelvic fracture).
- Remember cardiac tamponade in a rapidly deteriorating child where chest injury has occurred and where the cause of the deterioration is not clear (**refer to thoracic trauma guideline**).

Table 4.7 – NORMAL HEART RATES

Age	Heart rate
<1 year	110–160 beats per minute
1–2 years	100–150 beats per minute
2–5 years	95–140 beats per minute
5–11 years	80–120 beats per minute
>12 years	60–100 beats per minute

Significant blood losses are seen in long bone fractures with even greater losses (double the volume) seen when the fracture is open, when compared to a corresponding closed fracture: for example, in a closed femoral fracture 20% of the circulating blood volume may bleed into the surrounding tissues compared to losses of 40% from an open femoral shaft fracture.

Management

Splintage, traction and full immobilisation can reduce blood loss and pain.

Where possible, vascular access can be gained en-route to hospital, reducing the time spent on scene. Use the widest possible cannula for the veins available.

In paediatric trauma **5 ml/kg fluid boluses** are used and repeated as needed to improve clinical signs (e.g. RR, HR, capillary refill, conscious level) **towards normal.**

NB Hypotensive resuscitation practices (as used in adult trauma) should not be used in children.

(Due to their physiological reserves, children maintain their systolic blood pressures in the face of major blood loss, with hypotension only occurring at a very late stage. Significant cardiovascular compromise and even cardiac arrest may occur if volume resuscitation were to be delayed until a child had reached such an advanced state of hypovolaemia).

Following IV fluid resuscitation, in paediatric major trauma with catastrophic haemorrhage, a bolus of tranexamic acid should be given, if available (refer to tranexamic acid guideline).

9. Disability – Assessment

Record the initial level of consciousness using the AVPU Scale (below):

A Alert

V Responds to voice

P Responds to painful stimulus

U Unresponsive

as well as:

- The time of the AVPU assessment.
- Pupil size, shape, symmetry and response to light.
- Whether the child was moving some or all limbs. If there is no movement, then ask the child to 'wiggle' their fingers and toes, paying particular note to movements peripheral to any injury site.
- Any abnormalities of posture.

If the child is not **alert** they should be considered time critical. A formal GCS (see Appendix) en-route may be valuable to the receiving hospital but should only be recorded if it can be accurately done and does not delay transfer.

9.1 Stepwise disability management

Confusion or agitation in an injured child may result directly from a significant head injury, but equally may be secondary to hypoxia from an impaired airway or compromised breathing or else hypoperfusion due to blood loss and shock.

The management of any child with impaired consciousness is based on ensuring an adequate airway, oxygenation, ventilation and circulation.

Always measure the blood glucose level in any child with altered consciousness. If hypoglycaemia is detected **refer to the glycaemic emergencies in children guideline for treatment**.

10. Exposure

Children will lose heat rapidly when exposed for examination and immobilised during trauma care. Do protect the child from a cold environment during your assessment.

Expose children 'piecemeal' if possible, replacing a piece of clothing before removing the next as stripping a child may cause insecurity or embarrassment as well as exposing them to cold.

If the child is **TIME CRITICAL** they must be packaged appropriately (with full spinal immobilisation – or improvisation as tolerated – and pelvic splint if pelvic injury suspected) and transported rapidly to hospital.

An **alert/information call should be given for all TIME CRITICAL children** en-route.

If there is no apparent problem with the primary survey, a secondary survey may be commenced en-route. This should not delay the transfer to definitive care.

10.1 Secondary survey

This is a systematic and careful review of each part of the injured child looking for non-critical and/or occult injuries. It is rarely possible to complete this before hospital in a seriously injured child.

Any deterioration in the child's condition mandates an immediate return to the primary survey and the problem sought and treated.

Dress and immobilise any injuries found as required. Perform a simple **MSC** check of **ALL** 4 limbs (see below):

M	MOTOR	Test for movement
S	SENSATION	Apply light touch to evaluate sensation
C	CIRCULATION	Assess pulse and skin temperature

11. Analgesia in Trauma

As would happen for an adult, a child's pain must be addressed once their life-threatening problems have been attended to (**refer to pain management in children guideline**).

Note: Paediatric drug doses are expressed as mg/kg (refer to specific drug protocols/Page-for-Age for dosages and information). Drug doses **MUST** be checked prior to **ANY** drug administration, no matter how confident the practitioner may be.

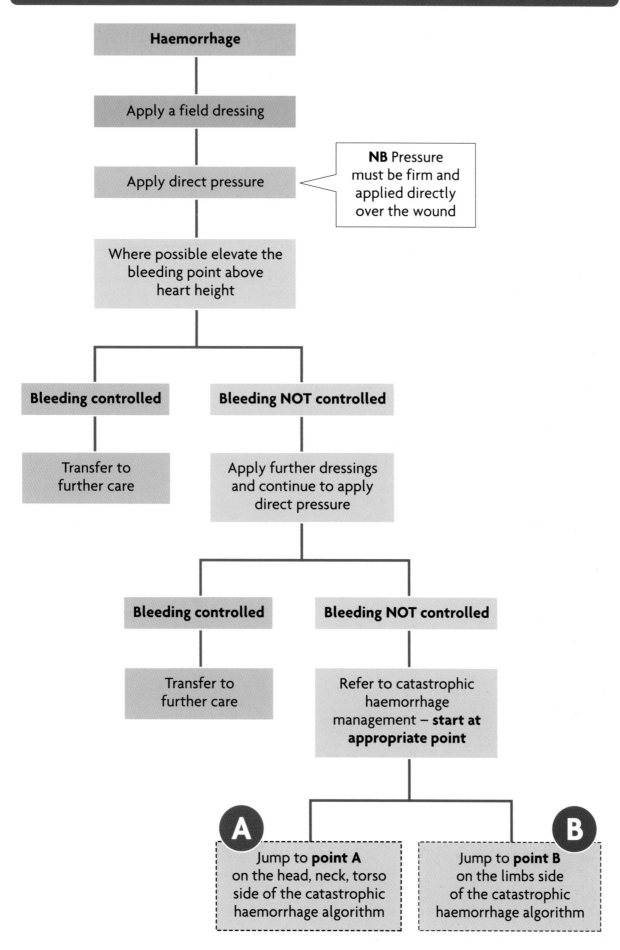

Figure 4.3 – The management of haemorrhage algorithm.

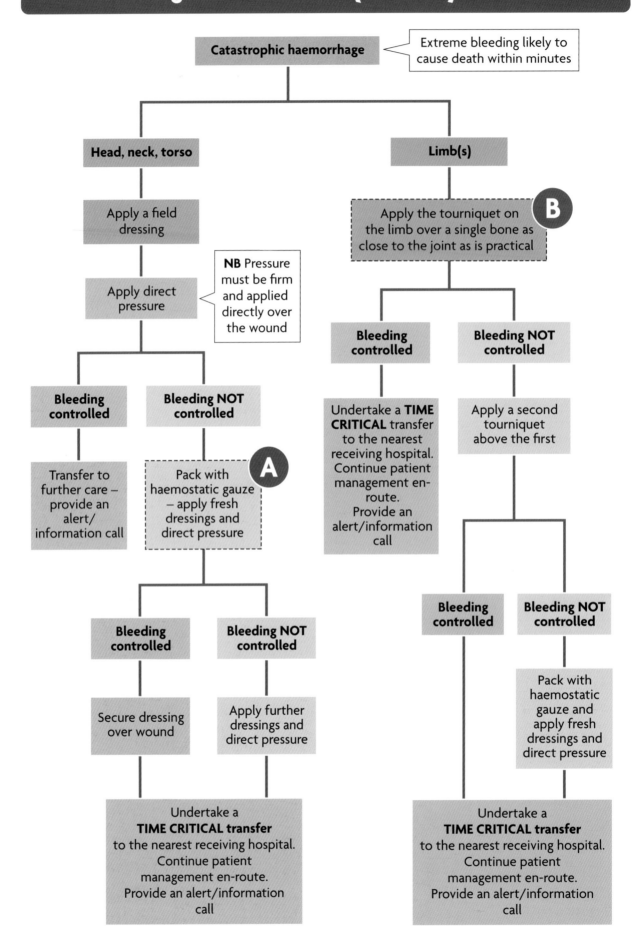

Catastrophic haemorrhage — Extreme bleeding likely to cause death within minutes

Head, neck, torso

Apply a field dressing

Apply direct pressure — NB Pressure must be firm and applied directly over the wound

Bleeding controlled

Transfer to further care – provide an alert/information call

Bleeding NOT controlled

Pack with haemostatic gauze – apply fresh dressings and direct pressure (A)

Bleeding controlled

Secure dressing over wound

Bleeding NOT controlled

Apply further dressings and direct pressure

Undertake a **TIME CRITICAL transfer** to the nearest receiving hospital. Continue patient management en-route. Provide an alert/information call

Limb(s)

Apply the tourniquet on the limb over a single bone as close to the joint as is practical (B)

Bleeding controlled

Undertake a **TIME CRITICAL** transfer to the nearest receiving hospital. Continue patient management en-route. Provide an alert/information call

Bleeding NOT controlled

Apply a second tourniquet above the first

Bleeding controlled

Bleeding NOT controlled

Pack with haemostatic gauze and apply fresh dressings and direct pressure

Undertake a **TIME CRITICAL transfer** to the nearest receiving hospital. Continue patient management en-route. Provide an alert/information call

Figure 4.4 – The management of catastrophic haemorrhage algorithm.

SECTION 4 Trauma

12. Summary

Read the scene for mechanism of injury and the presence of children.

Trauma emergencies in childhood are managed using similar priorities and techniques to those used in adult practice. Remember the important anatomical and physiological differences encountered in children whilst performing primary (and/or secondary) surveys.

Children may **conceal** serious underlying injuries using compensatory mechanisms so a high index of clinical suspicion is required. Agitation and/or confusion may indicate primary brain injury, but also be due to inadequate ventilation and/or cerebral perfusion.

KEY POINTS

Trauma Emergencies Overview (Children)

- Important anatomical and physiological differences exist between children and adults – a different approach will often be needed.

- Read the wreckage – toys or child seats may indicate that children have been involved in the incident.

- Assess and continuously re-assess <C>ABCDE.

- Detect time critical problems as part of the primary survey and transport urgently with a hospital pre-alert.

APPENDIX – Glasgow Coma Scale and Modified Glasgow Coma Scale

Table 4.8 – GLASGOW COMA SCALE

Item		Score
Eyes opening:		
	Spontaneously	4
	To speech	3
	To pain	2
	None	1
Motor response:		
	Obeys commands	6
	Localises pain	5
	Withdraws from pain	4
	Abnormal Flexion	3
	Extensor response	2
	No response to pain	1
Verbal response:		
	Orientated	5
	Confused	4
	Inappropriate words	3
	Incomprehensible sounds	2
	No verbal response	1

Table 4.9 – MODIFICATION OF GLASGOW COMA SCALE FOR CHILDREN AGED UNDER 4 YEARS OLD

Item	Score
Eyes opening:	As per adult scale
Motor response:	As per adult scale
Best verbal response:	
Appropriate words or social smiles, fixes on and follows objects	5
Cries, but is consolable	4
Persistently irritable	3
Restless, agitated	2
Silent	1

4 Trauma SECTION

1. Introduction

- Trauma to the abdomen can be extremely difficult to assess even in a hospital setting. In the field, identifying which abdominal structure(s) has been injured is less important than identifying that abdominal trauma itself has occurred.

- It is therefore, of major importance to note abnormal signs associated with blood loss and to establish that abdominal injury is the probable cause, rather than being concerned with, for example, whether the source of that abdominal bleeding originates from the spleen or liver.

- There may be significant intra-abdominal injury with very few, if any, initial indications of this at the time the abdomen is examined by the paramedic at the scene.

2. Severity and Outcome

The leading cause of morbidity and mortality is as a result of blunt trauma. Mortality from isolated abdominal stab wounds is approximately 1–2%.

3. Pathophysiology

The abdomen may be described as three anatomical areas:

i. **Abdominal cavity**
ii. **Pelvis**
iii. **Retro-peritoneal area.**

i. **Abdominal cavity** – extends from the diaphragm to the pelvis. It contains the stomach, small intestine, large intestine, liver, gall bladder and spleen.

The upper abdominal organs are partly in the lower thorax and lie under the lower ribs; therefore fractures of lower ribs may damage abdominal structures such as the liver and spleen.

ii. **Pelvis** – contains the bladder, the lower part of the large intestine and, in the female, the uterus and ovaries. The iliac artery and vein overlie the posterior part of the pelvic ring and may be torn in pelvic fractures, adding to already major bleeding.

iii. **Retro-peritoneal area** – lies against the posterior abdominal wall, and contains the kidneys and ureters, pancreas, abdominal aorta, vena cava and part of the duodenum. These structures are attached to the posterior abdominal wall, and are often injured by shearing due to rapid deceleration forces.

4. Abdominal Injuries

Blunt trauma – is the most common pattern of injury seen and results from direct blows to the abdomen or rapid deceleration. Blunt trauma may also result from all phases of a blast.

- The spleen, liver (hepatic tear) and 'tethered' structures such as duodenum are the most commonly injured. The small bowel, mesentery and aorta may also sustain injury.

Penetrating trauma – stab wounds, gunshot wounds, blast injuries and other penetrating injuries.

- **Stab wounds** – stab injures should be assumed to have caused serious damage until proved otherwise. Damage to liver, spleen or major blood vessels may cause massive haemorrhage. NB Upper abdominal stab wounds may have caused major intra-thoracic damage if the weapon was directed upwards (**refer to thoracic trauma guideline**). Similarly, chest stabbing injuries may also cause intra-abdominal injury.

- **Gunshot wounds** – tend to cause both direct and indirect injury, due to the forces involved and the chaotic paths that bullets may take. The same rules apply to associated intra-thoracic injuries.

- **Blast injuries** – can lead to both blunt and penetrating injuries. In an explosion in a confined space the blast wave can cause injuries to the bowel (perforation and haemorrhage) and penetrating ballistics can lead to organ damage.

5. Assesssment and Management

For the assessment and management of abdominal trauma refer to Table 4.10.

KEY POINTS

Abdominal Trauma
- Abdominal trauma can be difficult to assess.
- Identifying that abdominal trauma has occurred is more important than identifying which structure(s) has been injured, therefore note signs associated with blood loss.
- Observe mechanism of injury.
- Ensure <C>ABCs are assessed and managed; consider C-spine immobilisation.
- Transport to the nearest appropriate facility, providing an alert/information call en-route.

Abdominal Trauma

Table 4.10 – ASSESSMENT and MANAGEMENT of:

Abdominal Trauma

ASSESSMENT	MANAGEMENT

● **Assess <C>ABC**	● Control any external catastrophic haemorrhage – **refer to trauma emergencies overview**.
	● If any of the following **TIME CRITICAL** features are present:
	  – major **ABC** problems
	  – haemodynamic compromise
	  – decreased level of consciousness
	  – neck and back injuries – **refer to neck and back trauma guideline**, then:
	● Start correcting **A** and **B** problems.
	● Undertake a **TIME CRITICAL** transfer to nearest appropriate receiving hospital.
	● Provide an alert/information call.
	● Continue patient management en-route.

● Assess	● Ascertain the mechanism of injury: ● **Road traffic collision:** look for impact speed and severity of deceleration; seat belt and lap belt use are particularly associated with torn or perforated abdominal structures. ● **Stabbing and gunshot wound(s):** consider the length of the weapon used or the type of gun and the range. ● **Blast injuries:** blast wave injuries and penetrating ballistics. Assess the chest and abdomen – NB Some abdominal organs (e.g. liver and spleen) are covered by lower ribs/chest margins. **ABDOMEN:** ● Examine for signs of tenderness. ● Examine for external signs of injury (e.g. contusions, seat/lap belt abrasions). ● Evisceration (protruding abdominal organs). **GENTLY** palpate the four quadrants of the abdomen for signs of tenderness, guarding and rigidity. Shoulder-tip pain should increase suspicion of injury or internal bleeding. NB Significant **INTRA-ABDOMINAL TRAUMA** may show little or no evidence in the early stages, therefore **DO NOT** rule out injury if initial examination is normal. **CHEST:** ● Fractures of the lower ribs – if confirmed or suspected **refer to thoracic trauma guideline**.
● Evisceration	● **DO NOT** push protruding abdominal organs back into the abdominal cavity. ● Cover protruding abdominal organs with warm moist dressings.
● Impaling objects	● Leave impaling objects (e.g. a knife) **IN-SITU** ● Secure the object prior to transfer to further care. If the object(s) is pulsating, **DO NOT** completely immobilise it, but allow it to pulsate.
● Haemorrhage	● In the case of external haemorrhage apply a field dressing and direct pressure – **refer to trauma emergencies overview guideline**.
● Oxygen	● Administer high levels of supplemental oxygen (aim for SpO$_2$ 94–98%) – refer to oxygen guideline. ● Apply pulse oximeter.
● Ventilation	Consider assisted ventilation at a rate of 12–20 respirations per minute if: ● Oxygen saturation (SpO$_2$) is <90% on high levels of supplemental oxygen. ● Respiratory rate is <12 or >30bpm. ● Inadequate chest expansion. Refer to airway and breathing management guideline.
● Vital signs	● Monitor vital signs. ● Monitor ECG.
● Pelvic injuries	● Consider pelvic injuries – if suspected **refer to pelvic trauma guideline**.
● Thoracic injuries	● If the injury affects the chest **refer to thoracic trauma guideline**.
● Pain management	● If pain relief is indicated **refer to pain management guidelines**.
● Fluid	● If fluid resuscitation is indicated – refer to intravascular fluid therapy guideline. ● **DO NOT** delay on scene for fluid replacement.
● Transfer to further care	● Continue patient management en-route. ● Provide an alert/information call. ● Complete documentation.

4 Trauma
SECTION

1. Management of Traumatic Brain Injury (TBI) in the Pre-hospital Setting

Airway with C spine control

It is well recognised that airway obstruction or aspiration are major and often preventable causes of death in patients with severe traumatic brain injury [534]. Basic airway manoeuvres are essential to prevent primary airway obstruction and associated brain hypoxia. These should be instigated with consideration for protecting the cervical spine, as it is estimated that up to 10% of TBIs are complicated by a cervical spine injury [535–538]. However, there is also strong evidence to suggest that rigid cervical spinal immobilisation collars create a detrimental rise in ICP [539–541], which should be avoided where possible in TBI (probably due to compression of the jugular veins of the neck). Current practice involves loosening the collar once extrication is completed and the patient is secured in a position of neutral alignment with conventional head and body immobilisation. Be aware of the increased risk of cervical spine injury in frail or elderly patients or those with established musculoskeletal pathologies.

In addition to maintaining C-spine immobilisation, some evidence suggests that placing the patient in a 30° head up position reduces the effects of a raised ICP in patients with TBI [542], and this is traditionally employed once the cervical collar is removed on the Intensive Care Unit. The logistical challenges of elevating a patient to 30° whilst immobilised in the pre-hospital setting probably render this process all but redundant, however, clinicians should remain aware of the effect of positioning, and ensure the patient's head remains above, or at least level with the feet throughout extrication and transfer.

The most appropriate way of securing the airway in the pre-hospital setting is still contentious, with evidence highlighting a conflict between basic measures with a rapid extrication to a neurosurgical centre, or a delayed transport with endotracheal intubation. Current opinion leans towards Rapid Sequence Induction and intubation, with paralysing drugs by appropriately trained and qualified people (if available,) but the evidence of merit is still far from conclusive [540, 540].

Breathing and ventilation

Adequate ventilation is essential to the management of TBI through the avoidance of hypoxia and maintenance of 'normocapnia'. Numerous studies have demonstrated the correlation between arterial hypoxaemia and poor prognosis following TBI [543], with some even demonstrating increased mortality of up to 50% following only brief episodes of desaturation [544]. Current evidence suggests that oxygen should initially be administered at 10–15 l/min via a non-rebreathing mask, with a target saturation of 94–98% [545].

Evidence also demonstrates that those patients who remain normocapnic ($ETCO_2$ between 35 and 44 mmHg / 4.6 and 6 Kpa) following a TBI have significantly better outcomes [546]. Hyperventilation reduces arterial carbon dioxide (CO_2) concentrations, and leads to a consequent vasoconstriction within the cerebral vasculature, worsening both cerebral hypoxia and oedema [547]. Hypercapnia, associated with hypoventilation increases the vasodilatation of the cerebral blood vessels, which increases intracranial volumes and therefore ICP.

Circulation

Estimates have previously suggested that between 8% and 13% of patients with severe traumatic head injuries are hypotensive either at the scene of the injury, or in the Emergency Department [548]. In addition, a wealth of evidence demonstrates a strong correlation between hypotension and poor outcome in TBI, with some highlighting that a single episode of hypotension (SBP < 90 mmHg) is independently linked to a 100% increase in mortality rate [548–549]. This leads to the obvious conclusion that effective management of hypotension in the pre-hospital setting improves the outcomes of patients with TBI. Haemorrhage control (especially from the highly vascular scalp) should be established early to avoid the unnecessary consumption of coagulation products, and where hypotension is identified intravenous fluid resuscitation should be commenced. Unfortunately, there still remains a lack of clear research evidence to demonstrate the most appropriate fluid for resuscitation in TBI [550] and in most cases it will be dictated by local service interpretations and current formulary restrictions.

Disability

There is a high incidence of associated injuries found in patients with TBI, and an attempt to identify these during the secondary survey should be made, whilst remaining aware of the severe impacts of prolonged scene delays. The patient's GCS should be calculated, as this can be an important prognostic indicator and is useful for monitoring injury progression over time.

Over recent years there has been a growing interest in the potential benefits of therapeutic hypothermia in TBI, although to date, research has failed to demonstrate any statistical benefit in long-term outcome. A large meta-analysis demonstrated no statistical benefit for patients who underwent therapeutic cooling [551], and a more recent RCT examined another approach to cooling in the ED, and also demonstrated no beneficial outcome when compared to normothermia [552]. However, inadvertent hypothermia in patients with TBI has been demonstrated to have a strong correlation with death. In subgroup analysis (n=5,670) of an extremely large retrospective review of their trauma registry, one research group demonstrated that patients who had experienced accidental hypothermia were twice as likely to die as those who hadn't [553]. The key message therefore is that whilst investigations into the clinical benefit of therapeutic hypothermia are likely to continue, clinicians should strive to avoid inadvertent hypothermia in all victims of trauma, including those with TBI.

Pain and agitation

Agitation in TBI has a number of potential causes, several of which have already been addressed in this review. One commonly overlooked cause of agitation in patients with a TBI is pain, either from the head injury itself or associated injuries sustained at the time of the TBI. Managing pain in TBI poses a challenge for the pre-hospital clinician; whilst a patient in pain will be agitated, more difficult to manage and place themselves at risk of further cerebral hypoxia, the administration of opiates in severe TBI is a relative contraindication due to the potential for exaggerated respiratory depression, hypoventilation, hypercapnia and increased ICP [553]. The decision whether to use opiates in those with a TBI is therefore a clinical one, underpinned by careful assessment and close monitoring for adverse effects. Clinicians might consider requesting more senior assistance for patients whose TBI is complicated by agitation associated with acute pain.

Evacuation considerations

The underlying principles of effective pre-hospital management of TBI are rapid assessment; swift and appropriate management; and timely evacuation to a receiving centre with sufficient expertise to manage the patient. Clearly, this will be heavily dependent upon local resources and operational plans for those sustaining significant trauma, but clinicians should consider the most appropriate mode of evacuation early in the incident, to reduce on-scene delays as much as possible. HEMS services now operate across most of the UK and Ireland, and are often best placed to facilitate rapid evacuation to specialist centres. In any eventuality, a suitably detailed hand-over to the receiving unit is imperative for all patients with a significant TBI.

Special considerations

Head injuries in the elderly

Although significant head injury is predominantly a disease of the younger generation, a second peak in incidence occurs in those >65 years [554]. A number of age related structural changes in the cerebral architecture leaves elderly people at increased susceptibility to intracranial haemorrhage following what may be an apparently minor head injury [555]. In addition, elderly people are at increased risk of intracranial bleeding following head injury due to co-morbidities (such as clotting derangements) or polypharmacology. Finally, elderly patients may present to healthcare services in an atypical way following a head injury, due to altered intracranial anatomy or pre-existing cognitive decline. Clinicians should suspect TBI in all elderly patients identified to have sustained trauma of any significance, and ensure that they maintain a high index of suspicion when assessing and treating elderly patients with traumatic injuries.

2. Midazolam in Traumatic Brain Injury

Background

Patients with TBI can pose a challenge for management in the pre-hospital setting, and any associated hypoxia, hypercapnia and intracranial hypertension can contribute significantly to a poorer prognosis [556]. Although not robust, the evidence suggests that the therapeutic benefits of midazolam for these patients can include amnesia, anxiolysis and most critically, an ability to effectively provide oxygenation and ventilation, which may help reduce the detrimental secondary brain injury they incur [557]. However, sedating agents may reduce systemic blood pressure leading to a decrease in cerebral perfusion pressure (CPP), in addition to further jeopardising the patient's airway. Quite clearly therefore, the decision to use midazolam to facilitate safe patient management needs to be carefully considered.

Type

A short acting central nervous system depressant of the benzodiazepine class.

Pharmacokinetics / pharmacodynamics

Midazolam is a benzodiazepine derivative available in a stable and well tolerated solution for injection or infusion.

The pharmacological effect of midazolam is characterised by short duration because of a rapid metabolic transformation over a short time. Midazolam has a potent sedative and sleep-inducing effect. Furthermore, it has the effect of relieving anxiety and convulsions and of relaxing muscles.

Midazolam is eliminated primarily through the kidneys (60–80% of the dose injected) and in healthy test subjects, the elimination half-life of midazolam is 1.5–2.5 hours. The elimination half-life of midazolam is extended in obesity, hepatic, renal and cardiac insufficiency and critical illness

Indications

● Post intubation sedation.[a]

● Induction of conscious sedation to manage combativeness / agitation in order to enable effective oxygenation / ventilation.

● Management of emergence phenomenon following ketamine analgesia.

Contra-indications

● Known hypersensitivity to benzodiazepines.

● Severe respiratory distress / respiratory depression.

Cautions

As with all benzodiazepines, severe adverse cardiorespiratory events have been reported following the use of midazolam, including respiratory depression; respiratory arrest; apnoea and cardiac arrest. These may be associated with excessively rapid administration.

Special caution should be exercised when administering midazolam to high-risk patients:

● Adults over 60 years of age.

● Chronically ill, injured or debilitated patients.

● Patients with impaired renal, hepatic or cardiac function.

● Paediatric patients – of any age are particularly vulnerable to airway obstruction and hypoventilation.

● Concomitant alcohol use.

These high-risk patients require lower dosages and should be continuously monitored for early signs of alterations of vital functions. Titration with small increments to clinical effect, and careful respiratory rate and oxygen saturation monitoring are essential.

Special considerations

As with any substance with CNS depressant and/or muscle-relaxant properties, particular care should be taken when administering midazolam to a patient with myasthenia gravis.

---

[a] It is inappropriate for a clinician without senior anaesthetic capability to administer midazolam with the aim of facilitating intubation. However, in patients who are failing to tolerate an endotracheal tube already *in situ*, there may be clinical merit in the use of midazolam, as an alternative to removing the tube and further compromising the airway patency.

Amnesia

Midazolam causes anterograde amnesia (frequently this effect is very desirable in situations such as before and during surgical and diagnostic procedures), the duration of which is directly related to the administered dose.

Paradoxical reactions

Paradoxical reactions such as agitation, involuntary movements (including tonic/clonic convulsions and muscle tremor), hyperactivity, hostility, rage reaction, aggressiveness, paroxysmal excitement and assault, have been reported to occur with midazolam. These reactions may occur with high doses and/or when the injection is given rapidly. The highest incidence to such reactions has been reported among children and the elderly.

Table 4.11 – PREPARATION AND DOSING	
Adults <60 years	**Adults >60 years**
	High risk patients
IV	**I/V**
Initial dose: 0.5–1 mg	Initial dose: 0.5–1 mg
Titration doses: 0.5–1 mg	Titration doses: 0.5–1 mg
Total dose: 3.5–7.5 mg	Total dose: <3.5 mg

Adverse effects

- Reduced level of consciousness resulting in upper airway obstruction.

- Respiratory and cardiovascular depression.

Key considerations / additional information

- Midazolam should not be used to assist or facilitate intubation.

- Full ALS resuscitation equipment should be available to hand whenever midazolam is administered.

- Vital signs must be carefully monitored and equipment to support respiration must be available. Apnoea can occur following parenteral use (especially in the elderly and those with respiratory disease).

- Adverse effects are increased in the presence of other sedating drugs such as opiates and alcohol.

3. Pathophysiology

- Primary brain injury occurs at the time of injury. Prevention strategies include the wearing of motorcycle and cycle helmets, the use of vehicle restraint systems (e.g. seatbelts and airbags) and public education.

- Secondary brain injury occurs following the primary event as a result of hypoxia, hypercarbia or hypoperfusion.

- A reduced level of consciousness may lead to airway obstruction or inadequate ventilation resulting in poor oxygenation, carbon dioxide retention and acidosis.

- Blood loss from other injuries in a patient with multisystem trauma may lead to hypovolaemia, hence a fall in mean arterial pressure and consequently cerebral perfusion pressure.

- Cerebral perfusion pressure (CPP) needs to be maintained to ensure normal brain physiology and prevent oedema. It is determined by the relationship between the mean arterial pressure (MAP). This is the mean pressure during the cardiac pumping cycle pushing blood into the brain against the resistance of the intracranial pressure (ICP).

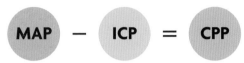

Figure 4.5 – Cerebral perfusion pressure.

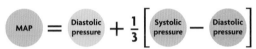

Figure 4.6 – Mean arterial pressure.

- The ICP is increased by the presence of anything that occupies the intracerebral space (haematoma, a neoplasm) or causes vasodilatation (hypoxia, hypercarbia) and consequent oedema.

Assessment

Management

C - Catastrophic haemorrhage
manage catastrophic haemorrhage (see management of catastrophic haemorrhage algorithm)

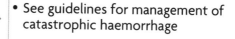

- See guidelines for management of catastrophic haemorrhage

A – Airway and C spine
Establish current or impending airway loss. Consider C spine status

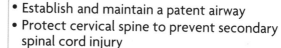

- Establish and maintain a patent airway
- Protect cervical spine to prevent secondary spinal cord injury

B – Breathing:
Assess rate, pattern and effectiveness of respiration. Obtain oxygen saturations and CRT

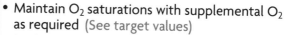

- Maintain O_2 saturations with supplemental O_2 as required (See target values)
- Instigate capnographic monitoring if available.
- Avoid hyper / hypoventilation of mechanically ventilated patients (See target values)

C – Circulation
Assess pulse rate, rhythm and volume. Assess BP. Confirm control of significant haemorrhage

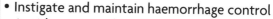

- Instigate and maintain haemorrhage control
- Avoid any episodes of unmanaged hypotension (See target values)
- Obtain IV access
- Adult: use 250ml boluses of selected fluid to ensure BP remains above 90 mmHg
- Children: avoid hypotension (see age specific systolic BP targets)
- Avoid excessive dilution of clotting factors through excessive fluid therapy

D – Disability
Assess GCS
Measure temperature and blood glucose
Identify associated injuries taking account of mechanism and injury patterns
Check pupil reaction

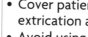

- Cover patients to prevent heat loss during extrication and evacuation
- Avoid using cool or cold infusions
- Correct abnormalities of blood glucose
- Manage pain in accordance with local or national guidelines
- Monitor level of consciousness and be prepared for impending management challenges in those with a diminishing GCS
- Treat seizures according to established JRCALC guidelines

Evacuation considerations

- Early referral to specialist neurosurgical
- centre*
- Monitor for deterioration Consider 30° head up tilt
- Early pre-alert call to receiving unit

Treatment Goals (Adults):
SPO$_2$: >94% [23]
Systolic Blood Pressure: >90 mmHg [24]
ETCO$_2$: 35–40 mmHg [25]

Treatment goals (children):
SPO$_2$: 95%
ETCO$_2$: 35–40 mmHg
Blood Pressure: see age-specific systolic BP targets

Age-specific systolic Blood Pressure targets (children)	
< 1 year	> 80 mmHg
1–5 years	> 90 mmHg
5–14 years	> 100 mmHg
> 14 years	> 110 mmHg

Figure 4.7 Assessment and management of significant head injury.

4 SECTION Trauma

1. Introduction

- There is one fundamental rule to apply to limb trauma cases and that is **NOT** to let limb injuries, however dramatic in appearance, distract the clinician from less visible but life-threatening problems such as airway obstruction, compromised breathing, poor perfusion and spinal injury

- Patients with limb trauma are likely to be in considerable pain and distress; therefore consider pain management as soon as clinically possible after arriving on scene (**refer to pain management guidelines**).

Table 4.12 – TYPES OF LIMB INJURY

Greenstick fracture

One side of the bone breaks, the other side bends – common accidental injury in children.

Transverse fracture

A fracture across the bone that occurs due to direct blow or force on the end of the bone (e.g. a fall on the hand may break the forearm bones or the distal humerus).

Spiral or oblique fracture

A fracture around the bone or at an angle across it, due to a twisting force.

Compound fracture (open)

A fracture in which the bone is broken into multiple (more than two) pieces.

Comminuted fracture

A fracture that comprises small fragmented ends.

Closed fracture

A fracture that is contained, that is skin is unbroken.

Dislocations

Dislocations are very painful and commonly affect the digits, elbow, shoulder, patella and occasionally the hip (high energy).

Compartment syndrome

A complication of limb fractures arising from increased pressure in muscular compartments due to contained haemorrhage. This can lead to ischaemia, with potentially catastrophic consequences for the limb.

Degloving

Degloving can accompany limb fractures and be to the superficial fasica or full depth down to the bone.

Amputations/partial amputations

Amputations most frequently involve digits, but can involve part or whole limbs. Amputations may still result in a viable limb, providing there is minimal crushing damage and survival of some vascular and nerve structures.

Neck of femur fractures

Such fractures commonly occur in the elderly and are one of the most common limb injuries encountered in the pre-hospital environment. Typical patients present with shortening and external rotation of the leg on the injured side, with pain in the hip and referred pain in the knee. The circumstances of the injury must be taken into account – often the elderly person has been on the floor for some time, which increases the possibility of hypothermia, dehydration, pressure sores and chest infection, so careful monitoring of vital signs is essential.

2. Pathophysiology

- The pathophysiology differs depending on the nature of the injury – refer to Table 4.12.

- Blood loss from femoral shaft fractures can be considerable, involving loss of 500–2,000 millilitres in volume. If the fracture is open, blood loss is increased.

- Nerves and blood vessels are placed at risk from sharp bony fragments, especially in very displaced fractures, hence the need to return fractured limbs to normal alignment as rapidly as possible. Fractures around the elbow and knee are especially likely to injure arteries and nerves.

- The five 'P's of ischaemia are shown in Table 4.13.

Table 4.13 – 'P's OF ISCHAEMIA

Sign	Symptom
Pain	Out of proportion to the apparent injury; often in the muscle, which may not ease with splinting/analgesia.
Pallor	Due to compromised blood flow to limb.
Paralysis	Loss of movement.
Paraesthesia	Changes in sensation.
Pulselessness	The loss of peripheral pulses is a grave late sign caused by swelling which can lead to the complete occlusion of circulation.
Perishing cold	The limb is cold to the touch.

3. Incidence

- Limb trauma is a common injury in high energy impacts. Causes can include but are not limited to falls, sports, traffic, occupational and intentional causes, and can occur at any age.

- In older people injuries can occur from relatively minor trauma (e.g. falls from a standing height can lead to femoral fractures).

4. Severity and Outcome

- The severity and outcome differ depending on the nature of the injury. However, limb trauma can have serious consequences, for example, infection following an open fracture can affect the future viability and long-term function of the limb.

Splinting

- Splinting will contribute to 'circulation' care by considerably reducing further blood loss and pain en-route to hospital.

- **Traction splint** – is a device for applying longitudinal traction to the femur, using the pelvis and the ankle as static points. Correct splintage technique using a traction splint reduces:

  – pain
  – haemorrhage and damage to blood vessels and nerves
  – bone fragment movement and the risk of a closed fracture becoming an open fracture

- the risk of fat embolisation (brain and lungs)
- muscle spasm by pulling thigh to a natural cylindrical shape
- blood loss by compression of bleeding sites.

● Traction splints such as the Sager, Trac 3, Donway splints and Kendrick are easy to apply and some now have quantifiable traction, measured on a scale in pounds. The correct amount of traction is best judged by the injured leg being the same length as the uninjured limb.

5. Assessment and Management

For the assessment and management of limb trauma refer to Table 4.15.

Table 4.14 – SPLINTING

Injury	Splintage type
Fractured neck of femur	Padding between legs. Figure of eight bandage around ankles. Broad bandage: two above, two below the knee.
Fractured shaft of femur	Traction splint. NB Fractures of the ankle, tibia, fibula, knee or pelvis on the same side as the femoral fracture may limit use of a traction splint, Trust guidelines should be followed.
Fracture or fracture dislocation around the knee	Long leg box splint. Vacuum splint. Traction splint without the application of traction.
Patella dislocation	Companion strapping (one leg to the other). Support on pillow. Contoured vacuum splint. If the leg is gently straightened the patella often spontaneously relocates, if resistance is felt, the leg should be splinted in the position of comfort.
Tibia/fibula shaft fracture	Long leg box splint. Long vacuum splint.
Ankle fracture	Short leg box splint. Short vacuum splint.
Foot fractures	Short box splint. Short vacuum splint.
Clavicle Humerus Radius Ulna	Self-splintage may be adequate and less painful than a sling. Sling. Vacuum splints may be well suited to immobilising forearm fractures. Short box splint.

KEY POINTS

Limb Trauma

● Ensure <C>ABCs are assessed and managed; consider C-spine immobilisation.

● DO NOT become distracted by the appearance of limb trauma, from assessing less visible but life-threatening problems, such as airway obstruction, compromised breathing, poor perfusion and spinal injury.

● Transfer to nearest appropriate hospital as per local trauma care pathway; provide an alert/information call.

● Limb trauma can cause life-threatening haemorrhage.

● Assess for intact circulation and nerve function distal to the fracture site.

● Any dislocation that threatens the neurovascular status of a limb must be treated with urgency.

● Splintage is fundamental to prevention of further blood loss and can reduce pain.

● Limb trauma can cause considerable pain and distress – consider pain management as soon as clinically possible after arriving on scene.

● In cases of life-threatening trauma commence a time critical transfer and perform any splinting en-route if possible.

Table 4.15 – ASSESSMENT and MANAGEMENT of:

Limb Trauma

ASSESSMENT	MANAGEMENT

● Assess **<C>ABCD**	Control any external catastrophic haemorrhage – **refer to trauma emergencies overview.**
	● If any of the following **TIME CRITICAL** features are present:
	  – major **ABC** problems
	  – haemodynamic compromise – refer to intravascular fluid management guideline
	  – altered level of consciousness – **refer to altered level of consciousness guideline**
	  – neck and back injuries – **refer to neck and back trauma guideline**
	  – threatened limb – loss of neurovascular function (e.g. as a result of a dislocation which requires prompt realignment), then:
	● Start correcting **A** and **B** problems.
	● Mid shaft femoral fracture – apply a traction splint if this can be applied quickly without delaying transfer, otherwise apply manual traction where sufficient personnel are available – once applied it should not be released.
	● Undertake a **TIME CRITICAL** transfer to nearest appropriate hospital as per local trauma care pathway.
	● Provide an alert/information call.
	● Continue patient management en-route.

● External haemorrhage	Control any external haemorrhage – **refer to trauma emergencies overview.**

● Specifically assess	● Ascertain the mechanism of injury and any factors indicating the forces involved (e.g. the pattern of fractures may indicate mechanism of injury):
	  – fractures of the heel in a fall from a height may be accompanied by pelvic and spinal crush fractures (**refer to pelvic trauma and neck and back trauma guidelines**)
	  – 'dashboard' injury to the knee may be accompanied by a fracture or dislocation of the hip
	  – humeral fractures from a side impact are associated with chest injuries (**refer to thoracic trauma guidelines**)
	  – tibial fractures are rarely isolated injuries and often associated with high energy trauma and other life-threatening injuries.
	● All four limbs for injury to long bones and joints – in suspected fracture – expose site(s) to assess swelling and deformity.
	● Assess neurovascular function – MSC × 4: motor, sensation and circulation, distal to the fracture site. Assess foot pulses; palpate dorsalis pedis as capillary refill time can be misleading.
	● Assess general skin colour.
	● Assess age of patient – consider greenstick fractures in children, and fractures of wrist and hip in the elderly.
	● For accompanying illnesses:
	  – some cancers can involve bones (e.g. breast, lung and prostate) and result in fractures from minor injuries
	  – osteoporosis in elderly females makes fractures more likely.
	NB Where possible avoid unnecessary pain stimulus.

● Oxygen	● Administer high levels of supplemental oxygen (aim for SpO$_2$ 94–98%) refer to oxygen guideline.
● Splintage	In pre-hospital care it is difficult to differentiate between ligament sprain and a fracture; therefore **ASSUME** a fracture and immobilise. ● Remove jewellery from the affected limbs before swelling occurs. ● Check and record the presence/absence of pulses, and muscle function distal to injury. ● Consider realignment of grossly deformed limbs, to a position, as close to normal anatomic alignment as possible. Where deformity is minor and both distal sensation and circulation are intact, then realignment may not be necessary. ● If the pulse disappears during realignment then reposition limb slowly to previous site until pulse returns. ● Apply splintage – refer to Table 4.14. NB Vacuum splints are used if limbs need to be immobilised in an abnormal alignment. Rigid splints may need to be padded to conform to anatomy.
● Compound fracture	● Irrigate grossly contaminated wounds with saline. ● Apply a moist field dressing. ● Any gross displacement from normal alignment must, where possible, be corrected, and splints applied (refer to Table 4.14). NB Document the nature of the contamination as contaminates may be drawn inside following realignment.

Table 4.15 – ASSESSMENT and MANAGEMENT of:

Limb Trauma *continued*

ASSESSMENT	MANAGEMENT
● Amputations, partial amputations and degloving	● Irrigate grossly contaminated wounds with saline. ● Immobilise a partially amputated limb in a position of normal anatomical alignment. ● Where possible dress the injured limb to prevent further contamination. ● Apply a moist field dressing. NB Reimplantation following amputation or partial amputation may be possible; in order that the amputated parts are maintained and transported in the best condition possible: ● Remove any gross contamination. ● Cover the part(s) with a moist field dressing. ● Secure in a sealed plastic bag. ● Place the bag on ice – do not place body parts in direct contact with ice as this can cause tissue damage; the aim is to keep the temperature low but not freezing.
Neck of femur fractures	● Assess for shortening and external rotation of the leg on the injured side, with pain in the hip and referred pain in the knee. ● Ascertain whether the patient has been on the floor for some time, assess for signs of hypothermia, dehydration, pressure sores and chest infection (refer to relevant guidelines). ● Monitor vital signs. ● Immobilise by strapping the injured leg to the normal one with foam padding between the limbs – extra padding with blankets and strapping around the hips and pelvis can be used to provide additional support whilst moving the patient (refer to Table 4.14).
● Compartment syndrome	Consider the need for rapid transfer to nearest appropriate hospital as per local trauma care pathway as the patient may require immediate surgery, elevate limb and consider pain relief en-route.
● Pain management	● Pain management is an important intervention – if indicated **refer to pain management guidelines**.
● Fluid	● If fluid resuscitation is indicated – refer to intravascular fluid therapy guideline. ● DO NOT delay on scene for fluid replacement if peripheral pulses are present.
● Non-accidental injury	When assessing an injury in a child, consider the possibility of non-accidental injury – **refer to safeguarding children guideline**.

● Transfer to further care	● Transfer to nearest appropriate hospital as per local trauma care pathway.
	● Continue patient management en-route.
	● Provide an alert/information call.
	● **At hospital inform staff of:**
	  – any skin wound relating to a fracture
	  – an underlying fracture(s) that was initially open.
	● Complete documentation.

Neck and Back Trauma

1. Introduction

- There are a number of injuries that can lead to spinal cord injury (SCI) (see below).

- Effective management from the time of injury is important to ensure good outcomes. This guideline provides guidance for the assessment and management of neck and back trauma including indicators to guidance for related conditions.

2. Pathophysiology

- The spinal cord runs in the spinal canal down to the level of the second lumbar vertebra in adults.

- The amount of space in the spinal canal in the upper neck is relatively large, and risk of secondary injury in this area can be reduced if adequate immobilisation is applied. In the thoracic area, the cord is wide, and the spinal canal relatively narrow and injury in this area is more likely to completely disrupt and damage the spinal cord.

- Spinal shock is a state of complete loss of motor function and often sensory function found sometimes after SCI. This immediate reaction may go on for some considerable time, but some recovery may well be possible.

- Neurogenic shock is the state of poor tissue perfusion caused by sympathetic tone loss after spinal cord injury.

3. Incidence

- SCI most commonly affects young and fit people and will continue to affect them to a varying degree for the rest of their lives.

- Road traffic collisions, falls and sporting injuries are the most common causes of SCI – as a group, motorcyclists occupy more spinal injury unit beds than any other group involved in road traffic collisions. Roll-over road traffic collisions where occupants are not wearing seatbelts, and the head comes into contact with the vehicle body, and pedestrians struck by vehicles are likely to suffer SCI. Ejection from a vehicle increases the risk of injury significantly.

Risk factors

Road traffic collisions (RTC):

- Rollover RTC.
- Non-wearing of seatbelts.
- Ejection from vehicle.
- Struck by a vehicle.

Sporting injuries:

- Diving into shallow water.
- Horse riding.
- Rugby.
- Gymnastics and trampolining.

Falls:

- Older people.
- Rheumatoid arthritis.
- Certain sporting accidents, especially diving into shallow water, horse riding, rugby, gymnastics and

trampolining have a higher than average risk of SCI. Rapid deceleration injury such as gliding and light aircraft accidents also increase the risk of SCI.

- Older people and those with rheumatoid arthritis are prone to odontoid peg fractures, that may be difficult to detect clinically. Such injuries can occur from relatively minor trauma (e.g. falls from a standing height).

4. Severity and Outcome

- Injury most frequently occurs at junctions of mobile and fixed sections of the spine. Hence fractures are more commonly seen in the lower cervical vertebrae where the cervical and thoracic spine meets (C5, 6, 7/ T1 area) and the thoracolumbar junction (T12/L1) (refer to Figure 4.6). Of patients with one identified spinal fracture, 10–15% will be found to have another.

- In the extreme, SCI may prove immediately fatal where the upper cervical cord is damaged, paralysing the diaphragm and respiratory muscles.

- Partial cord damage, however, may solely affect individual sensory or motor nerve tracts producing varying long-term disability. It is important to note that there is an increasing percentage of cases where the cord damage is only partial and some considerable recovery is possible, providing the condition is recognised and managed appropriately.

5. Immobilisation

- All patients with the possibility of spinal injury should have manual immobilisation commenced at the earliest time, whilst initial assessment is undertaken.

- If immobilisation is indicated then the whole spine must be immobilised.

Only **two** methods are acceptable:

1. Manual immobilisation whilst the back is supported.
2. Collar, head blocks and back support.

NB There are several acceptable means of back support and the optimal method will vary according to circumstances. The following techniques may be used:

1. Patient lying supine:

- Use a scoop stretcher and head immobilisation. This can be achieved with a minimal amount of log rolling, and is preferable.

- Log roll patient with manual immobilisation of the neck to enable long extrication board to be used. Log rolling can result in lateral movement throughout the spinal column as well as disrupting clots and caution is advised.

- Directly lift patient using a spinal lift if there are adequately trained personnel on scene or use a scoop stretcher then insert a vacuum mattress underneath patient.

- Patients should be transported on the scoop stretcher unless there is a prolonged journey time where a vacuum mattress should be utilised.

2. Patient lying prone:

- Log roll patient with manual immobilisation of the neck to enable scoop stretcher to be used. This can be achieved with a minimal amount of log rolling as is preferable.

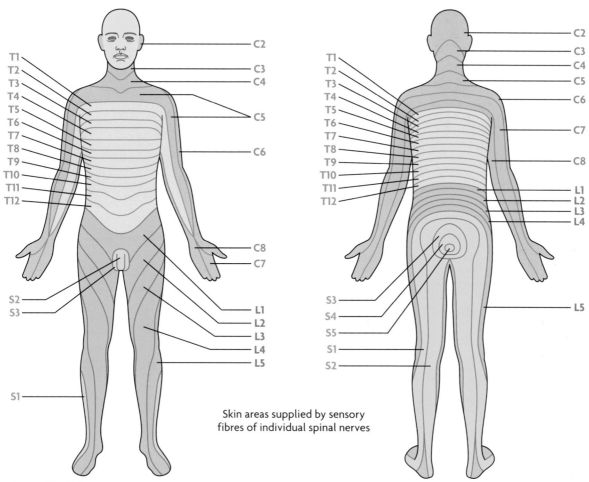

Figure 4.6 – Spinal nerves.

Skin areas supplied by sensory fibres of individual spinal nerves

- 2-stage log roll on to a vacuum mattress.

3. Patient requiring extrication:

- Extrication devices should be used if there is any risk of rotational movement.

- Rearward extrication on an extrication board.

- Side extrication invariably involves some rotational component and therefore has higher risks in many circumstances.

The techniques for use of devices are described in Prehospital Trauma Life Support (PHTLS) and other manuals.

5.1 Cautions/precautions

Vomiting

- Vomiting and consequent aspiration are serious consequences of immobilisation. Ambulance clinicians must always have a plan of action in case vomiting should occur.

- The collar will usually need to be removed and manual in-line immobilisation instituted. This may include:
  - suction
  - head-down tilt of the immobilisation device
  - rolling onto side on the immobilisation device.

Restless/combative patients

- There are many reasons for the patient to be restless and it is important to rule out reversible causes (e.g. hypoxia, pain, fear).

- If, despite appropriate measures, the patient remains restless then immobilisation techniques may need to be modified. A struggling patient is more likely to increase any injury, so a compromise between full immobilisation and degree of agitation/movement is appropriate.

- The use of restraint can increase forces on the injured spine and therefore a 'best possible' approach should be adopted.

Head injury

- Patients with a head injury may have raised intracranial pressure which restraint can increase; therefore, a 'best possible' approach should be adopted.

Special cases

- Some older patients, and those with cervical spine abnormalities (e.g. ankylosing spondylitis), may not be able to breathe adequately when positioned absolutely flat or tolerate a collar. Therefore a 'best possible' approach should be adopted which may include manual in-line immobilisation or maintenance of the pre-existing spinal deformity where putting the patient in the in-line neutral position is unsafe.

Immobilisation – evidence for how to immobilise

A recent Cochrane review found no randomised controlled trials comparing out of hospital spinal immobilisation techniques:

4 Trauma

SECTION

- Soft collars do not limit movement and should not be used.
- There is variable difference between the various types of semi-rigid collars.
- Addition of side supports and tapes increases immobilisation.
- Combining collar with extrication board improves immobilisation.
- The application of devices is more important than the variation of devices.
- Neutral position needs slight flexion of the neck and the occiput should be raised by 2 cm in an adult.
- Extrication devices are better than extrication boards at reducing rotational movement.
- Patients should spend no longer than 30 minutes on a rigid extrication board, but padding can extend this time.
- Vacuum mattress is more comfortable, and gives better immobilisation.
- Vacuum mattresses cannot be used for extrication and are vulnerable to damage.
- Log rolling is not without risk and use of the scoop stretcher may be safer for lifting patients.
- Long extrication/spinal board should only be used as an extrication device. Usually patients should be immobilised using a scoop. Once on a scoop they should remain on a scoop unless they are placed on a vacuum mattress when there is a prolonged journey time.

Emergency extrication

- If there is an immediate threat to life, for example, fire or airway obstruction, that cannot be resolved in situ, then the ambulance clinicians must decide on the relative risks of spinal immobilisation and the other factors.
- Rapid extrication techniques with manual immobilisation of the cervical spine are appropriate in these circumstances; this includes side extrication.

5.2 Immobilisation – when not to apply immobilisation

- Penetrating injury to the head has not been shown to be an indication for spinal immobilisation, and even penetrating injuries of the neck only rarely need selective immobilisation.
- A small prospective pre-hospital study indicated that the presence of **ALL** the following criteria can exclude significant spinal injury:
  - normal mental status with ability to appreciate pain
  - no neurological deficit
  - no spinal pain or tenderness
  - no evidence of intoxication
  - no evidence of distracting injury (e.g. extremity fracture).
- The few patients missed with SCI are often at the extremes of age. Such criteria can be reproducibly used in the pre-hospital environment. Mechanism of injury was not shown to be an independent predictor of injury.
- Use of such guidelines can significantly reduce the use of unnecessary immobilisation.

- Some patients may sustain thoracic or lumbar injuries in addition to, or in isolation from, cervical spine injuries. If you suspect thoracic or lumbar injuries whether the cervical spine has been cleared, then full spinal immobilisation should be undertaken whenever possible.

5.3 Immobilisation – hazards

The value of routine pre-hospital spinal immobilisation remains uncertain and any benefits may be outweighed by the risks of rigid collar immobilisation, including:

1. airway difficulties
2. increased intracranial pressure
3. increased risk of aspiration
4. restricted ventilation
5. dysphagia
6. skin ulceration
7. can induce pain, even in those with no injury.

5.4 Sequence for immobilisation

- All patients should be initially immobilised if the mechanism of injury suggests the possibility of SCI.

Blunt trauma

- Following assessment it is possible to remove the immobilisation if **ALL** the criteria are met (refer to the immobilisation algorithm Figure 4.7).
- Spinal pain does not include tenderness isolated to the muscles of the side of the neck.

Penetrating trauma

- Those with isolated penetrating injuries to limbs or the head do not require immobilisation.
- Those with truncal or neck trauma should be immobilised if there is new neurology and/or the trajectory of the penetrating wound could pass near or through the spinal column.

5.5 Children

- None of the studies have been validated in children. It is recommended that these guidelines are interpreted with caution in children, although there is some evidence to support similar principles.
- In children it is difficult to assess the neutral position but a padded board, head blocks, straps and collar appear to be the optimal method.

6. Assessment and Management

For assessment and management of neck and back trauma refer to Table 4.16 and Figure 4.7.

Table 4.16 – ASSESSMENT and MANAGEMENT of:

Neck and Back Trauma

ASSESSMENT	MANAGEMENT
• Assess **<C>ABCD** whilst controlling the spine	• Control any external catastrophic haemorrhage – **refer to trauma emergencies overview guideline** • All patients with the possibility of spinal injury should have manual immobilisation commenced at the earliest time, whilst initial assessment is undertaken.
• Evaluate whether the patient is **TIME CRITICAL** or **NON-TIME CRITICAL**	• Follow criteria in trauma emergencies overview. • If the patient is **TIME CRITICAL:** 　– control the airway 　– immobilise the spine 　– transfer to the nearest suitable receiving hospital 　– provide a hospital alert/information message 　– continue patient management en-route (see below).
• Assess oxygen saturation (refer to oxygen guideline)	• Adults – administer high levels of supplemental oxygen and aim for target saturation within the range of 94–98% – except for patients with COPD. • Children – administer high levels of supplemental oxygen.
• Determine mechanism of injury – forces causing injury include	• Hyperflexion. • Hyperextension. • Rotation. • Compression. • One or more of these.
• Specific symptoms of SCI	The patient may complain of: • Neck or back pain. • Loss of sensation in the limbs. • Loss of movement in the limbs. • Sensation of burning in the trunk or limbs. • Sensation of electric shock in the trunk or limbs.
• Rapidly assess to determine presence and estimate level of spinal cord injury	The following signs may indicate injury: • Diaphragmatic or abdominal breathing. • Hypotension (BP often <80–90 mmHg) with bradycardia. • Warm peripheries or vasodilatation in presence of low blood pressure. • Flaccid (floppy) muscles with absent reflexes. • Priapism – partial or full erection of the penis. **In a conscious patient** – assess sensory and motor function. • Use light touch and response to pain. • Examine upper limbs and hands. • Examine lower limbs and feet. • Examine both sides. • Undertake the examination in the **MID-AXILLARY** line **NOT** the **MID-CLAVICULAR** line as **C2, C3** and **C4** all supply sensation to the nipple line; use the forehead as the reference point to guide what is normal sensation. NB Always presume SCI in the unconscious trauma victim.
• If the patient is non-time critical, perform a more thorough assessment with a brief secondary survey	
• Assess for neurogenic shock	Diagnosis is difficult in pre-hospital care – the aim is to: • Maintain blood pressure of approximately 90 mmHg systolic. • Obtain IV access. • Determine need for fluid replacement but **DO NOT** delay on scene (refer to intravascular fluid therapy guideline) • In neurogenic shock, a few degrees of head-down tilt may improve the circulation, but remember that in cases of abdominal breathing, this manoeuvre may further worsen respiration and ventilation. This position is also unsuitable for a patient who has, or may have, a head injury. • If bradycardia is present consider atropine (refer to atropine guideline) – but it is important to rule out other causes (e.g. hypoxia, severe hypovolaemia).
• Assess the need for assisted ventilation	• Refer to airway management guideline.

4 SECTION Trauma

Table 4.16 – ASSESSMENT and MANAGEMENT of:

Neck and Back Trauma *continued*

ASSESSMENT	MANAGEMENT
● Steroids	● Evidence is conflicting on the use of early high dose steroids in acute spinal cord injury. If benefit exists then steroids need to be given within 8 hours of injury and therefore can be delayed until arrival at hospital.
● At hospital	● In addition to the usual information given at the time of hand-over it is important to inform the hospital staff of the duration period of immobilisation. ● Assist in the early removal from the extrication board. ● Complete documentation.

ADDITIONAL INFORMATION

Transportation of spinal patients:

- Driving should balance the advantages of smooth driving and time to arrival at hospital. No immobilisation technique eliminates movement from vehicle swaying and jarring. The technique of loosening the collar is not supported by evidence.
- There is no evidence to show advantage of direct transport to a spinal injury centre.
- Patients can tolerate 30 minutes on a long extrication board. The receiving ED should be told how long the patient has already been on the board so they can make an appropriate judgement on the timing of its removal. The duration of time on the extrication board should be recorded on the clinical record. The extrication board should be removed as soon as possible on arrival in hospital.
- If a journey time of greater than 30 minutes is anticipated, the patient should be transferred from the extrication board using an orthopaedic ('scoop') stretcher to a vacuum mattress. It may be appropriate to immobilise the patient using a vacuum mattress in the first instance in non-extrication situations.
- If there is a clear paralysing injury to the spinal cord then the benefits of the back board may be limited, while the risk of pressure sores may be very high. In these circumstances, the use of a vacuum mattress is often preferred.
- However, as half of cases of spinal injuries have other serious injuries, any unnecessary delay at scene or in transit should be avoided.

KEY POINTS

Neck and Back Trauma

- **Immobilise the spine until it is positively cleared.**
- **Immobilise the spine of all unconscious blunt trauma victims.**
- **If the neck is immobilised the thoracic and lumbar spine also need immobilisation.**
- **Standard immobilisation is by means of collar, headblocks, tapes and scoop or long board where patients require extrication.**
- **Aspiration of vomit, pressure sores and raised intracranial pressure are major complications of immobilisation.**

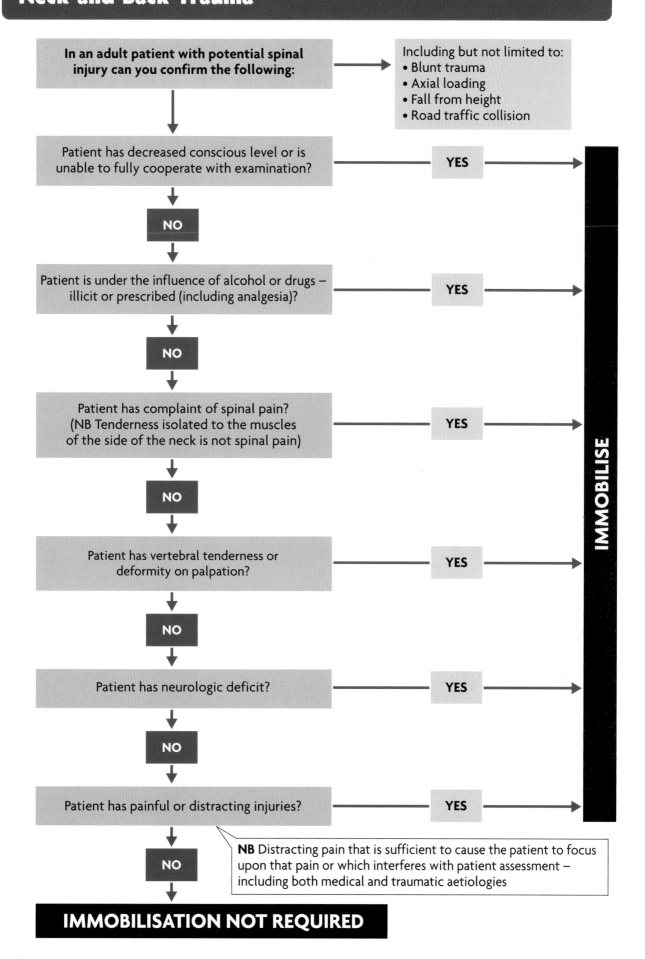

Figure 4.7 – Immobilisation algorithm.

1. Introduction

Major pelvic injuries are predominantly observed where there is a high-energy transfer to the patient such as might occur following road traffic collision, pedestrian accident, fall from height or crush injury.

Less serious pelvic injuries may also occur following low-energy transfer events, particularly in the elderly (such as a simple fall), amongst patients with degenerative bone disease or receiving radiotherapy and rarely as a direct consequence of seizure activity.

The majority of pelvic injuries do not result in major disruption of the pelvic ring, but rather involve fractures of the pubic ramus or acetabulum. Presentation of these injuries is very similar to neck of femur fractures; therefore please **refer to the limb trauma guideline** for management of these less serious pelvic injuries.

Mechanism of injury

- High-energy transfer
- Fall from height
- Crush injury

Risk factors

- Advancing age
- Degenerative bone disease
- Radiotherapy

2. Incidence

Pelvic fractures represent 3–6% of all fractures in adults and occur in up to 20% of all polytrauma cases. They display a bimodal distribution of age with most injuries occurring in the age ranges 15–30 and over 60 years; up to 75% of all pelvic injuries occur in men.

Unstable pelvic fracture is estimated to occur in up to 20% of pelvic fractures; a further 22% of pelvic fractures will remain stable despite significant damage to the pelvic ring. The remaining 58% of pelvic fractures are less serious retaining both haemodynamic and structural stability.

The incidence of pelvic fracture resulting from blunt trauma ranges from 5% to 11.9%; with obese patients more likely to sustain a pelvic fracture from blunt trauma than non-obese patients. Pelvic fracture associated with penetrating trauma is far less frequent. Open pelvic fractures are rare and account for only 2.7–4% of all pelvic fractures.

3. Severity and Outcome

Major pelvic injuries can be devastating and are often associated with a number of complications that may require extensive rehabilitation. Pelvic trauma deaths frequently occur as a result of associated injuries and complications rather than the pelvic injury itself.

Haemorrhage is the cause of death in 40% of all pelvic trauma victims and the leading cause of death (60% of fatal cases) in unstable pelvic fracture. Bleeding is usually retroperitoneal; the volume of blood loss correlates with the degree and type of pelvic disruption.

Reported mortality rates range from 6.4% to 30% depending on the type of pelvic fracture, haemodynamic status, and the nature of concomitant injuries and their complications.

The mortality rate among haemodynamically stable patients is around 10%, whereas the mortality rate amongst haemodynamically unstable patients approaches 20–30% but has been reported to be as high as 50% in cases of unstable open fracture; combined mortality approaches 16%.

4. Pathophysiology

4.1 Skeletal anatomy

Increasing pelvic volume allows for increased haemorrhage; conversely, reducing pelvic volume reduces potential for bleeding by realignment of broken bone ends.

4.2 Classification of injury

As with other fractures, pelvic fractures may be classified as open or closed, and benefit from being further described as either haemodynamically stable or unstable. Patients who are haemodynamically unstable are at greater risk of death and would benefit greatly from a suitable pre-hospital alert message.

Pelvic ring disruptions (as identified by in-hospital imaging) can be subdivided into four classes by mechanism of injury: antero-posterior compression (APC), lateral compression (LC), vertical shear (VS) and combined mechanical injury (CMI), a combination of the aforementioned classes.

4.3 Vascular injury

The arteries most frequently injured are the iliolumbar arteries, the superior gluteal and the internal pudendal because of their proximity to the bone, the sacro-iliac joint and the inferior ligaments of the pelvis. Bleeding from the venous network after a pelvic fracture is more frequent than arterial bleeding because the walls of the veins are more fragile than arteries. Blood may pool in the retroperitoneal space and haemostasis may occur spontaneously in closed fractures, especially if there is no concomitant arterial haemorrhage.

4.4 Other injuries

The incidence of urogenital injury ranges from 23% to 57%. Urethral and vaginal injuries are the most common injuries. Vaginal lacerations result from either penetration of a bony fragment or from indirect forces from diastasis of the symphysis pubis. Injuries to the cervix, uterus and ovaries are rare. Bladder rupture occurs in up to 10% of pelvic fractures.

The incidence of rectal injury ranges from 17% to 64% dependent upon type of fracture. Bowel entrapment is rare.

Pelvic injury is commonly associated with concomitant intra-thoracic and/or intra-abdominal injury.

Table 4.17 – ASSESSMENT and MANAGEMENT of:

Major Pelvic Trauma

ASSESSMENT
- Assess: **<C> ABCD; <C> catastrophic haemorrhage**
  - Airway
  - Breathing
  - Disability (mini neurological examination).
- Evaluate whether patient is **TIME CRITICAL** or **NON-TIME CRITICAL** following criteria as per trauma emergencies guideline. If patient is **TIME CRITICAL, correct A and B problems, stabilise the pelvis on scene and rapidly transport to nearest suitable receiving hospital. Provide an alert/information call.** En-route, continue patient management of pelvic trauma (see below).
- In **NON-TIME CRITICAL** patients perform a more thorough patient assessment with a brief secondary survey.

Specifically consider
- Pelvic fracture should be considered based upon the mechanism of injury.
- Clinical assessment of the pelvis includes observation for physical injury such as bruising, bleeding, deformity or swelling to the pelvis. Shortening of a lower limb may be present (see also **limb trauma guideline**)
- Assessment by compression or distraction (e.g. springing) of the pelvis is unreliable and may both dislodge clots and exacerbate any injury and should not be performed. Any patient with a relevant mechanism of injury and concomitant hypotension **MUST** be managed as having a **time critical pelvic injury** until proven otherwise.

MANAGEMENT
- Control any external catastrophic haemorrhage – **refer to trauma emergencies overview**.

Oxygen therapy
- Major pelvic injury falls into the category of critical illness and requires high levels of supplemental oxygen regardless of initial oxygen saturation reading (SpO_2). Maintain high flow oxygen (15 litres per minute) until vital signs are normal; thereafter reduce flow rate, titrating to maintain oxygen saturations (SpO_2) in the 94–98% range (refer to oxygen guideline).

Pelvic stabilisation
There is currently no evidence to suggest that any particular pelvic immobilisation device or approach is superior in terms of outcome in pelvic trauma and a number of methods have been reported. Effective stabilisation of the pelvic ring should be instigated at the earliest possible opportunity, preferably before moving the patient, and may be achieved by:
- Use of an appropriate pelvic splint.
- Apply the pelvic splint directly to skin, if this can be done easily with minimal handling.
- Expert consensus suggests the use of an appropriate pelvic splint is preferable to improvised immobilisation techniques. In all methods, circumferential pressure is applied over the greater trochanters and not the iliac crests. Care must be exercised so as to ensure that the pelvis is not reduced beyond its normal anatomical position.
- Pressure sores and soft tissue injuries may occur when immobilisation devices are incorrectly fitted.
- Reduction and stabilisation of the pelvic ring should occur as soon as is practicable whilst still on scene, as stabilisation helps to reduce blood loss by realigning fracture surfaces, thereby limiting active bleeding and additionally helping to stabilise clots. Reduction of the pelvis may have a tamponade effect, particularly for venous bleeding; however, there is little evidence to support this belief.
- Log rolling of the patient with possible pelvic fracture should be avoided as this may exacerbate any pelvic injury; where possible utilise an orthopaedic scoop stretcher to lift patients off the ground and limit movement to a 15° tilt.

Fluid therapy
- There is little evidence to support the routine use of IV fluids in adult trauma patients; refer to the intravascular fluid therapy guideline.

Pain management
- Patients' pain should be managed appropriately (**refer to pain management guidelines**); analgesia in the form of entonox (refer to entonox drug guidelines for administration and information) or morphine sulphate may be appropriate (refer to morphine drug guidelines for dosages and information).

5. Referral Pathway

5.1 The following cases should ALWAYS be transferred to further care:

- Any patient with hypotension and potential pelvic injury **MUST** be treated as a **TIME CRITICAL** pelvic injury until proven otherwise.
- Any patient with sufficient mechanism of injury to cause a pelvic injury.

5.2 The following cases MAY be considered suitable/ safe to be left at home:

- None.

6. Special Considerations for Children

(**See also** paediatric trauma guideline.)

- Pelvic fractures represent 1–3% of all fractures in children, thus there is a lower incidence compared with adults.

- In children, pelvic injuries have a lower mortality accounting for 3.6–5.7% of trauma deaths, with fewer deaths occurring as a direct result of pelvic haemorrhage; blood loss is more likely to be from solid visceral injury than the pelvis.

- Different injury patterns – multi-system injuries in 60%; greater incidence of diaphragmatic injury.

Major Pelvic Trauma

- Principles of management are the same, with the exception of fluid and oxygen therapy (refer to fluid therapy and oxygen guidelines).
- Clinical findings in small children can be unreliable.

7. Audit Information

- Incidence of suspected/actual pelvic fracture.
- Incidence of concomitant hypotension.
- Frequency of pelvic immobilisation when pelvic fracture suspected.
- Method of pelvic immobilisation.

KEY POINTS

Major Pelvic Trauma

- Pelvic fracture should be considered based upon mechanism of injury.
- The majority of pelvic fractures are stable pubic ramus or acetabular fractures.
- Any patient with hypotension and potentially relevant mechanism of injury MUST be considered to have a TIME CRITICAL pelvic injury.
- 'Springing' or distraction of the pelvis must not be undertaken.
- Pelvic stabilisation should be implemented as soon as is practicable whilst still on scene.
- Consider appropriate pain management.
- The use of a scoop stretcher is recommended to avoid log rolling the patient unless extrication is required.

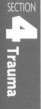

SECTION

4

Trauma

Thoracic Trauma [29, 178, 677–692]

1. Introduction

- In pre-hospital care, the most common problem associated with severe thoracic injuries is hypoxia, either from impaired ventilation or secondary to hypovolaemia from massive bleeding into the chest (haemothorax) or major vessel disruption (e.g. ruptured thoracic aorta).

2. Incidence

- Severe thoracic injuries are one of the most common causes of death from trauma accounting for approximately 25% of such deaths.

3. Severity and Outcome

- Despite the very high percentage of serious thoracic injuries, the vast majority of them can be managed in hospital with chest drainage and resuscitation and only 10–15% require surgical intervention.

4. Pathophysiology

- The mechanism of injury is an important guide to the likelihood of significant thoracic injuries. Injuries to the chest wall usually arise from direct contact, for example, intrusion of wreckage in a road traffic collision or blunt trauma arising from direct blow. Seat belt injuries fall into this category and may cause fractures of sternum, ribs and clavicle.

- If the force is sufficient, the deformity and the damage to the chest wall structures may induce tearing and contusion to the underlying lung and other structures. This may produce a combination of severe pain on breathing (pleuritic pain) and a damaged lung, both of which will significantly reduce the ability to ventilate adequately. This combination is a common cause of **hypoxia.**

- Blunt trauma to the sternum may cause myocardial contusion which may result in cardiac rhythm disturbances (ECG rhythm disturbances).

- Penetrating trauma may well damage the heart, the lungs and great vessels both in isolation or combination. It must be remembered that **penetrating wounds to the upper abdomen and neck may well have caused injuries within the chest remote from the entry wound.** Conversely, penetrating wounds to the chest may well involve the liver, kidneys and spleen.

- The lung may be damaged with bleeding causing a haemothorax or an air-leak causing a pneumothorax. Penetrating or occasionally a blunt injury may result in cardiac injuries. Blood can leak into the non-elastic surrounding pericardial sac and build up pressure to an extent that the heart is incapable of refilling to pump blood into circulation. This is known as **cardiac tamponade** and can be fatal if not rapidly relieved at hospital (see additional information in Table 4.19).

- Rapid deceleration injuries may result in sheering forces sufficient to rupture great vessels such as the aorta, caused by compressing the vessels between the sternum and spine.

- The six major thoracic injuries encountered in the pre-hospital setting include:
  i.   a tension pneumothorax,
  ii. massive haemothorax (following uncontrolled haemorrhage into the chest cavity),
  iii. open chest wounds,
  iv. flail chest,
  v.   cardiac tamponade
  vi. air embolism.

5. Assessment/Management

For the assessment and management of thoracic trauma refer to Tables 4.18 and 4.19.

KEY POINTS

Thoracic Trauma

- **Thoracic injury is commonly associated with hypoxia, either from impaired ventilation or secondary to hypovolaemia from massive bleeding into the chest (haemathorax) or major vessel disruption.**

- **Count respiratory rate and look for asymmetrical chest movement.**

- **Pulse oximetry MUST BE used as this will assist in recognising hypoxia.**

- **The mechanism of injury is an important guide to the likelihood of significant thoracic injury.**

- **Blunt trauma to the sternum may induce myocardial contusion which may result in ECG rhythm disturbances.**

- **ECG monitoring.**

- **Impaling objects should be adequately secured. If the object is pulsating do not completely immobilise, but allow the object to pulsate.**

- **Do not probe or explore penetrating injuries.**

Table 4.18 – ASSESSMENT and MANAGEMENT of:

Thoracic Trauma

ASSESSMENT	MANAGEMENT

● Assess <C>ABCD	● Control any external catastrophic haemorrhage – **refer to trauma emergencies overview guideline**.
	● If any of the following **TIME CRITICAL** features are present:
	  – major ABCD problems
	  – penetrating chest injury
	  – flail chest
	  – tension pneumothorax
	  – air embolism
	  – cardiac tamponade
	  – surgical emphysema
	  – blast injury to the lungs, then:
	● Correct **A** and **B** problems.
	● Undertake a **TIME CRITICAL** transfer to the nearest appropriate receiving hospital.[a]
	● Provide an alert/information call.
	● Continue patient management en-route.

● If the patient is **NON-TIME CRITICAL** undertake a brief secondary survey	

● Specifically consider:
  – tension pneumothorax
  – open chest wounds
  – flail chest
  – surgical emphysema
  – cardiac tamponade
  – air embolism
  – impaling objects.
	Refer to Table 4.19 for the assessment and management of these conditions/situations.

● Monitor SpO₂ and assess for signs of hypoxia – NB Normal readings **DO NOT** exclude hypoxia	● Administer high levels of supplemental oxygen until the vital signs are normal then aim for a target saturation within the range of 94–98% (refer to oxygen guideline).
● Monitor heart rate and rhythm	● Attach ECG monitor.
● Assess breathing adequacy, respiratory rate, effort and volume, and equality of air entry	Consider assisted ventilation at a rate of 12–20 respirations per minute, if any of the following are present: ● SpO₂ <90% on high levels of supplemental oxygen. ● Respiratory rate is <12 or >30 breaths per minute. ● Inadequate chest expansion. NB Exercise caution as any positive pressure ventilation may increase the size of a pneumothorax.
● Consider the need for IV fluids	● Refer to the fluid therapy guideline – **DO NOT delay on scene.** ● Obtain IV access.
● Assess patient's level of pain	**Refer to the pain management guideline**. NB Avoid **entonox** in a patient with chest injury as there is a significant risk of enlarging a pneumothorax. NB Adequate morphine analgesia may improve ventilation by allowing better chest wall movement, but high doses may induce respiratory depression. Careful titration of doses is therefore required (refer to morphine drug guideline for dosage and information). ● Transfer to further care. ● Provide an alert/information call. ● Continue patient management en-route.
Assessment (children) ● Assess as above	Management (children) Manage as above but consider: ● Children can have severe internal chest injuries with minimal or no external evidence of chest injuries.

a Patients should normally be transported in a semi-recumbent or upright posture; however, this may often not be possible due to other injuries present or suspected.

SECTION **4** Trauma

Table 4.18 – ASSESSMENT and MANAGEMENT of:

Thoracic Trauma *continued*

ASSESSMENT	MANAGEMENT
Assessment (children) *continued* ● Assess as above	Management (children) *continued* ● Children show signs of shock late due to good compensatory mechanisms. ● Always consider multiple injuries in children with rib fractures as this suggests a significant mechanism of injury and isolated chest injuries are rare in children. ● Consider non-accidental injury.
	ADDITIONAL INFORMATION ● Chest trauma is treated with difficulty in the field and prolonged treatment before transportation is **NOT** indicated if significant chest injury is suspected. ● Penetrating trauma – in particular where lung or cardiac wounds are suspected, patients must be transferred to further care immediately to the nearest appropriate receiving hospital, with resuscitation en-route and an alert/information call. **Open chest wounds**– seal the wound with a non-occlusive dressing. ● Specifically consider the need for thoracic surgery intervention. ● **Impaling objects** – handle carefully, secure the object with dressing and if the object is pulsating do not completely immobilise it but allow the object to pulsate. NB Be vigilant – the patient may try to remove the object and this could be used as a weapon. ● Remember any stab or bullet wound to the chest, abdomen or back may penetrate the heart. ● Patients with significant chest trauma may often insist on sitting upright and this is especially common in patients with diaphragmatic injury who may get extremely breathless when lying down. In this instance a decision will have to be made as to whether a patient is best managed sitting upright or whether spinal immobilisation should be continued. ● In the rare incident of gunshot/stab injury to personnel wearing protection vests (e.g. ballistic and stab), these may protect from penetrating injury. However, serious underlying blunt trauma (e.g. pulmonary contusion) may be caused to the thorax. ● **NEVER UNDERESTIMATE THESE INJURIES**. There is a strong link between serious chest wall injury and thoracic spine injury. Maintain a high index of suspicion.

Table 4.19 – ASSESSMENT and MANAGEMENT of:

Specific Thoracic Trauma

Flail Chest

Flail chest is usually the result of a significant blunt chest injury, causing two or more rib fractures in two or more places. A sternal flail can also occur where the ribs or costal cartilages are fractured on both sides of the chest. This results in a flail segment that moves independently of the rest of the chest during respiration leading to inadequate ventilation. The ensuing pulmonary insufficiency is caused by three pathophysiological processes:

1. The negative pressure required for effective ventilation is disrupted due to the paradoxical motion of the flail segment.
2. The underlying pulmonary contusion which causes haemorrhage and oedema of the lung.
3. The pain associated with the multiple rib fractures will result in a degree of hypoventilation.
● Small flail segments may not be detectable.
● Large flail segments may impair ventilation considerably as a result of pain.

ASSESSMENT	MANAGEMENT
● Assess for signs of a flail chest	● Flail segments should not be immobilised and efforts to maintain ventilation are the priority. NB Traditionally, the patient has been turned onto the affected side for transportation, but this **CANNOT** be achieved on a long board.
● Assess patient's level of pain	● Consider the need for analgesia – if indicated refer to the **pain management guidelines**.
	● Undertake a **TIME CRITICAL** transfer to the nearest appropriate receiving hospital. ● Provide an alert/information call. ● Continue patient management en-route.

Table 4.19 – ASSESSMENT and MANAGEMENT of:

Specific Thoracic Trauma *continued*

Tension pneumothorax

- This is a rare respiratory emergency which may require immediate action at the scene or en-route to further care. A tension pneumothorax occurs when a damaged area of lung leaks air out into the pleural space on each inspiration, but does not permit the air to exit from the chest via the lung on expiration.
- This progressively builds up air under tension on the affected side collapsing that lung and putting increasing pressure on the heart and great vessels and the opposite lung. Decreased venous return is significantly affected by the kinking of the vessels, especially the inferior vena cava, as the mediastinum is pushed towards the contralateral side. Coughing and shouting can make a situation worse. If this air is not released externally, the heart will be unable to fill and the other lung will no longer be able to ventilate inducing cardiac arrest.
- Tension pneumothorax is most related to penetrating trauma but can arise spontaneously from blunt or crushing injuries to the chest and as the result of a blast wave. This will present rapidly with an increase in breathlessness and extreme respiratory distress (respiratory rate often >30 breaths per minute). Subsequently the patient may deteriorate and the breathing rate may rapidly slow to <10 breaths per minute before the patient arrests.
- **Signs and symptoms:** the chest on the affected side may appear to be moving poorly or not at all; at the same time, the affected chest wall may appear to be over-expanded (hyperexpansion); air entry will be greatly reduced or absent on the affected side. In the absence of shock, the neck veins may become distended. Later, the trachea and apex beat of the heart may become displaced away from the side of the pneumothorax and cyanosis and breathlessness may appear. Hyperresonance may be present. Occasionally, the patient will only present with rapidly deteriorating respiratory distress. The patient may appear shocked as a result of decreased cardiac output. They are usually tachycardic and hypotensive.
- Ventilation of a patient with a chest injury is a common cause of tension pneumothorax in the pre-hospital setting. Forcing oxygenated air down into the lung under positive pressure will progressively expand a small, undetected simple pneumothorax into a tension pneumothorax. This will take some minutes and may well be several minutes after ventilation has commenced. It is usually noticed by increasing back pressure during ventilation; either by the bag becoming harder to squeeze or the ventilator alarms sounding.

ASSESSMENT	MANAGMENT
- Assess breathing adequacy, respiratory rate and volume, and equality of air entry **FEEL, LOOK, AUSCULTATE and PERCUSS** - View both sides of the chest and check they are moving; auscultate to ensure air entry is present and percuss on both sides	- If a tension pneumothorax is confirmed, decompress rapidly by needle thoracocentesis.
- Closely monitor the patient to ensure the procedure was successful	- If the procedure was unsuccessful repeat the thoracocentesis. Consider the use of a thicker needle in patients with a thicker chest wall, following Trust guidelines.
	- Undertake a **TIME CRITICAL** transfer to the nearest appropriate receiving hospital. - Provide an alert/information call. NB Needle thoracocentesis may not always decompress pneumothoraces in large patients. In such cases, a thoracostomy with or without a chest drain may need to be performed. This needs to be done either in hospital or by appropriately skilled practitioners (e.g. BASICS or HEMS doctors on scene or in hospital).

Air embolism

Air embolism is a rare fatal complication of penetrating injury involving the central chest. It can also occur if an IV line is left open.

ASSESSMENT	MANAGEMENT
- Assess for signs of air embolism – if a conscious patient becomes unconscious or develops neurological signs in the absence of a head injury, the possibility of an air embolism must be raised	- The patient should be transported in the head down position. - Undertake a **TIME CRITICAL** transfer to the nearest appropriate receiving hospital. - Provide an alert/information call.

Table 4.19 – ASSESSMENT and MANAGEMENT of:

Specific Thoracic Trauma *continued*

Cardiac tamponade

The heart is enclosed in a tough, non-elastic membrane, called the pericardium. A potential space exists between the pericardium and the heart itself. If a penetrating wound injures the heart, the blood may flow under pressure into the pericardial space. As the pericardium cannot expand, a leak of as little as 20–30 ml of blood can cause compression of the heart! This decreases cardiac output and causes tachycardia and hypotension. Further compression reduces cardiac output and cardiac arrest may occur.

ASSESSMENT	MANAGEMENT
• Assess for signs of cardiac tamponade • Signs of hypovolaemic shock, tachycardia and hypotension, accompanied by blunt or penetrating chest trauma may be an indication of cardiac tamponade • Note presence of distended neck veins and muffled heart sounds when with a stethoscope	• Cardiac tamponade is a **TIME CRITICAL LIFE-THREATENING** condition that requires rapid surgical intervention in an open chest operation to evacuate the compressing blood. • **DO NOT** delay on scene inserting cannulae or commencing fluid therapy.
• Transfer	• Undertake a **TIME CRITICAL** transfer to the nearest appropriate receiving hospital. • Provide an alert/information call.
• Re-assess ABC	NB Pericardiocentesis is not recommended in the pre-hospital setting as it is rarely successful and has significant complications and delays definitive care.

Surgical emphysema

Surgical emphysema produces swelling of the chest wall, neck and face with a cracking feeling under the fingers when the skin is pressed. This indicates an air leak from within the chest, either from a pneumothorax, a ruptured large airway or a fractured larynx. Normally it requires no specific treatment but it does indicate potentially **SERIOUS** underlying chest trauma. Sometimes the surgical emphysema might be extensive and cause the patient to swell up. Where the emphysema is progressively increasing, look for a possible underlying tension pneumothorax.

In some cases, surgical emphysema may become so severe as to tighten the overlying skin and restrict chest movement. A tension pneumothorax must be excluded as above. If there is no improvement, the patient must be transferred to hospital as soon as possible.

ASSESSMENT	MANAGEMENT
• Assess for signs of surgical emphysema, swelling of the chest wall, neck and face with a cracking feeling under the fingers when the skin is pressed	
• Consider possible underlying tension pneumothorax	• Refer to tension pneumothorax for guidance.
	• Undertake a **TIME CRITICAL** transfer to the nearest appropriate receiving hospital. • Provide an alert/information call.

Blast injury

Blast injury is caused by three mechanisms:
1. Rupture of air-filled organs
2. Missiled debris
3. Contact injury.

NB Although rare in survivors, strongly suspect a blast lung injury if the patient is suffering from tympanic injury. However the absence of a tympanic injury **DOES NOT** exclude lung injury.
NB Being shielded from blast debris **DOES NOT** exclude lung injury.

ASSESSMENT	MANAGEMENT
• Assess for blast injury	• Pre-hospital management is supportive.
	• Undertake a **TIME CRITICAL** transfer to the nearest appropriate receiving hospital. • Provide an alert/information call.

1. Introduction

- The management of obstetric patients with major injuries requires a special approach.

- Mechanism of injury may indicate possible trauma to enlarged internal organs and structures especially trauma occurring in the third trimester. For example, trauma to the gravid uterus during domestic violence can be linked to placental abruption.

- It is important to remember that resuscitation of the mother facilitates resuscitation of the fetus.

2. Incidence

- In the UK 5% of maternal deaths are as a result of trauma with a high proportion related to domestic violence and road traffic collisions.

Mechanism of injury
- Domestic violence.
- High energy transfer.
- Fall from height.

3. Severity and Outcome

- Managing an obstetric patient with major trauma is rare; both blunt and penetrating trauma causing catastrophic haemorrhage, and significant burns are the likely causes.

4. Pathophysiology

- There are a number of physiological and anatomical changes during pregnancy that may influence the management of the obstetric patient (**refer to obstectric and gynaecology overview guideline**).

Table 4.20 – ASSESSMENT and MANAGEMENT of:

Trauma in Pregnancy

ASSESSMENT	MANAGEMENT
• Quickly scan the patient and scene as you approach. • Undertake a primary survey **<C>ABCDEF** – specifically assess for: • Abdominal pain – should be presumed to be significant and may be associated with internal unseen blood loss. • Vaginal blood loss. • Abruption may occur 3–4 days after the initial incident. • Stage of the pregnancy. • Any problems with the pregnancy. • Fetal movements (**refer to obstetric and gynaecology overview guideline**). • Whether the mother has her pregnancy record card available.	• Control external catastrophic haemorrhage using direct and indirect pressure or tourniquets where indicated – **refer to trauma emergencies overview.** • Open, maintain and protect the airway in accordance with the patient's clinical need. • Administer high levels of supplemental oxygen and aim for a target saturation within the range of 94–98% (refer to oxygen guideline). Provide assisted ventilation as indicated (refer to airway management guideline). • If the patient is unable to position herself (e.g. in trauma cases or if she is unconscious), the patient should be tilted 15–30° to the left (right side up) or the uterus manually displaced (and this must be recorded on the patient record). • Provide cervical spine protection as necessary (**refer to neck and back trauma guideline**). • Manage thoracic injuries (**refer to thoracic trauma guideline**). NB The management of thoracic injuries are the same as for the non-obstetric patient. • Insert a **large bore** IV cannula – do not delay transfer. • Administer intravascular fluids as indicated to maintain a systolic blood pressure of 90 mmHg (refer to intravascular fluid therapy guideline).
• Undertake a secondary survey **<C>ABCDEF.**	
• Assess patient's level of pain.	• Pain management (**refer to adult pain management guidelines**) NB Administer morphine cautiously if the patient is hypotensive. • Apply splints as appropriate, for example pelvis (**refer to pelvic trauma guideline**), long bone fractures (**refer to limb trauma guideline**).
• Assess blood glucose.	• Measure blood glucose en-route.
	• Nil by mouth.
• Assess for burns and scalds.	• For the management of burns treat as non-obstetric patient (**refer to the burns and scalds guideline** / refer to intravascular fluid therapy guideline).

KEY POINTS

Trauma in Pregnancy

- Main principle of treatment is that resuscitation of the mother facilitates resuscitation of the fetus.
- Compression of the inferior vena cava by the pregnant uterus (>20 weeks) is a serious potential complication; tilt the patient 15–30° to the left side or manually displace the uterus.
- Signs of shock appear very late and hypotension is an extremely late sign. Any signs of hypovolaemia during pregnancy are likely to indicate a 35% (class III) blood loss and must be treated aggressively.
- All trauma is significant.
- If the mother is found in cardiac arrest or develops cardiac/respiratory arrest en-route, commence life support and alert the hospital so that an obstetrician can be on standby in the ED for emergency Caesarean section.
- Abruption may occur 3–4 days after the initial incident.

SECTION 4 Trauma

1. Introduction

- Burns arise in a number of accident situations, and may have a variety of presentations (refer to Table 4.21), accompanying injuries or pre-existing medical problems associated with the burn injury. Scalds, flame or thermal burns, chemical and electrical burns will all produce a different burn pattern, and inhalation of smoke or toxic chemicals from the fire may cause serious accompanying complications.

- A number of burn patients will also be seriously injured following falls from a height in fires, or injuries sustained as a result of road traffic collision where a vehicle ignites after a collision or crash.

- Explosions will often induce flash burns, and other serious injuries due to the effect of the blast wave or flying debris.

- Inhalation of superheated smoke, steam or gases in a fire, will induce major airway swelling and respiratory obstruction – refer to Table 4.22 for signs of airway burns. The likelihood of an airway injury increases with the presence of multiple risk factors or signs.

- Non-accidental injury should always be considered when burns have occurred in vulnerable adults including the elderly, in particular where the mechanism of injury described does not match the injury sustained, or there is inconsistency in the history (**refer to safeguarding adults guideline**).

Table 4.21 – BURNS/SCALDS

Electrical

Search for entry and exit sites. Assess ECG rhythm. The extent of burn damage in electrical burns is often impossible to assess fully at the time of injury (refer to guidelines).

Thermal

The skin contact time and temperature of the source determines the depth of the burn. Scalds with boiling water are frequently of short duration as the water flows off the skin rapidly. Record the type of clothing (e.g. wool retains the hot water). Those resulting from hot fat and other liquids that remain on the skin may cause significantly deeper and more serious burns. Also the time to cold water and removal of clothing is of significant impact.

Chemical

It is vital to note the nature of the chemical. Alkalis in particular may cause deep, penetrating burns, sometimes with little initial discomfort. Certain chemicals such as phenol or hydrofluoric acid can cause poisoning by absorption through the skin and therefore must be irrigated with COPIOUS amounts of water for a minimum of 15 minutes (this should be continued until definitive care is available if patient condition and water supply allows) (**refer to CBRNE guideline**).

Table 4.22 – SIGNS/INCREASED RISK OF AIRWAY BURNS

Signs

- Facial or neck burns.
- Soot in the nasal and oral cavities.
- Coughing up blackened sputum.
- Cough and hoarseness.
- Difficulty with breathing and swallowing.
- Blistering around the mouth and tongue.
- Scorched hair, eyebrows or facial hair.
- Stridor or altered breath sounds such as wheezing.
- Loss of consciousness.
- Fires/blasts in enclosed spaces.

- Preceding long-term illness, especially chronic bronchitis and emphysema, will seriously worsen the outcome from airway burns.

- Remember that a burn injury may be preceded by a medical condition causing a collapse (e.g. elderly patient with a stroke collapsing against a radiator).

- Burns can be very painful (**refer to pain management in adults guideline**).

2. Burn Severity

- Refer to Wallace's Rule of Nines or the Lund and Browder chart to assess total body surface area (TBSA).

- For small or large burns (<15% or > 85%) it is acceptable to use the patient's palmar surface including the fingers as a size estimate. This equates to approximately 1% TBSA.

- Be aware of the risk of underestimating the size of burns with patients with large breasts or the obese patient. These factors can significantly affect the proportion of total body surface area using standardised charts.

- Use all of the burn area, but do not consider areas of erythema as this is often transient in the initial phases of a burn. Do not try to differentiate between levels of burn (superficial, partial thickness, full thickness etc.) as it is impractical to estimate the depth of burns in the initial hours following injury.

- Only a rough estimate is required; an accurate measure is not possible in the early stages; however, the size of a burn may well influence referral and management pathways.

3. Assessment and Management

- For the assessment and management of burns and scalds in adults refer to Table 4.23.

Burns and Scalds (Adults)

Table 4.23 – ASSESSMENT and MANAGEMENT of:

Burns and Scalds in Adults

ASSESSMENT	MANAGEMENT
● Ensure scene safety for rescuer and patient	**If safe to do so, stop the burning process:** ● Remove from the burn source. ● Brush off dry chemical.

● Assess **ABCD**	● If any of the following **TIME CRITICAL** features present:
	  – major ABCD problems
	  – airway burns (soot or oedema around the mouth and nose)
	  – history of hot air or gas inhalation; these patients may initially appear well but can deteriorate very rapidly and need complex airway intervention
	  – respiratory distress
	  – evidence of circumferential (completely encircling) burns of the chest, neck, limb
	  – significant facial burns
	  – burns >15% total body surface area (TBSA)
	  – presence of other major injuries, then:
	● Start correcting A and B and undertake a **TIME CRITICAL** transfer to nearest appropriate hospital according to local care pathways.
	● Continue patient management en-route.
	● Provide an alert/information call.

● Specifically assess	● Airway patency as early intervention may be required with inhalational burns; if intubation is impossible, needle cricothyroidotomy is the management of choice. ● Intubation can only be performed if capnography is available. ● Breathing for rate, depth and any breathing difficulty – refer to airway management guideline. ● Evidence of trauma – for neck and back trauma **refer to neck and back trauma guideline**. ● Co-existing or precipitating medical conditions.
● Oxygen	● Administer supplemental **oxygen** via a non-rebreathing mask – SpO$_2$ readings may be false due to carboxyhaemoglobin.
● Cool/irrigate the burn	● Irrigate with copious amounts of water (minimum 15 mins chemical burns; maximum of 20 mins for all other burns to avoid hypothermia) – as soon as is practicable, this can still be effective up to 3 hours after the injury. ● Cut off burning, or smouldering clothing, providing it is not adhering to the skin. ● Remove any constricting jewellery including rings. ● **DO NOT** use ice or ice water as this can worsen the burn injury. ● Use saline if no other irrigant available. ● Gel based dressings may be used but water treatment is preferred. ● Alkali burns require prolonged irrigation – continue until definitive care.
● Assess burn size	● Rule of Nines or Lund and Browder Chart. ● Patient's palmar surface including adducted fingers. ● Consider obesity and large breasts when estimating burn size.
● Dress the burn	● Use small sheets of clingfilm – do not wrap around limbs but layer the film. ● In the absence of clingfilm use a wet non-adherent dressing. NB Do not apply creams/ointments; they interfere with the assessment process.
● Fluid resuscitation	● If indicated refer to intravascular fluid therapy guideline.
● Wheezing	If the patient is wheezing as a result of smoke inhalation: ● Administer nebulised **salbutamol** (refer to salbutamol guideline) 6–8 litres of O$_2$ per minute.
● Assess the need for analgesia	If indicated: **refer to pain management guideline in adults**. NB Cooling and application of dressings frequently eases pain.
● Documentation	● How the patient was burned. ● Time the burn occurred and how long patient was exposed to source of burning. ● Temperature of the source of burning (e.g. boiling water, hot fat etc). ● Whether first aid was undertaken? ● Time and volume of infusions.
● Transfer to further care	● Consider receiving service; refer to local guidance. ● Complete documentation.

4 Trauma

SECTION

Burns and Scalds (Adults)

Table 4.23 – ASSESSMENT and MANAGEMENT of:

Burns and Scalds in Adults *continued*

ASSESSMENT	MANAGEMENT
● **Alkali burns** to the skin and eye(s)[a]	● Irrigate with water and continue en-route to hospital – it may take hours of irrigation to neutralise the alkali – this also applies to eyes which require copious and continual irrigation ideally with water or saline in the absence of a water source.
● **Acid/chemical burns** to the skin and eye(s)[a]	● Irrigate copiously; ideally with water, or saline if no water source available. NB Specific treatment agents may be available in industrial settings with on-site medical/ first aid.
● **Chemical burns**	● **DO NOT** wrap in clingfilm. ● Cover with wet dressings (refer to CBRNE guideline).
● **Circumferential burns**	● Encircling completely a limb or digit. Full thickness burns may be 'limb threatening', and require early in-hospital incision/release of the burn area along the length of the burnt area of the limb (surgical escharotomy).

[a] When irrigating the eyes ensure that the fluid runs away from the contralateral eye to avoid contamination.

KEY POINTS

Burns and Scalds (Adults)

● Airway status can deteriorate rapidly and may need complex interventions available at the emergency departments.

● Stopping the burning process is essential.

● The time from burning is an essential piece of information.

● Pain relief is important.

● Consider non-accidental injury in vulnerable adults including the elderly.

Burns and Scalds (Children)

[29, 699–705, 707–719, 723–726, 735–775, 776–779]

1. Introduction

- Burns and scalds are relatively common in children and can arise from a number of accidental situations. They have a variety of presentations (refer to Table 4.24) and children may present with accompanying injuries or pre-existing medical problems associated with the burn injury. Scalds, flame or thermal burns, chemical and electrical burns will all produce a different burn pattern, and inhalation of smoke or toxic chemicals from the fire may cause serious accompanying complications.

- A number of burn cases will also be seriously injured following falls from a height in fires, or injuries sustained as a result of road traffic collision where a vehicle ignites after an accident.

- Explosions will often induce flash burns, and other serious injuries due to the effect of the blast wave or flying debris.

- Inhalation of superheated smoke, steam or gases in a fire, will induce major airway swelling and may lead to fatal airway obstruction – refer to Table 4.25 for signs of airway burns. The likelihood of an airway injury increases with the presence of multiple risk factors or signs.

- Non-accidental injury should always be borne in mind when burns have occurred in small children, in particular where the mechanism of injury described does not match the injury sustained, or there is inconsistency in the history (**refer to safeguarding children guideline**).

Table 4.24 – BURNS/SCALDS

Electrical

Search for entry and exit sites.

Assess ECG rhythm.

The extent of burn damage in electrical burns is often impossible to assess fully at the time of injury.

Thermal

The skin contact time and temperature of the burning fluid determines the depth of the burn.

Scalds with boiling water are frequently of extremely short duration as the water flows off the skin rapidly. Record the type of clothing (e.g. wool retains the hot water).

Scalds resulting from hot fat and other liquids that remain on the skin may cause significantly deeper and more serious burns.

Times of contact, the application of cold water and the removal of clothing determine tissue damage.

Chemical

It is vital to note the nature of the chemical. Alkalis cause deep, penetrating burns, sometimes with little initial discomfort. Certain chemicals such as phenol or hydrofluoric acid can cause poisoning by absorption through the skin and therefore must be irrigated with **copious** amounts of water for a minimum of 15 minutes (this should be continued until definitive care if patient condition and water supply allows).

Table 4.25 – SIGNS/INCREASED RISK OF AIRWAY BURNS

Signs

- Facial or neck burns.
- Soot in the nasal and oral cavities.
- Coughing up blackened sputum.
- Cough and hoarseness.
- Difficulty with breathing and swallowing.
- Blistering around the mouth and tongue.
- Scorched hair, eyebrows or facial hair.
- Stridor or altered breath sounds such as wheezing.
- Loss of consciousness.
- Fires/blasts in enclosed spaces.

- Preceding long-term illness, especially respiratory disease, will seriously worsen outcome.

- Burns can be very painful (**refer to pain management in children guideline**).

2. Burn Severity

Calculation of burn area

- Wallace's Rule of Nines does not work in children under the age of 14 because of different body proportions.

- Local guidance or charts such as the Lund and Browder Paediatric Chart should be used; a rough guide is to assume that the size of the palmar surface of the child's hand, including the digits equates to approximately 1% of the total body surface area (TBSA) of the child.

- Use all of the burn area, but do not consider areas of erythema as this is often transient in the initial phases of a burn injury. Attempts to differentiate burn depths (e.g. superficial, partial thickness, full thickness etc) in the initial hours following injury are not helpful.

3. Assessment and Management

For the assessment and management of burns and scalds in children refer to Table 4.26.

4 Trauma

SECTION

Table 4.26 – ASSESSMENT and MANAGEMENT of:

Burns and Scalds in Children

ASSESSMENT	MANAGEMENT
● Ensure scene safety for rescuer and patient	**If safe to do so, stop the burning process** ● Remove from the burn source. ● Brush off dry chemical.

● Assess **ABCD**	● Identify **TIME CRITICAL** features such as:
	  – major ABCD problems
	  – airway burns (soot or oedema around the mouth and nose)
	  – history of hot air or gas inhalation; these patients may initially appear well but can deteriorate very rapidly and need complex airway intervention
	  – respiratory distress
	  – evidence of circumferential (completely encircling) burns of the chest, neck, limb
	  – significant facial burns
	  – burns >10% total body surface area (TBSA)
	  – presence of other major injuries (e.g. possible C-spine injury in explosions), then:
	● Start correcting **A** and **B** and undertake a **TIME CRITICAL** transfer to nearest appropriate hospital according to local care pathways.
	● Continue patient management en-route.
	● Provide an alert/information call.

● Specifically assess	● Airway patency as early intervention may be required with inhalational burns; if intubation is impossible, needle cricothyroidotomy is the management of choice. ● Intubation can only be performed if capnography is available. ● Breathing for rate, depth and any breathing difficulty – *refer to airway and breathing management guideline*. ● Evidence of trauma – for neck and back trauma **refer to neck and back trauma guideline**. ● Co-existing or precipitating medical conditions.
● Oxygen	● Administer supplemental oxygen via a non-rebreathing mask – SpO$_2$ readings may be false due to carboxyhaemoglobin.
● Cool/irrigate the burn	● Irrigate with copious amounts of water (chemical burns: minimum 15 minutes); all other burns: 20 minutes but **NO LONGER as this may cause hypothermia.** This can still be beneficial up to 3 hours after the injury. ● Cut off burning, or smouldering clothing, providing it is not adhering to the skin. ● **DO NOT** use ice or ice water as this can worsen the burn injury and exagerate hypothermia. ● Use saline if no other irrigant available. ● Gel based dressings may be used but water treatment is preferred. ● Alkali burns require prolonged irrigation – continue until definitive care.
● Assess burn size	● Lund and Browder Paediatric Chart. ● Child's palmar surface including adducted fingers. NB Consider obesity when estimating burn size.
● Dress the burn	● Use small sheets of clingfilm – do not wrap around limbs but layer the film. ● In the absence of clingfilm use a wet non-adherent dressing. NB Do not apply creams/ointments as they compromise assessment.
● Assess the need for fluid resuscitation	Large burns (>10%) require intravenouse fluids *refer to intravascular fluid therapy in children guideline*. ● If IV access is required, obtain on a non-affected limb, where possible.
● Wheezing	If the patient is wheezing as a result of smoke inhalation: ● Administer nebulised salbutamol (*refer to salbutamol guideline*) 6–8 litres of O$_2$ per minute.
● Assess the need for child's pain score	If indicated: ● Obtain IV access. ● **Refer to pain management guideline in children**. NB Cooling and application of dressings frequently eases pain.
● Documentation	● How the patient was burned. ● Time the burn occurred and how long patient was exposed to source of burning. ● Temperature of the source of burning (e.g. boiling water, hot fat etc). ● What treatments have been undertaken. ● Time and volume of infusions.
● Transfer to further care	● Consider receiving service; refer to local guidance.

SECTION **4** Trauma

Table 4.26 – ASSESSMENT and MANAGEMENT of:

Burns and Scalds in Children *continued*

ASSESSMENT	MANAGEMENT
● **Chemical burns**	● Cover in clingfilm; **DO NOT** wrap in clingfilm. ● Cover with wet dressings (refer to CBRNE guideline).
● **Alkali burns** to the skin and eye(s)[a]	● Irrigate with water and continue en-route to hospital. It may take hours of irrigation to neutralise the alkali. ● Alkali burns to the eyes require copious and continual irrigation ideally with water (saline can be used in the absence of a water source).
● **Acid/chemical burns** to the skin and eye(s)[a]	● Irrigate copiously ideally with water or saline if no water source available. NB Specific treatment agents may be available on site (e.g. medical kit or first aid boxes).
● **Circumferential burns**	● Encircling completely a limb or digit. Full thickness burns, may be 'limb threatening', and require early in-hospital incision/release of the burn area along the length of the burnt area of the limb (a surgical escharotomy).

[a] When irrigating the eyes ensure that the fluid runs away from the contralateral eye to avoid contamination.

KEY POINTS

Burns and Scalds (Children)

● **Warm the child and cool the burn.**

● **Consider the possibility of other injuries including inhalational injury and spinal injury.**

● **Give early adequate analgesia.**

● **Large burns (>10%) require intravenous fluids (see** intravascular fluid therapy in children guideline**).**

● **Consider non-accidental injury when burns have occurred in small children; in particular where the mechanism of injury does not match the injury sustained, or there is inconsistency in the history.**

4 Trauma SECTION

1. Introduction

- Electrical injury is potentially life-threatening.
- In adults incidents generally occur in the workplace, involving high voltage electricity (415 volts).
- In children incidents generally occur in the home and involve lower voltage electricity (240 volts).
- Electrical injury may also result from a lightning strike which may deliver up to 300kV.

2. Incidence

- In the UK, approximately 1,000 people at work are injured following contact with an electrical supply; of these 25 will die from their injuries (HSE).
- Electrical injuries resulting from a lightning strike lead to approximately 1,000 deaths per annum worldwide.

3. Severity and Outcome

- Electrical injury can cause serious multi-system damage leading to morbidity and mortality. This is caused by electric shock and tissue damage from the thermal effects along the current pathway.

The nature and extent of injury depends on:

- The voltage and whether it is alternating (AC) or direct (DC).
- The magnitude of the current.
- Resistance to current flow.
- Duration of exposure to the current.
- The pathway of the current – current traversing the myocardium is more likely to be fatal and hand-to-hand travel is more dangerous than hand-to-foot or foot-to-foot.

4. Pathophysiology

Injury occurs when electricity passes through the body causing:

- **Cardiac** arrhythmias (e.g. ventricular fibrillation); cardiorespiratory arrest can arise from the direct effects of the current on cell membranes and smooth muscle as it traverses the myocardium. Myocardial ischaemia can occur due to spasm of the coronary artery.

- **Burns** to the skin at the point of contact (entry and exit) and in deeper tissues, including viscera, muscles and nerves as thermal energy traverses the body and tends to follow neurovascular bundles. Unusual burn patterns may be left on the body following a lightning strike.
- **Trauma** including joint dislocation, fractures and compartment syndrome can arise from sustained tetanic muscle contraction, falling or being thrown.
- **Muscular paralysis** may occur from contact with high voltage electricity affecting the central respiratory control system or respiratory muscles.
- **Pregnancy** can be affected depending on the magnitude and duration of contact with the current.

5. Assessment and Management

For the assessment and management of electrical injuries refer to Table 4.27 and Figure 4.8.

KEY POINTS

Electrical Injuries
- **Scene safety.**
- **Manage cardiac/respiratory arrest.**
- **Consider trauma.**
- **Severe tissue damage may be present despite apparently minor injury.**
- **Exposure to domestic voltage may not require hospitalisation.**

SECTION

4

Trauma

Table 4.27 – ASSESSMENT and MANAGEMENT of:

Electrical Injuries

ASSESSMENT	MANAGEMENT
⚠ Ensure scene safety for rescuer and patient	⚠ **DO NOT** approach the patient until the electricity supply is cut off and you are certain it is safe to approach.
	NOTE: Attach defibrillator pad at the earliest opportunity and keep defibrillator with the patient until hand-over to hospital staff.

● Assess **ABCD**	● If any of the following **TIME CRITICAL** features present:
	  – major **ABCD** problems
	  – cardiorespiratory arrest – refer to advanced life support guideline
	  – facial/airway burns – refer to airway management guideline
	  – cardiac arrhythmia – **refer to cardiac rhythm disturbance guideline**
	  – significant trauma – **refer to appropriate trauma guideline**
	  – extensive burns – **refer to burns and scalds guideline**, then:
	● Start correcting A and B and undertake a **TIME CRITICAL** transfer to nearest receiving hospital or specialist burns unit if appropriate.
	● Continue patient management en-route.
	● Provide an alert/information call.

● Burn process	● Remove smouldering clothing and shoes to prevent further thermal injury – **refer to burns and scalds guideline**.

● Specifically assess:	● Airway patency as early intervention may be required.
	● Breathing for rate, depth and any breathing difficulty – refer to airway management guideline.
	● Heart rate/rhythm – undertake a 12-lead ECG:
	  – arrhythmias are unlikely to develop in cases of contact with domestic low voltage sources once the patient is isolated from the current
	  – in cases of contact with high voltage sources arrhythmias may develop later.
	● Evidence of trauma (e.g. neck and back, burns) – **refer to appropriate trauma guideline**.
	● Magnitude of the current, that is domestic low voltage (≤240 volts)/industrial high voltage (>480 volts).

● Oxygen	● Administer supplemental oxygen and aim for a target saturation within the range of 94–98%.
● Fluid	● If fluid resuscitation indicated – refer to intravascular fluid therapy guideline.
● Assess the need for pain relief	● If pain relief indicated – **refer to pain management guideline**.
● Transfer to further care	● **ALL** patients exposed to high voltage current. ● Patients exposed to a domestic or low voltage electrical source, who are asymptomatic, with no injuries and have normal initial 12-lead ECG may not require hospital assessment.

SECTION 4 Trauma

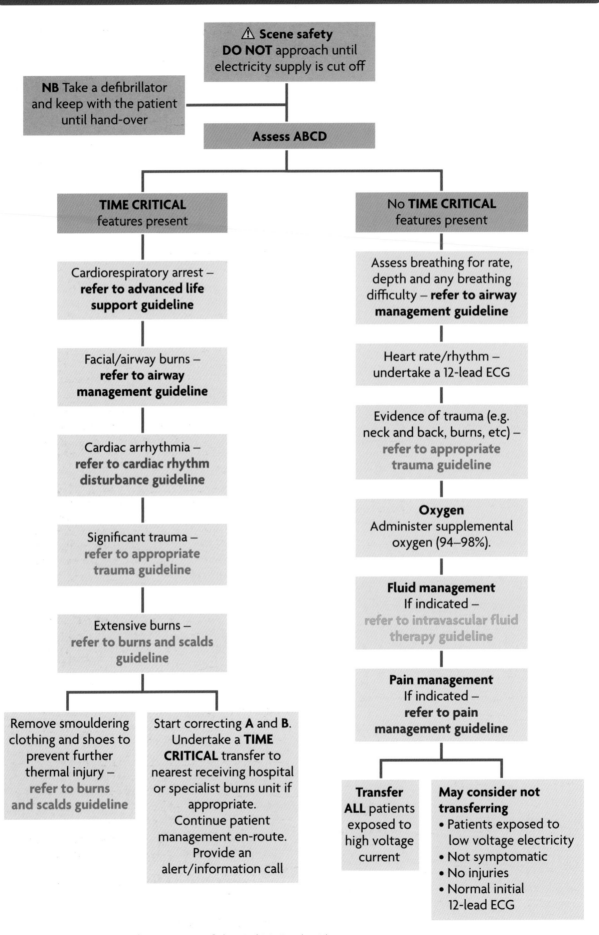

Figure 4.8 – Assessment and management of electrical injuries algorithm.

SECTION
4
Trauma

1. Introduction

- Drowning is a common cause of accidental death.
- **Drowning** refers to the 'process resulting in primary respiratory impairment from submersion/immersion in a liquid medium'. Thus the person is prevented from breathing air due to liquid medium at the entrance of the airway. NB Drowning does not infer that the patient has died.
- **Immersion** refers to being covered in a liquid medium and the main problems will be hypothermia and cardiovascular collapse from the hydrostatic pressure of the surrounding water on the lower limbs.
- **Submersion** refers to the entire body, including the airway being under the liquid medium and the main problems are asphyxia and hypoxia.
- **Exacerbating factors** – intoxication from alcohol or drugs may often accompany incidents. Occasionally, an immersion incident may be precipitated by a medical cause such as a convulsion.

2. Incidence

- Worldwide there are approximately 450,000 deaths per year with 205 deaths from accidental drowning occurring in England and Wales in 2009; with many more near-drownings. A high percentage of deaths will involve young males and children.

3. Severity and Outcome

- The extent of hypoxia and hypothermia, resulting from duration of immersion and/or submersion and/or the temperature of the liquid medium will determine severity and outcome.
- Concomitant trauma may result; for example, 0.5% of patients may suffer neck and/or head injury; diving into shallow water is a common cause.

4. Pathophysiology

- Following submersion, the patient will initially try to hold their breath. They may develop laryngospasm as water irritates the vocal cords or may aspirate large quantities of water. Both processes result in rapid hypoxia and hypercapnia.
- If rescue is not made, the patient will aspirate water into their lungs, exacerbating hypoxia. The patient will become bradycardic and sustain a cardiac arrest; thus correction of hypoxaemia is critical to obtaining a return of spontaneous circulation. In 10–15% of cases, the laryngeal spasm is so intense, none of the liquid medium enters the lungs.
- Changes in haemodynamics after immersion (the 'hydrostatic squeeze effect') make positional hypotension likely. If the patient is raised vertically from the water their blood pressure will fall – 'after-drop' – which may lead to cardiovascular collapse. Therefore it is recommended that rescuers must always attempt to maintain the patient flat and avoid vertical removal from water.

5. Rescue and Resuscitation

- ⚠ Safety first – **DO NOT** put yourself in danger. Carry out a dynamic risk assessment and undertake measures to preserve your own safety and that of other rescuers.
- Establish the number of patients involved.
- History is often incomplete at the scene, both relating to the incident and the patient.

5.1 Aquatic rescue

- When the patient is rescued, attempt to maintain the patient flat and avoid vertical removal from water.
- If neck and back trauma is suspected, wait until the patient has been rescued before attempting to apply spinal immobilisation, but limit neck flexion and extension.

5.2 Airway and breathing

- Alleviate hypoxaemia as soon as possible, as adequate ventilation and oxygenation may restore cardiac activity.
- In patients in cardiac arrest clear airway and commence CPR as soon as the patient is rescued.
- Administer supplemental oxygen, preferably via bag-valve-mask. Apply pulse oximeter. If the patient does not respond to oxygen therapy consider assisted ventilation.
- Mechanical drainage of water from the lungs should not be carried out. The lungs can be ventilated even with large volumes of water inside them, although ventilation may be difficult due to reduced lung compliance.
- Approximately 80% of patients will aspirate water into their stomach. There is a high risk of regurgitation of the stomach contents, especially if the patient has ingested alcohol/drugs – have suction at hand. Tilting to drain aspirated water simply empties water from the stomach into the pharynx, risking further airway contamination.

5.3 Chest compression

- Commence chest compressions when the patient is on a firm surface (it's usually impossible to perform CPR in a boat) and commence CPR appropriate to patient's age.
- Apply ECG monitoring to aid diagnosis.

5.4 Hypothermia

- If the patient's core body temperature is <30°C, limit defibrillation attempts to 3.
- In the presence of hypothermia, drugs are less effective; withhold intravenous drugs until the patient's body temperature reaches ≥30°C. When at this temperature, double the dose interval until the patient's temperature reaches 35°C.
- If the patient is hypothermic, the heart rate may be extremely slow and external cardiac compression may be required – **refer to cardiac rhythm disturbance guideline**. NB Bradycardia often responds to improved ventilation.

5.5 Intravascular fluid therapy

- Following prolonged immersion patients may become hypovolaemic – if fluid resuscitation indicated refer to intravascular fluid therapy guideline.

Table 4.28 – ASSESSMENT and MANAGEMENT of:

Immersion Incident

⚠ Safety First – DO NOT put yourself in danger – carry out a dynamic risk assessment and undertake measures to preserve your own safety, and where possible that of the patient, bystanders and other rescuers.

- Take a defibrillator at the earliest opportunity.
- Ascertain how many patients are involved.
  NB Information may be incomplete at the scene.
- Note the environment – in certain circumstances hair may become entangled in a drain/filter (e.g. pools/hot tubs).

- If the patient has been submerged (entire body, including the airway under the liquid medium) for >60 minutes? Refer to ROLE guideline unless the water is ICY COLD when a decision may be made to attempt resuscitation in a witnessed submersion time of 90 minutes.

NB The duration of hypoxia is the most important factor in determining outcome. Oxygenate and restore circulation at the earliest opportunity.

ASSESSMENT	MANAGEMENT

● Assess <C>ABCDE	● If any of the following **TIME CRITICAL** features present:
	  – major **<C>ABCDE** problems – **refer to trauma emergencies overview**
	  – pulseless and apnoeic – refer to relevant resuscitation guideline
	  – major life-threatening trauma – **refer to relevant trauma guideline**
	  – neck and back injuries – **refer to neck and back trauma guideline**, then:
	● Start correcting **A** and **B** and undertake a **TIME CRITICAL** transfer to nearest receiving hospital.
	● Administer high levels of supplemental oxygen – refer to oxygen guideline.
	● Prevent further heat loss/consider warming the patient – **refer to hypothermia guideline**.
	● Continue patient management en-route.
	● Provide an alert/information call.

● Airway	● Clear airway. ● There is a high risk of regurgitation of the stomach contents, especially if the patient has ingested alcohol/drugs – have suction at hand.

● Ventilation	● Adequate ventilation and oxygenation may restore cardiac activity. Consider assisted ventilation if:
	  – SpO$_2$ is <90% with oxygen therapy
	  – respiratory rate <12 or >30 breaths per minute
	  – expansion is inadequate.
	NB Ventilation may be difficult due to reduced lung compliance if water has been inhaled
	– refer to airway and breathing management guideline.

● Oxygen	● Administer supplemental oxygen – refer to oxygen guideline.
	● Apply pulse oximeter – NB the measurement may be unreliable in patients with cold peripheries.
	  – **children** – administer high levels of supplemental oxygen
	  – **adults** – aim for a target saturation within the range of 94–98%.

● Heart rate	● In the presence of hypothermia the heart rate may be extremely slow and external cardiac compression may be required – **refer to cardiac rhythm disturbance guideline**. NB Bradycardia often responds to improved ventilation and oxygenation.
● Concomitant injuries	● Consider concomitant injuries. ● Consider neck and back injuries – **refer to neck and back trauma guideline**. ● Treat associated injuries – refer to specific guideline(s).
● ECG	● Undertake a 12-lead ECG.
● Fluid	● In cases of prolonged immersion patients may become hypovolaemic – if fluid resuscitation indicated refer to intravascular fluid therapy guideline.
● Pain	● If pain management indicated **refer to pain management guideline**.
● Position	● If possible, the patient should be removed from the water and managed in a horizontal position, especially in rescue involving a helicopter or large vessel, where the patient is lifted more than a few metres – however, in **TIME CRITICAL** conditions speed of removal from the water takes precedence over method of removal.

Table 4.28 – ASSESSMENT and MANAGEMENT of:

Immersion Incident *continued*

ASSESSMENT	MANAGEMENT
● Transfer to further care	● Transfer all patients to further care. ● If neck and back injury not suspected transfer in the recovery position. ● If the patient is immobilised prepare for side-tilt. ● Prevent further heat loss/consider warming the patient – **refer to hypothermia guideline**. ● Provide an alert/information call. ● Continue patient management en-route.
● Discontinuation of resuscitative efforts	● Refer to ROLE guideline.

5.6 Discontinuing resuscitative efforts

If the patient has been submerged for **60** minutes (or 90 minutes in ICY COLD water). In all other cases for guidance on discontinuation of resuscitative efforts refer to recognition of life extinct (**ROLE**).

5.7 Survival and submersion

Research has shown that there is little accurate data on which factors predict survival, following submersion. Submersion time is a significant factor but there is little accurate data. In order to obtain more accurate data on the factors associated with good outcomes following submersion, data will be collected on a number of parameters, such as:

● Time of the incident.

● Time the patient was rescued.

● Time of first effective CPR.

● Duration of submersion.

● Water temperature.

● Type (salt, fresh, contaminated).

● Precipitating factors (e.g. intoxication from alcohol or drugs, convulsion etc).

As it is often difficult to obtain accurate time information from witnesses, for the purpose of deciding whether to commence resuscitation the submersion time is measured from the time of initial call to ambulance control centre.

6. Assessment and Management

For the assessment and management of the immersion incident refer to Table 4.28.

KEY POINTS

Immersion and Drowning

● **Ensure own personal safety.**

● **Successful resuscitations have occurred after prolonged submersion/immersion.**

● **Hypothermia is a condition often associated with the immersion incident.**

● **Special considerations in cardiac arrest treatment in the presence of hypothermia.**

● **Severe complications may develop several hours after submersion/immersion.**

5

Obstetrics and Gynaecology

Obstetrics and Gynaecology

Obstetrics and Gynaecology
Emergencies Overview   277

Birth Imminent: Normal Delivery and
Delivery Complications   280

Care of the Newborn   288

Haemorrhage During Pregnancy
(including Miscarriage and Ectopic
Pregnancy)   292

Pregnancy-Induced Hypertension
(including Eclampsia)   295

Vaginal Bleeding: Gynaecological
Causes   298

1. Introduction

- Any female of childbearing age **MAY** be pregnant, and, unless there is a history of hysterectomy, even the slightest doubt must make one consider if any abdominal pain or vaginal bleeding may be pregnancy related.

- There are three fundamental rules which must be followed at all times when dealing with the pregnant patient:
  - the maternal well-being is essential to the survival of the fetus and thus resuscitation of the mother must always be the priority
  - compression of the inferior vena cava by the pregnant uterus (beyond 20 weeks) is a serious potential complication and suitable positioning or manual displacement must be employed (see displacement below)
  - signs of shock appear very late during pregnancy and hypotension is an extremely late sign. Any signs of hypovolaemia during pregnancy are likely to indicate a 35% (class III) blood loss and must be treated aggressively. **ESTABLISH LARGE BORE IV CANNULATION EARLY.**

If the mother is in cardiac arrest it is important to undertake a **TIME CRITICAL** transfer immediately to the nearest suitable receiving hospital and provide an alert/information call to ask for an **OBSTETRICIAN ON STANDBY IN THE EMERGENCY DEPARTMENT** for an emergency Caesarean section – delivering the fetus **MAY** facilitate maternal resuscitation. NB Effective resuscitation of the mother will provide effective resuscitation of the fetus.

2. Pathophysiology

Pregnancy is timed from the FIRST day of the last period, and from that date lasts up to **42** weeks. The pregnancy is divided into **first** (1–12 weeks), **second** (13–23+6) and **third** (24+) trimesters. These terms are used on shared care antenatal records, that is the patient's personal maternity plan.

There are a multitude of physiological and anatomical changes during pregnancy that may influence the management of the obstetric patient. These changes include:

- An increase in cardiac output by 20–30% in the first 10 weeks of pregnancy.

- An increase in average maternal heart rate by 10–15 beats per minute.

- A decrease in systolic and diastolic blood pressure by an average of 10–15 mmHg.

- Uterine pressure may cause compression of the inferior vena cava, reducing venous return, and lowering cardiac output, by up to 40%, for patients in the supine position; this in turn will reduce blood pressure.

- An increase in breathing rate and effort and a decrease in vital capacity, as the fetus enlarges and the diaphragm becomes splinted.

- An increase in blood volume (↑45%) and the numbers of red cells; but not in proportion, so the patient becomes **relatively anaemic**. Due to the increase in blood volume the obstetric patient is able to tolerate greater blood or plasma loss before showing signs of hypovolaemia. This compensation is at the expense of shunting blood away from the uterus and placenta and therefore fetus.

- An increase in the acidity of the stomach contents, due to a delay in gastric emptying, caused by progesterone-like effects of the placental hormones.

- Relaxation of the cardiac sphincter makes regurgitation of the stomach contents more likely.

- Oedema of the larynx.

- Enlargement of the breasts.

3. Procedures

- In medical cases the patient can either position themselves to avoid compression of the vena cava or if the patient is unable to position herself (e.g. in trauma cases or if she is unconscious), the patient should be tilted 15–30° to the left (right side up) or the uterus manually displaced (and this must be recorded on the patient record) (**refer to trauma in pregnancy guideline**).

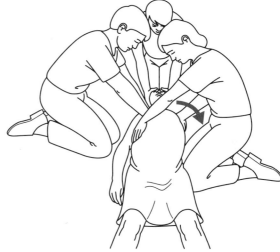

Figure 5.1 – Manual tilt.

4. Assessment

4.1 Quickly assess the patient and scene as you approach

4.2 Primary survey

- It is important to remember there are two patients: neither the mother nor a newly born baby should be overlooked whilst assessing and caring for the other. Both may be at risk, or one may need more urgent attention than the other – it is unlikely to be possible to determine which until a primary survey has been completed on both patients.

- The aim of the primary survey is to identify the existence of life-threatening problems, to enable management to be commenced as rapidly as possible and to reach an early determination of the priority for transportation. The primary survey should be modified in the presence of actual or suspected trauma (**refer to trauma in pregnancy guideline**).

Circulation/massive external haemorrhage

Is there a significant volume of blood visible without the need to disturb the patient's clothing?

- On the floor?
- Is the patient's clothing soaked?
- Are there a number of blood-soaked pads in evidence?

Airway

- Is the patient able to talk? (yes = airway open).
- Is the patient making unusual sounds? (gurgling = fluid in the airway).
- Requiring suction (snoring = tongue/swelling/foreign body obstruction).
- If the patient is unresponsive, open the airway and look in – suction for fluids, manually remove solid obstructions.

Breathing

- Document respiratory rate and effort (are accessory muscles being used?).
- Obtain oxygen saturations as soon as possible.
- Auscultate for added sounds (wheeze bronchospasm; coarse sounds = pulmonary oedema).
- Assess for the presence of cyanosis.
- Give oxygen based on clinical findings (not routinely).

Circulation

- Document radial pulse rate and volume (capillary refill time (CRT) may be used if neither the radial nor carotid pulses can be palpated).
- Assess skin colour and temperature (to touch) (pallor, or cold or damp skin = an adrenergic reaction to shock).
- Assess for bleeding – check underwear, pads, the surface the patient is sitting on, and briefly examine the vaginal opening with the patient's consent and considering their privacy. Ask the patient about bleeding during this problem – if they have discarded pads, how saturated were they? How many pads have they used in what time period?
- Check for visible blood loss again and feel under any clothing or bed linen the patient is sitting or lying on, as this can absorb significant volumes of blood. Look at your gloved hands to see if they are stained with blood. Check the vaginal opening for evidence of bleeding (soaked pads or underwear, wounds).
- Check the abdominal area for evidence of internal bleeding (tenderness, guarding, firm woody uterus).
- Document blood pressure measurement – the systolic is most valuable if you suspect shock.

Disability

- Perform an AVPU assessment of conscious level (is the patient Alert, responding only to Voice, responding only to Pain or Unresponsive?).
- Document the patient's posture (normal, convulsing (state whether focal or generalised), abnormal flexion, abnormal extension).
- Document pupil size and reaction (PEaRL – Pupils Equal and Reacting to Light).

Expose/environment/evaluate

- If you haven't already done so, briefly examine the vaginal opening:
  - is there any evidence of bleeding? Can you see a presenting part of the baby?
  - is there a prolapsed loop of cord? Have the waters broken?
  - does the perineum bulge with each contraction?
  - if the baby has been delivered, is there a significant perineal tear? Can you see part of the uterus?
- Is the room warm – is a newborn at risk of hypothermia? Are the surroundings as clean as you can make them if you are going to deliver on-site? Are there other children present (indicates previous pregnancy with live birth)?
- Make an early evaluation about how time critical the patient's problem is. If the patient is time critical, decide immediately whether you need to transport the patient urgently to hospital, with a hospital obstetric pre-alert, or whether it is more prudent to treat them at the scene – remember to call for skilled obstetric help if this is the case.

Fundus

- Make a quick assessment of fundal height: a fundus at the level of the umbilicus equates to a gestation of approximately 22 weeks. By definition, fundal height below the umbilicus suggests that if the fetus is delivered it is unlikely to survive.

4.3 Obstetric secondary survey

If any critical problems are identified during the primary survey the secondary survey should only be undertaken when any ABCDE problems have been addressed and transportation to definitive care has commenced (if this is possible). In many cases where critical problems are identifed it will not be possible or appropriate to undertake a secondary survey in the pre-hospital phase of care.

Obstetrics and Gynaecology Emergencies Overview

Table 5.1

Glossary

ABBREVIATION	TERM
LMP	Last menstrual period.
EDD	Estimated date of delivery – the timing of the pregnancy is written in the notes in the format 12/40, i.e. 12 weeks have elapsed out of the 40 weeks pregnancy.
T	Term or expected end of pregnancy, therefore T+3 in the notes is 3 days over the EDD.
CEPH	Cephalic (head).
BR	Breech.
G	Gravida, the number of times a woman has been pregnant.
P	Parity, the number of times a woman has given birth.
Colposcopy	An outpatient test where the cervix is inspected following an abnormal smear. Treatment such as cone biopsy for the abnormal smear may have been undertaken. Heavy colposcopy bleeding affects very few women in this situation.

KEY POINTS

Obstetrics and Gynaecology Emergencies Overview

- Any female of childbearing age MAY be pregnant.
- Due to the increase in blood volume the obstetric patient is able to tolerate greater blood or plasma loss before showing signs of hypovolaemia.
- Any signs of hypovolaemia during pregnancy are likely to indicate a 35% (class III) blood loss and must be treated aggressively – ESTABLISH LARGE BORE IV CANNULATION EARLY.

1. Introduction

The best clinical management for a mother who is experiencing an abnormal labour or delivery is to be transferred to further care without delay.

When there is a midwife on scene it is their responsibility to manage the delivery, and crews should work under their direction. If the midwife is not present, the decision on whether to move the mother should be based on the principle that any situation which deviates from a normal uncomplicated delivery should result in the mother being transported immediately to hospital.

In this situation the crew must alert the hospital via control en-route. Ambulance clinicians should make an early assessment of the need for additional assistance from an additional ambulance and ensure that the request is made as soon as possible.

The most important feature of managing an obstetric incident is a rapid and accurate assessment of the mother to ascertain whether there is anything abnormal taking place.

The following maternal assessment process **MUST** be followed in order to decide whether to:

- **STAY ON SCENE AND REQUEST A MIDWIFE** (if not already present).
- **TRANSFER TO FURTHER CARE IMMEDIATELY.**

In maternity cases where delivery is not imminent and there are no complications (refer to maternal assessment flowchart) the mother may be transported to the unit into which she is booked.

The assessment should be repeated en-route and, if any complications occur, the condition should be treated appropriately and the woman's destination revised if necessary. If the mother is booked into a unit that is not within a reasonable distance or travelling time, crews should base their judgements on the maternal assessment, and take the mother to the most appropriate unit.

Table 5.2 – ASSESSMENT and MANAGEMENT of:

Normal Delivery

ASSESSMENT	MANAGEMENT
<ul><li>Quickly assess the patient and scene as you approach</li><li>Undertake a primary survey **\<C\>ABCDEF**</li></ul>	<ul><li>If any time critical features are present correct **\<C\>ABC** and transport to nearest suitable receiving hospital (**refer to medical emergencies guideline**).</li><li>Provide an alert/information call.</li></ul>
<ul><li>Ascertain the period of gestation</li><li>Ask to see the patient-held record for indications of multiple births, breech presentation, obstetric complications</li></ul>	
Assess for: – show – waters broken – contractions – and/or bleeding **(refer to obstetric and gynaecology overview for guidance)**	If **NONE** of these indications are present **AND** there is no other medical/traumatic condition discuss the mother's management with the **BOOKED OBSTETRIC UNIT** – informing of: <ul><li>Mother's name.</li><li>Mother's age and date of birth.</li><li>Hospital registration number.</li><li>Name of lead clinician.</li><li>History of this pregnancy.</li><li>Estimated date of delivery (EDD).</li><li>Previous obstetric history.</li></ul>
If **ANY** of the above indications are present assess: <ul><li>Contraction interval</li><li>The urge to push or bear down</li><li>Crowning/top of the baby's head/breech presentation visible at the vulva</li></ul>	<ul><li>Undertake a visual inspection if there are regular contractions (1–2 minute intervals) and an urge to push or bear down.</li></ul>
<ul><li>If delivery is imminent, that is regular contractions (1–2 minute intervals) and an urge to push or bear down and or crowning/top of the baby's head/breech presentation visible at the vulva</li></ul>	<ul><li>Remain on scene, request a midwife, an additional ambulance with a paramedic if not present and prepare for delivery (see below).</li></ul>

Table 5.2 – ASSESSMENT and MANAGEMENT of:

Normal Delivery *continued*

Second stage of labour (10 cm cervical dilatation – delivery) ● Continue assessing the mother's level of pain.	Reassure the mother, tell her what you are doing and include her partner if present. ● Prepare delivery area: 　– **incontinence pads** – cover the ambulance stretcher or delivery area 　– **maternity pack** – open and set out 　– **towels** – enough to dry and wrap the baby 　– **blanket(s)** – cover the mother for warmth and modesty 　– **heat** – turn the heat up in the delivery area (aim for 25°C). ● Support the mother in a semi-recumbent (or other comfortable) position with padding under her buttocks – discourage her from lying flat on her back because of the risk of supine hypotension.
	● Encourage the mother to continue taking entonox to relieve pain/discomfort. ● **CAUTION – morphine** should only be administered in exceptional circumstances due to the risk of neonatal respiratory depression. ● As the baby's head is delivering, help the mother to avoid pushing by telling her to concentrate on panting or breathing out in little puffs – entonox may help. ● Instruct the mother to pant or puff, allowing the head to advance slowly with the contraction. Consider applying gentle pressure to the top of the baby's head as it advances through the vaginal entrance to prevent very rapid delivery of the head. ● Check to see if the umbilical cord is around the baby's neck. If it is, gently attempt to loop it over the head. If it is too tight, it is better to deliver the rest of the baby with the cord left in place. A tight cord will not prevent the baby delivering. ● Hold the baby as it is born and lift it towards the mother's abdomen. ● Wipe any obvious large collections of mucous from the baby's mouth and nose.
● Undertake an initial ABCD assessment of the baby – include head, trunk, axilla and groin	● Newborns are at risk of hypothermia. ● **CAUTION** – premature babies lose heat even faster than full term babies ● Quickly and thoroughly dry the baby using a warm towel while you make your initial assessment. ● Remove the now wet towel and wrap the baby in dry towelling to minimise heat losses.
● Assess the baby's airway	● If the baby is crying they have a clear airway. ● If the baby is not breathing, confirm that the airway is open – the head is ideally placed in the 'neutral' position – i.e. not the extended 'sniffing position' used in older children and adults. 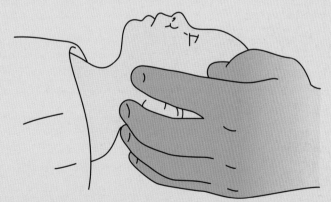 Figure reproduced with the kind permission of the Resuscitation Council (UK). ● **SUCTION IS NOT USUALLY NECESSARY** – if required, use the suction unit on low power (around 150 mm Hg) with a CH12–14 catheter and then only within the oral cavity. ● If the baby is not breathing refer to newborn life support guideline. ● Once the baby is breathing adequately, cyanosis will gradually improve over several minutes – if the cyanosis is not clearing, enrich the atmosphere near the baby's face with low flow of oxygen. ● **Refer to care of the newborn guideline.**

Birth Imminent: Normal Delivery and Delivery Complications

Table 5.2 – ASSESSMENT and MANAGEMENT of:

Normal Delivery *continued*

ASSESSMENT	MANAGEMENT
Cutting the cord ● Assess whether the cord has stopped pulsating	1. Wait until the cord has stopped pulsating; apply two cord clamps securely 3 cm apart and about 15 cm from the umbilicus. Cut the cord between the two clamps. **CAUTION:** ensure the newborn's fingers and genitals are clear of the scissors. 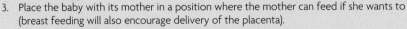 2. Ensure the baby remains wrapped and keep the baby warm. 3. Place the baby with its mother in a position where the mother can feed if she wants to (breast feeding will also encourage delivery of the placenta). 4. Reassure the mother. 5. Await the midwife and third stage (delivery of the placenta and membranes). 6. If delivery has occurred en-route proceed to the nearest obstetric unit. It is not necessary to await delivery of the placenta before continuing with the transfer. 7. Provide an alert/information call.
Third stage of labour (delivery of the placenta and membranes) – may take 15–20 minutes	● Assist the mother in expelling the placenta naturally by encouraging her to adopt a squatting, upright position, but only if there has been no delay in delivery of the placenta and **NOT IF THERE IS ANY SIGNIFICANT BLEEDING**. ● Do not pull the cord during delivery of the placenta as this could rupture the cord, making delivery of the placenta difficult and cause excessive bleeding or inversion of uterus. ● Deliver the placenta straight into a bowl or plastic bag. Keep it, together with any blood and membranes, for inspection by a doctor or midwife. NB If the placenta has not been delivered within 20 minutes after delivery insert a **LARGE BORE** cannula, as patients are at increased risk of haemorrhage and may require intravascular fluid and medication.
● Assess how much blood has accompanied the delivery of the placenta and membranes – this should not exceed 200–300 ml	● If bleeding continues after delivery of the placenta, palpate the abdomen and feel for the top of the uterus (fundus) usually at the level of the umbilicus and massage gently with a cupped hand in a circular motion. ● The fundus will become firm as massage is applied and this may be quite uncomfortable so entonox (refer to the entonox drug guideline for administration and information) can be offered.
● Assess blood loss – if bleeding is severe	● Obtain IV access – insert **LARGE BORE** cannulae. ● Administer fluid replacement (refer to fluid therapy guideline). ● Administer syntometrine if available (refer to syntometrine guideline). ● If syntometrine is **NOT** available or the patient is hypertensive (≥140/90) administer misoprostol (refer to misoprostol guideline).
● Assess and monitor respiration rate, pulse and blood pressure	● Administer O_2 to aim for a target saturation within the range of 94–98%.
	A number of complications may arise during pregnancy and/or labour. Refer to Table 5.3 for the assessment and management of: 1. Pre-term delivery 2. Maternal seizures 3. Prolapsed umbilical cord 4. Post-partum haemorrhage 5. Continuous severe/sudden abdominal/back pain/placental abruption 6. Multiple births – delayed delivery of second or subsequent baby 7. Malpresentation 8. Shoulder dystocia.

Birth Imminent: Normal Delivery and Delivery Complications

Table 5.3 – ASSESSMENT and MANAGEMENT of:

Delivery complications
1. Pre-term delivery – delivery before the completion of 37 weeks

ASSESSMENT	MANAGEMENT
• Ascertain the period of gestation	• **<22 weeks gestation** – transfer the mother and baby to the **NEAREST GYNAECOLOGY UNIT or follow local protocols**. • **22–37 weeks gestation** – every effort should be made to transport the mother to a **CONSULTANT-LED UNIT** without delay as the baby will need specialist care once delivered.
• Re-assess the mother constantly en-route	• Manage as circumstances change. • Should delivery take place en-route assess the baby and take appropriate action. Convey mother and baby to the **NEAREST ED or CONSULTANT-LED UNIT**[a] depending on local arrangements. • Provide an alert/information call to the receiving hospital.
	• If transfer to further care is not possible because the birth is so advanced, request a midwife plus an additional ambulance and inform control (**refer to birth imminent guideline**). • Once the baby is born, utilise the additional ambulance to transport the infant **IMMEDIATELY** to the **NEAREST ED or OBSTETRIC UNIT**[a] depending on local arrangements. • The infant should be transported even if the midwife has not yet arrived. • Provide an alert/information call to the hospital, giving an ETA and description of the baby's condition. • The mother should then be transferred to the **OBSTETRIC UNIT** of the **same hospital as the baby**.

2. Maternal seizures

ASSESSMENT	MANAGEMENT
• Quickly assess the patient and scene as you approach	• Correct A and B problems and transfer to **CONSULTANT-LED UNIT**. • If the patient is convulsing **refer to convulsion guideline**.
• Undertake a primary survey **<C>ABCDEF** • Assess for **TIME CRITICAL** features	
	• Refer to pregnancy-induced hypertension (including pre-eclampsia).

3. Prolapsed umbilical cord

ASSESSMENT	MANAGEMENT
The descent of the umbilical cord into the lower uterine segment. This is a TIME CRITICAL EMERGENCY requiring immediate intervention, rapid removal and transfer to a CONSULTANT-LED UNIT	• Use two fingers to replace the cord **GENTLY** in the vagina. Only make **ONE** attempt to replace the cord. • Handle the cord as little as possible to prevent spasm. • If it is not possible to replace the cord easily in the vagina (particularly if a large loop has prolapsed): – use dry padding to prevent further prolapse (this will keep the cord warm and moist within the vagina and prevent cord spasm) – position the mother on her side with padding placed under her hips to raise the pelvis and reduce pressure on the cord.
	• Determine the best means of removal – ideally the ambulance stretcher should be used, but where necessary and expedient the mother may be helped to walk to the nearest point of access for the ambulance stretcher. Use of the service carrying chair should be avoided if at all possible and if used should only be to convey the mother to the nearest point of access for the stretcher. • Administer entonox to help prevent the urge to push, which increases pressure on the cord.
	• Transfer to the nearest **CONSULTANT-LED UNIT** with the mother positioned on her side, with padding under the pelvis to reduce pressure on the cord. • Provide an alert/information call. • Alert the hospital that the mother has a prolapsed cord.

[a] When placing the alert call ask what the arrangements are for units receiving distressed neonates where this is not the obstetric unit.

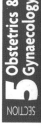

Table 5.3 – ASSESSMENT and MANAGEMENT of:

Delivery complications continued
4. Post-partum haemorrhage (PPH)[b]

ASSESSMENT	MANAGEMENT
Primary PPH: blood loss of 500 ml or more within 24 hours of delivery **Massive PPH: blood loss of 50% of the blood volume within 3 hours of delivery**	**NOTE** – If severe haemorrhage occurs following delivery (post-partum) follow one of the two treatment regimens below en-route to further care if possible. **1. IF THE PLACENTA HAS DELIVERED:** ● Palpate the abdomen and feel for the top of the uterus (fundus) usually at the level of the umbilicus and massage gently with a cupped hand in a circular motion. ● The fundus will become firm as massage is applied and this may be quite uncomfortable and entonox can be offered (refer to the entonox drug guideline for administration and information). ● Administer a bolus of syntometrine (refer to syntometrine guideline) – if **syntometrine** or other oxytocics are unavailable, have been ineffective at reducing haemorrhage after 15 minutes or the patient is hypertensive (BP >140/90) administer **misoprostol** (refer to misoprostol guideline).
	2. IF THE PLACENTA HAS NOT DELIVERED: ● In the presence of haemorrhage, **DO NOT** massage the top of the uterus (fundus) when the placenta is undelivered. This may provoke **partial separation** of the placenta and cause further haemorrhage. ● Administer a bolus of **syntometrine** (refer to syntometrine guideline) – if **syntometrine** or other oxytocics are unavailable, have been ineffective at reducing haemorrhage after 15 minutes or if the patient is hypertensive (BP >140/90), administer **misoprostol** (refer to misoprostol guideline). NB Administration of **syntometrine** or **misoprostol** may cause the placenta to separate and deliver. If the placenta delivers ensure there is no further bleeding. If bleeding continues after the placenta is delivered – commence massage of uterine fundus (**see 1 above**).
● Assess blood loss – if bleeding is >500 ml ● Re-assess prior to further fluid replacement ● If bleeding continues check for bleeding from tears at the vaginal entrance	● Obtain IV access – insert a **LARGE BORE** cannula. ● Administer fluid replacement (refer to intravascular fluid therapy guideline) ● Apply direct pressure to a tear using a gauze or maternity pad. ● If not in transit transfer the mother and baby to the **NEAREST OBSTETRIC UNIT** immediately. Provide an alert/information call. Include details as to whether the placenta has been delivered or is still in situ.

5. Continuous severe abdominal pain/placental abruption[c]

ASSESSMENT	MANAGEMENT
● Quickly assess the patient and scene as you approach NB In the presence of severe/sudden continuous abdominal/back pain consider abruption ● Undertake a primary survey **<C>ABCDEF** ● Assess for **TIME CRITICAL** features	● Correct A and B problems and transfer to the **CONSULTANT-LED UNIT WITHOUT DELAY.**
● Assess for signs of shock **A separation of a normally sited placenta from the uterine wall**	● Obtain IV access – insert a **LARGE BORE** cannula. ● If fluid therapy indicated refer to intravascular fluid therapy guideline. ● Encourage the mother to lie on her side or sit when in transit, whichever position is the more comfortable for her. ● Provide an alert/information call. ● Commence the appropriate resuscitation regimen as soon as possible.

[b] The commonest cause of severe haemorrhage immediately after delivery is uterine atony (i.e. poor uterine contraction).

[c] Major placental abruption is when a large part of the placenta detaches from the uterine wall. Bleeding occurs under the placenta causing significant abdominal, back and/or epigastric pain. There may be no visible vaginal bleeding ('concealed' abruption). Alternatively there may be a variable amount of vaginal bleeding ('concealed' abruption). Despite little or no visible bleeding, there may be signs of hypovolaemic shock.

Table 5.3 – ASSESSMENT and MANAGEMENT of:

Delivery complications *continued*
6. Multiple births – delayed delivery of second or subsequent baby[d]

ASSESSMENT	MANAGEMENT
NOTE – with a twin delivery, the mother is at increased risk of immediate post-partum haemorrhage due to poor uterine tone **(refer to 4 above)**. **It is now very unusual for a mother expecting a multiple birth to deliver outside hospital. However, twin pregnancies are at much higher risk of delivering pre-term (i.e. before 37 weeks) – the babies may therefore need resuscitation**	If delivery is **NOT** in progress: ● Transfer mother to the **CONSULTANT-LED UNIT** without delay. ● Constantly re-assess en-route and take appropriate action if the circumstances change.
	If delivery **IS** in progress or occurs en-route: ● Request back up following local guidelines (as not every area can request a midwife). ● Follow the normal delivery process and management of the newborn for each baby.
	● Once the first baby has been born and assessed transfer, mother and baby to the **NEAREST OBSTETRIC UNIT IMMEDIATELY** if delivery of the second baby is not imminent. If there are any complications, transfer to a **CONSULTANT-LED UNIT** – it is not necessary to await the arrival of the midwife. ● Provide an alert/information call.
	● If the delivery of the second baby occurs en-route, park the ambulance and make a request via control for an **ADDITIONAL AMBULANCE**. ● Once the second baby has been delivered, utilise both vehicles to transfer mother and babies to the nearest consultant-led obstetric unit. ● Provide an alert/information call.
Assess if any/either baby requires resuscitation	● Refer to the appropriate newborn resuscitation guideline.

7. Malpresentation[e]

ASSESSMENT	MANAGEMENT
Breech birth is where the feet or buttocks present first during delivery rather than the baby's head **NB Cord prolapse is more common with a breech presentation (refer to 3 – prolapsed umbilical cord). Follow local guidelines**	**Breech birth** – If delivery is **NOT** in progress: ● Transfer mother to the **BOOKED OBSTETRIC UNIT** without delay. ● Constantly re-assess en-route and take appropriate action if the circumstances change.
	Breech Birth – If delivery **IS** in progress treat as for a normal delivery except: ● If the mother is on the bed or sofa etc, encourage her to move to the edge. This will enable gravity to help deliver the baby. The mother's legs should be supported (this may look like the McRoberts Position – page 284). ● Do not touch the baby or the umbilical cord until the body is free of the birth canal and the nape of the neck is visible. The only exception is when the baby's back rotates to face the mother's anus (the umbilicus should always face the anus). Gently hold the baby by its pelvis and rotate the baby's back – the baby's umbilicus must face the mother's anus (take care **NOT** to squeeze the infant's abdomen which could damage internal organs). ● Do not clamp or cut the cord until the **HEAD** is free of the birth canal. ● Once the body of the baby is born and the nape of the neck is visible, gently lift the baby by its feet to facilitate delivery of the head. This should be undertaken as the head is delivering and so as not to over-extend the baby's neck. Care should be taken not to pull the baby. ● Once the baby is born treat as for a normal delivery. Breech babies are more likely to be covered in meconium and may require resuscitation. If the baby requires resuscitation, refer to the appropriate newborn resuscitation guideline.
	Any presenting body part other than the head, buttocks or feet (e.g. one foot or a hand/arm) ● Transfer the mother **immediately** to a **CONSULTANT-LED OBSTETRIC UNIT** ● Provide an alert/information call.

[d] It is now very unusual for a mother expecting a multiple birth to deliver outside hospital. However, twin pregnancies are at much higher risk of delivering pre-term (i.e. before 37 weeks) – the babies may therefore need resuscitation.

[e] Breech birth is where the feet or buttocks present first during delivery rather than the baby's head. Cord prolapse is more common with a breech presentation (refer to 3 – prolapsed umbilical cord). Follow local guidelines.

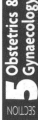

5 Obstetrics & Gynaecology
SECTION

Table 5.3 – ASSESSMENT and MANAGEMENT of:

Delivery complications *continued*
8. Shoulder dystocia[f]

ASSESSMENT

An arrest of spontaneous delivery; when delivery of the baby's shoulders is delayed because the baby's anterior shoulder is stuck behind the symphysis pubis

MANAGEMENT

- **DO NOT** cut the cord before the baby's head is delivered.
- **DO NOT** press on the uterine fundus.
- If the shoulders are not delivered within two contractions following the birth of the head a further attempt must be made to deliver the shoulders using the McRoberts manoeuvre (see below).

McRoberts manoeuvre (increases the pelvic diameters/alters the angle of the pelvis)

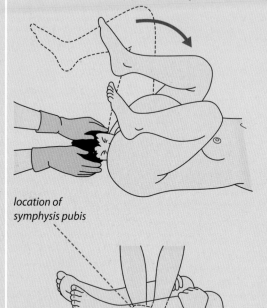

location of symphysis pubis

1. Ask the mother to lie flat with only one pillow under her head.
2. Bring the mother's knees up towards her chest and outwards slightly.
3. During the next two contractions, attempt to deliver the baby's shoulders with gentle traction applied to the baby's head (both outward and downward), while the mother is encouraged to push.
4. **If after two contractions the shoulders have not delivered, attempt suprapubic pressure.**

Suprapubic pressure

1. Identify the side where the fetal back lies. This will often be the opposite side to the direction the baby is facing. NB The mother should be flat with a maximum of one pillow under her head.
2. Ask the assistant to:
   - Stand on the side of the baby's back (if the baby is facing left, stand on the mother's right or vice versa).
   - Use their hands in CPR grip and place the heel of their hand two finger breadths above the symphysis pubis behind the baby's shoulder.
   - Use suprapubic pressure in conjunction with gentle traction of the baby's head (pressure alone is unlikely to be successful).
   - Apply moderate pressure on the baby's shoulder pushing downwards and away from them.
   - This will hopefully dislodge and rotate the shoulder from behind the symphysis pubis.
3. Encourage the mother to push and during the next two contractions attempt to deliver the baby's shoulders with gentle traction applied to the baby's head (both outward and downward), while the mother continues to push.
4. **If after two attempts the shoulders have not delivered, apply intermittent pressure.**

[f] This is when delivery of the baby's shoulders is delayed. The baby's anterior shoulder is stuck behind the symphysis pubis.

Table 5.3 – ASSESSMENT and MANAGEMENT of:

Delivery complications *continued*
8. Shoulder dystocia

ASSESSMENT	MANAGEMENT
	Intermittent pressure
	1. Encourage the mother to empty her bladder.
	2. Ask the assistant to apply intermittent pressure on the shoulder by rocking gently backwards and forwards.
	3. Encourage the mother to push and during the next two contractions attempt to deliver the baby's shoulders using gentle traction applied to the baby's head (both outward and downward).
	4. **If after two attempts the shoulders have not delivered, place the mother in the all-fours position.**

All-fours position
1. Position the mother on her hands and knees with her hips well flexed, bottom elevated and her head as low as possible (see diagram below).
2. While the mother pushes, apply gentle traction to the baby's head (both outward and downward towards the floor), to try and deliver the shoulder nearer the maternal back first.
3. **If after two attempts the shoulders have not delivered:**
   a. Undertake a **TIME CRITICAL** transfer to a **CONSULTANT-LED UNIT**.
   b. Administer high levels of supplemental oxygen.
   c. In this situation do not await the arrival of the midwife.
   d. Provide an alert/information call.
   e. Ideally, the mother should be removed from scene using the ambulance stretcher. However, if necessary, the mother may be helped to walk a **SHORT** distance to the nearest point of access for the stretcher, but crews should be prepared to deliver the baby as this may precipitate birth. Once on the stretcher and during transportation the mother should be placed on her side with padding placed under her hips to raise the pelvis.

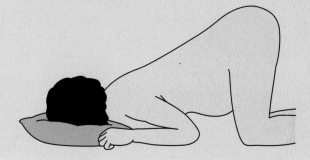

KEY POINTS

Birth Imminent: Normal Delivery and Delivery Complications
- For a patient experiencing an abnormal labour or delivery, transfer to further care without delay.
- Undertake a rapid assessment of the patient to ascertain whether there is anything abnormal taking place.
- If the mother presents with an obvious medical or traumatic condition that puts her life in imminent danger treat appropriately.
- The period of gestation is important in informing the appropriate course of action.
- Severe vaginal bleeding, prolapsed cord, continuous severe abdominal/epigastric pain and presentation of part of the baby other than the head (e.g. an arm or leg) warrant IMMEDIATE transfer to the CONSULTANT-LED UNIT.
- Do not allow the baby to become cold during transfer.
- Using McRoberts manoeuvre (+/- suprapubic pressure) will also require gentle traction on the baby's head while the mother pushes, to complete delivery.

1. Introduction

- Ambulance personnel may become involved in the care of the newborn as some deliveries occur at home, or on the way to hospital. Hence it is important to be aware of the differences in physiology of the newborn baby. The newborn baby has emerged from dependence on the protective uterine environment to independent life. Physiology is changing within the first few hours to weeks after birth. Hence what may apply to infants and children may not necessarily be applicable to newborn babies. Additionally, different management issues arise in premature babies.

- Some babies may deliver at home and a proportion of these may need to be transported to hospital because of unexpected problems.

A newborn baby or mother will need to be transferred to hospital for the reasons listed below.

Reasons in the baby

- Any baby that required resuscitation.
- Birth asphyxia (pale floppy apnoeic baby or APGAR score below 5).
- Meconium staining or aspiration.
- Baby of a diabetic mother.
- Small for dates/growth-retarded baby.
- Prematurity (gestation <36 weeks).
- Any baby that required naloxone at birth.
- Major congenital abnormalities, even if the baby appears well at birth.
- Red flags ⚑ suggesting a high risk of early onset neonatal bacterial infection.

Reasons in the the mother

- Severe maternal blood loss from either antepartum or post-partum haemorrhage.
- Retained products of conception.
- Maternal drugs (especially opiates).
- Suspected or confirmed invasive bacterial infection within 24 hours of birth.

2. Pathophysiology

Birth asphyxia

- Birth asphyxia can occur for various reasons including cord prolapse, the cord being tightly wrapped around the neck, significant placental or umbilical bleeds, or prolonged second stage of labour.

- Birth asphyxia has a poor outlook and is often associated with neurological deficits and cerebral palsy. A low APGAR score at 10 minutes suggests a high possibility of long-term neurological problems.

- Recent studies have shown that in babies born at >36 weeks gestation with birth asphyxia, moderate hypothermia results in a better neurological outcome. The multicentre CoolCap, ICE and TOBY trials showed that cooling to 33.5°C within 6 hours of birth for 72 hours was associated with a decreased death rate, less neurodevelopmental disability and less cerebral palsy in survivors. This controlled cooling was done without adverse effects being seen in the babies. A meta-analysis of all the neonatal cooling trials strongly supports the use of therapeutic hypothermia in newborn infants with hypoxic ischaemic encephalopathy to reduce the risk of death and neurological impairment at 18 months.

- Researchers are currently studying the benefits of controlled therapeutic cooling using special blankets or suits during interhospital transfers when taking asphyxiated babies to tertiary neonatal units. The transfer of these babies between neonatal intensive care units is, however, the only situation when babies can be transferred without ensuring the ambulance is well heated, and it will be made clear by the medical staff if this is required. Unless the specific equipment is available and requested by hospital staff then the ambulance should be as warm as possible for transfer.

Hypothermia

- Babies have a large body surface area relative to their weight, and heat loss occurs easily by convection. Premature babies are at particular risk. A wet baby will also lose heat by evaporation, especially if in a draught. Babies lose heat as a result of their proportionately large heads when compared to their bodies. Bonnets, towels and blankets can be used to significantly reduce these heat losses. Transfer the baby in a POD if this is available.

- The body temperature of the baby should be kept at about 36–37°C. The ambulance should therefore be kept well heated to prevent cooling during the transfer to hospital. Accidental hypothermia, especially in the premature baby, can be harmful. A cold baby has increased oxygen consumption, and is at risk of hypoglycaemia and acidosis. It is therefore important that the baby is kept warm during the transfer in the ambulance, to prevent hypoglycaemia and these complications.

Hypoglycaemia

- The newborn baby has a relatively immature liver with limited glycogen stores and so low blood sugars are not an uncommon problem.

- In a baby without any abnormal signs and symptoms (see below) and no risk factors (see page 287 for list) hypoglycaemia is any single blood glucose reading with a value of <1.0 mmol/l even if a subsequent reading is normal. In a baby who is at-risk (see page 287 for list) hypoglycaemia is two consecutive blood glucose readings of <2.0 mmol/l. In a baby with abnormal signs and symptoms, a single reading of <2.5 mmol/l can be used to diagnose hypoglycaemia. Glucose is the main energy source for the fetus and neonate, and the newborn brain depends almost exclusively on glucose for energy metabolism.

- Hypoglycaemia can therefore lead to seizures and brain injury. Severe and prolonged hypoglycaemia may result in long-term neurological damage. It is therefore important to prevent and treat a low blood sugar level as soon as it is detected.

- Signs and symptoms of hypoglycaemia include:
  - jitteriness
  - irritability
  - lethargy
  - apnoeic episodes
  - seizures.

NB Many hypoglycaemic babies are asymptomatic, hence the importance of routine blood glucose checks in babies at risk. Babies at risk of hypoglycaemia include:

- premature babies
- small for gestational age babies
- baby of a diabetic mother due to high circulating insulin levels
- birth asphyxia
- hypothermia
- infection
- delayed feeding.

After birth, give a feed as soon as possible (or at least within the first hour). Failing this, intravenous glucose may be needed, depending on i) the baby's condition and ii) the blood glucose level. The newborn baby's liver has very limited glycogen stores, so hypoglycaemia must not be treated using intramuscular glucagon (glucagon works by stimulating the liver to convert glycogen into glucose). A baby found to have hypoglycaemia (as previously defined) must be transported to hospital for further investigation and management.

Neonatal jaundice

- Jaundice refers to the yellow colouration of the skin and sclera caused by a raised bilirubin level. About 60% of term and 80% of pre-term babies develop jaundice in the first week of life. Physiological jaundice occurs around day 2–7, although 10% of breast fed babies are still jaundiced at 1 month of age. Physiological jaundice is due to increased breakdown of haemoglobin in red blood cells to bilirubin, and the immature liver is unable to handle the conversion of bilirubin to a form that can be excreted in the gut. Jaundice is harmless unless the bilirubin level is very high, when this can cross the blood-brain barrier.

- Unconjugated bilirubin is potentially toxic to brain tissue causing kernicterus and brain damage. Different treatment thresholds are recommended for different gestations and age (see graphs published by National Institute for Health and Clinical Excellence). Jaundice is treated with phototherapy or exchange transfusion depending on the level of bilirubin and the cause. Early jaundice (occurring before day 2) or prolonged jaundice (after day 14) may be due to other pathological causes or underlying diseases and requires investigation. Babies with early jaundice occurring <2 days of age must be referred for an urgent medical review.

Pre-term delivery

- Prematurity is defined as <36 weeks gestation. Premature infants are more likely to need help with ventilation. Spontaneous breathing will be inadequate for babies born at <32 weeks gestation. Additionally they are likely to be deficient in surfactant. (Surfactant reduces alveolar surface tension and keeps the lung alveoli open during expiration.) They are therefore likely to need a higher inflation pressure with bag and mask ventilation than term infants to open up their lungs. They are also likely to need surfactant replacement and/or ventilatory support, and require immediate hospital transfer even if apparently well; they are also at particular risk of hypothermia.

- The other complications of prematurity include hypothermia, hypoglycaemia and a higher risk of infection. Pre-term infants <32 weeks gestation are also at risk of intracranial bleeds.

- Improving neonatal intensive care has seen better outcomes for babies born pre-term (especially in babies born after 28 weeks gestation). However, the EPICure study following up babies born in the UK at the limits of viability before 26 weeks gestation showed a high mortality and morbidity. Overall survival was only 39% and survivors commonly have severe disabilities. Hypothermia was one of the factors associated with death.

Congenital abnormalities

- The outcome of babies born with congenital abnormalities varies but is improving with advancement in medical therapies and interventions. The abnormality may have been detected on previous antenatal scans or may have been undiagnosed until birth. Hence all babies who are known to have a congenital abnormality should be transferred to hospital where the abnormality can be assessed and treated, even when the baby appears to be normal at birth.

- Babies with abdominal wall defects should be transferred with food grade clingfilm covering the defect to reduce fluid and heat losses.

  NB Do not wrap the clingfilm circumferentially around the newborn's body as this will inhibit breathing.

Early onset neonatal infection

- Early onset neonatal bacterial infection can be life-threatening and it is important that it is recognised and treated early. The following **red flags** ⚑ suggest a high risk of early onset neonatal bacterial infection:

  ⚑ systemic antibiotic treatment given to the mother for confirmed or suspected invasive bacteria

  ⚑ seizures in the baby

  ⚑ signs for shock in the baby

  ⚑ need for mechanical ventilation in a term baby

  ⚑ suspected or confirmed infection in a co-twin.

3. Assessment and Management

- For the assessment and management of the newborn see below and refer to Table 5.5.

APGAR score

- The condition of the baby at birth is assessed using the APGAR score. Dr Virginia Apgar first devised these scores to assess the effect of obstetric anaesthesia on the baby, but it has been used universally to assess the condition of the baby after birth. APGAR is an easy to use mnemonic to remember what needs to be assessed:

  A appearance (skin colour)
  P pulse rate
  G grimace (response to stimulation)
  A activity or tone (whether active or floppy)
  R respiratory rate.

- A healthy term baby normally takes the first breath or cries within 1 minute after the umbilical cord is clamped. The newborn's condition should be assessed

5 Obstetrics & Gynaecology SECTION

at 1 and 5 minutes after birth (refer to Table 5.5). This helps inform resuscitation decisions. (NB Resuscitation should not be delayed whilst calculating the APGAR score (refer to Table 5.4).) The baby's condition can be assessed quickly just from their colour, heart rate and breathing effort.

- A pink baby with a lusty cry and a heart rate >100/min will need no further treatment, and just needs to be dried, and given to the mother to hold. Most babies fall into this category and only require drying, warming and some gentle stimulation.

- A blue baby with a heart rate >80/min, who has some tone and some response to stimulation may begin to breathe spontaneously after a short wait (not >1 minute) if given some gentle stimulation and 'blow by' oxygen.

- A pale, floppy and apnoeic baby with a heart rate <80/min will need bag-and-mask ventilation, followed by cardiac compression if the heart rate does not improve or breathing does not start (**refer to newborn life support guidelines**) and undertake **TIME CRITICAL** transfer.

- Use gentle suctioning of the mouth and nose with a soft suction catheter to remove excess secretions. Avoid deep pharyngeal suctioning as this can cause bradycardia (from vagal stimulation) or laryngospasm.

- If there has been either meconium staining of the liquor or baby, or evidence of meconium aspiration,

the baby will need to be transferred to hospital quickly, as this indicates foetal distress and possible foetal hypoxia. Meconium aspiration can lead to respiratory distress and the need for ventilatory support. The baby may additionally have associated complications from birth asphyxia.

KEY POINTS

Care of the Newborn
- **The need for resuscitation can be made from a quick assessment of the baby's condition at birth.**
- **Keep the baby warm and dry.**
- **Treat hypoglycaemia as soon as it is detected to prevent seizures or long-term neurological damage.**
- **Pre-term babies require further management in hospital.**
- **All babies with congenital abnormalities should be transferred to hospital for assessment.**
- **Be aware of red flags in mother or baby which might suggest a high risk of early onset neonatal bacterial infection.**

Table 5.4 – APGAR SCORE

Score	0	1	2
Appearance	blue or pale all over	blue at extremities body pink	body and extremities pink
Pulse rate	absent	<100	≥100
Grimace or response to stimulation	no response to stimulation	grimace/feeble cry when stimulated	cry or pull away when stimulated
Activity or muscle tone	none	some flexion	flexed arms and legs that resist extension
Respiration	absent	weak, irregular, gasping	strong, lusty cry

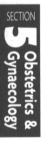

Care of the Newborn

Table 5.5 – ASSESSMENT and MANAGEMENT of:

The Newborn

ASSESSMENT	MANAGEMENT

● Assess **ABCD**	● If any of the following **TIME CRITICAL** features present:
	  – major **ABCD** problems
	  – birth asphyxia
	  – major congenital abnormalities
	  – prematurity
	  – hypoglycaemia.
	● Start correcting **A** and **B** problems.
	● Undertake a **TIME CRITICAL** transfer to a hospital where there is a neonatal unit.
	● Continue patient management en-route.
	● Provide an alert/information call.

● Assess need for resuscitation at birth	● Use a quick assessment observing:
	  – the colour
	  – heart rate, and
	  – respiratory effort.
	● If time permits, perform an APGAR score at 1 and 5 minutes after birth.
	● Pre-term babies require ongoing hospital care and should be transferred as soon as possible to a hospital with a neonatal unit.

● Birth asphyxia	● If resuscitation required at birth or there is evidence of asphyxia, transfer to a hospital with a neonatal unit for ongoing care. ● Consider controlled cooling of the baby during the transfer as there is evidence from clinical trials of improved neurological outcome.
● Suspected hypoglycaemia	● Check blood sugar level from a heel prick. ● If hypoglycaemia confirmed, treatment is **TIME CRITICAL** to prevent seizures and brain damage. ● Consider early feed. ● IM glucagon will **NOT** work due to poor glycogen stores in the newborn. ● If transferring the baby to hospital keep baby warm during the transfer unless there has been evidence of birth asphyxia (**see above**).
● Assess temperature	● Heat loss occurs readily because of the large body surface area. ● Ensure the newborn baby is dried after birth, as heat loss also occurs by evaporation if the baby is wet.
● Transfer to further care	

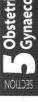

Haemorrhage During Pregnancy (including Miscarriage and Ectopic Pregnancy) [103, 373, 832, 695–696, 698]

1. Introduction

- This guidance is for the assessment and management of patients with bleeding during early and late pregnancy (including miscarriage and ectopic pregnancy). For postpartum haemorrhage **refer to birth imminent: normal delivery and delivery complications guideline**. For complications associated with abortion **refer to vaginal bleeding: gynaecological causes (including abortion) guideline**.

Haemorrhage may be:

- **Revealed** with evident vaginal loss of blood (e.g. miscarriage and placenta praevia).

- **Concealed** where bleeding occurs within the abdomen or uterus. This presents with little or no external loss, but pain and signs of hypovolaemic shock (e.g. ruptured ectopic pregnancy and placental abruption). **REMEMBER,** pregnant women may appear well even with a large amount of concealed blood loss. Tachycardia may not appear until 30% or more of the circulating volume has been depleted.

Haemorrhage during pregnancy is broadly divided into two types:

1. Haemorrhage occurring in early pregnancy (≤22 weeks).

2. Haemorrhage occurring in late pregnancy (>22 weeks).

SECTION 1 – Haemorrhage Occurring in Early Pregnancy (≤22 weeks) May Indicate Miscarriage or Ectopic Pregnancy

1. Incidence

- Miscarriage is more common in the first 12 weeks.

2. Pathophysiology

- **Miscarriage (previously known as spontaneous abortion)** is the loss of pregnancy before 23 completed weeks; commonly seen at 6–14 weeks of gestation but can occur after 14 weeks.

- This occurs when some products of conception are partly passed through the cervix and become trapped, leading to blood loss. The level of shock is often out of proportion to the amount of blood loss.

> **Risk factors – miscarriage**
> - Previous history of miscarriage.
> - Previously identified potential miscarriage at scan.
> - Smoker.
> - Obesity.

Symptoms:

- Bleeding – light or heavy, often with clots and or jelly-like tissue.

- Pain – central, crampy, suprapubic, or backache.

- Signs of pregnancy may be subsiding (e.g. nausea or breast tenderness).

- Significant symptoms (including hypotension) without obvious external blood loss may indicate 'cervical shock' due to retained miscarriage tissue stuck in the cervix. Symptomatic bradycardia may arise due to vagal stimulation.

- **Ectopic pregnancy/ruptured ectopic pregnancy** usually presents at around 6–8 weeks gestation, so usually only one period has been missed.

Symptoms characteristic of a ruptured ectopic pregnancy:

- Acute lower abdominal pain.

- Slight bleeding or brownish vaginal discharge.

- Signs of blood loss within the abdomen with tachycardia and skin coolness.

Other suspicious symptoms:

- Unexplained fainting.

- Shoulder-tip pain.

- Unusual bowel symptoms.

> **Risk factors – ectopic pregnancy**
> - An intra-uterine contraceptive device fitted.
> - A previous ectopic pregnancy.
> - Tubal surgery.
> - Sterilisation or reversal of sterilisation.
> - Endometriosis.
> - Pelvic inflammatory disease.

SECTION 2 – Haemorrhage Occurring in Late Pregnancy – Antepartum Haemorrhage or Prepartum (>22weeks) May Indicate Placenta Praevia or Placental Abruption

1. Incidence

Placenta praevia occurs in 1 in 200 pregnancies and usually presents at 24–32 weeks with small episodes of painless bleeding.

2. Pathophysiology

- **Placenta praevia:** the placenta develops low down in the uterus and completely or partially covers the cervical canal; this can lead to severe haemorrhage during the pregnancy (i.e. painless bleed) or when labour begins.

- **Placental abruption** is any vaginal bleeding in late pregnancy or during labour which is accompanied by severe/sudden continuous abdominal/back pain; signs of shock may be due to placental abruption.

Bleeding occurs between the placenta and the wall of the uterus, detaching an area of the placenta from the uterine wall. It can be associated with severe pregnancy-induced hypertension (PIH). Placental abruption causes continuous severe/sudden abdominal/back pain, tightening of the uterus, signs of hypovolaemic shock

Haemorrhage During Pregnancy (including Miscarriage and Ectopic Pregnancy)

and puts the baby at immediate risk. There may be some external blood loss, but more commonly the haemorrhage is concealed behind the placenta. Where there is a combination of revealed (external) blood loss and concealed haemorrhage, this can be particularly dangerous, as it can lead to an underestimation of the amount of total blood lost. The woman's abdomen will be tender when felt and the uterus will feel rigid or 'woody' with no signs of relaxation.

NOTE:

- **OVERALL, ABRUPTION IS OFTEN MORE OMINOUS THAN BLEEDING FROM PLACENTA PRAEVIA** because the true amount of bleeding is concealed. It is also associated with disseminated intravascular coagulation (DIC) which can worsen the tendency to bleed.

- It can be very difficult to differentiate between **placenta praevia and placental abruption**.

Table 5.6 – ASSESSMENT and MANAGEMENT of:

Haemorrhage during Pregnancy

ASSESSMENT	MANAGEMENT
• Quickly assess the patient and scene as you approach • Undertake a primary survey **<C>ABCDEF** • Assess for **TIME CRITICAL** features	• If any time critical features are present correct **<C>ABC** and transport to nearest suitable receiving hospital (**refer to medical emergencies guideline**). • Provide an alert/information call.
• Monitor SpO₂	• If **oxygen** (O₂) <94% administer O₂ to aim for a target saturation within the range of 94–98%.
• Assess volume of blood loss[a,b]	• Obtain IV access – insert **LARGE BORE** cannulae.
• In the event of **LIFE-THREATENING HAEMORRHAGE** AND a confirmed diagnosis of miscarriage (e.g. where a patient has gone home with medical management and starts to bleed)	• Administer syntometrine if available (refer to syntometrine guideline). • If syntometrine is **NOT** available or the patient is hypertensive (≥140/90) administer misoprostol (refer to misoprostol guideline). **CAUTION: DO NOT** administer **syntometrine** or **misoprostol** with a fetus in situ.
• Assess for signs of shock (e.g. tachycardia >100 bpm, SBP <90 mmHg with cool sweaty skin) • Undertake a capillary refill test **NOTE** – hypovolaemia is manifested late in pregnant women; the patient may be very unwell and the fetus may be compromised therefore **ADMINISTER** fluid replacement early (refer to intravascular therapy guideline)	• If >20 weeks the gravid uterus may compress the inferior vena cava in a patient who is supine, therefore, it is important to ensure adequate venous return before determining the need for fluid resuscitation; this can be achieved by placing the patient in left lateral tilt, or manually displacing the uterus. • Administer 250 ml of **sodium chloride 0.9%** IV to maintain SBP of 90 mmHg (refer to intravascular therapy guideline). • Re-assess vital signs prior to further fluid therapy. • Take any blood-soaked pads to hospital. NB Symptoms of hypovolaemic shock occur very late in otherwise fit young women; tachycardia may not appear until 30% of circulating volume has been lost, by which stage the patient is very unwell.
Ask 'When did you last feel the baby move?'	• Be particularly tactful, so as not to cause alarm, as anxiety in the mother will only exacerbate the situation.
• If no **TIME CRITICAL** features, perform a more thorough patient assessment with secondary survey including fetal assessment (**refer to obstetrics and gynaecology overview**) • Check the patient-carried notes for scan results confirming a 'low-lying' placenta	
• Assess patient's level of pain	Titrate pain relief against pain (refer to pain management guideline): – **Paracetamol** – **Entonox** – **Morphine: NOTE** administer cautiously if the patient is hypotensive.
	• Nil by mouth.
	• Symptomatic bradycardia due to vagal stimulation can be treated with atropine (refer to atropine and **cardiac rhythm disturbance guidelines**).
	• Adjust patient's position as required.
	• Transfer to further care.

[a] Large sanitary towel can absorb 50 ml of blood.
[b] Blood loss will appear greater if mixed with amniotic fluid.

KEY POINTS

Haemorrhage During Pregnancy (including Miscarriage and Ectopic Pregnancy)

- Haemorrhage during pregnancy is broadly divided into two categories, occurring in early and late pregnancy.

- Haemorrhage may be revealed (evident vaginal blood loss) or concealed (little or no loss).

- Pregnant women may appear well even when a large amount of blood has been lost.

- Obtain venous access with large bore cannulae.

- Tachycardia may not appear until 30% of circulating volume has been lost. In otherwise fit young women, symptoms of hypovolaemic shock occur very late, by which stage the patient is very unwell.

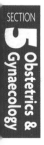
SECTION 5 Obstetrics & Gynaecology

SECTION 1 – Pregnancy-induced Hypertension and Severe Pre-eclampsia

1. Introduction

- Pregnancy-induced hypertension (PIH) is a generic term used to define a significant rise in blood pressure after 22 weeks, in the absence of proteinuria or other features of pre-eclampsia.

- Remember that treating and resuscitating the mother is also assisting the baby.

2. Incidence

- Hypertension from all causes is a common medical problem affecting 10–15% of all pregnancies.

- Approximately 15% of women who present with pregnancy-induced hypertension will develop pre-eclampsia.

3. Severity and Outcome

- PIH is usually mild (i.e. blood pressure (BP) 140/90 mmHg) and there is only a 10% risk of developing pre-eclampsia with mild rises in BP beyond 37 weeks.

- Earlier onset of PIH (i.e. 20–24 weeks) results in a 40% risk of developing pre-eclampsia. If PIH is uncomplicated by pre-eclampsia, then maternal and fetal outcomes are good; however, pre-eclampsia accounted for 13.6% of maternal deaths related to pregnancy causes.

4. Pathophysiology

Pre-eclampsia

- Pre-eclampsia is PIH associated with proteinuria. It commonly occurs beyond 24–28 weeks gestation, but can occur as early as 22 weeks.

- Although the underlying pathophysiology is not fully understood, pre-eclampsia is primarily a placental disorder associated with poor placental perfusion which often results in a fetus which is growth-restricted (i.e. smaller than expected because of the poor placental blood flow).

- In the UK the diagnosis of pre-eclampsia includes an increase in BP above 140/90 mmHg, oedema and detection of protein in the patient's urine.

- Pre-eclampsia is usually diagnosed at routine antenatal visits and may require admission to hospital and early delivery.

- The disease may be of mild, moderate or severe degree.

Severe pre-eclampsia

- May present in a patient with known mild pre-eclampsia or may present with little prior warning.

Symptoms of severe pre-eclampsia:

- The BP is significantly raised (i.e. 160/110 mmHg) with proteinuria and often one or more of the following symptoms:

  – headache – severe and frontal
  – visual disturbances
  – epigastric pain – often mistaken for heartburn
  – right-sided upper abdominal pain – due to stretching of the liver capsule
  – muscle twitching or tremor
  – nausea
  – vomiting
  – confusion
  – rapidly progressive oedema.

> **Risk factors – pre-eclampsia**
> - Primiparity or first child with a new partner.
> - Previous severe pre-eclampsia.
> - Essential hypertension.
> - Diabetes.
> - Obesity.
> - Twins of higher multiples.
> - Renal disease.
> - Advanced maternal age (over 40 years).
> - Young maternal age (less than 16 years).
> - Pre-existing cardiovascular disease.

Severe pre-eclampsia is:

- a 'multi-organ' disease; although hypertension is a cardinal feature, other complications include:

  – intracranial haemorrhage
  – stroke
  – renal failure
  – liver failure
  – abnormal blood clotting (e.g. disseminated intravascular coagulation (DIC)).

5. Assessment and Management

- For the assessment and management of mild/moderate pre-eclampsia refer to Table 5.7.

- For the assessment and management of severe pre-eclampsia refer to Table 5.8.

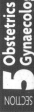

Table 5.7 – ASSESSMENT and MANAGEMENT of:

Mild/Moderate Pre-eclampsia

Definition – raised blood pressure >140/90 mmHg, detection of proteinuria, and sometimes oedema.

ASSESSMENT	MANAGEMENT
● Undertake a quick scan assessment ● Undertake a primary survey **ABCDEF** ● Assess for **TIME CRITICAL** features (see definition and symptoms of severe pre-eclampsia below)	● If any time critical features are present correct A and B and transport to nearest suitable receiving hospital (**refer to medical emergencies guideline**). ● Provide an alert/information call.
● If no **TIME CRITICAL** features perform a more thorough patient assessment with secondary survey including fetal assessment (**refer to obstetric and gynaecology overview for guidance**)	
● Measure blood pressure	Transfer to further care: ● If pregnancy >22 weeks and systolic blood pressure is >140/90 mmHg discuss management directly with the **BOOKED OBSTETRIC UNIT** or **MIDWIFE**.

Table 5.8 – ASSESSMENT and MANAGEMENT

Severe Pre-eclampsia

Definition and symptoms – raised blood pressure >160/110 mmHg, detection of proteinuria, and with one or more of the following: headache (severe and frontal), visual disturbances, epigastric pain, right-sided upper abdominal pain, muscle twitching or tremor, nausea, vomiting, confusion, rapidly progressive oedema.

ASSESSMENT	MANAGEMENT
● Undertake a quick scan assessment ● Undertake a primary survey **ABCDEF** ● Assess for signs of severe pre-eclampsia (see definition and symptoms above). Signs of severe pre-eclampsia are **TIME CRITICAL FEATURES**	● If any time critical features are present correct A and B problems (**refer to medical emergencies guideline**) and transfer to a consultant-led obstetric unit. NB Caution with 'lights and sirens' as strobe lights and noise may precipitate convulsions. ● If the patient is convulsing **refer to convulsion guideline**. ● Provide an alert/information call. ● If the convulsion is **NOT** self-limiting transfer to consultant-led obstetric unit.
● Monitor SpO$_2$ (94–98%)	● Attach pulse oximeter; if O$_2$ <94% administer O$_2$ to aim for a target saturation within the range of 94–98%.
	● Obtain IV access – insert a **LARGE BORE** cannula en-route. ● **DO NOT** administer intravenous fluid boluses because of the risk of provoking pulmonary oedema.
● Measure blood glucose level	**Refer to glycaemic emergencies.**

SECTION 2 – Eclampsia

1. Introduction

● Eclampsia is generalised tonic/clonic 'grand mal' convulsion and identical to an epileptic convulsion.

● Many patients will have had pre-existing pre-eclampsia (of mild, moderate or severe degree), but cases of eclampsia can present acutely with no prior warning – **ONE-THIRD** of cases present for the **FIRST TIME** post-delivery (usually in the first 48 hours). **THE BP MAY ONLY BE MILDLY ELEVATED AT PRESENTATION** (i.e. 140/80–90 mmHg).

● A convulsion is usually 'self-limiting' and will end after 2–3 minutes and can present for up to 6 weeks post partum (**refer to convulsion guideline**).

2. Incidence

● Eclampsia occurs in approximately 2.7:10,000 deliveries, usually beyond 24 weeks.

3. Severity and Outcome

● Eclampsia is one of the most dangerous complications of pregnancy and is a significant cause of maternal mortality with a mortality rate of 2% in the UK.

- Convulsions are usually self-limiting, but may be severe and repeated.
- Other complications associated with eclampsia include renal failure, hepatic failure and DIC.

4. Pathophysiology

- The hypoxia caused during a tonic/clonic convulsion may lead to significant fetal compromise and even death.

5. Assessment and Management

- For the assessment and management mild/moderate eclampsia and eclamptic convulsion refer to Table 5.9.

Risk factors – eclampsia
- Known pre-eclampsia.
- Primiparity or first child with a new partner.
- Previous severe pre-eclampsia.
- Essential hypertension.
- Diabetes.
- Obesity.
- Twins or higher multiples.
- Renal disease.
- Advanced maternal age (over 40 years).
- Young maternal age (less than 16 years).

Table 5.9 – ASSESSMENT and MANAGEMENT of:

Eclampsia

Definition – Eclampsia is generalised tonic/clonic 'grand mal' convulsion and identical to an epileptic convulsion.

ASSESSMENT	MANAGEMENT
- Undertake a primary survey **ABCDEF** - Assess for **TIME CRITICAL** features such as recurrent convulsions	- Correct A and B and transport to a consultant-led obstetric unit (**refer to medical emergencies guideline**). - Obtain IV (**LARGE BORE** cannulae) or IO access. **DO NOT** administer fluid boluses because of the risk of provoking pulmonary oedema. - Provide an alert/information call.
- If no **TIME CRITICAL** features perform a more thorough patient assessment with secondary survey including fetal assessment (**refer to obstetric and gynaecology overview for guidance**)	NOTE: epileptic patients may suffer tonic/clonic convulsions. - If >20 weeks gestation with a history of hypertension or pre-eclampsia treat as for eclampsia – refer to Tables 5.4 and 5.5. - If there is no history of hypertension or pre-eclampsia and blood pressure is normal treat as for epilepsy (**refer to convulsion guideline**). - Position the patient in 15–30° **LEFT LATERAL TILT** or left lateral (recovery) position.
- Monitor SpO₂ (94–98%)	- Attach pulse oximeter; if O₂ <94% administer O₂ to aim for a target saturation within the range of 94–98%.
- Continuous or recurrent convulsion	- If the patient convulses for longer than 2–3 minutes or has a second or subsequent convulsion administer diazepam IV/PR titrated against effect (refer to diazepam guideline for dosages and information). NOTE: in hospital, IV magnesium sulphate will be given and it is better to avoid multiple drugs if possible.

KEY POINTS

Pregnancy-Induced Hypertension (including Eclampsia)

- **Pregnancy-induced hypertension commonly occurs beyond 24–28 weeks but can occur as early as 22 weeks.**
- **Can present up to 6 weeks post delivery.**
- **Diagnosis includes an increase in blood pressure above 140/90 mmHg, oedema and detection of protein in the patient's urine.**
- **Eclampsia is one of the most dangerous complications of pregnancy.**
- **Eclampsia patients present with generalised tonic/clonic convulsions which are usually self-limiting.**
- **Only administer diazepam if the convulsions are prolonged or recurrent.**
- **Severe pre-eclampsia and eclampsia are TIME CRITICAL EMERGENCIES for both mother and unborn child.**

5 Obstetrics & Gynaecology SECTION

Vaginal Bleeding: Gynaecological Causes [693–694, 832]

1. Introduction

- A number of conditions can cause vaginal bleeding that is different from normal menstruation. Such conditions may result in a call to the ambulance service, including:
  - excessive menstrual period
  - normal or excessive menstrual period associated with severe abdominal pain
  - surgical or medical therapeutic abortion (may occur up to 10 days after treatment)
  - following gynaecological surgery (e.g. hysterectomy) (may occur up to 10 days after surgery)
  - colposcopy (may occur up to 10 days after a colposcopy)
  - gynaecological cancers, either before diagnosis or after treatment (i.e. cervix, uterus or vagina).

- This guideline provides guidance for the assessment and management of gynaecological vaginal bleeding. For causes of bleeding in early or late pregnancy, **refer to haemorrhage during pregnancy (including miscarriage and ectopic pregnancy) guideline**.

2. Incidence

- Women over 50 years are more at risk of cancers of the uterus and cervix.

3. Severity and Outcome

- The majority of causes of vaginal bleeding do not compromise the circulation, but blood loss can be alarming.

4. Pathophysiology

- Various pathophysiology.

Table 5.10 – ASSESSMENT and MANAGEMENT of:

Vaginal Bleeding

ASSESSMENT	MANAGEMENT
• Quickly scan the patient and scene as you approach • Undertake a primary survey **<C>ABCDEF** • Evaluate whether the patient has any **TIME CRITICAL** features or any signs of hypovolaemic shock	• If any **TIME CRITICAL** features are present correct **A** and **B** and transport to nearest suitable receiving hospital (**refer to medical emergencies guidance**). • Provide an alert/information call.
• Assess blood loss – ask about clots, blood-soaked clothes, bed sheets, number of soaked tampons/towels/pads NB Blood under the feet or between toes implies significant bleeding.	• Obtain IV access – insert a **LARGE BORE** cannula. • If there is visible external blood loss >500 ml refer to intravascular fluid therapy guideline.
• If no TIME CRITICAL features, perform a more through patient assessment with brief secondary survey for lower abdominal tenderness or guarding	
• Measure temperature	

• Check the patient's age:
  – >50 years – more at risk of cancers of the uterus/cervix
  – <50 years may be pregnant	

• Monitor SpO₂ (94–98%)	• If oxygen (O₂) <94% administer O₂ to aim for a target saturation within the range of 94–98%.

• Assess patient's level of pain	Titrate pain relief against pain (**refer to pain management guideline**):
	  – Paracetamol
	  – Entonox
	  – Morphine NB administer cautiously if the patient is hypotensive.

• Assess patient's comfort	• Nil by mouth.
	• Adjust patient's position as required.
	• Transfer to further care.

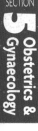

SECTION

5

Obstetrics & Gynaecology

KEY POINTS

Vaginal Bleeding: Gynaecological Causes

- The majority of vaginal bleeding episodes do not compromise circulation, but blood loss can be alarming.
- Assess blood loss; ask about number of soaked tampons/towels/pads.
- Provide pain management.
- **If you suspect a miscarriage or ectopic pregnancy** refer to haemorrhage during pregnancy (including miscarriage and ectopic pregnancy) guideline.

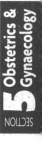

SECTION **5** Obstetrics & Gynaecology

6

Drugs

Drugs

Drugs Overview — 303

Adrenaline — 308

Amiodarone — 310

Aspirin — 311

Atropine — 312

Benzylpenicillin (Penicillin G) — 315

Chlorphenamine — 317

Clopidogrel — 320

Dexamethasone — 321

Diazepam — 322

Entonox — 326

Furosemide — 327

Glucagon (Glucagen) — 328

Glucose 10% — 330

Glucose 40% Oral Gel — 331

Glyceryl Trinitrate (GTN, Suscard) — 332

Heparin — 333

Hydrocortisone — 334

Ibuprofen — 338

Ipratropium Bromide (Atrovent) — 340

Metoclopramide (Maxolon) — 342

Midazolam — 343

Patient's Own Buccal Midazolam for Convulsions — 345

Misoprostol — 346

Morphine Sulphate — 347

Naloxone Hydrochloride (Narcan) — 351

Ondansetron — 355

Oxygen — 357

Paracetamol — 363

Reteplase — 367

Salbutamol — 370

0.9% Sodium Chloride — 373

Sodium Lactate Compound (Hartmann's/Ringer's Lactate) — 380

Syntometrine — 386

Tenecteplase — 387

Tetracaine 4% — 390

Tranexamic Acid — 391

Intravascular Fluid Therapy (Adults) — 392

Intravascular Fluid Therapy (Children) — 397

Page for Age — 400

Drugs Overview

1. Introduction

- The guidelines contained in this section are the current medicines that can be administered by registered paramedics[a].

- The Medicines Act 1968 governs what paramedics can administer and this is regulated by The Medicines and Healthcare Products Regulatory Agency (MHRA).

- Where a Prescription-Only Medicines (POMs) exemption exists, the MHRA has agreed a Patient Group Direction (PGD) is no longer required for paramedics to administer drugs where a JRCALC drug protocol is issued. Currently POMs exemptions have not been issued for tranexamic acid, therefore a PGD is required. A POMs exemption is not required for dexamethasone as the intravenous preparation is administered orally.

- The drugs administered by ambulance clinicians fall into two categories:
1. **Non-prescription drugs** (e.g. aspirin)
2. **Prescription-only medicines (POMs)** (e.g. morphine). POMs can only be prescribed by a qualified doctor (or dentist) and non-medical prescribers but exemptions exist under Part III of Schedule 5 to the Prescription Only Medicines (Human Use) Order 1997, which allows suitably trained paramedics to administer these drugs in specified circumstances.

1.1 Safety aspects

- Always check the following:
  - the drug type
  - the drug strength
  - whether the packaging is intact
  - the clarity of fluid
  - the expiry date.

1.2 Prescribing terms

In the case of prescription medicines, a variety of abbreviations are used, some of which are described – refer to Table 6.2.

NB Internationally recognised units and symbols should be used where possible.

Table 6.2 – COMMON ABBREVIATIONS

Abbreviation	Translation
ac	ante cibum (before food)
approx	approximately
bd	twice daily
CD	controlled drug preparation subject to prescription requirements control – The Misuse of Drugs Act
ec	enteric-coated (termed gastro-resistant in British Pharmacopoeia)
f/c	film-coated
IM	intramuscular
IV	intravenous
m/r	modified-release
MAOI	monoamine-oxidase inhibitors
max	maximum
NSAID	non-steroidal anti-inflammatory drug
o.d	omni die (every day)
o.m	omni mane (every morning)
o.n	omni nocte (every night)
p.c	post cibum (after food)
PGD	patient group direction
POM	prescription only medicine
pr	per rectum (rectally)
prn	when required
q.d.s	quater die sumendus (to be taken four times daily)
q.q.h	quarta quaque hora (every four hours)
s/c	sugar-coated
SSRI	selective serotonin re-uptake inhibitor
SOS	when required
SR	slow release
stat	immediately
t.d.s	ter die sumendus (to be taken three times daily)
t.i.d	ter in die (three times daily)
top	topical

Table 6.1 – DOCUMENTATION

Note the following:	✔	✘
● Avoid unnecessary use of decimal points	3 mg	3.0 mg
● Quantities of 1 gram or more should be written as	1 g	-
● Quantities less than 1 gram should be written in milligrams	500 mg	0.5 g
● Quantities less than 1 mg should be written in micrograms	100 micrograms	0.1 mg
● When decimals are unavoidable a zero should be written in front of the decimal point where there is no other figure	0.5 ml	not .5 ml
● Use of the decimal point is acceptable to express a range	0.5 to 1 g	-
● 'Micrograms' and 'nanograms' should not be abbreviated nor should 'units'	-	-
● The term 'millilitre' is used	ml or mL	cubic centimetre, c.c., or cm³

[a] Paramedic is defined as being on the register of paramedics maintained by the Health and Care Professions Council pursuant to paragraph 11 of Schedule 2 to the Health Professions Order 2001.

Drugs

SECTION 6 Drugs

1.3 Drug routes

- Drug routes are classified as **parenteral** and **non-parenteral**:
  - **Parenteral routes** are those where a physical breach of the skin or mucous membrane is made, for example, by injection
  - **Non-parenteral routes** are those where the drug is absorbed passively, for example, via the gastrointestinal tract, mucous membranes or skin.

- Drugs can be administered via a number of routes – refer to Table 6.3. It is important that the most appropriate route is selected – refer to Table 6.4 – taking into account the patient's condition and the urgency of the situation.

- Drugs and their possible routes of administration are listed in Table 6.4. In cases of parenteral administration, where at all possible, intravenous (IV) cannulation should be attempted, except for children in cardiac arrest where intraosseous cannulation is the preferred method. NB If a vein cannot be found it is not necessary to attempt IV cannulation. With intramuscular and subcutaneous routes, absorption may be erratic or incomplete if the patient is hypovolaemic or clinically unstable.

1.4 Drug codes

The drug codes listed in Table 6.5 are provided for **INFORMATION ONLY** and represent drugs that may be commonly encountered in the emergency/urgent care environment. **ONLY** the drugs listed in the guidelines are for use by registered paramedics; the remaining drugs are for use by physicians or under patient group directions by paramedics who have undertaken extended training.

Table 6.3 – DRUG ROUTES

Parenteral routes

Intramuscular – Injection of the drug into muscle, which is then absorbed into the blood. Absorption may be decreased in poor perfusion states.

Intraosseous – A rigid needle inserted directly into the bone marrow. Resuscitation drugs and fluid replacement may be administered by this route. Absorption is as quick as by the intravenous route.

Intravenous – Direct introduction of the drug into the cardiovascular system that normally delivers the drug to the target organs very quickly.

Subcutaneous – Injection of the drug into subcutaneous tissue. This usually has a slower rate of absorption than from intramuscular injection and may be decreased in poor perfusion states.

Non-parenteral routes

Inhaled – Gaseous drugs that are absorbed via the lungs.

Nebulisation – Liquid drugs agitated in a stream of gas such as oxygen to create fine droplets that are absorbed rapidly from the lungs.

Oral – The drug is swallowed and is absorbed into the blood from the gut. In serious trauma or illness, absorption may be delayed.

Rectal – The drug is absorbed from the wall of the rectum. This route is used for patients who are having seizures and who cannot be cannulated without risk to themselves or ambulance personnel. Effects usually occur 5–15 minutes after administration.

Sub-lingual – Tablet or aerosol spray is absorbed from the mucous membrane beneath the tongue. Effects usually occur within 2–3 minutes.

Transdermal – Absorption of a drug through the skin.

Buccal – Absorption via the mucous membrane.

Intranasal – Aerosol spray absorbed from the mucous membrane

KEY POINTS

Drugs Overview

- Check the drug type, strength, whether the packaging is intact, the clarity of fluid and the expiry date.
- Select the most appropriate route taking into account the patient's condition and the urgency of the situation.
- Only administer drugs via the routes you have been trained for.
- The drug codes are provided for INFORMATION ONLY.
- Complete documentation.

Table 6.4 – SUGGESTED DRUG ROUTES

Drug/Route	IV	IO	IM	SC	Oral	Sub-lingual	Buccal	Intranasal	Rectal	Inhaled	Nebulised	Transdermal	Flush
Adrenaline	✔	✔	✔	✔	N/A	N/A	N/A	N/A	N/A	N/A	N/A	N/A	N/A
Amiodarone	✔	✔	N/A	N/A	N/A	N/A	N/A	N/A	N/A	N/A	N/A	N/A	N/A
Aspirin	N/A	N/A	N/A	N/A	✔	N/A	N/A	N/A	N/A	N/A	N/A	N/A	N/A
Atropine	✔	✔	N/A	N/A	N/A	N/A	N/A	N/A	N/A	N/A	N/A	N/A	N/A
Atropine (CBRNE)	N/A	N/A	✔	N/A	N/A	N/A	N/A	N/A	N/A	N/A	N/A	N/A	N/A
Benzylpenicillin	✔	✔	✔	N/A	N/A	N/A	N/A	N/A	N/A	N/A	N/A	N/A	N/A
Chlorphenamine	✔	✔	✔	N/A	✔	N/A	N/A	N/A	N/A	N/A	N/A	N/A	N/A
Ciprofloxacin (CBRNE)	N/A	N/A	N/A	N/A	✔	N/A	N/A	N/A	N/A	N/A	N/A	N/A	N/A
Clopidogrel	N/A	N/A	N/A	N/A	✔	N/A	N/A	N/A	N/A	N/A	N/A	N/A	N/A
Dexamethasone	✔	✔	✔	N/A	✔	N/A	N/A	N/A	N/A	N/A	N/A	N/A	N/A
Diazepam	✔	✔	N/A	N/A	N/A	N/A	N/A	N/A	✔	N/A	N/A	N/A	N/A
Dicobalt (CBRNE)	✔	✔	N/A	N/A	N/A	N/A	N/A	N/A	N/A	N/A	N/A	N/A	N/A
Doxycycline (CBRNE)	N/A	N/A	N/A	N/A	✔	N/A	N/A	N/A	N/A	N/A	N/A	N/A	N/A
Entonox	N/A	N/A	N/A	N/A	N/A	N/A	N/A	N/A	N/A	✔	N/A	N/A	N/A
Furosemide	✔	✔	N/A	N/A	N/A	N/A	N/A	N/A	N/A	N/A	N/A	N/A	N/A
Glucagon	N/A	N/A	✔	N/A	N/A	N/A	N/A	N/A	N/A	N/A	N/A	N/A	N/A
Glucose 10%	✔	✔	N/A	N/A	N/A	N/A	N/A	N/A	N/A	N/A	N/A	N/A	N/A
Glucose 40% gel	N/A	N/A	N/A	N/A	N/A	N/A	✔	N/A	N/A	N/A	N/A	N/A	N/A
Glyceryl trinitrate	N/A	N/A	N/A	N/A	N/A	✔	✔	N/A	N/A	N/A	N/A	N/A	N/A
Heparin	✔	✔	N/A	N/A	N/A	N/A	N/A	N/A	N/A	N/A	N/A	N/A	N/A
Hydrocortisone	✔	✔	✔	N/A	N/A	N/A	N/A	N/A	N/A	N/A	N/A	N/A	N/A
Ibuprofen	N/A	N/A	N/A	N/A	✔	N/A	N/A	N/A	N/A	N/A	N/A	N/A	N/A
Ipratropium bromide	N/A	N/A	N/A	N/A	N/A	N/A	N/A	N/A	N/A	N/A	✔	N/A	N/A
Ketamine	✔	✔	✔	N/A	N/A	N/A	N/A	N/A	N/A	N/A	N/A	N/A	N/A
Metoclopramide	✔	✔	✔	N/A	N/A	N/A	N/A	N/A	N/A	N/A	N/A	N/A	N/A
Patient's own midazolam	N/A	N/A	N/A	N/A	N/A	✔	✔	N/A	N/A	N/A	N/A	N/A	N/A
Misoprostol	N/A	N/A	N/A	N/A	✔	N/A	N/A	N/A	✔	N/A	N/A	N/A	N/A
Morphine sulphate	✔	✔	✔	✔	✔	N/A	N/A	N/A	N/A	N/A	N/A	N/A	N/A
Naloxone hydrochloride	✔	✔	✔	✔	N/A	N/A	N/A	✔	N/A	N/A	N/A	N/A	N/A
Obidoxime (CBRNE)	✔	✔	N/A	N/A	N/A	N/A	N/A	N/A	N/A	N/A	N/A	N/A	N/A
Ondansetron	✔	✔	✔	N/A	N/A	N/A	N/A	N/A	N/A	N/A	N/A	N/A	N/A
Oxygen	N/A	N/A	N/A	N/A	N/A	N/A	N/A	N/A	N/A	✔	N/A	N/A	N/A
Paracetamol	✔	✔	N/A	N/A	✔	N/A	N/A	N/A	N/A	N/A	N/A	N/A	N/A
Potassium iodate (CBRNE)	N/A	N/A	N/A	N/A	✔	N/A	N/A	N/A	N/A	N/A	N/A	N/A	N/A
Pralidoxime mesylate (CBRNE)	✔	✔	N/A	N/A	N/A	N/A	N/A	N/A	N/A	N/A	N/A	N/A	N/A
Reteplase	✔	N/A	N/A	N/A	N/A	N/A	N/A	N/A	N/A	N/A	N/A	N/A	N/A
Salbutamol	N/A	N/A	N/A	N/A	N/A	N/A	N/A	N/A	N/A	✔	✔	N/A	N/A
0.9% Sodium chloride	✔	✔	N/A	N/A	N/A	N/A	N/A	N/A	N/A	N/A	N/A	N/A	✔
Sodium lactate	✔	✔	N/A	N/A	N/A	N/A	N/A	N/A	N/A	N/A	N/A	N/A	N/A
Syntometrine	N/A	N/A	✔	N/A	N/A	N/A	N/A	N/A	N/A	N/A	N/A	N/A	N/A
Tenecteplase	✔	N/A	N/A	N/A	N/A	N/A	N/A	N/A	N/A	N/A	N/A	N/A	N/A
Tetracaine	N/A	N/A	N/A	N/A	N/A	N/A	N/A	N/A	N/A	N/A	N/A	✔	N/A
Tranexamic acid	✔	N/A	N/A	N/A	N/A	N/A	N/A	N/A	N/A	N/A	N/A	N/A	N/A

Table 6.5 – JRCALC DRUG CODES

Drug	Code	Drug	Code
Adenosine	ADE	Glucose 50%	GLL
Adrenaline (epinephrine) 1:1,000	ADM	Glycerol suppositories	GLS
Adrenaline (epinephrine) 1:10,000	ADX	Glucagon	GLU
Aminophylline	AMN	Dextrose 5%	GLV
Amiodarone	AMO	Glucose 5%	GLX
Amoxicillin	AMX	Glucose 10%	GLX
Alteplase	APL	Glyceryl trinitrate (GTN)	GTN
Aspirin	ASP	Heparin (standard unfractionated)	HEP
Atracurium	ATC	Haloperidol	HPD
Atropine	ATR	Hydrocortisone	HYC
Benzylpenicillin	BPN	Ibuprofen	IBP
Co-dydramol	CDY	Ipratropium bromide	IPR
Cefalexin	CEF	Ketamine	KET
Cefotaxime	CFT	Lidocaine	LID
Ceftriaxone	CFX	Lidocaine gel (mucocutaneous anaesthesia)	LDU
Chlorpromazine	CHZ	Lorazepam	LRZ
Clopidogrel	CLO	Levonorgestrel	LVG
Clarithromycin	CMY	Midazolam (patient,s own midazolam)	MDZ
Codeine	COD	Midazolam	MDZ
Colloid gel solution	COL	Misoprostol	MIS
Codeine-paracetamol combination	CPC	Morphine sulphate	MOR
Chlorphenamine	CPH	Metoclopramide	MTC
Chloramphenicol eye preparation	CPL	Methylprednisolone	MTP
Cetirizine	CTZ	Metronidazole	MTZ
Ciprofloxacin	CXN	Nitrofurantoin	NFT
Co-amoxiclav	CXV	Naloxone hydrochloride	NLX
Cyclimorph	CYM	Entonox	NOO
Cyclizine	CYZ	Naproxen	NPN
Clotrimazole	CZL	Nystatin	NST
Diclofenac	DCF	Oxybuprocaine benoxinate	OBP
Dicobalt edetate	DCO	Obidoxime chloride	ODC
Dexamethasone	DEX	Ondansetron	ODT
Dihydrocodeine	DHC	Oral rehydration salts	ORS
Diamorphine	DMO	Oseltamivir	OSV
Domperidone	DMP	Otosporin ear drops	OTS
Doxycycline	DXN	Oxygen	OXG
Diazepam	DZP	Oxytetracycline	OXL
Enoxaparin (low molecular weight heparin)	ENP	Oxytocin	OXT
Ergometrine maleate	ERG	Paracetamol	PAR
Erythromycin	ERY	Procyclidine	PCY
Etomidate	ETO	Prochlorperazine	PCZ
Flucloxacillin	FCX	Pralidoxime mesylate	PDM
Fluorescein sodium	FLR	Potassium iodate	PIO
Flumazenil	FLZ	Penicillin V	PNV
Furosemide	FRM	Propofol	PPL
Fusidic acid eye preparation	FUA	Prednisolone	PRD
Glucose 40% gel	GLG	Pethidine	PTH

Drugs Overview

Table 6.5 – JRCALC DRUG CODES

Drug	Code	Drug	Code
Rocuronium	**RCR**	Terbutaline	**TER**
Reteplase	**RPA**	Tetanus immunoglobulin	**TIG**
0.9% Sodium chloride	**SCP**	Trimethoprim	**TMP**
Salbutamol	**SLB**	Tramadol	**TRM**
Sodium lactate compound	**SLC**	Tetracaine (amethocaine)	**TTC**
Sodium thiopentone	**STP**	Tetanus/low dose diphtheria vaccine	**TTD**
Suxamethonium	**SUX**	Tranexamic acid	**TXA**
Syntometrine	**SYN**	Vecuronium	**VEC**
Tenecteplase	**TNK**	Water for injection	**WFI**

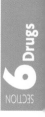

Adrenaline [839]

Presentation

Pre-filled syringe or ampoule containing 1 milligram of adrenaline (epinephrine) in 1 ml (1:1,000) ADM.

Pre-filled syringe containing 1 milligram of adrenaline (epinephrine) in 10 ml (1:10,000) ADX.

Indications

Cardiac arrest.

Anaphylaxis.

Life-threatening asthma with failing ventilation and continued deterioration despite nebuliser therapy.

Actions

Adrenaline is a sympathomimetic that stimulates both alpha- and beta-adrenergic receptors. As a result myocardial and cerebral blood flow is enhanced during CPR and CPR becomes more effective due to increased peripheral resistance which improves perfusion pressures.

Reverses allergic manifestations of acute anaphylaxis.

Relieves bronchospasm in acute severe asthma.

Contra-Indications

Do not give repeated doses of adrenaline in hypothermic patients.

Cautions

Severe hypertension may occur in patients on non-cardioselective beta-blocker, (e.g. Propranolol).

Dosage and Administration

1. Cardiac arrest:

● **Shockable rhythms:** administer adrenaline after the 3rd shock and then after alternate shocks (i.e. 5th, 7th etc).

● **Non-shockable rhythms:** administer adrenaline immediately IV access is achieved then alternate loops.
Route: Intravenous/intraosseous – **administer as a rapid bolus.**

AGE	INITIAL DOSE	REPEAT DOSE	DOSE INTERVAL	CONCENTRATION	VOLUME	MAXIMUM DOSE
Adult	1 milligram	1 milligram	3–5 minutes	1 milligram in 10 ml (1:10,000)	10 ml	No limit
11 years	350 micrograms	350 micrograms	3–5 minutes	1 milligram in 10 ml (1:10,000)	3.5 ml	No limit
10 years	320 micrograms	320 micrograms	3–5 minutes	1 milligram in 10 ml (1:10,000)	3.2 ml	No limit
9 years	300 micrograms	300 micrograms	3–5 minutes	1 milligram in 10 ml (1:10,000)	3 ml	No limit
8 years	260 micrograms	260 micrograms	3–5 minutes	1 milligram in 10 ml (1:10,000)	2.6 ml	No limit
7 years	230 micrograms	230 micrograms	3–5 minutes	1 milligram in 10 ml (1:10,000)	2.3 ml	No limit
6 years	210 micrograms	210 micrograms	3–5 minutes	1 milligram in 10 ml (1:10,000)	2.1 ml	No limit
5 years	190 micrograms	190 micrograms	3–5 minutes	1 milligram in 10 ml (1:10,000)	1.9 ml	No limit
4 years	160 micrograms	160 micrograms	3–5 minutes	1 milligram in 10 ml (1:10,000)	1.6 ml	No limit
3 years	140 micrograms	140 micrograms	3–5 minutes	1 milligram in 10 ml (1:10,000)	1.4 ml	No limit
2 years	120 micrograms	120 micrograms	3–5 minutes	1 milligram in 10 ml (1:10,000)	1.2 ml	No limit
18 months	110 micrograms	110 micrograms	3–5 minutes	1 milligram in 10 ml (1:10,000)	1.1 ml	No limit
12 months	100 micrograms	100 micrograms	3–5 minutes	1 milligram in 10 ml (1:10,000)	1 ml	No limit
9 months	90 micrograms	90 micrograms	3–5 minutes	1 milligram in 10 ml (1:10,000)	0.9 ml	No limit
6 months	80 micrograms	80 micrograms	3–5 minutes	1 milligram in 10 ml (1:10,000)	0.8 ml	No limit
3 months	60 micrograms	60 micrograms	3–5 minutes	1 milligram in 10 ml (1:10,000)	0.6 ml	No limit
1 month	50 micrograms	50 micrograms	3–5 minutes	1 milligram in 10 ml (1:10,000)	0.5 ml	No limit
Birth	35 micrograms	35 micrograms	3–5 minutes	1 milligram in 10 ml (1:10,000)	0.35 ml	No limit

Adrenaline

2. Anaphylaxis and **life-threatening asthma.**

Route: Intramuscular – antero-lateral aspect of thigh or upper arm.

AGE	INITIAL DOSE	REPEAT DOSE	DOSE INTERVAL	CONCENTRATION	VOLUME	MAXIMUM DOSE
Adult	500 micrograms	500 micrograms	5 minutes	1 milligram in 1 ml (1:1,000)	0.5 ml	No limit
11 years	300 micrograms	300 micrograms	5 minutes	1 milligram in 1 ml (1:1,000)	0.3 ml	No limit
10 years	300 micrograms	300 micrograms	5 minutes	1 milligram in 1 ml (1:1,000)	0.3 ml	No limit
9 years	300 micrograms	300 micrograms	5 minutes	1 milligram in 1 ml (1:1,000)	0.3 ml	No limit
8 years	300 micrograms	300 micrograms	5 minutes	1 milligram in 1 ml (1:1,000)	0.3 ml	No limit
7 years	300 micrograms	300 micrograms	5 minutes	1 milligram in 1 ml (1:1,000)	0.3 ml	No limit
6 years	300 micrograms	300 micrograms	5 minutes	1 milligram in 1 ml (1:1,000)	0.3 ml	No limit
5 years	150 micrograms	150 micrograms	5 minutes	1 milligram in 1 ml (1:1,000)	0.15 ml	No limit
4 years	150 micrograms	150 micrograms	5 minutes	1 milligram in 1 ml (1:1,000)	0.15 ml	No limit
3 years	150 micrograms	150 micrograms	5 minutes	1 milligram in 1 ml (1:1,000)	0.15 ml	No limit
2 years	150 micrograms	150 micrograms	5 minutes	1 milligram in 1 ml (1:1,000)	0.15 ml	No limit
18 months	150 micrograms	150 micrograms	5 minutes	1 milligram in 1 ml (1:1,000)	0.15 ml	No limit
12 months	150 micrograms	150 micrograms	5 minutes	1 milligram in 1 ml (1:1,000)	0.15 ml	No limit
9 months	150 micrograms	150 micrograms	5 minutes	1 milligram in 1 ml (1:1,000)	0.15 ml	No limit
6 months	150 micrograms	150 micrograms	5 minutes	1 milligram in 1 ml (1:1,000)	0.15 ml	No limit
3 months	150 micrograms	150 micrograms	5 minutes	1 milligram in 1 ml (1:1,000)	0.15 ml	No limit
1 months	150 micrograms	150 micrograms	5 minutes	1 milligram in 1 ml (1:1,000)	0.15 ml	No limit
Birth	150 micrograms	150 micrograms	5 minutes	1 milligram in 1 ml (1:1,000)	0.15 ml	No limit

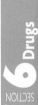

Amiodarone [840]

AMO

Presentation

Pre-filled syringe containing 300 milligrams amiodarone in 10 ml.

Indications

Cardiac arrest

- **Shockable rhythms:** if unresponsive to defibrillation administer amiodarone after the 3rd shock and an additional bolus depending on age to unresponsive VF or pulseless VT following the 5th shock.

Actions

Antiarrhythmic; lengthens cardiac action potential and therefore effective refractory period. Prolongs QT interval on ECG.

Blocks sodium and potassium channels in cardiac muscle. Acts to stabilise and reduce electrical irritability of cardiac muscle.

Contra-Indications

No contra-indications in the context of the treatment of cardiac arrest.

Side Effects

Bradycardia.

Vasodilatation causing hypotension, flushing.

Bronchospasm.

Arrhythmias – Torsades de pointes.

Dosage and Administration

- Administer into large vein as extravasation can cause burns.
- Follow administration with a 0.9% sodium chloride flush – **refer to sodium chloride guideline**.
- Cardiac arrest – Shockable rhythms: if unresponsive to defibrillation administer amiodarone after the 3rd shock.

Route: intravenous/intraosseous – administer as a rapid bolus.

AGE	INITIAL DOSE	REPEAT DOSE	DOSE INTERVAL	CONCENTRATION	VOLUME	MAXIMUM DOSE
Adult	300 milligrams	150 milligrams	After 5th shock	300 milligrams in 10 ml	10 ml	450 milligrams
11 years	180 milligrams	180 milligrams	After 5th shock	300 milligrams in 10 ml	6 ml	360 milligrams
10 years	160 milligrams	160 milligrams	After 5th shock	300 milligrams in 10 ml	5.3 ml	320 milligrams
9 years	150 milligrams	150 milligrams	After 5th shock	300 milligrams in 10 ml	5 ml	300 milligrams
8 years	130 milligrams	130 milligrams	After 5th shock	300 milligrams in 10 ml	4.3 ml	260 milligrams
7 years	120 milligrams	120 milligrams	After 5th shock	300 milligrams in 10 ml	4 ml	240 milligrams
6 years	100 milligrams	100 milligrams	After 5th shock	300 milligrams in 10 ml	3.3 ml	200 milligrams
5 years	100 milligrams	100 milligrams	After 5th shock	300 milligrams in 10 ml	3.3 ml	200 milligrams
4 years	80 milligrams	80 milligrams	After 5th shock	300 milligrams in 10 ml	2.7 ml	160 milligrams
3 years	70 milligrams	70 milligrams	After 5th shock	300 milligrams in 10 ml	2.3 ml	140 milligrams
2 years	60 milligrams	60 milligrams	After 5th shock	300 milligrams in 10 ml	2 ml	120 milligrams
18 months	55 milligrams	55 milligrams	After 5th shock	300 milligrams in 10 ml	1.8 ml	110 milligrams
12 months	50 milligrams	50 milligrams	After 5th shock	300 milligrams in 10 ml	1.7 ml	100 milligrams
9 months	45 milligrams	45 milligrams	After 5th shock	300 milligrams in 10 ml	1.5 ml	90 milligrams
6 months	40 milligrams	40 milligrams	After 5th shock	300 milligrams in 10 ml	1.3 ml	80 milligrams
3 months	30 milligrams	30 milligrams	After 5th shock	300 milligrams in 10 ml	1 ml	60 milligrams
1 month	25 milligrams	25 milligrams	After 5th shock	300 milligrams in 10 ml	0.8 ml	50 milligrams
Birth	18 milligrams	18 milligrams	After 5th shock	300 milligrams in 10 ml	0.6 ml	36 milligrams

Aspirin [841]

ASP

Presentation

300 milligrams aspirin (acetylsalicylic acid) in tablet form (dispersible).

Indications

Adults with:

- Clinical or ECG evidence suggestive of myocardial infarction or ischaemia.

Actions

Has an antiplatelet action which reduces clot formation.

Contra-Indications

- Known aspirin allergy or sensitivity.
- Children under 16 years (see additional information).
- Active gastrointestinal bleeding.
- Haemophilia or other known clotting disorders.
- Severe hepatic disease.

Cautions

As the likely benefits of a single 300 milligram aspirin outweigh the potential risks, aspirin may be given to patients with:

- Asthma
- Pregnancy
- Kidney or liver failure
- Gastric or duodenal ulcer
- Current treatment with anticoagulants.

Side Effects

- Gastric bleeding.
- Wheezing in some asthmatics.

Additional Information

In suspected myocardial infarction a 300 milligram aspirin tablet should be given regardless of any previous aspirin taken that day.

Clopidogrel may be indicated in acute ST segment elevation myocardial infarction – refer to clopidogrel guideline.

Aspirin is contra-indicated in children under the age of 16 years as it may precipitate Reye's syndrome. This syndrome is very rare and occurs in young children, damaging the liver and brain. It has a mortality rate of 50%.

Dosage and Administration

Route: Oral – chewed or dissolved in water.

AGE	INITIAL DOSE	REPEAT DOSE	DOSE INTERVAL	CONCENTRATION	VOLUME	MAXIMUM DOSE
Adults	300 milligrams	NONE	N/A	300 milligrams per tablet	1 tablet	300 milligrams

Atropine [842]

Presentation

Pre-filled syringe containing 1 milligram atropine in 10 ml.

Pre-filled syringe containing 1 milligram atropine in 5 ml.

Pre-filled syringe containing 3 milligrams atropine in 10 ml.

An ampoule containing 600 micrograms in 1 ml.

Indications

Symptomatic bradycardia in the presence of **ANY** of these adverse signs:

- Absolute bradycardia (pulse <40 beats per minute).
- Systolic blood pressure below expected for age (refer to page-for-age guideline for age related blood pressure readings in children).
- Paroxysmal ventricular arrhythmias requiring suppression.
- Inadequate perfusion causing confusion, etc.

NB Hypoxia is the most common cause of bradycardia in children, therefore interventions to support ABC and oxygen therapy should be the first-line therapy.

Contra-Indications

Should **NOT** be given to treat bradycardia in suspected hypothermia.

Actions

May reverse effects of vagal overdrive.

May increase heart rate by blocking vagal activity in sinus bradycardia, second or third degree heart block.

Enhances A-V conduction.

Side Effects

Dry mouth, visual blurring and pupil dilation.

Confusion and occasional hallucinations.

Tachycardia.

In the elderly retention of urine may occur.

Do not use small (<100 micrograms) doses as they may cause paradoxical bradycardia.

Additional Information

May induce tachycardia when used after myocardial infarction, which will increase myocardial oxygen demand and worsen ischaemia. Hence, bradycardia in a patient with an MI should **ONLY** be treated if the low heart rate is causing problems with perfusion.

Dosage and Administration

SYMPTOMATIC BRADYCARDIA

NB BRADYCARDIA in children is most commonly caused by **HYPOXIA,** requiring immediate ABC care, **NOT** drug therapy; therefore **ONLY** administer atropine in cases of bradycardia caused by vagal stimulation (e.g. suction).

Route: Intravenous/intraosseous administer as a rapid bolus.

AGE	INITIAL DOSE	REPEAT DOSE	DOSE INTERVAL	CONCENTRATION	VOLUME	MAXIMUM DOSE
≥12 years	600 micrograms[a]	600 micrograms[a]	3–5 minutes	600 micrograms per ml	1 ml	3 milligrams
11 years	500 micrograms	NONE	N/A	600 micrograms per ml	0.8 ml	500 micrograms
10 years	500 micrograms	NONE	N/A	600 micrograms per ml	0.8 ml	500 micrograms
9 years	500 micrograms	NONE	N/A	600 micrograms per ml	0.8 ml	500 micrograms
8 years	500 micrograms	NONE	N/A	600 micrograms per ml	0.8 ml	500 micrograms
7 years	400 micrograms	NONE	N/A	600 micrograms per ml	0.7 ml	400 micrograms
6 years	400 micrograms	NONE	N/A	600 micrograms per ml	0.7 ml	400 micrograms
5 years	300 micrograms	NONE	N/A	600 micrograms per ml	0.5 ml	300 micrograms
4 years	300 micrograms	NONE	N/A	600 micrograms per ml	0.5 ml	300 micrograms
3 years	240 micrograms	NONE	N/A	600 micrograms per ml	0.4 ml	240 micrograms
2 years	240 micrograms	NONE	N/A	600 micrograms per ml	0.4 ml	240 micrograms
18 months	200 micrograms	NONE	N/A	600 micrograms per ml	0.3 ml	200 micrograms
12 months	200 micrograms	NONE	N/A	600 micrograms per ml	0.3 ml	200 micrograms
9 months	120 micrograms	NONE	N/A	600 micrograms per ml	0.2 ml	120 micrograms
6 months	120 micrograms	NONE	N/A	600 micrograms per ml	0.2 ml	120 micrograms
3 months	120 micrograms	NONE	N/A	600 micrograms per ml	0.2 ml	120 micrograms
1 month	90 micrograms	NONE	N/A	600 micrograms per ml	0.15 ml	90 micrograms
Birth	60 micrograms	NONE	N/A	600 micrograms per ml	0.1 ml	60 micrograms

[a] The adult dosage can be given as 500 or 600 micrograms to a maximum of 3 milligrams depending on presentation available.

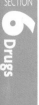

SECTION 6 Drugs

Atropine

Route: Intravenous/intraosseous **administer as a rapid bolus.**

AGE	INITIAL DOSE	REPEAT DOSE	DOSE INTERVAL	CONCENTRATION	VOLUME	MAXIMUM DOSE
≥12 years	600 micrograms[a]	600 micrograms[a]	3–5 minutes	300 micrograms per ml	2 ml	3 milligrams
11 years	500 micrograms	NONE	N/A	300 micrograms per ml	1.7 ml	500 micrograms
10 years	500 micrograms	NONE	N/A	300 micrograms per ml	1.7 ml	500 micrograms
9 years	500 micrograms	NONE	N/A	300 micrograms per ml	1.7 ml	500 micrograms
8 years	500 micrograms	NONE	N/A	300 micrograms per ml	1.7 ml	500 micrograms
7 years	400 micrograms	NONE	N/A	300 micrograms per ml	1.3 ml	400 micrograms
6 years	400 micrograms	NONE	N/A	300 micrograms per ml	1.3 ml	400 micrograms
5 years	300 micrograms	NONE	N/A	300 micrograms per ml	1 ml	300 micrograms
4 years	300 micrograms	NONE	N/A	300 micrograms per ml	1 ml	300 micrograms
2 years	240 micrograms	NONE	N/A	300 micrograms per ml	0.8 ml	240 micrograms
18 months	200 micrograms	NONE	N/A	300 micrograms per ml	0.7 ml	200 micrograms
12 months	200 micrograms	NONE	N/A	300 micrograms per ml	0.7 ml	200 micrograms
9 months	120 micrograms	NONE	N/A	300 micrograms per ml	0.4 ml	120 micrograms
6 months	120 micrograms	NONE	N/A	300 micrograms per ml	0.4 ml	120 micrograms
3 months	120 micrograms	NONE	N/A	300 micrograms per ml	0.4 ml	120 micrograms
1 month	90 micrograms	NONE	N/A	300 micrograms per ml	0.3 ml	90 micrograms
Birth	60 micrograms	NONE	N/A	300 micrograms per ml	0.2 ml	60 micrograms

Route: Intravenous/intraosseous **administer as a rapid bolus.**

AGE	INITIAL DOSE	REPEAT DOSE	DOSE INTERVAL	CONCENTRATION	VOLUME	MAXIMUM DOSE
≥12 years	600 micrograms[a]	600 micrograms[a]	3–5 minutes	200 micrograms per ml	3 ml	3 milligrams
11 years	500 micrograms	NONE	N/A	200 micrograms per ml	2.5 ml	500 micrograms
10 years	500 micrograms	NONE	N/A	200 micrograms per ml	2.5 ml	500 micrograms
9 years	500 micrograms	NONE	N/A	200 micrograms per ml	2.5 ml	500 micrograms
8 years	500 micrograms	NONE	N/A	200 micrograms per ml	2.5 ml	500 micrograms
7 years	400 micrograms	NONE	N/A	200 micrograms per ml	2 ml	400 micrograms
6 years	400 micrograms	NONE	N/A	200 micrograms per ml	2 ml	400 micrograms
5 years	300 micrograms	NONE	N/A	200 micrograms per ml	1.5 ml	300 micrograms
4 years	300 micrograms	NONE	N/A	200 micrograms per ml	1.5 ml	300 micrograms
3 years	240 micrograms	NONE	N/A	200 micrograms per ml	1.2 ml	240 micrograms
2 years	240 micrograms	NONE	N/A	200 micrograms per ml	1.2 ml	240 micrograms
18 months	200 micrograms	NONE	N/A	200 micrograms per ml	1 ml	200 micrograms
12 months	200 micrograms	NONE	N/A	200 micrograms per ml	1 ml	200 micrograms
9 months	120 micrograms	NONE	N/A	200 micrograms per ml	0.6 ml	120 micrograms
6 months	120 micrograms	NONE	N/A	200 micrograms per ml	0.6 ml	120 micrograms
3 months	120 micrograms	NONE	N/A	200 micrograms per ml	0.6 ml	120 micrograms
1 month	100 micrograms	NONE	N/A	200 micrograms per ml	0.5 ml	100 micrograms
Birth[b]	80 micrograms	NONE	N/A	200 micrograms per ml	0.4 ml	80 micrograms

[a] The adult dosage can be given as 500 or 600 micrograms to a maximum of 3 milligrams depending on presentation available.
[b] **NB** BRADYCARDIA in children is most commonly caused by **HYPOXIA,** requiring immediate ABC care, **NOT** drug therapy; therefore **ONLY** administer atropine in cases of bradycardia caused by vagal stimulation (e.g. suction).

6 Drugs
SECTION

Atropine

Route: Intravenous/Intraosseous **administer as a rapid bolus**.

AGE	INITIAL DOSE	REPEAT DOSE	DOSE INTERVAL	CONCENTRATION	VOLUME	MAXIMUM DOSE
≥12 years	600 micrograms[a]	600 micrograms[a]	3–5 minutes	100 micrograms per ml	6 ml	3 milligrams
11 years	500 micrograms	NONE	N/A	100 micrograms per ml	5 ml	500 micrograms
10 years	500 micrograms	NONE	N/A	100 micrograms per ml	5 ml	500 micrograms
9 years	500 micrograms	NONE	N/A	100 micrograms per ml	5 ml	500 micrograms
8 years	500 micrograms	NONE	N/A	100 micrograms per ml	5 ml	500 micrograms
7 years	400 micrograms	NONE	N/A	100 micrograms per ml	4 ml	400 micrograms
6 years	400 micrograms	NONE	N/A	100 micrograms per ml	4 ml	400 micrograms
5 years	300 micrograms	NONE	N/A	100 micrograms per ml	3 ml	300 micrograms
4 years	300 micrograms	NONE	N/A	100 micrograms per ml	3 ml	300 micrograms
3 years	240 micrograms	NONE	N/A	100 micrograms per ml	2.4 ml	240 micrograms
2 years	240 micrograms	NONE	N/A	100 micrograms per ml	2.4 ml	240 micrograms
18 months	200 micrograms	NONE	N/A	100 micrograms per ml	2 ml	200 micrograms
12 months	200 micrograms	NONE	N/A	100 micrograms per ml	2 ml	200 micrograms
9 months	120 micrograms	NONE	N/A	100 micrograms per ml	1.2 ml	120 micrograms
6 months	120 micrograms	NONE	N/A	100 micrograms per ml	1.2 ml	120 micrograms
3 months	120 micrograms	NONE	N/A	100 micrograms per ml	1.2 ml	120 micrograms
1 month	90 micrograms	NONE	N/A	100 micrograms per ml	0.9 ml	90 micrograms
Birth	70 micrograms	NONE	N/A	100 micrograms per ml	0.7 ml	70 micrograms

[a] The adult dosage can be given as 500 or 600 micrograms to a maximum of 3 milligrams depending on presentation available.

Benzylpenicillin (Penicillin G) [843]

Presentation

Ampoule containing 600 milligrams of benzylpenicillin as powder.

Administered intravenously, intraosseously or intramuscularly.

NB Different concentrations and volumes of administration (refer to dosage and administration tables).

Indications

Suspected meningococcal disease in the presence of:

1. a non-blanching rash (the classical, haemorrhagic, non-blanching rash (may be petechial or purpuric) – seen in approximately 40% of infected children)

and

2. signs/symptoms suggestive of meningococcal septicaemia (refer to meningococcal meningitis and septicaemia guideline for signs/symptoms).

Actions

Antibiotic: broad-spectrum.

Contra-Indications

Known severe penicillin allergy (more than a simple rash alone).

Additional Information

- Meningococcal septicaemia is commonest in children and young adults.
- It may be rapidly progressive and fatal.
- Early administration of benzylpenicillin improves outcome.

Dosage and Administration

Administer en-route to hospital (unless already administered).

NB IV/IO and IM concentrations are different and have different volumes of administration.

Route: Intravenous/intraosseous – by slow injection.

AGE	INITIAL DOSE	REPEAT DOSE	DOSE INTERVAL	CONCENTRATION	VOLUME	MAXIMUM DOSE
Adult	1.2 grams	NONE	N/A	1.2 grams dissolved in 19.2 ml water for injection	20 ml	1.2 grams
11 years	1.2 grams	NONE	N/A	1.2 grams dissolved in 19.2 ml water for injection	20 ml	1.2 grams
10 years	1.2 grams	NONE	N/A	1.2 grams dissolved in 19.2 ml water for injection	20 ml	1.2 grams
9 years	600 milligrams	NONE	N/A	600 milligrams dissolved in 9.6 ml water for injection	10 ml	600 milligrams
8 years	600 milligrams	NONE	N/A	600 milligrams dissolved in 9.6 ml water for injection	10 ml	600 milligrams
7 years	600 milligrams	NONE	N/A	600 milligrams dissolved in 9.6 ml water for injection	10 ml	600 milligrams
6 years	600 milligrams	NONE	N/A	600 milligrams dissolved in 9.6 ml water for injection	10 ml	600 milligrams
5 years	600 milligrams	NONE	N/A	600 milligrams dissolved in 9.6 ml water for injection	10 ml	600 milligrams
4 years	600 milligrams	NONE	N/A	600 milligrams dissolved in 9.6 ml water for injection	10 ml	600 milligrams
3 years	600 milligrams	NONE	N/A	600 milligrams dissolved in 9.6 ml water for injection	10 ml	600 milligrams
2 years	600 milligrams	NONE	N/A	600 milligrams dissolved in 9.6 ml water for injection	10 ml	600 milligrams
18 months	600 milligrams	NONE	N/A	600 milligrams dissolved in 9.6 ml water for injection	10 ml	600 milligrams
12 months	600 milligrams	NONE	N/A	600 milligrams dissolved in 9.6 ml water for injection	10 ml	600 milligrams
9 months	300 milligrams	NONE	N/A	600 milligrams dissolved in 9.6 ml water for injection	5 ml	300 milligrams
6 months	300 milligrams	NONE	N/A	600 milligrams dissolved in 9.6 ml water for injection	5 ml	300 milligrams
3 months	300 milligrams	NONE	N/A	600 milligrams dissolved in 9.6 ml water for injection	5 ml	300 milligrams
1 month	300 milligrams	NONE	N/A	600 milligrams dissolved in 9.6 ml water for injection	5 ml	300 milligrams
Birth	300 milligrams	NONE	N/A	600 milligrams dissolved in 9.6 ml water for injection	5 ml	300 milligrams

March 2016

SECTION 6 Drugs

Benzylpenicillin (Penicillin G)

Route: Intramuscular (antero-lateral aspect of thigh or upper arm – preferably in a well perfused area) if rapid intravascular access cannot be obtained.

AGE	INITIAL DOSE	REPEAT DOSE	DOSE INTERVAL	CONCENTRATION	VOLUME	MAXIMUM DOSE
Adult	1.2 grams	NONE	N/A	1.2 grams dissolved in 3.2 ml water for injection	4 ml	1.2 grams
11 years	1.2 grams	NONE	N/A	1.2 grams dissolved in 3.2 ml water for injection	4 ml	1.2 grams
10 years	1.2 grams	NONE	N/A	1.2 grams dissolved in 3.2 ml water for injection	4 ml	1.2 grams
9 years	600 milligrams	NONE	N/A	600 milligrams dissolved in 1.6 ml water for injection	2 ml	600 milligrams
8 years	600 milligrams	NONE	N/A	600 milligrams dissolved in 1.6 ml water for injection	2 ml	600 milligrams
7 years	600 milligrams	NONE	N/A	600 milligrams dissolved in 1.6 ml water for injection	2 ml	600 milligrams
6 years	600 milligrams	NONE	N/A	600 milligrams dissolved in 1.6 ml water for injection	2 ml	600 milligrams
5 years	600 milligrams	NONE	N/A	600 milligrams dissolved in 1.6 ml water for injection	2 ml	600 milligrams
4 years	600 milligrams	NONE	N/A	600 milligrams dissolved in 1.6 ml water for injection	2 ml	600 milligrams
3 years	600 milligrams	NONE	N/A	600 milligrams dissolved in 1.6 ml water for injection	2 ml	600 milligrams
2 years	600 milligrams	NONE	N/A	600 milligrams dissolved in 1.6 ml water for injection	2 ml	600 milligrams
18 months	600 milligrams	NONE	N/A	600 milligrams dissolved in 1.6 ml water for injection	2 ml	600 milligrams
12 months	600 milligrams	NONE	N/A	600 milligrams dissolved in 1.6 ml water for injection	2 ml	600 milligrams
9 months	300 milligrams	NONE	N/A	600 milligrams dissolved in 1.6 ml water for injection	1 ml	300 milligrams
6 months	300 milligrams	NONE	N/A	600 milligrams dissolved in 1.6 ml water for injection	1 ml	300 milligrams
3 months	300 milligrams	NONE	N/A	600 milligrams dissolved in 1.6 ml water for injection	1 ml	300 milligrams
1 month	300 milligrams	NONE	N/A	600 milligrams dissolved in 1.6 ml water for injection	1 ml	300 milligrams
Birth	300 milligrams	NONE	N/A	600 milligrams dissolved in 1.6 ml water for injection	1 ml	300 milligrams

Presentation

Ampoule containing 10 milligrams of chlorphenamine maleate in 1 ml.

Tablet containing 4 milligrams of chlorphenamine maleate.

Oral solution containing 2 milligrams of chlorphenamine maleate in 5 ml.

Indications

Severe anaphylactic reactions (when indicated, should follow initial treatment with IM adrenaline).

Symptomatic allergic reactions falling short of anaphylaxis but causing patient distress (e.g. severe itching).

Actions

An antihistamine that blocks the effect of histamine released during a hypersensitivity (allergic) reaction.

Also has anticholinergic properties.

Contra-Indications

Known hypersensitivity.

Children less than 1 year of age.

Cautions

Hypotension.

Epilepsy.

Glaucoma.

Hepatic disease.

Prostatic disease.

Side Effects

Sedation.

Dry mouth.

Headache.

Blurred vision.

Psychomotor impairment.

Gastrointestinal disturbance.

Transient hypotension.

Convulsions (rare).

The elderly are more likely to suffer side effects.

Warn anyone receiving chlorphenamine against driving or undertaking any other complex psychomotor task, due to the sedative and psychomotor side effects.

Dosage and Administration

Route: Intravenous/intraosseous (IV preferred route) – **SLOWLY** over 1 minute/intramuscularly.

AGE	INITIAL DOSE	REPEAT DOSE	DOSE INTERVAL	CONCENTRATION	VOLUME	MAXIMUM DOSE
Adult	10 milligrams	NONE	N/A	10 milligrams in 1 ml	1 ml	10 milligrams
11 years	5–10 milligrams	NONE	N/A	10 milligrams in 1 ml	0.5 ml–1 ml	5–10 milligrams
10 years	5–10 milligrams	NONE	N/A	10 milligrams in 1 ml	0.5–1 ml	5–10 milligrams
9 years	5–10 milligrams	NONE	N/A	10 milligrams in 1 ml	0.5–1 ml	5–10 milligrams
8 years	5–10 milligrams	NONE	N/A	10 milligrams in 1 ml	0.5–1 ml	5–10 milligrams
7 years	5–10 milligrams	NONE	N/A	10 milligrams in 1 ml	0.5–1 ml	5–10 milligrams
6 years	5–10 milligrams	NONE	N/A	10 milligrams in 1 ml	0.5–1 ml	5–10 milligrams
5 years	2.5 milligrams	NONE	N/A	10 milligrams in 1 ml	0.25 ml	2.5 milligrams
4 years	2.5 milligrams	NONE	N/A	10 milligrams in 1 ml	0.25 ml	2.5 milligrams
3 years	2.5 milligrams	NONE	N/A	10 milligrams in 1 ml	0.25 ml	2.5 milligrams
2 years	2.5 milligrams	NONE	N/A	10 milligrams in 1 ml	0.25 ml	2.5 milligrams
18 months	2.5 milligrams	NONE	N/A	10 milligrams in 1 ml	0.25 ml	2.5 milligrams
12 months	2.5 milligrams	NONE	N/A	10 milligrams in 1 ml	0.25 ml	2.5 milligrams
9 months	N/A	N/A	N/A	N/A	N/A	N/A
6 months	N/A	N/A	N/A	N/A	N/A	N/A
3 months	N/A	N/A	N/A	N/A	N/A	N/A
1 month	N/A	N/A	N/A	N/A	N/A	N/A
Birth	N/A	N/A	N/A	N/A	N/A	N/A

Section 6 Drugs

Chlorphenamine

Route: Oral (tablet).

AGE	INITIAL DOSE	REPEAT DOSE	DOSE INTERVAL	CONCENTRATION	VOLUME	MAXIMUM DOSE
Adult	4 milligrams	NONE	N/A	4 milligrams per tablet	1 tablet	4 milligrams
11 years	2 milligrams	NONE	N/A	4 milligrams per tablet	$\frac{1}{2}$ of one tablet	2 milligrams
10 years	2 milligrams	NONE	N/A	4 milligrams per tablet	$\frac{1}{2}$ of one tablet	2 milligrams
9 years	2 milligrams	NONE	N/A	4 milligrams per tablet	$\frac{1}{2}$ of one tablet	2 milligrams
8 years	2 milligrams	NONE	N/A	4 milligrams per tablet	$\frac{1}{2}$ of one tablet	2 milligrams
7 years	2 milligrams	NONE	N/A	4 milligrams per tablet	$\frac{1}{2}$ of one tablet	2 milligrams
6 years	2 milligrams	NONE	N/A	4 milligrams per tablet	$\frac{1}{2}$ of one tablet	2 milligrams
5 years	1 milligram	NONE	N/A	4 milligrams per tablet	$\frac{1}{4}$ of one tablet	1 milligram
4 years	1 milligram	NONE	N/A	4 milligrams per tablet	$\frac{1}{4}$ of one tablet	1 milligram
3 years	1 milligram	NONE	N/A	4 milligrams per tablet	$\frac{1}{4}$ of one tablet	1 milligram
2 years	1 milligram	NONE	N/A	4 milligrams per tablet	$\frac{1}{4}$ of one tablet	1 milligram
18 months	1 milligram	NONE	N/A	4 milligrams per tablet	$\frac{1}{4}$ of one tablet	1 milligram
12 months	1 milligram	NONE	N/A	4 milligrams per tablet	$\frac{1}{4}$ of one tablet	1 milligram
9 months	N/A	N/A	N/A	N/A	N/A	N/A
6 months	N/A	N/A	N/A	N/A	N/A	N/A
3 months	N/A	N/A	N/A	N/A	N/A	N/A
1 month	N/A	N/A	N/A	N/A	N/A	N/A
Birth	N/A	N/A	N/A	N/A	N/A	N/A

SECTION **6** Drugs

Chlorphenamine

Route: Oral (solution).

AGE	INITIAL DOSE	REPEAT DOSE	DOSE INTERVAL	CONCENTRATION	VOLUME	MAXIMUM DOSE
Adult	4 milligrams	NONE	N/A	2 milligrams in 5 ml	10 ml	4 milligrams
11 years	2 milligrams	NONE	N/A	2 milligrams in 5 ml	5 ml	2 milligrams
10 years	2 milligrams	NONE	N/A	2 milligrams in 5 ml	5 ml	2 milligrams
9 years	2 milligrams	NONE	N/A	2 milligrams in 5 ml	5 ml	2 milligrams
8 years	2 milligrams	NONE	N/A	2 milligrams in 5 ml	5 ml	2 milligrams
7 years	2 milligrams	NONE	N/A	2 milligrams in 5 ml	5 ml	2 milligrams
6 years	2 milligrams	NONE	N/A	2 milligrams in 5 ml	5 ml	2 milligrams
5 years	1 milligram	NONE	N/A	2 milligrams in 5 ml	2.5 ml	1 milligram
4 years	1 milligram	NONE	N/A	2 milligrams in 5 ml	2.5 ml	1 milligram
3 years	1 milligram	NONE	N/A	2 milligrams in 5 ml	2.5 ml	1 milligram
2 years	1 milligram	NONE	N/A	2 milligrams in 5 ml	2.5 ml	1 milligram
18 months	1 milligram	NONE	N/A	2 milligrams in 5 ml	2.5 ml	1 milligram
12 months	1 milligram	NONE	N/A	2 milligrams in 5 ml	2.5 ml	1 milligram
9 months	N/A	N/A	N/A	N/A	N/A	N/A
6 months	N/A	N/A	N/A	N/A	N/A	N/A
3 months	N/A	N/A	N/A	N/A	N/A	N/A
1 month	N/A	N/A	N/A	N/A	N/A	N/A
Birth	N/A	N/A	N/A	N/A	N/A	N/A

Clopidogrel [845]

Presentation

Tablet containing clopidogrel:

- 75 milligrams
- 300 milligrams.

Indications

Acute ST-elevation myocardial infarction (STEMI):

- In patients not already taking clopidogrel.
- Receiving thrombolytic treatment.
- Anticipated thrombolytic treatment.
- Anticipated primary percutaneous coronary intervention (PPCI).

Actions

Inhibits platelet aggregation.

Contra-Indications

- Known allergy or hypersensitivity to clopidogrel.
- Known severe liver impairment.
- Active pathological bleeding such as peptic ulcer or intracranial haemorrhage.

Cautions

As the likely benefits of a single dose of clopidogrel outweigh the potential risks, clopidogrel may be administered in:

- Pregnancy.
- Patients taking non-steroidal anti-inflammatory drugs (NSAIDs).
- Patients with renal impairment.

Side Effects

- Dyspepsia.
- Abdominal pain.
- Diarrhoea.
- Bleeding (gastrointestinal and intracranial) – the occurrence of severe bleeding is similar to that observed with the administration of aspirin.

Dosage and Administration

Adults aged 18–75 years with acute ST-elevation myocardial infarction (STEMI) receiving thrombolysis or anticipated primary PCI, as per locally agreed STEMI care pathways.

NOTE: To be administered in conjunction with aspirin unless there is a known aspirin allergy or sensitivity (refer to aspirin protocol for administration and dosage).

Route: Oral.

Patient care pathway: Thrombolysis.

AGE	INITIAL DOSE	REPEAT DOSE	DOSE INTERVAL	CONCENTRATION	VOLUME	MAXIMUM DOSE
Adult	300 milligrams	NONE	N/A	75 milligrams per tablet	4 tablets	300 milligrams
Adult	300 milligrams	NONE	N/A	300 milligrams per tablet	1 tablet	300 milligrams

Patient care pathway: Primary percutaneous coronary intervention.

AGE	INITIAL DOSE	REPEAT DOSE	DOSE INTERVAL	CONCENTRATION	VOLUME	MAXIMUM DOSE
Adult	600 milligrams	NONE	N/A	75 milligrams per tablet	8 tablets	600 milligrams
Adult	600 milligrams	NONE	N/A	300 milligrams per tablet	2 tablets	600 milligrams

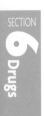

Presentation

Ampoules of **intravenous** preparation 3.8 mg/ml.

Indications

Moderate/severe croup.

Actions

Corticosteroid – reduces subglottic inflammation.

Contra-Indications

Previously diagnosed hypertension.

Systemic infection/sepsis.

Cautions

Upper airway compromise can be worsened by any procedure distressing the child – including the administration of medication and measuring blood pressure.

Side Effects

None.

Additional Information

Additional doses given acutely do not have additional benefits.

Dosage and Administration

Route: Oral.

The intravenous preparation is administered ORALLY.

AGE	INITIAL DOSE	REPEAT DOSE	DOSE INTERVAL	CONCENTRATION	VOLUME	MAXIMUM DOSE
11 years	N/A	N/A	N/A	N/A	N/A	N/A
10 years	N/A	N/A	N/A	N/A	N/A	N/A
9 years	N/A	N/A	N/A	N/A	N/A	N/A
8 years	N/A	N/A	N/A	N/A	N/A	N/A
7 years	N/A	N/A	N/A	N/A	N/A	N/A
6 years	3.8 milligrams	NONE	N/A	3.8 milligrams per ml	1 ml	3.8 milligrams
5 years	3.8 milligrams	NONE	N/A	3.8 milligrams per ml	1 ml	3.8 milligrams
4 years	3.8 milligrams	NONE	N/A	3.8 milligrams per ml	1 ml	3.8 milligrams
3 years	3.8 milligrams	NONE	N/A	3.8 milligrams per ml	1 ml	3.8 milligrams
2 years	3.8 milligrams	NONE	N/A	3.8 milligrams per ml	1 ml	3.8 milligrams
18 months	3.8 milligrams	NONE	N/A	3.8 milligrams per ml	1 ml	3.8 milligrams
12 months	1.9 milligrams	NONE	N/A	3.8 milligrams per ml	0.5 ml	1.9 milligrams
9 months	1.9 milligrams	NONE	N/A	3.8 milligrams per ml	0.5 ml	1.9 milligrams
6 months	1.9 milligrams	NONE	N/A	3.8 milligrams per ml	0.5 ml	1.9 milligrams
3 months	1.9 milligrams	NONE	N/A	3.8 milligrams per ml	0.5 ml	1.9 milligrams
1 month	1.9 milligrams	NONE	N/A	3.8 milligrams per ml	0.5 ml	1.9 milligrams
Birth	N/A	N/A	N/A	N/A	N/A	N/A

Presentation

Ampoule containing 10 milligrams diazepam in an oil-in-water emulsion making up 2 ml.

Rectal tube containing 2.5 milligrams, 5 milligrams or 10 milligrams diazepam.

Indications

Fits longer than 5 minutes and **STILL FITTING.**

Repeated fits – not secondary to an uncorrected hypoxia or hypoglycaemic episode.

Status epilepticus.

Eclamptic fits (initiate treatment if fit lasts >2–3 minutes or if it is recurrent).

Symptomatic cocaine toxicity (severe hypertension, chest pain or fitting).

Actions

Central nervous system depressant, acts as an anticonvulsant and sedative.

Cautions

Respiratory depression.

Should be used with caution if alcohol, antidepressants or other CNS depressants have been taken as side effects are more likely.

Recent doses by carers/relatives should be taken into account when calculating the maximum cumulative dose.

Contra-Indications

None.

Side Effects

Respiratory depression may occur, especially in the presence of alcohol, which enhances the depressive side effect of diazepam. In addition, opioid drugs also enhance the cardiac and respiratory depressive effect of diazepam.

Hypotension may occur. This may be significant if the patient has to be moved from a horizontal position to allow for extrication from an address. Caution should therefore be exercised and consideration given to either removing the patient flat or, if fitting has stopped and it is considered safe, allowing a 10 minute recovery period prior to removal.

Drowsiness and light-headedness, confusion and unsteadiness.

Occasionally amnesia may occur.

Additional Information

The intravenous route is preferred for terminating fits and thus, where IV access can be gained rapidly, this should be the first choice. Early consideration should be given to using the PR route when IV access cannot be rapidly and safely obtained, **which is particularly likely in the case of children.** In small children the PR route should be considered the first choice treatment and IV access sought subsequently.

NB If a **SINGLE** dose of diazepam has been administered via the PR route and IV access is subsequently available, a **SINGLE** dose of IV diazepam may be administered where required.

The earlier the drug is given the more likely the patient is to respond, which is why the rectal route is preferred in children, while the IV route is sought.

Diazepam should only be used if the patient has been fitting for >5 minutes (and is still fitting), or if fits recur in rapid succession without time for full recovery in between. There is no value in giving this drug 'preventatively' if the fit has ceased. **In any clearly sick or ill child, there must be no delay at the scene** while administering the drug, and if it is essential to give diazepam, this should be done en-route to hospital.

Care must be taken when inserting the rectal tube and this should be inserted no more than 2.5 cm in children and 4–5 cm in adults. (All tubes have an insertion marker on nozzle.)

Diazepam

Dosage and Administration

Route: Intravenous/intraosseous – administer **SLOWLY** titrated to response.

AGE	INITIAL DOSE	REPEAT DOSE	DOSE INTERVAL	CONCENTRATION	VOLUME	MAXIMUM DOSE
Adult	10 milligrams	10 milligrams	5 minutes	10 milligrams in 2 ml	2 ml	20 milligrams
11 years	10 milligrams	NONE	N/A	10 milligrams in 2 ml	2 ml	10 milligrams
10 years	10 milligrams	NONE	N/A	10 milligrams in 2 ml	2 ml	10 milligrams
9 years	9 milligrams	NONE	N/A	10 milligrams in 2 ml	1.8 ml	9 milligrams
8 years	8 milligrams	NONE	N/A	10 milligrams in 2 ml	1.6 ml	8 milligrams
7 years	7 milligrams	NONE	N/A	10 milligrams in 2 ml	1.4 ml	7 milligrams
6 years	6.5 milligrams	NONE	N/A	10 milligrams in 2 ml	1.3 ml	6.5 milligrams
5 years	6 milligrams	NONE	N/A	10 milligrams in 2 ml	1.2 ml	6 milligrams
4 years	5 milligrams	NONE	N/A	10 milligrams in 2 ml	1 ml	5 milligrams
3 years	4.5 milligrams	NONE	N/A	10 milligrams in 2 ml	0.9 ml	4.5 milligrams
2 years	3.5 milligrams	NONE	N/A	10 milligrams in 2 ml	0.7 ml	3.5 milligrams
18 months	3.5 milligrams	NONE	N/A	10 milligrams in 2 ml	0.7 ml	3.5 milligrams
12 months	3 milligrams	NONE	N/A	10 milligrams in 2 ml	0.6 ml	3 milligrams
9 months	2.5 milligrams	NONE	N/A	10 milligrams in 2 ml	0.5 ml	2.5 milligrams
6 months	2.5 milligrams	NONE	N/A	10 milligrams in 2 ml	0.5 ml	2.5 milligrams
3 months	2 milligrams	NONE	N/A	10 milligrams in 2 ml	0.4 ml	2 milligrams
1 month	1.5 milligrams	NONE	N/A	10 milligrams in 2 ml	0.3 ml	1.5 milligrams
Birth	1 milligram	NONE	N/A	10 milligrams in 2 ml	0.2 ml	1 milligram

Diazepam

Route: Rectal (smaller dose).[a]

AGE	INITIAL DOSE	REPEAT DOSE	DOSE INTERVAL	CONCENTRATION	RECTAL TUBE	MAXIMUM DOSE
>12 years-Adult	10 milligrams	NONE	N/A	10 milligrams in 2.5 ml	1 × 10 milligram tube	10 milligrams
11 years	5 milligrams	NONE	N/A	5 milligrams in 2.5 ml	1 × 5 milligram tube	5 milligrams
10 years	5 milligrams	NONE	N/A	5 milligrams in 2.5 ml	1 × 5 milligram tube	5 milligrams
9 years	5 milligrams	NONE	N/A	5 milligrams in 2.5 ml	1 × 5 milligram tube	5 milligrams
8 years	5 milligrams	NONE	N/A	5 milligrams in 2.5 ml	1 × 5 milligram tube	5 milligrams
7 years	5 milligrams	NONE	N/A	5 milligrams in 2.5 ml	1 × 5 milligram tube	5 milligrams
6 years	5 milligrams	NONE	N/A	5 milligrams in 2.5 ml	1 × 5 milligram tube	5 milligrams
5 years	5 milligrams	NONE	N/A	5 milligrams in 2.5 ml	1 × 5 milligram tube	5 milligrams
4 years	5 milligrams	NONE	N/A	5 milligrams in 2.5 ml	1 × 5 milligram tube	5 milligrams
3 years	5 milligrams	NONE	N/A	5 milligrams in 2.5 ml	1 × 5 milligram tube	5 milligrams
2 years	5 milligrams	NONE	N/A	5 milligrams in 2.5 ml	1 × 5 milligram tube	5 milligrams
18 months	5 milligrams	NONE	N/A	5 milligrams in 2.5 ml	1 × 5 milligram tube	5 milligrams
12 months	5 milligrams	NONE	N/A	5 milligrams in 2.5 ml	1 × 5 milligram tube	5 milligrams
9 months	5 milligrams	NONE	N/A	5 milligrams in 2.5 ml	1 × 5 milligram tube	5 milligrams
6 months	5 milligrams	NONE	N/A	5 milligrams in 2.5 ml	1 × 5 milligram tube	5 milligrams
3 months	5 milligrams	NONE	N/A	5 milligrams in 2.5 ml	1 × 5 milligram tube	5 milligrams
1 month	5 milligrams	NONE	N/A	5 milligrams in 2.5 ml	1 × 5 milligram tube	5 milligrams
Birth	1.25 milligrams	NONE	N/A	2.5 milligrams in 1.25 ml	$\frac{1}{2}$ × 2.5 milligram tube	1.25 milligrams

NB If a **SINGLE** dose of diazepam has been given by the PR route and IV access is subsequently available, a **SINGLE** dose of IV diazepam may be given where required.

[a] The doses for rectal diazepam show all concentrations as listed in the BNF.

Diazepam

Route: Rectal (larger dose).[a]

AGE	INITIAL DOSE	REPEAT DOSE	DOSE INTERVAL	CONCENTRATION	RECTAL TUBE	MAXIMUM DOSE
>12 years – Adult	20 milligrams	NONE	N/A	10 milligrams in 2.5 ml	2 × 10 milligram tube	20 milligrams
11 years	10 milligrams	NONE	N/A	10 milligrams in 2.5 ml	1 × 10 milligram tube	10 milligrams
10 years	10 milligrams	NONE	N/A	10 milligrams in 2.5 ml	1 × 10 milligram tube	10 milligrams
9 years	10 milligrams	NONE	N/A	10 milligrams in 2.5 ml	1 × 10 milligram tube	10 milligrams
8 years	10 milligrams	NONE	N/A	10 milligrams in 2.5 ml	1 × 10 milligram tube	10 milligrams
7 years	10 milligrams	NONE	N/A	10 milligrams in 2.5 ml	1 × 10 milligram tube	10 milligrams
6 years	10 milligrams	NONE	N/A	10 milligrams in 2.5 ml	1 × 10 milligram tube	10 milligrams
5 years	10 milligrams	NONE	N/A	10 milligrams in 2.5 ml	1 × 10 milligram tube	10 milligrams
4 years	10 milligrams	NONE	N/A	10 milligrams in 2.5 ml	1 × 10 milligram tube	10 milligrams
3 years	10 milligrams	NONE	N/A	10 milligrams in 2.5 ml	1 × 10 milligram tube	10 milligrams
2 years	10 milligrams	NONE	N/A	10 milligrams in 2.5 ml	1 × 10 milligram tube	10 milligrams
12 months	5 milligrams	NONE	N/A	5 milligrams in 2.5 ml	1 × 5 milligram tube	5 milligrams
9 months	5 milligrams	NONE	N/A	5 milligrams in 2.5 ml	1 × 5 milligram tube	5 milligrams
6 months	5 milligrams	NONE	N/A	5 milligrams in 2.5 ml	1 × 5 milligram tube	5 milligrams
3 months	5 milligrams	NONE	N/A	5 milligrams in 2.5 ml	1 × 5 milligram tyube	5 milligrams
1 months	5 milligrams	NONE	N/A	5 milligrams in 2.5 ml	1 × 5 milligram tube	5 milligrams
Birth	2.5 milligrams	NONE	N/A	2.5 milligrams in 1.25 ml	1 × 2.5 milligram tube	2.5 milligrams

NB If a **SINGLE** dose of diazepam has been given by the PR route and IV access is subsequently available, a **SINGLE** dose of IV diazepam may be given where required.

[a] The doses for rectal diazepam show all concentrations as listed in the BNF.

Presentation

Entonox is a combination of nitrous oxide 50% and oxygen 50%. It is stored in medical cylinders that have a blue body with white shoulders.

Indications

Moderate to severe pain.

Labour pains.

Actions

Inhaled analgesic agent.

Contra-Indications

- Severe head injuries with impaired consciousness.
- Decompression sickness (the bends) where entonox can cause nitrogen bubbles within the blood stream to expand, aggravating the problem further. Consider anyone that has been diving within the previous 24 hours to be at risk.
- Violently disturbed psychiatric patients.

Cautions

Any patient at risk of having a pneumothorax, pneumomediastinum and/or a pneumoperitoneum (e.g. polytrauma, penetrating torso injury).

Dosage and Administration

Adults:

- Entonox should be self-administered via a facemask or mouthpiece, after suitable instruction. It takes about **3–5 minutes** to be effective, but it may be **5–10 minutes** before maximum effect is achieved.

Children:

- Entonox is effective in children provided they are capable of following the administration instructions and can activate the demand valve.

Side Effects

Minimal side effects.

Additional Information

Administration of entonox should be in conjunction with pain score monitoring.

Entonox's advantages include:

- Rapid analgesic effect with minimal side effects.
- No cardiorespiratory depression.
- Self-administered.
- Analgesic effect rapidly wears off.
- The 50% oxygen concentration is valuable in many medical and trauma conditions.
- Entonox can be administered whilst preparing to deliver other analgesics.

The usual precautions must be followed with regard to caring for the entonox equipment and the cylinder MUST be inverted several times to mix the gases when temperatures are low.

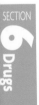

Furosemide [850]

Presentation

Ampoules containing furosemide 50 milligrams in 5 ml.

Ampoules containing furosemide 40 milligrams in 2 ml.

Pre-filled syringe containing furosemide 80 milligrams.

Indications

Pulmonary oedema secondary to left ventricular failure.

Actions

Furosemide is a potent diuretic with a rapid onset (within 30 minutes) and short duration.

Contra-Indications

Pre-comatose state secondary to liver cirrhosis.

Severe renal failure with anuria.

Children under 18 years old.

Cautions

Hypokalaemia (low potassium) could induce arrhythmias.

Pregnancy.

Hypotensive patient.

Side Effects

Hypotension.

Gastrointestinal disturbances.

Additional Information

Glyceryl trinatrate is the first-line treatment for acute pulmonary oedema. Use furosemide secondary to nitrates in the treatment of acute pulmonary oedema where transfer times to hospital are prolonged.

Dosage and Administration

Route: Intravenous – administer **SLOWLY OVER** 2 minutes.

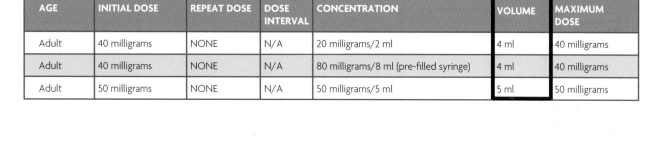

AGE	INITIAL DOSE	REPEAT DOSE	DOSE INTERVAL	CONCENTRATION	VOLUME	MAXIMUM DOSE
Adult	40 milligrams	NONE	N/A	20 milligrams/2 ml	4 ml	40 milligrams
Adult	40 milligrams	NONE	N/A	80 milligrams/8 ml (pre-filled syringe)	4 ml	40 milligrams
Adult	50 milligrams	NONE	N/A	50 milligrams/5 ml	5 ml	50 milligrams

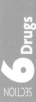

Presentation

Glucagon injection, 1 milligram of powder in vial for reconstitution with water for injection.

Indications

- Hypoglycaemia (blood glucose <4.0 millimoles per litre), especially in known diabetics.
- Clinically suspected hypoglycaemia where oral glucose administration is not possible.
- The unconscious patient, where hypoglycaemia is considered a likely cause.

Actions

Glucagon is a hormone that induces the conversion of glycogen to glucose in the liver, thereby raising blood glucose levels.

Contra-Indications

- Low glycogen stores (e.g. recent use of glucagon).
- Hypoglycaemic seizures – glucose 10% IV is the preferred intervention.

Cautions

Avoid intramuscular administration of any drug when a patient is likely to require thrombolysis.

Side Effects

- Nausea, vomiting.
- Diarrhoea.
- Acute hypersensitivity reaction (rare).
- Hypokalaemia.
- Hypotension.

Additional Information

- Glucagon should NOT be given by IV injection because of increased vomiting associated with IV use.
- Confirm effectiveness by checking blood glucose 5–10 minutes after administration (i.e. blood sugar >5.0 millimoles per litre).
- When treating hypoglycaemia, use all available clinical information to help decide between glucagon IM, glucose 40% oral gel, or glucose 10% IV (see advice below):
  - glucagon is relatively ineffective once body glycogen stores have been exhausted (especially hypoglycaemic, non-diabetic children). In such patients, use oral glucose gel smeared round the mouth or glucose 10% IV as first-line treatments
  - the newborn baby's liver has very limited glycogen stores, so hypoglycaemia may not be effectively treated using intramuscular glucagon (glucagon works by stimulating the liver to convert glycogen into glucose)
  - glucagon may also be ineffective in some instances of alcohol-induced hypoglycaemia
  - consider oral glucose gel or glucose 10% IV as possible alternatives
  - hypoglycaemic patients who fit should **preferably** be given glucose 10% IV.

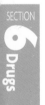

Glucagon (Glucagen)

Dosage and Administration

Route: Intramuscular – antero-lateral aspect of thigh or upper arm.

AGE	INITIAL DOSE	REPEAT DOSE	DOSE INTERVAL	CONCENTRATION	VOLUME	MAXIMUM DOSE
Adult	1 milligram	NONE	N/A	1 milligram per vial	1 vial	1 milligram
11 years	1 milligram	NONE	N/A	1 milligram per vial	1 vial	1 milligram
10 years	1 milligram	NONE	N/A	1 milligram per vial	1 vial	1 milligram
9 years	1 milligram	NONE	N/A	1 milligram per vial	1 vial	1 milligram
8 years	1 milligram	NONE	N/A	1 milligram per vial	1 vial	1 milligram
7 years	500 micrograms	NONE	N/A	1 milligram per vial	0.5 vial	500 micrograms
6 years	500 micrograms	NONE	N/A	1 milligram per vial	0.5 vial	500 micrograms
5 years	500 micrograms	NONE	N/A	1 milligram per vial	0.5 vial	500 micrograms
4 years	500 micrograms	NONE	N/A	1 milligram per vial	0.5 vial	500 micrograms
3 years	500 micrograms	NONE	N/A	1 milligram per vial	0.5 vial	500 micrograms
2 years	500 micrograms	NONE	N/A	1 milligram per vial	0.5 vial	500 micrograms
18 months	500 micrograms	NONE	N/A	1 milligram per vial	0.5 vial	500 micrograms
12 months	500 micrograms	NONE	N/A	1 milligram per vial	0.5 vial	500 micrograms
9 months	500 micrograms	NONE	N/A	1 milligram per vial	0.5 vial	500 micrograms
6 months	500 micrograms	NONE	N/A	1 milligram per vial	0.5 vial	500 micrograms
3 months	500 micrograms	NONE	N/A	1 milligram per vial	0.5 vial	500 micrograms
1 month	500 micrograms	NONE	N/A	1 milligram per vial	0.5 vial	500 micrograms
Birth	100 micrograms	NONE	N/A	1 milligram per vial	0.1 vial	100 micrograms

NB If no response within 10 minutes, administer intravenous glucose – refer to glucose 10% guideline.

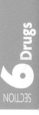

Glucose 10% [853]

Presentation

500 ml pack of 10% glucose solution (50 grams).

Indications

Hypoglycaemia (blood glucose <4.0 millimoles per litre), especially in known diabetics.

Clinically suspected hypoglycaemia where oral glucose administration is not possible.

The unconscious patient, where hypoglycaemia is considered a likely cause.

Actions

Reversal of hypoglycaemia.

Cautions

Administer via a large gauge cannula into a large vein – a 10% concentration of glucose solution is an irritant to veins (especially in extravasation).

Additional Information

When treating hypoglycaemia, use all available clinical information to help decide between glucose 10% IV, glucose 40% oral gel, or glucagon IM.

Side Effects

None.

Contra-Indications

None.

Dosage and Administration

- If the patient has shown no response, the dose may be repeated after 5 minutes.

- If the patient has shown a **PARTIAL** response then a further infusion may be necessary, titrated to response to restore a normal GCS.

- If after the second dose there has been **NO** response, pre-alert and transport rapidly to further care. Consider an alternative diagnosis or the likelihood of a third dose en-route benefiting the patient.

Route: Intravenous infusion.

AGE	INITIAL DOSE	REPEAT DOSE	DOSE INTERVAL	CONCENTRATION	VOLUME	MAXIMUM DOSE
Adult	10 grams	10 grams	5 minutes	50 grams in 500 ml	100 ml	30 grams
11 years	7 grams	7 grams	5 minutes	50 grams in 500 ml	70 ml	21 grams
10 years	6.5 grams	6.5 grams	5 minutes	50 grams in 500 ml	65 ml	19.5 grams
9 years	6 grams	6 grams	5 minutes	50 grams in 500 ml	60 ml	18 grams
8 years	5 grams	5 grams	5 minutes	50 grams in 500 ml	50 ml	15 grams
7 years	5 grams	5 grams	5 minutes	50 grams in 500 ml	50 ml	15 grams
6 years	4 grams	4 grams	5 minutes	50 grams in 500 ml	40 ml	12 grams
5 years	4 grams	4 grams	5 minutes	50 grams in 500 ml	40 ml	12 grams
4 years	3 grams	3 grams	5 minutes	50 grams in 500 ml	30 ml	9 grams
3 years	3 grams	3 grams	5 minutes	50 grams in 500 ml	30 ml	9 grams
2 years	2.5 grams	2.5 grams	5 minutes	50 grams in 500 ml	25 ml	7.5 grams
18 months	2 grams	2 grams	5 minutes	50 grams in 500 ml	20 ml	6 grams
12 months	2 grams	2 grams	5 minutes	50 grams in 500 ml	20 ml	6 grams
9 months	2 grams	2 grams	5 minutes	50 grams in 500 ml	20 ml	6 grams
6 months	1.5 grams	1.5 grams	5 minutes	50 grams in 500 ml	15 ml	4.5 grams
3 months	1 gram	1 gram	5 minutes	50 grams in 500 ml	10 ml	3 grams
1 month	1 gram	1 gram	5 minutes	50 grams in 500 ml	10 ml	3 grams
Birth[a]	0.9 grams	0.9 grams	5 minutes	50 grams in 500 ml	9 ml	2.7 grams

[a] **NB** Neonatal doses are intentionally larger per kilo than those used in older children.

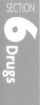

Glucose 40% Oral Gel [853]

GLG

Presentation

Plastic tube containing 25g glucose 40% oral gel.

Indications

Known or suspected hypoglycaemia in a conscious patient where there is no risk of choking or aspiration.

Actions

Rapid increase in blood glucose levels via buccal absorption.

Cautions

Altered consciousness – risk of choking or aspiration (in such circumstances glucose gel can be administered by soaking a gauze swab and placing it between the patient's lip and gum to aid absorption).

Side Effects

None.

Additional Information

Can be repeated as necessary in the hypoglycaemic patient.

Treatment failure should prompt the use of an alternative such as glucagon IM or glucose 10% IV.

(Refer to glucagon guideline or glucose 10% guideline).

Contra-Indications

None.

Dosage and Administration

Route: Buccal – Measure blood glucose level after each dose.

AGE	INITIAL DOSE	REPEAT DOSE	DOSE INTERVAL	CONCENTRATION	VOLUME	MAXIMUM DOSE[a]
Adults	10 grams	10 grams	5 minutes	10 grams in 25 grams of gel	1 tube	No limit
Children ≥12 years	10 grams	10 grams	5 minutes	10 grams in 25 grams of gel	1 tube	No limit
Children <12 years	An appropriate amount should be given, considering the child's age – NB Protect the airway.					

NB Assess more frequently in children who require a smaller dose for a response.

a Consider IM glucagon or IV glucose 10% if no clinical improvement.

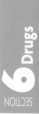

Presentation

Metered dose spray containing 400 micrograms glyceryl trinitrate per dose.

Tablets containing glyceryl trinitrate 2, 3 or 5 milligrams for buccal administration (depends on local ordering).

Indications

Cardiac chest pain due to angina or myocardial infarction.

Acute cardiogenic pulmonary oedema.

Actions

A potent vasodilator drug resulting in:

- Dilatation of coronary arteries/relief of coronary spasm.
- Dilatation of systemic veins resulting in lower pre-load.
- Reduced blood pressure.

Contra-Indications

Hypotension (actual or estimated systolic blood pressure <90 mmHg).

Hypovolaemia.

Head trauma.

Cerebral haemorrhage.

Sildenafil (Viagra) and other related drugs – glyceryl trinitrate must not be given to patients who have taken sildenafil or related drugs within the previous 24 hours. Profound hypotension may occur.

Unconscious patients.

Side Effects

Headache.

Dizziness.

Hypotension.

Dosage and Administration

The oral mucosa must be moist for GTN absorption, moisten if necessary.

Route: Buccal/sub-lingual (spray under the patient's tongue and close mouth).

AGE	INITIAL DOSE	REPEAT DOSE[a]	DOSE INTERVAL	CONCENTRATION	TABLETS	MAXIMUM DOSE[a]
Adult	1–2 spray	1–2 spray	5–10 minutes	400 micrograms per dose spray	400–800 micrograms	No limit
Adult	2 milligrams	2 milligrams	5–10 minutes	2 milligrams per tablet	1 tablet	No limit
Adult	3 milligrams	3 milligrams	5–10 minutes	3 milligrams per tablet	1 tablet	No limit
Adult	5 milligrams	5 milligrams	5–10 minutes	5 milligrams per tablet	1 tablet	No limit

[a] **The effect of the first dose should be assessed over 5 minutes;** further doses can be administered provided the systolic blood pressure is >90 mmHg. Remove the tablet if side effects occur, for example, hypotension.

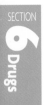

Presentation

An ampoule of unfractionated heparin containing 5,000 units per ml.

Indications

ST-elevation myocardial infarction (STEMI) where heparin is required as adjunctive therapy with reteplase or tenecteplase to reduce the risk of re-infarction.

It is extremely important that the initial bolus dose is given at the earliest opportunity prior to administration of thrombolytic agents and a heparin infusion is commenced immediately on arrival at hospital.

A further intravenous bolus dose of 1,000 units heparin may be required if a heparin infusion **HAS NOT** commenced within 45 minutes of the original bolus of thrombolytic agent.

Actions

Anticoagulant.

Side Effects

Haemorrhage – major or minor.

Contra-Indications

- **Haemophilia and other haemorrhagic disorders.**
- Thrombocytopenia.
- Recent cerebral haemorrhage.
- Severe hypertension.
- Severe liver disease.
- Oesophageal varices.
- Peptic ulcer.
- Major trauma.
- Recent surgery to eye or nervous system.
- Acute bacterial endocarditis.
- Spinal or epidural anaesthesia.

Additional Information

Analysis of MINAP data suggests inadequate anticoagulation following pre-hospital thrombolytic treatment is associated with increased risks of re-infarction.

AT HOSPITAL it is essential that the care of the patient is handed over as soon as possible to a member of hospital staff qualified to administer the second bolus (if not already given) and commence a heparin infusion.

Dosage and Administration

Heparin dosage when administered with **RETEPLASE.**

Route: Intravenous single bolus unfractionated heparin.

AGE	INITIAL DOSE	REPEAT DOSE	DOSE INTERVAL	CONCENTRATION	VOLUME	MAXIMUM DOSE
≥18	5,000 units	ªSee footnote	N/A	5,000 units/ml	1 ml	5,000 units

ª A further intravenous bolus dose of 1,000 units heparin may be required if a heparin infusion **HAS NOT** commenced within 45 minutes of the original bolus of thrombolytic agent.

Heparin dosage when administered with **TENECTEPLASE.**

AGE	WEIGHT	INITIAL DOSE	REPEAT DOSE	DOSE INTERVAL	CONCENTRATION	VOLUME	MAXIMUM DOSE
≥18	<67 kg	4,000 units	ªSee footnote	N/A	5,000 units/ml	0.8 ml	4,000 units
≥18	≥67 kg	5,000 units	ªSee footnote	N/A	5,000 units/ml	1 ml	5,000 units

ª A further intravenous bolus dose of 1,000 units heparin may be required if a heparin infusion **HAS NOT** commenced within 45 minutes of the original bolus of thrombolytic agent.

SECTION **6** Drugs

Hydrocortisone [856]

Presentation

An ampoule containing 100 milligrams hydrocortisone as either sodium succinate or sodium phosphate in 1 ml.

An ampoule containing 100 milligrams hydrocortisone sodium succinate for reconstitution with up to 2 ml of water.

Indications

Severe or life-threatening asthma.

Anaphylaxis.

Adrenal crisis (including Addisonian crisis) – sudden severe deficiency of steroids (occurs in patients on long-term steroid therapy for whatever reason) producing circulatory collapse with or without hypoglycaemia. Administer hydrocortisone to:

1. Patients in an established adrenal crisis.
2. Steroid-dependent patients who have become unwell to prevent them having an adrenal crisis – if in doubt, it is better to administer hydrocortisone.

Actions

Glucocorticoid drug that reduces inflammation and suppresses the immune response.

Contra-Indications

Known allergy (which will be to the sodium succinate or sodium phosphate rather than the hydrocortisone itself).

Cautions

None relevant to a single dose.

Avoid intramuscular administration if patient likely to require thrombolysis.

Side Effects

Sodium phosphate may cause burning or itching sensation in the groin if administered too quickly.

Dosage and Administration

1. **Asthma and adrenal crisis.** NB If there is any doubt about previous steroid administration, it is better to administer hydrocortisone.

Route: Intravenous (**SLOW** injection over a minimum of 2 minutes to avoid side effects)/intraosseous OR intramuscular (when IV access is impossible).

AGE	INITIAL DOSE	REPEAT DOSE	DOSE INTERVAL	CONCENTRATION	VOLUME	MAXIMUM DOSE
Adult	100 milligrams	NONE	N/A	100 milligrams in 1 ml	1 ml	100 milligrams
11 years	100 milligrams	NONE	N/A	100 milligrams in 1 ml	1 ml	100 milligrams
10 years	100 milligrams	NONE	N/A	100 milligrams in 1 ml	1 ml	100 milligrams
9 years	100 milligrams	NONE	N/A	100 milligrams in 1 ml	1 ml	100 milligrams
8 years	100 milligrams	NONE	N/A	100 milligrams in 1 ml	1 ml	100 milligrams
7 years	100 milligrams	NONE	N/A	100 milligrams in 1 ml	1 ml	100 milligrams
6 years	100 milligrams	NONE	N/A	100 milligrams in 1 ml	1 ml	100 milligrams
5 years	50 milligrams	NONE	N/A	100 milligrams in 1 ml	0.5 ml	50 milligrams
4 years	50 milligrams	NONE	N/A	100 milligrams in 1 ml	0.5 ml	50 milligrams
3 years	50 milligrams	NONE	N/A	100 milligrams in 1 ml	0.5 ml	50 milligrams
2 years	50 milligrams	NONE	N/A	100 milligrams in 1 ml	0.5 ml	50 milligrams
18 months	50 milligrams	NONE	N/A	100 milligrams in 1 ml	0.5 ml	50 milligrams
12 months	50 milligrams	NONE	N/A	100 milligrams in 1 ml	0.5 ml	50 milligrams
9 months	50 milligrams	NONE	N/A	100 milligrams in 1 ml	0.5 ml	50 milligrams
6 months	50 milligrams	NONE	N/A	100 milligrams in 1 ml	0.5 ml	50 milligrams
3 months	25 milligrams	NONE	N/A	100 milligrams in 1 ml	0.25 ml	25 milligrams
1 month	25 milligrams	NONE	N/A	100 milligrams in 1 ml	0.25 ml	25 milligrams
Birth	10 milligrams	NONE	N/A	100 milligrams in 1 ml	0.1 ml	10 milligrams

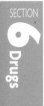

Hydrocortisone

Route: Intravenous (**SLOW** injection over a minimum of 2 minutes to avoid side effects)/intraosseous OR intramuscular (when IV access is impossible).

AGE	INITIAL DOSE	REPEAT DOSE	DOSE INTERVAL	CONCENTRATION	VOLUME	MAXIMUM DOSE
Adult	100 milligrams	NONE	N/A	100 milligrams in 2 ml	2 ml	100 milligrams
11 years	100 milligrams	NONE	N/A	100 milligrams in 2 ml	2 ml	100 milligrams
10 years	100 milligrams	NONE	N/A	100 milligrams in 2 ml	2 ml	100 milligrams
9 years	100 milligrams	NONE	N/A	100 milligrams in 2 ml	2 ml	100 milligrams
8 years	100 milligrams	NONE	N/A	100 milligrams in 2 ml	2 ml	100 milligrams
7 years	100 milligrams	NONE	N/A	100 milligrams in 2 ml	2 ml	100 milligrams
6 years	100 milligrams	NONE	N/A	100 milligrams in 2 ml	2 ml	100 milligrams
5 years	50 milligrams	NONE	N/A	100 milligrams in 2 ml	1 ml	50 milligrams
4 years	50 milligrams	NONE	N/A	100 milligrams in 2 ml	1 ml	50 milligrams
3 years	50 milligrams	NONE	N/A	100 milligrams in 2 ml	1 ml	50 milligrams
2 years	50 milligrams	NONE	N/A	100 milligrams in 2 ml	1 ml	50 milligrams
18 months	50 milligrams	NONE	N/A	100 milligrams in 2 ml	1 ml	50 milligrams
12 months	50 milligrams	NONE	N/A	100 milligrams in 2 ml	1 ml	50 milligrams
9 months	50 milligrams	NONE	N/A	100 milligrams in 2 ml	1 ml	50 milligrams
6 months	50 milligrams	NONE	N/A	100 milligrams in 2 ml	1 ml	50 milligrams
3 months	25 milligrams	NONE	N/A	100 milligrams in 2 ml	0.5 ml	25 milligrams
1 month	25 milligrams	NONE	N/A	100 milligrams in 2 ml	0.5 ml	25 milligrams
Birth	10 milligrams	NONE	N/A	100 milligrams in 2 ml	0.2 ml	10 milligrams

2. **Anaphylaxis**

Route: Intravenous (**SLOW** injection over a minimum of 2 minutes to avoid side effects)/intraosseous OR intramuscular (when IV access is impossible).

AGE	INITIAL DOSE	REPEAT DOSE	DOSE INTERVAL	CONCENTRATION	VOLUME	MAXIMUM DOSE
Adult	200 milligrams	NONE	N/A	100 milligrams in 1 ml	2 ml	200 milligrams
11 years	100 milligrams	NONE	N/A	100 milligrams in 1 ml	1 ml	100 milligrams
10 years	100 milligrams	NONE	N/A	100 milligrams in 1 ml	1 ml	100 milligrams
9 years	100 milligrams	NONE	N/A	100 milligrams in 1 ml	1 ml	100 milligrams
8 years	100 milligrams	NONE	N/A	100 milligrams in 1 ml	1 ml	100 milligrams
7 years	100 milligrams	NONE	N/A	100 milligrams in 1 ml	1 ml	100 milligrams
6 years	100 milligrams	NONE	N/A	100 milligrams in 1 ml	1 ml	100 milligrams
5 years	50 milligrams	NONE	N/A	100 milligrams in 1 ml	0.5 ml	50 milligrams
4 years	50 milligrams	NONE	N/A	100 milligrams in 1 ml	0.5 ml	50 milligrams
3 years	50 milligrams	NONE	N/A	100 milligrams in 1 ml	0.5 ml	50 milligrams
2 years	50 milligrams	NONE	N/A	100 milligrams in 1 ml	0.5 ml	50 milligrams
18 months	50 milligrams	NONE	N/A	100 milligrams in 1 ml	0.5 ml	50 milligrams
12 months	50 milligrams	NONE	N/A	100 milligrams in 1 ml	0.5 ml	50 milligrams
9 months	50 milligrams	NONE	N/A	100 milligrams in 1 ml	0.5 ml	50 milligrams
6 months	50 milligrams	NONE	N/A	100 milligrams in 1 ml	0.5 ml	50 milligrams
3 months	25 milligrams	NONE	N/A	100 milligrams in 1 ml	0.25 ml	25 milligrams
1 month	25 milligrams	NONE	N/A	100 milligrams in 1 ml	0.25 ml	25 milligrams
Birth	10 milligrams	NONE	N/A	100 milligrams in 1 ml	0.1 ml	10 milligrams

SECTION **6** Drugs

Hydrocortisone

Route: Intravenous (**SLOW** injection over a minimum of 2 minutes to avoid side effects)/intraosseous OR intramuscular (when IV access is impossible).

AGE	INITIAL DOSE	REPEAT DOSE	DOSE INTERVAL	CONCENTRATION	VOLUME	MAXIMUM DOSE
Adult	200 milligrams	NONE	N/A	100 milligrams in 2 ml	4 ml	200 milligrams
11 years	100 milligrams	NONE	N/A	100 milligrams in 2 ml	2 ml	100 milligrams
10 years	100 milligrams	NONE	N/A	100 milligrams in 2 ml	2 ml	100 milligrams
9 years	100 milligrams	NONE	N/A	100 milligrams in 2 ml	2 ml	100 milligrams
8 years	100 milligrams	NONE	N/A	100 milligrams in 2 ml	2 ml	100 milligrams
7 years	100 milligrams	NONE	N/A	100 milligrams in 2 ml	2 ml	100 milligrams
6 years	100 milligrams	NONE	N/A	100 milligrams in 2 ml	2 ml	100 milligrams
5 years	50 milligrams	NONE	N/A	100 milligrams in 2 ml	1 ml	50 milligrams
4 years	50 milligrams	NONE	N/A	100 milligrams in 2 ml	1 ml	50 milligrams
3 years	50 milligrams	NONE	N/A	100 milligrams in 2 ml	1 ml	50 milligrams
2 years	50 milligrams	NONE	N/A	100 milligrams in 2 ml	1 ml	50 milligrams
18 months	50 milligrams	NONE	N/A	100 milligrams in 2 ml	1 ml	50 milligrams
12 months	50 milligrams	NONE	N/A	100 milligrams in 2 ml	1 ml	50 milligrams
9 months	50 milligrams	NONE	N/A	100 milligrams in 2 ml	1 ml	50 milligrams
6 months	50 milligrams	NONE	N/A	100 milligrams in 2 ml	1 ml	50 milligrams
3 months	25 milligrams	NONE	N/A	100 milligrams in 2 ml	0.5 ml	25 milligrams
1 month	25 milligrams	NONE	N/A	100 milligrams in 2 ml	0.5 ml	25 milligrams
Birth	10 milligrams	NONE	N/A	100 milligrams in 2 ml	0.2 ml	10 milligrams

Ibuprofen [857]

Presentation

Solution or suspension containing ibuprofen 100 milligrams in 5 ml.

Tablet containing 200 milligrams or 400 milligrams.

Indications

Relief of mild to moderate pain and/or high temperature.

Soft tissue injuries.

Best when used as part of a balanced analgesic regimen.

Actions

Analgesic (relieves pain).

Antipyretic (reduces temperature).

Anti-inflammatory (reduces inflammation).

Contra-Indications

Do **NOT** administer if the patient is:

● Dehydrated.

● Hypovolaemic.

● Known to have renal insufficiency.

● Suffering active upper gastrointestinal disturbance (e.g. oesophagitis, peptic ulcer, dyspepsia).

● Pregnant.

Avoid giving further non-steroidal anti-inflammatory drugs (NSAIDs) (i.e. ibuprofen), if an NSAID containing product (e.g. diclofenac, naproxen) has been used within the previous 4 hours or if the maximum cumulative daily dose has already been given.

Cautions

Asthma: Use cautiously in asthmatic patients due to the possible risk of hypersensitivity and bronchoconstriction. If an asthmatic has not used NSAIDs previously, do not use acutely in the pre-hospital setting.

Elderly: Exercise caution in older patients (>65 years old) that have not used and tolerated NSAIDs recently.

Side Effects

May cause nausea, vomiting and tinnitus.

SECTION
6
Drugs

Dosage and Administration

Route: Oral.

AGE	INITIAL DOSE	REPEAT DOSE	DOSE INTERVAL	CONCENTRATION	VOLUME	MAXIMUM DOSE
12 years – Adult	400 milligrams	400 milligrams	8 hours	Various	Varies	1.2 grams per 24 hours
11 years	300 milligrams	300 milligrams	8 hours	100 milligrams in 5 ml	15 ml	900 milligrams per 24 hours
10 years	300 milligrams	300 milligrams	8 hours	100 milligrams in 5 ml	15 ml	900 milligrams per 24 hours
9 years	200 milligrams	200 milligrams	8 hours	100 milligrams in 5 ml	10 ml	600 milligrams per 24 hours
8 years	200 milligrams	200 milligrams	8 hours	100 milligrams in 5 ml	10 ml	600 milligrams per 24 hours
7 years	200 milligrams	200 milligrams	8 hours	100 milligrams in 5 ml	10 ml	600 milligrams per 24 hours
6 years	150 milligrams	150 milligrams	8 hours	100 milligrams in 5 ml	7.5 ml	450 milligrams per 24 hours
5 years	150 milligrams	150 milligrams	8 hours	100 milligrams in 5 ml	7.5 ml	450 milligrams per 24 hours
4 years	150 milligrams	150 milligrams	8 hours	100 milligrams in 5 ml	7.5 ml	450 milligrams per 24 hours
3 years	100 milligrams	100 milligrams	8 hours	100 milligrams in 5 ml	5 ml	300 milligrams per 24 hours
2 years	100 milligrams	100 milligrams	8 hours	100 milligrams in 5 ml	5 ml	300 milligrams per 24 hours
18 months	100 milligrams	100 milligrams	8 hours	100 milligrams in 5 ml	5 ml	300 milligrams per 24 hours
12 months	100 milligrams	100 milligrams	8 hours	100 milligrams in 5 ml	5 ml	300 milligrams per 24 hours
9 months	50 milligrams	50 milligrams	8 hours	100 milligrams in 5 ml	2.5 ml	150 milligrams per 24 hours
6 months	50 milligrams	50 milligrams	8 hours	100 milligrams in 5 ml	2.5 ml	150 milligrams per 24 hours
3 months	50 milligrams	50 milligrams	8 hours	100 milligrams in 5 ml	2.5 ml	150 milligrams per 24 hours
1 month	N/A	N/A	N/A	N/A	N/A	N/A
Birth	N/A	N/A	N/A	N/A	N/A	N/A

NB

- Combinations of both paracetamol and ibuprofen should not be given together. Only consider alternating these agents if the distress persists or recurs before the next dose is due.
- Given up to 3 times a day, preferably following food.

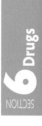

Presentation

Nebules containing ipratropium bromide 250 micrograms in 1 ml or 500 micrograms in 2 ml.

Indications

Acute severe or life-threatening asthma.

Acute asthma unresponsive to salbutamol.

Exacerbation of chronic obstructive pulmonary disease (COPD), unresponsive to salbutamol.

Actions

1. Ipratropium bromide is an antimuscarinic bronchodilator drug. It may provide short-term relief in acute asthma, but beta2 agonists (such as salbutamol) generally work more quickly.
2. Ipratropium is considered of greater benefit in:
   a. children suffering acute asthma
   b. adults suffering with COPD.

Contra-Indications

None in the emergency situation.

Cautions

Ipratropium should be used with care in patients with:

- Glaucoma (protect the eyes from mist).
- Pregnancy and breastfeeding.
- Prostatic hyperplasia.

If COPD is a possibility limit nebulisation to 6 minutes.

Side Effects

Nausea.

Dry mouth (common).

Tachycardia/arrhythmia.

Paroxysmal tightness of the chest.

Allergic reaction.

Dosage and Administration

- **In life-threatening or acute severe asthma:** undertake a **TIME CRITICAL** transfer to the **NEAREST SUITABLE RECEIVING HOSPITAL** and provide nebulisation en-route.

- If COPD is a possibility limit nebulisation to 6 minutes.

Route: Nebuliser with 6–8 litres per minute oxygen (refer to oxygen guideline).

AGE	INITIAL DOSE	REPEAT DOSE	DOSE INTERVAL	CONCENTRATION	VOLUME	MAXIMUM DOSE
Adult	500 micrograms	NONE	N/A	250 micrograms in 1 ml	2 ml	500 micrograms
11 years	250 micrograms	NONE	N/A	250 micrograms in 1 ml	1 ml	250 micrograms
10 years	250 micrograms	NONE	N/A	250 micrograms in 1 ml	1 ml	250 micrograms
9 years	250 micrograms	NONE	N/A	250 micrograms in 1 ml	1 ml	250 micrograms
8 years	250 micrograms	NONE	N/A	250 micrograms in 1 ml	1 ml	250 micrograms
7 years	250 micrograms	NONE	N/A	250 micrograms in 1 ml	1 ml	250 micrograms
6 years	250 micrograms	NONE	N/A	250 micrograms in 1 ml	1 ml	250 micrograms
5 years	250 micrograms	NONE	N/A	250 micrograms in 1 ml	1 ml	250 micrograms
4 years	250 micrograms	NONE	N/A	250 micrograms in 1 ml	1 ml	250 micrograms
3 years	250 micrograms	NONE	N/A	250 micrograms in 1 ml	1 ml	250 micrograms
2 years	250 micrograms	NONE	N/A	250 micrograms in 1 ml	1 ml	250 micrograms
18 months	250 micrograms	NONE	N/A	250 micrograms in 1 ml	1 ml	250 micrograms
12 months	125–250 micrograms	NONE	N/A	250 micrograms in 1 ml	0.5 ml–1 ml	125–250 micrograms
9 months	125–250 micrograms	NONE	N/A	250 micrograms in 1 ml	0.5 ml–1 ml	125–250 micrograms
6 months	125–250 micrograms	NONE	N/A	250 micrograms in 1 ml	0.5 ml–1 ml	125–250 micrograms
3 months	125–250 micrograms	NONE	N/A	250 micrograms in 1 ml	0.5 ml–1 ml	125–250 micrograms
1 month	125–250 micrograms	NONE	N/A	250 micrograms in 1 ml	0.5 ml–1 ml	125–250 micrograms
Birth	N/A	N/A	N/A	N/A	N/A	N/A

SECTION

6

Drugs

Ipratropium Bromide (Atrovent)

Route: Nebuliser with 6–8 litres per minute oxygen (refer to oxygen guideline).

AGE	INITIAL DOSE	REPEAT DOSE	DOSE INTERVAL	CONCENTRATION	VOLUME	MAXIMUM DOSE
Adult	500 micrograms	NONE	N/A	500 micrograms in 2 ml	2 ml	500 micrograms
11 years	250 micrograms	NONE	N/A	500 micrograms in 2 ml	1 ml	250 micrograms
10 years	250 micrograms	NONE	N/A	500 micrograms in 2 ml	1 ml	250 micrograms
9 years	250 micrograms	NONE	N/A	500 micrograms in 2 ml	1 ml	250 micrograms
8 years	250 micrograms	NONE	N/A	500 micrograms in 2 ml	1 ml	250 micrograms
7 years	250 micrograms	NONE	N/A	500 micrograms in 2 ml	1 ml	250 micrograms
6 years	250 micrograms	NONE	N/A	500 micrograms in 2 ml	1 ml	250 micrograms
5 years	250 micrograms	NONE	N/A	500 micrograms in 2 ml	1 ml	250 micrograms
4 years	250 micrograms	NONE	N/A	500 micrograms in 2 ml	1 ml	250 micrograms
3 years	250 micrograms	NONE	N/A	500 micrograms in 2 ml	1 ml	250 micrograms
2 years	250 micrograms	NONE	N/A	500 micrograms in 2 ml	1 ml	250 micrograms
18 months	250 micrograms	NONE	N/A	500 micrograms in 2 ml	1 ml	250 micrograms
12 months	125–250 micrograms	NONE	N/A	500 micrograms in 2 ml	0.5 ml–1 ml	125–250 micrograms
9 months	125–250 micrograms	NONE	N/A	500 micrograms in 2 ml	0.5 ml–1 ml	125–250 micrograms
6 months	125–250 micrograms	NONE	N/A	500 micrograms in 2 ml	0.5 ml–1 ml	125–250 micrograms
3 months	125–250 micrograms	NONE	N/A	500 micrograms in 2 ml	0.5 ml–1 ml	125–250 micrograms
1 month	125–250 micrograms	NONE	N/A	500 micrograms in 2 ml	0.5 ml–1 ml	125–250 micrograms
Birth	N/A	N/A	N/A	N/A	N/A	N/A

Presentation

Ampoule containing metoclopramide 10 milligrams in 2 ml.

Indications

The treatment of nausea or vomiting in adults aged 20 and over.

Prevention and treatment of nausea and vomiting following administration of morphine sulphate.

Actions

An anti-emetic which acts centrally as well as on the gastrointestinal tract.

Contra-Indications

- Age less than 20 years.
- Renal failure.
- Phaeochromocytoma.
- Gastrointestinal obstruction.
- Perforation/haemorrhage/3–4 days after GI surgery.
- Cases of drug overdose.

Cautions

If patient is likely to require thrombolysis then intramuscular administration of any drug should be avoided.

Side Effects

Severe extra-pyramidal effects are more common in children and young adults.

- Drowsiness and restlessness.
- Cardiac conduction abnormalities following IV administration.
- Diarrhoea.
- Rash.

Additional Information

Metoclopramide should always be given in a separate syringe to morphine sulphate. The drugs must not be mixed.

Dosage and Administration

Route: Intravenous – administer over 2 minutes.

AGE	INITIAL DOSE	REPEAT DOSE	DOSE INTERVAL	CONCENTRATION	VOLUME	MAXIMUM DOSE
Adult	10 milligrams	NONE	N/A	10 milligrams in 2 ml	2 ml	10 milligrams

NB Monitor pulse, blood pressure, respiratory rate and cardiac rhythm before, during and after administration.

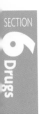

Midazolam

Presentation

Ampoule containing Midazolam 5 mg in 5 ml (1 mg/ml)

Oromucosal (Buccal) solutions are available as 4 different pre-filled syringes (2.5 mg, 5 mg, 7.5 mg and 10 mg respectively), all with a concentration of 5 milligrams in 1 ml – take care to ensure the correct milligram dose is given.

Indications

Convulsion lasting 5 minutes or more and STILL FITTING.

Three or more focal or generalised convulsions in an hour.

Convulsion continuing 10 minutes after first dose of medication.

Traumatic brain injury with combativeness or agitation where sedation is required to facilitate effective oxygenation.

Actions

Benzodiazepine derivative.

Onset of action within 2 minutes with peak effect at 5–10 mins.

Short acting with sedative effect decreasing from 15 minutes onwards.

There is a large variability in how sensitive patients are to the sedative effects of Midazolam so when used for sedation the dose needs to be titrated according to response taking into account time taken to reach peak effect.

Cautions

Rapid administration can lead to respiratory depression leading to respiratory arrest. Susceptible patients are children, adults over 60yrs, chronic illness (renal, hepatic or cardiac).

Under the age of 6 months, infants are more prone to midazolam drug accumulation (due to hepatic immaturity) and therefore at greater risk of respiratory depression.

Enhanced side effects when alcohol or other sedative drugs are present.

Contra-indications

None.

Side effects

- Respiratory depression.
- Hypotension.
- Reduced level of consciousness leading to impaired airway control.
- Confusion leading to increased agitation.
- Amnesia in some patients.

Additional Information

When administered for convulsions in known epileptic patients ask/look to see if the patient has an individualised treatment plan or an Epilepsy Passport. Aim to follow patient's own treatment plan when possible and effective.

Carefully monitor vital signs for delayed respiratory or cardiovascular side effects as the effect of the Midazolam and other drugs such as rectal diazepam reach a peak effect.

When used for sedation ensure that any reversible factors contributing to the agitation such as hypoxia, hypovolaemia, hypoglycaemia are assessed and treated.

Dosage and Administration

Convulsions

Route: Intravenous/intra-osseous.

AGE	INITIAL DOSE	REPEAT DOSE	DOSE INTERVAL	CONCENTRATION	VOLUME	MAXIMUM DOSE
Adult (17 years and over)	2 milligrams	2 milligrams	2 mins	1 milligram in 1 ml	2 ml	10 milligrams
0–16 years	N/A	N/A	N/A	N/A	N/A	N/A

Midazolam

Convulsions

Route: Buccal.

AGE	INITIAL DOSE	REPEAT DOSE	DOSE INTERVAL	CONCENTRATION	VOLUME	MAXIMUM DOSE
Adult	10 milligrams	10 milligrams	10 mins	5 milligrams in 1 ml	2 ml pre-filled syringe	20 milligrams
11 years	10 milligrams	10 milligrams	10 mins	5 milligrams in 1 ml	2 ml pre-filled syringe	20 milligrams
10 years	10 milligrams	10 milligrams	10 mins	5 milligrams in 1 ml	2 ml pre-filled syringe	20 milligrams
9 years	7.5 milligrams	7.5 milligrams	10 mins	5 milligrams in 1 ml	1.5 ml pre-filled syringe	15 milligrams
8 years	7.5 milligrams	7.5 milligrams	10 mins	5 milligrams in 1 ml	1.5 ml pre-filled syringe	15 milligrams
7 years	7.5 milligrams	7.5 milligrams	10 mins	5 milligrams in 1 ml	1.5 ml pre-filled syringe	15 milligrams
6 years	7.5 milligrams	7.5 milligrams	10 mins	5 milligrams in 1 ml	1.5 ml pre-filled syringe	15 milligrams
5 years	7.5 milligrams	7.5 milligrams	10 mins	5 milligrams in 1 ml	1.5 ml pre-filled syringe	15 milligrams
4 years	5 milligrams	5 milligrams	10 mins	5 milligrams in 1 ml	1 ml pre-filled syringe	10 milligrams
3 years	5 milligrams	5 milligrams	10 mins	5 milligrams in 1 ml	1 ml pre-filled syringe	10 milligrams
2 years	5 milligrams	5 milligrams	10 mins	5 milligrams in 1 ml	1 ml pre-filled syringe	10 milligrams
18 months	5 milligrams	5 milligrams	10 mins	5 milligrams in 1 ml	1 ml pre-filled syringe	10 milligrams
12 months	5 milligrams	5 milligrams	10 mins	5 milligrams in 1 ml	1 ml pre-filled syringe	10 milligrams
9 months	2.5 milligrams	2.5 milligrams	10 mins	5 milligrams in 1 ml	0.5 ml pre-filled syringe	5 milligrams
6 months	2.5 milligrams	2.5 milligrams	10 mins	5 milligrams in 1 ml	0.5 ml pre-filled syringe	5 milligrams
3 months	See Epilepsy Passport	See Epilepsy Passport	10 mins	5 milligrams in 1 ml	See Epilepsy Passport	See Epilepsy Passport
1 month	See Epilepsy Passport	See Epilepsy Passport	10 mins	5 milligrams in 1 ml	See Epilepsy Passport	See Epilepsy Passport
Birth	See Epilepsy Passport	See Epilepsy Passport	10 mins	5 milligrams in 1 ml	See Epilepsy Passport	See Epilepsy Passport

Sedation

Route: Intravenous/intra-osseous – administer **SLOWLY** titrated to response.

AGE	INITIAL DOSE	REPEAT DOSE	DOSE INTERVAL	CONCENTRATION	VOLUME	MAXIMUM DOSE
Adult <60yrs	0.5–1 milligrams	0.5–1 milligram	2 mins	1 milligram in 1 ml	0.5–1 ml	7.5 milligrams
Adult >60yrs	0.5–1 milligrams	0.5–1 milligram	2 mins	1 milligram in 1 ml	0.5–1 ml	3.5 milligrams
0–18 years	N/A	N/A	N/A	N/A	N/A	N/A

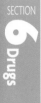

Presentation

Buccolam oromucosal solution (concentration 5 milligrams in 1 millilitre) comes in 4 pre-filled syringes containing either 2.5 mg, 5 mg, 7.5 mg or 10 mg respectively. The child's Individualised Treatment Plan/ 'Epilepsy passport' should specify the correct prescribed dose for that child.

Indications

Buccal midazolam can be used as an anticonvulsant for generalised **convulsions** lasting **more than 5 minutes,** as they may not stop spontaneously.

Ambulance paramedics and technicians can administer the patient's own prescribed midazolam provided they are competent to administer buccal medication and are familiar with midazolam's indications, actions and side effects. Those that are not familiar with the use of this medication should use rectal (PR) or intravenous (IV) diazepam instead.

NB If the convulsion is continuing 10 minutes after this first anticonvulsant, one dose of an intravenous or intra-osseous anticonvulsant should be given e.g. diazepam IV/IO (refer to diazepam guideline).

Where a generalised convulsion continues 10 minutes after the second anticonvulsant, senior medical advice should be sought.

Contra-indications

None.

Actions

Midazolam has a sedative action similar to that of diazepam but of shorter duration. The onset of action usually occurs within 5 minutes, but is dependent on the route of administration. In 80% of episodes convulsions have stopped after 10 minutes.

Side Effects

The side effects of buccal midazolam are similar in effect to IV administration, although the timings may differ:

● Respiratory depression.

● Hypotension.

● Drowsiness.

● Muscle weakness.

● Slurred speech.

● Occasionally agitation, restlessness and disorientation may occur.

Additional Information

● **Midazolam is a benzodiazepine drug, which is now being administered by carers to treat convulsions as an alternative to rectal diazepam.**

● Some patients may have a Patient Specific Direction (PSD) drawn up by their specialist, customised to the specific nature of their convulsions. This is especially true of patients with learning disabilities living in residential care homes. Whenever possible check with the carers for the existence of a PSD for the patient, as this will normally give further guidance on treatment and when the patient should be further assessed.

Dosage and Administration

Route: buccal (administered by carers).

Dosage – individual tailored dose as per the patient's individualised treatment plan.

Administration

The required dose is drawn up and divided equally between each side of the lower buccal cavity (between the cheek and gum).

NB If a generalised convulsion continues 10 minutes after the second dose, senior medical advice should be sought.

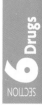

Presentation

Tablet containing misoprostol:

- 200 micrograms.

Indications

Post-partum haemorrhage within 24 hours of delivery of the infant where bleeding from the uterus is uncontrollable by uterine massage.

Miscarriage with life-threatening bleeding and a confirmed diagnosis (e.g. where a patient has gone home with medical management and starts to bleed).

Both syntometrine and ergometrine are contra-indicated in hypertension (BP >140/90); in this case misoprostol (or preferably syntocinon if available) should be administered instead.

In all other circumstances misoprostol should only be used if syntometrine or other oxytocics are unavailable or if they have been ineffective at reducing haemorrhage after 15 mins.

Actions

Stimulates contraction of the uterus.

Onset of action 7–10 minutes.

Contra-Indications

- Known hypersensitivity to misoprostol.
- Active labour.
- Possible multiple pregnancy/known or suspected fetus in utero.

Side Effects

- Abdominal pain.
- Nausea and vomiting.
- Diarrhoea.
- Pyrexia.
- Shivering.

Additional Information

Syntometrine and misoprostol reduce bleeding from a pregnant uterus through different pathways; therefore if one drug has not been effective after 15 mins, the other may be administered in addition.

Dosage and Administration

- Administer orally unless the patient is unable to swallow.
- The vaginal route is not appropriate in post-partum haemorrhage.

Route: Oral.

AGE	INITIAL DOSE	REPEAT DOSE	DOSE INTERVAL	CONCENTRATION	TABLETS	MAXIMUM DOSE
Adult	600 micrograms	None	N/A	200 micrograms per tablet	3 tablets	600 micrograms

Route: Rectal.

NB At the time of publication there is no rectal preparation of misoprostol – therefore the same tablets can be administered orally or rectally.

AGE	INITIAL DOSE	REPEAT DOSE	DOSE INTERVAL	CONCENTRATION	TABLETS	MAXIMUM DOSE
Adult	1 mg	None	N/A	200 micrograms per tablet	5 tablets	1 mg

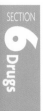

SECTION 6 Drugs

Presentation

Parenteral – ampoules containing morphine sulphate 10 milligrams in 1 ml.

Oral – vials containing morphine sulphate 10 milligrams in 5 ml.

Indications

Pain associated with suspected myocardial infarction (analgesic of first choice).

Severe pain as a component of a balanced analgesia regimen.

The decision about which analgesia and which route should be guided by clinical judgement (**refer to adult and child pain management guidelines**).

Actions

Morphine is a strong opioid analgesic. It is particularly useful for treating continuous, severe musculoskeletal and soft tissue pain.

Morphine produces sedation, euphoria and analgesia; it may both depress respiration and induce hypotension.

Histamine is released following morphine administration and this may contribute to its vasodilatory effects. This may also account for the urticaria and bronchoconstriction that are sometimes seen.

Contra-Indications

Do **NOT** administer morphine in the following circumstances:

- Children under 1 year of age.
- Respiratory depression (adult <10 breaths per minute, child <20 breaths per minute).
- Hypotension (actual, not estimated, systolic blood pressure <90 mmHg in adults, <80 mmHg in school children, <70 mmHg in pre-school children).
- Head injury with significantly impaired level of consciousness (e.g. below P on the AVPU scale or below 9 on the GCS).
- Known hypersensitivity to morphine.
- Severe headache.

Cautions

Known severe renal or hepatic impairment – smaller doses may be used carefully and titrated to effect.

Use with **extreme** caution (minimal doses) during pregnancy. **NOTE:** Not to be used for labour pain where entonox is the analgesic of choice.

Use morphine **WITH GREAT CAUTION** in patients with chest injuries, particularly those with any respiratory difficulty, although if respiration is inhibited by pain, analgesia may actually improve respiratory status.

Any patients with other respiratory problems (e.g. asthma, COPD).

Head injury. Agitation following head injury may be due to acute brain injury, hypoxia or pain. The decision to administer analgesia to an agitated head injured patient is a clinical one. It is vital that if such a patient receives opioids they are closely monitored since opioids can cause disproportionate respiratory depression, which may ultimately lead to an elevated intracranial pressure through a raised arterial pCO_2.

Acute alcohol intoxication. All opioid drugs potentiate the central nervous system depressant effects of alcohol and they should therefore be used with great caution in patients who have consumed significant quantities of alcohol.

Medications. Prescribed antidepressants, sedatives or major tranquillisers may potentiate the respiratory and cardiovascular depressant effects of morphine.

Side Effects

- Respiratory depression.
- Cardiovascular depression.
- Nausea and vomiting.
- Drowsiness.
- Pupillary constriction.

Additional Information

Morphine is a Class A controlled drug under Schedule 2 of the Misuse of Drugs Regulations 1985, and must be stored and its prescription and administration documented in accordance with these regulations.

Morphine is not licensed for use in children but its use has been approved by the Medicines and Healthcare Products Regulatory Agency (MHRA) for 'off label' use. This means that it can legally be administered under these guidelines by paramedics.

Unused morphine in open vials or syringes must be discarded in the presence of a witness.

Special Precautions

Naloxone can be used to reverse morphine related respiratory or cardiovascular depression. It should be carefully titrated after assessment and appropriate management of ABC for that particular patient and situation (refer to naloxone guideline).

Morphine frequently induces nausea or vomiting which may be potentiated by the movement of the ambulance. Titrating to the lowest dose to achieve analgesia will reduce the risk of vomiting. The use of an anti-emetic should also be considered whenever administering any opioid analgesic (refer to ondansetron and metoclopramide guidelines).

Morphine Sulphate

Dosage and Administration

Administration must be in conjunction with pain score monitoring (**refer to pain management guidelines**).

Intravenous morphine takes a minimum of 2–3 minutes before starting to take effect, reaching its peak between 10 and 20 minutes.

The absorption of intramuscular, subcutaneous or oral morphine is variable, particularly in patients with major trauma, shock and cardiac conditions; these routes should preferably be avoided if the circumstances favour intravenous or intraosseous administration.

Morphine **should be** diluted with sodium chloride 0.9% to make a concentration of 10 milligrams in 10 ml (1 milligram in 1 ml) unless it is being administered by the intramuscular or subcutaneous route when it should not be diluted.

ADULTS – If pain is not reduced to a tolerable level after 10 milligrams of IV/IO morphine, then further **2 milligram** doses may be administered by slow IV/IO injection every 5 minutes to **20 milligrams maximum.** The patient should be closely observed throughout the remaining treatment and transfer. Care should be taken with elderly patients who may be more susceptible to complications and in whom smaller doses of morphine may be adequate.

CHILDREN – The doses and volumes given below are for the initial and maximum doses. Administer **0.1 ml/kg** (equal to **0.1 milligrams/kg**) as an initial slow IV injection over 2 minutes. If pain is not reduced to a tolerable level after 5 minutes then a further dose of up to **0.1 milligrams/kg,** titrated to response, may be repeated (**maximum dose 0.2 milligrams/kg**).

NOTE: Peak effect of each dose may not occur until 10–20 minutes after administration.

Route: Intravenous/intraosseous – administer by slow IV injection (rate of approximately 2 milligrams per minute up to appropriate dose for age). Observe the patient for at least 5 minutes after completion of initial dose before repeating the dose if required.

AGE	INITIAL DOSE	REPEAT DOSE	DOSE INTERVAL	DILUTED CONCENTRATION	VOLUME	MAXIMUM DOSE
Adult	10 milligrams	10 milligrams	5 minutes	10 milligrams in 10 ml	10 ml	20 milligrams
11 years	3.5 milligrams	3.5 milligrams	5 minutes	10 milligrams in 10 ml	3.5 ml	7 milligrams
10 years	3 milligrams	3 milligrams	5 minutes	10 milligrams in 10 ml	3 ml	6 milligrams
9 years	3 milligrams	3 milligrams	5 minutes	10 milligrams in 10 ml	3 ml	6 milligrams
8 years	2.5 milligrams	2.5 milligrams	5 minutes	10 milligrams in 10 ml	2.5 ml	5 milligrams
7 years	2.5 milligrams	2.5 milligrams	5 minutes	10 milligrams in 10 ml	2.5 ml	5 milligrams
6 years	2 milligrams	2 milligrams	5 minutes	10 milligrams in 10 ml	2 ml	4 milligrams
5 years	2 milligrams	2 milligrams	5 minutes	10 milligrams in 10 ml	2 ml	4 milligrams
4 years	1.5 milligrams	1.5 milligrams	5 minutes	10 milligrams in 10 ml	1.5 ml	3 milligrams
3 years	1.5 milligrams	1.5 milligrams	5 minutes	10 milligrams in 10 ml	1.5 ml	3 milligrams
2 years	1 milligram	1 milligram	5 minutes	10 milligrams in 10 ml	1 ml	2 milligrams
18 months	1 milligram	1 milligram	5 minutes	10 milligrams in 10 ml	1 ml	2 milligrams
12 months	1 milligram	1 milligram	5 minutes	10 milligrams in 10 ml	1 ml	2 milligrams
9 months	N/A	N/A	N/A	N/A	N/A	N/A
6 months	N/A	N/A	N/A	N/A	N/A	N/A
3 months	N/A	N/A	N/A	N/A	N/A	N/A
1 month	N/A	N/A	N/A	N/A	N/A	N/A
Birth	N/A	N/A	N/A	N/A	N/A	N/A

Morphine Sulphate

Route: Oral.

AGE	INITIAL DOSE	REPEAT DOSE	DOSE INTERVAL	CONCENTRATION	VOLUME	MAXIMUM DOSE
Adult	20 milligrams	20 milligrams	60 minutes	10 milligrams in 5 ml	10 ml	40 milligrams
11 years	7 milligrams	NONE	N/A	10 milligrams in 5 ml	3.5 ml	7 milligrams
10 years	6 milligrams	NONE	N/A	10 milligrams in 5 ml	3 ml	6 milligrams
9 years	6 milligrams	NONE	N/A	10 milligrams in 5 ml	3 ml	6 milligrams
8 years	5 milligrams	NONE	N/A	10 milligrams in 5 ml	2.5 ml	5 milligrams
7 years	5 milligrams	NONE	N/A	10 milligrams in 5 ml	2.5 ml	5 milligrams
6 years	4 milligrams	NONE	N/A	10 milligrams in 5 ml	2 ml	4 milligrams
5 years	4 milligrams	NONE	N/A	10 milligrams in 5 ml	2 ml	4 milligrams
4 years	3 milligrams	NONE	N/A	10 milligrams in 5 ml	1.5 ml	3 milligrams
3 years	3 milligrams	NONE	N/A	10 milligrams in 5 ml	1.5 ml	3 milligrams
2 years	2 milligrams	NONE	N/A	10 milligrams in 5 ml	1 ml	2 milligrams
18 months	2 milligrams	NONE	N/A	10 milligrams in 5 ml	1 ml	2 milligrams
12 months	2 milligrams	NONE	N/A	10 milligrams in 5 ml	1 ml	2 milligrams
9 months	N/A	N/A	N/A	N/A	N/A	N/A
6 months	N/A	N/A	N/A	N/A	N/A	N/A
3 months	N/A	N/A	N/A	N/A	N/A	N/A
1 month	N/A	N/A	N/A	N/A	N/A	N/A
Birth	N/A	N/A	N/A	N/A	N/A	N/A

NB Only administer via the oral route in patients with major trauma, shock or cardiac conditions if the IV/IO routes are not accessible.

Morphine Sulphate

Route: Intramuscular/subcutaneous.

AGE	INITIAL DOSE	REPEAT DOSE	DOSE INTERVAL	CONCENTRATION	VOLUME	MAXIMUM DOSE
Adult	10 milligrams	10 milligrams	60 minutes	10 milligrams in 1 ml	1 ml	20 milligrams
11 years	3.5 milligrams	3.5 milligrams	60 minutes	10 milligrams in 1 ml	0.35 ml	7 milligrams
10 years	3 milligrams	3 milligrams	60 minutes	10 milligrams in 1 ml	0.30 ml	6 milligrams
9 years	3 milligrams	3 milligrams	60 minutes	10 milligrams in 1 ml	0.30 ml	6 milligrams
8 years	2.5 milligrams	2.5 milligrams	60 minutes	10 milligrams in 1 ml	0.25 ml	5 milligrams
7 years	2.5 milligrams	2.5 milligrams	60 minutes	10 milligrams in 1 ml	0.25 ml	5 milligrams
6 years	2 milligrams	2 milligrams	60 minutes	10 milligrams in 1 ml	0.20 ml	4 milligrams
5 years	2 milligrams	2 milligrams	60 minutes	10 milligrams in 1 ml	0.20 ml	4 milligrams
4 years	1.5 milligrams	1.5 milligrams	60 minutes	10 milligrams in 1 ml	0.15 ml	3 milligrams
3 years	1.5 milligrams	1.5 milligrams	60 minutes	10 milligrams in 1 ml	0.15 ml	3 milligrams
2 years	1 milligram	1 milligram	60 minutes	10 milligrams in 1 ml	0.10 ml	2 milligrams
18 months	1 milligram	1 milligram	60 minutes	10 milligrams in 1 ml	0.10 ml	2 milligrams
12 months	1 milligram	1 milligram	60 minutes	10 milligrams in 1 ml	0.10 ml	2 milligrams
9 months	N/A	N/A	N/A	N/A	N/A	N/A
6 months	N/A	N/A	N/A	N/A	N/A	N/A
3 months	N/A	N/A	N/A	N/A	N/A	N/A
1 months	N/A	N/A	N/A	N/A	N/A	N/A
Birth	N/A	N/A	N/A	N/A	N/A	N/A

NB Only administer via the intramuscular or subcutaneous route in patients with major trauma, shock or cardiac conditions if the IV/IO routes are not accessible.

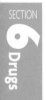

Naloxone Hydrochloride (Narcan) [861]

Presentation

Naloxone hydrochloride 400 micrograms per 1 ml ampoule.

Indications

Opioid overdose producing respiratory, cardiovascular and central nervous system depression.

Overdose of either an opioid analgesic (e.g. dextropropoxyphene, codeine), or a compound analgesic (refer to Table 6.6, e.g. co-codamol, combination of codeine and paracetamol).

Unconsciousness, associated with respiratory depression of unknown cause, where opioid overdose is a possibility, **refer to altered level of consciousness guideline**.

Reversal of respiratory and central nervous system depression in a neonate following maternal opioid use during labour.

Actions

Antagonism of the effects (including respiratory depression) of opioid drugs.

Contra-Indications

Neonates born to opioid addicted mothers – produces serious withdrawal effects. Emphasis should be on bag-valve-mask ventilation and oxygenation – as with all patients.

Side Effects

In patients who are physically dependent on opiates, naloxone may precipitate violent withdrawal symptoms, including cardiac dysrrhythmias. It is better, in these cases, to titrate the dose of naloxone as described (see dosing charts below), to effectively reverse the cardiac and respiratory depression, but still leave the patient in a 'groggy' state with regular re-assessment of ventilation and circulation.

Additional information

When indicated, naloxone should be administered via the intravenous route.

If IV access is impossible, naloxone may be administered intramuscularly, **undiluted** (into the outer aspect of the thigh or upper arm), but absorption may be unpredictable.

Opioid induced respiratory and cardiovascular depression can be fatal.

When used, naloxone's effects are **short lived** and once its effects have worn off respiratory and cardiovascular depression can recur with fatal consequences. **All** cases of opioid overdose should be transported to hospital, even if the initial response to naloxone has been good. If the patient refuses hospitalisation, consider, if the patient consents, a loading dose of **800 micrograms IM** to minimise the risk described above.

Table 6.6 – EXAMPLES OF PRESCRIPTION OPIOID DRUGS

Buprenorphine	Temgesic
Codeine	Used in combination in Codis, Diarrest, Migraleve, Paracodol, Phensedyl, Solpadeine, Solpadol, Syndol, Terpoin, Tylex, Veganin
Dextromoramide	Palfium
Dipipanone	Dicanol
Dextropropoxyphene	Used in combination in Distalgesic/co-proxamol
Diamorphine	'Heroin'
Dihydrocodeine	Co-dydramol, DF 118
Meptazinol	Meptid
Methadone	Physeptone, Methadose
Morphine	Oramorph, Sevredol, MST Continus, SRM Rhotard
Oxycodone	Oxycontin
Pentazocine	Fortral
Pethidine	Pamergan
Phenazocine	Narphen

NB This list is not comprehensive; other opioid drugs are available.

Naloxone Hydrochloride (Narcan)

Dosage and Administration

Respiratory arrest/extreme respiratory depression.

- If there is no response after the initial dose, repeat every 3 minutes, up to the maximum dose, until an effect is noted. NB The half-life of naloxone is short.
- Known or potentially aggressive adults suffering respiratory depression: dilute up to 800 micrograms (2 ml) of naloxone into 8 ml of water for injections or sodium chloride 0.9% to a total volume of 10 ml and administer **SLOWLY,** titrating to response, 1 ml at a time.

Route: Intravenous/intraosseous – administer **SLOWLY** 1 ml at a time. Titrated to response relieving respiratory depression but maintain patient in 'groggy' state.

AGE	INITIAL DOSE	REPEAT DOSE	DOSE INTERVAL	CONCENTRATION	VOLUME	MAXIMUM DOSE
12 years–adult	400 micrograms	400 micrograms	3 minutes	400 micrograms in 1 ml	1 ml	4,400 micrograms
11 years	350 micrograms	350 micrograms	3 minutes	400 micrograms in 1 ml	0.9 ml	3,850 micrograms
10 years	320 micrograms	320 micrograms	3 minutes	400 micrograms in 1 ml	0.8 ml	3,520 micrograms
9 years	280 micrograms	280 micrograms	3 minutes	400 micrograms in 1 ml	0.7 ml	3,080 micrograms
8 years	280 micrograms	280 micrograms	3 minutes	400 micrograms in 1 ml	0.7 ml	3,080 micrograms
7 years	240 micrograms	240 micrograms	3 minutes	400 micrograms in 1 ml	0.6 ml	2,640 micrograms
6 years	200 micrograms	200 micrograms	3 minutes	400 micrograms in 1 ml	0.5 ml	2,200 micrograms
5 years	200 micrograms	200 micrograms	3 minutes	400 micrograms in 1 ml	0.5 ml	2,200 micrograms
4 years	160 micrograms	160 micrograms	3 minutes	400 micrograms in 1 ml	0.4 ml	1,760 micrograms
3 years	160 micrograms	160 micrograms	3 minutes	400 micrograms in 1 ml	0.4 ml	1,760 micrograms
2 years	120 micrograms	120 micrograms	3 minutes	400 micrograms in 1 ml	0.3 ml	1,320 micrograms
18 months	120 micrograms	120 micrograms	3 minutes	400 micrograms in 1 ml	0.3 ml	1,320 micrograms
12 months	100 micrograms	100 micrograms	3 minutes	400 micrograms in 1 ml	0.25 ml	1,100 micrograms
9 months	80 micrograms	80 micrograms	3 minutes	400 micrograms in 1 ml	0.2 ml	880 micrograms
6 months	80 micrograms	80 micrograms	3 minutes	400 micrograms in 1 ml	0.2 ml	880 micrograms
3 months	60 micrograms	60 micrograms	3 minutes	400 micrograms in 1 ml	0.15 ml	660 micrograms
1 month	40 micrograms	40 micrograms	3 minutes	400 micrograms in 1 ml	0.1 ml	440 micrograms
Birth	40 micrograms	40 micrograms	3 minutes	400 micrograms in 1 ml	0.1 ml	440 micrograms

Naloxone Hydrochloride (Narcan)

Respiratory arrest/extreme respiratory depression where the IV/IO route is unavailable or the ambulance clinician is not trained to administer drugs via the IV/IO route.

- If there is no response after the initial dose, repeat every 3 minutes, up to the maximum dose, until an effect is noted. NB The half-life of naloxone is short.

- **For adults when administering naloxone via the intramuscular route:** administering large volumes intramuscularly could lead to poor absorption and/or tissue damage; therefore divide the dose where necessary and practicable. Vary the site of injection for repeated doses; appropriate sites include: buttock (gluteus maximus), thigh (vastus lateralis), lateral hip (gluteus medius) and upper arm (deltoid).

Route: Intramuscular – initial dose.

AGE	INITIAL DOSE	REPEAT DOSE	DOSE INTERVAL	CONCENTRATION	VOLUME	MAXIMUM DOSE
12 years–adult	400 micrograms	See repeat dose	3 minutes	400 micrograms in 1 ml	1 ml	See below
11 years	350 micrograms	See repeat dose	3 minutes	400 micrograms in 1 ml	0.9 ml	See below
10 years	320 micrograms	See repeat dose	3 minutes	400 micrograms in 1 ml	0.8 ml	See below
9 years	280 micrograms	See repeat dose	3 minutes	400 micrograms in 1 ml	0.7 ml	See below
8 years	280 micrograms	See repeat dose	3 minutes	400 micrograms in 1 ml	0.7 ml	See below
7 years	240 micrograms	See repeat dose	3 minutes	400 micrograms in 1 ml	0.6 ml	See below
6 years	200 micrograms	See repeat dose	3 minutes	400 micrograms in 1 ml	0.5 ml	See below
5 years	200 micrograms	See repeat dose	3 minutes	400 micrograms in 1 ml	0.5 ml	See below
4 years	160 micrograms	See repeat dose	3 minutes	400 micrograms in 1 ml	0.4 ml	See below
3 years	160 micrograms	See repeat dose	3 minutes	400 micrograms in 1 ml	0.4 ml	See below
2 years	120 micrograms	See repeat dose	3 minutes	400 micrograms in 1 ml	0.3 ml	See below
18 months	120 micrograms	See repeat dose	3 minutes	400 micrograms in 1 ml	0.3 ml	See below
12 months	100 micrograms	See repeat dose	3 minutes	400 micrograms in 1 ml	0.25 ml	See below
9 months	80 micrograms	See repeat dose	3 minutes	400 micrograms in 1 ml	0.2 ml	See below
6 months	80 micrograms	See repeat dose	3 minutes	400 micrograms in 1 ml	0.2 ml	See below
3 months	60 micrograms	See repeat dose	3 minutes	400 micrograms in 1 ml	0.15 ml	See below
1 month	40 micrograms	See repeat dose	3 minutes	400 micrograms in 1 ml	0.1 ml	See below
Birth	40 micrograms	See repeat dose	3 minutes	400 micrograms in 1 ml	0.1 ml	See below

Naloxone Hydrochloride (Narcan)

Route: Intramuscular – repeat dose.

AGE	INITIAL DOSE	REPEAT DOSE	DOSE INTERVAL	CONCENTRATION	VOLUME	MAXIMUM DOSE
12 years–adult	See initial dose	400 micrograms	3 minutes	400 micrograms in 1 ml	1 ml	4,400 micrograms
11 years	See initial dose	400 micrograms	3 minutes	400 micrograms in 1 ml	1 ml	750 micrograms
10 years	See initial dose	400 micrograms	3 minutes	400 micrograms in 1 ml	1 ml	720 micrograms
9 years	See initial dose	400 micrograms	3 minutes	400 micrograms in 1 ml	1 ml	680 micrograms
8 years	See initial dose	400 micrograms	3 minutes	400 micrograms in 1 ml	1 ml	680 micrograms
7 years	See initial dose	400 micrograms	3 minutes	400 micrograms in 1 ml	1 ml	640 micrograms
6 years	See initial dose	400 micrograms	3 minutes	400 micrograms in 1 ml	1 ml	600 micrograms
5 years	See initial dose	400 micrograms	3 minutes	400 micrograms in 1 ml	1 ml	600 micrograms
4 years	See initial dose	400 micrograms	3 minutes	400 micrograms in 1 ml	1 ml	560 micrograms
3 years	See initial dose	400 micrograms	3 minutes	400 micrograms in 1 ml	1 ml	560 micrograms
2 years	See initial dose	400 micrograms	3 minutes	400 micrograms in 1 ml	1 ml	520 micrograms
18 months	See initial dose	400 micrograms	3 minutes	400 micrograms in 1 ml	1 ml	520 micrograms
12 months	See initial dose	400 micrograms	3 minutes	400 micrograms in 1 ml	1 ml	500 micrograms
9 months	See initial dose	400 micrograms	3 minutes	400 micrograms in 1 ml	1 ml	480 micrograms
6 months	See initial dose	400 micrograms	3 minutes	400 micrograms in 1 ml	1 ml	480 micrograms
3 months	See initial dose	400 micrograms	3 minutes	400 micrograms in 1 ml	1 ml	460 micrograms
1 month	See initial dose	400 micrograms	3 minutes	400 micrograms in 1 ml	1 ml	440 micrograms
Birth	See initial dose	400 micrograms	3 minutes	400 micrograms in 1 ml	1 ml	440 micrograms

NB In the event of IV access being unavailable for the administration of naloxone in children it is advised that the initial IM dose be given dependent on age and, if required, a single subsequent IM dose of 400 micrograms to be given once only. If IV access becomes available and further doses of naloxone are clinically indicated then revert to the IV dosage table.

Reversal of respiratory and central nervous system depression in a neonate following maternal opioid use during labour.

● Administer a single dose only.

Route: Intramuscular

AGE	INITIAL DOSE	REPEAT DOSE	DOSE INTERVAL	CONCENTRATION	VOLUME	MAXIMUM DOSE
Birth	200 micrograms	NONE	N/A	400 micrograms in 1 ml	0.5 ml	200 micrograms

The dose of 200 micrograms is for the reversal of respiratory and central nervous system depression in a newborn following confirmed opioid administration to the mother during labour (e.g. the administration of pethidine). This dose is deliberately higher than the recommended doses of naloxone for respiratory arrest or depression in children aged from birth to 4 years. In the first case the use of an opioid would have been confirmed so the diagnosis is certain and as naloxone is short acting this larger dose treats the problem and partially overcomes the need for repeat doses in the newborn baby. In the second case it is usually not possible to know if this is a chronic situation where the mother has been giving opioids regularly to the child to keep them quiet, or an acute poisoning event where the child drinks the whole bottle of morphine or methadone in the fridge by accident. In the chronic addicted situation it is possible that the child would suffer seizures and other violent physiological withdrawal effects if given a large dose of naloxone. Therefore it is safer to administer the smaller dose to start with, and then make arrangements to get the child to a hospital setting where withdrawal symptoms can be treated appropriately.

Ondansetron [862–864]

ODT

Presentation

Ampoule containing 4 milligrams of ondansetron (as hydrochloride) in 2 ml.

Ampoule containing 8 milligrams of ondansetron (as hydrochloride) in 4 ml.

NB Both these preparations share the same concentration (2 milligrams in 1 ml).

Indications

Adults:

- Prevention and treatment of opiate-induced nausea and vomiting (e.g. morphine sulphate).
- Treatment of nausea or vomiting.

Children:

- Prevention and treatment of opiate-induced nausea and vomiting (e.g. morphine sulphate).
- For travel associated nausea or vomiting.

Actions

An anti-emetic that blocks 5HT receptors both centrally and in the gastrointestinal tract.

Contra-Indications

Known sensitivity to ondansetron.

Infants <1 month old.

Cautions

QT interval prolongation (avoid concomitant administration of drugs that prolong QT interval).

Hepatic impairment.

Pregnancy.

Breastfeeding.

Side Effects

Hiccups.

Constipation.

Flushing.

Hypotension.

Chest pain.

Arrhythmias.

Bradycardia.

Headache.

Seizures.

Movement disorders.

Injection site reactions.

Additional Information

Ondansetron should always be given in a separate syringe to morphine sulphate – the drugs must **NOT** be mixed.

Ondansetron should **NOT** be routinely administered in the management of childhood gastroenteritis (**refer to gastroenteritis in children guideline**).

Ondansetron

Dosage and Administration

Note: Two preparations exist (4 mg in 2 ml and 8 mg in 4 ml). They share the same concentration, that is 2 milligrams in 1 ml.

Route: Intravenous (**SLOW** IV injection over 2 minutes)/intramuscular.

AGE	INITIAL DOSE	REPEAT DOSE	DOSE INTERVAL	CONCENTRATION	VOLUME	MAXIMUM DOSE
12 years – Adult	4 milligrams	NONE	N/A	2 milligrams in 1 ml	2 ml	4 milligrams
11 years	3 milligrams	NONE	N/A	2 milligrams in 1 ml	1.5 ml	3 milligrams
10 years	3 milligrams	NONE	N/A	2 milligrams in 1 ml	1.5 ml	3 milligrams
9 years	3 milligrams	NONE	N/A	2 milligrams in 1 ml	1.5 ml	3 milligrams
8 years	2.5 milligrams	NONE	N/A	2 milligrams in 1 ml	1.3 ml	2.5 milligrams
7 years	2.5 milligrams	NONE	N/A	2 milligrams in 1 ml	1.3 ml	2.5 milligrams
6 years	2 milligrams	NONE	N/A	2 milligrams in 1 ml	1 ml	2 milligrams
5 years	2 milligrams	NONE	N/A	2 milligrams in 1 ml	1 ml	2 milligrams
4 years	1.5 milligrams	NONE	N/A	2 milligrams in 1 ml	0.75 ml	1.5 milligrams
3 years	1.5 milligrams	NONE	N/A	2 milligrams in 1 ml	0.75 ml	1.5 milligrams
2 years	1 milligram	NONE	N/A	2 milligrams in 1 ml	0.5 ml	1 milligram
18 months	1 milligram	NONE	N/A	2 milligrams in 1 ml	0.5 ml	1 milligram
12 months	1 milligram	NONE	N/A	2 milligrams in 1 ml	0.5 ml	1 milligram
9 months	1 milligram	NONE	N/A	2 milligrams in 1 ml	0.5 ml	1 milligram
6 months	1 milligram	NONE	N/A	2 milligrams in 1 ml	0.5 ml	1 milligram
3 months	0.5 milligrams	NONE	N/A	2 milligrams in 1 ml	0.25 ml	0.5 milligrams
1 month	0.5 milligrams	NONE	N/A	2 milligrams in 1 ml	0.25 ml	0.5 milligrams
Birth	N/A	N/A	N/A	N/A	N/A	N/A

NB Monitor pulse, blood pressure, respiratory rate and cardiac rhythm before, during and after administration.

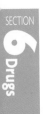

Presentation

Oxygen (O_2) is a gas provided in compressed form in a cylinder. It is also available in liquid form, in a system adapted for ambulance use. It is fed via a regulator and flow meter to the patient by means of plastic tubing and an oxygen mask/nasal cannulae.

Indications

Children

- Significant illness and/or injury.

Adults

- Critical illnesses requiring high levels of supplemental oxygen (refer to Table 6.7).
- Serious illnesses requiring moderate levels of supplemental oxygen if the patient is hypoxaemic (refer to Table 6.8).
- COPD and other conditions requiring controlled or low-dose oxygen therapy (refer to Table 6.9).
- Conditions for which patients should be monitored closely but oxygen therapy is not required unless the patient is hypoxaemic (refer to Table 6.10).

Actions

Essential for cell metabolism. Adequate tissue oxygenation is essential for normal physiological function.

Oxygen assists in reversing hypoxia, by raising the concentration of inspired oxygen. Hypoxia will, however, only improve if respiratory effort or ventilation and tissue perfusion are adequate.

If ventilation is inadequate or absent, assisting or completely taking over the patient's ventilation is essential to reverse hypoxia.

Contra-Indications

Explosive environments.

Cautions

Oxygen increases the fire hazard at the scene of an incident.

Defibrillation – ensure pads firmly applied to reduce spark hazard.

Side Effects

Non-humidified O_2 is drying and irritating to mucous membranes over a period of time.

In patients with COPD there is a risk that even moderately high doses of inspired oxygen can produce increased carbon dioxide levels which may cause respiratory depression and this may lead to respiratory arrest. Refer to Table 6.9 for guidance.

Dosage and Administration

- Measure oxygen saturation (SpO_2) in all patients using pulse oximetry.
- For the administration of **moderate** levels of supplemented oxygen nasal cannulae are recommended in preference to simple face mask as they offer more flexible dose range.
- Patients with tracheostomy or previous laryngectomy may require alternative appliances (e.g. tracheostomy masks).
- Entonox may be administered when required.
- Document oxygen administration.

Children

- **ALL** children with significant illness and/or injury should receive **HIGH** levels of supplementary oxygen.

Adults

- Administer the initial oxygen dose until a reliable oxygen saturation reading is obtained.
- If the desired oxygen saturation cannot be maintained with simple face mask change to reservoir mask (non-rebreathe mask).
- For dosage and administration of supplemental oxygen refer to Tables 6.7–6.10.
- For conditions where **NO** supplemental oxygen is required unless the patient is hypoxaemic refer to Table 6.10.

Table 6.7 – High levels of supplemental oxygen for adults with critical illnesses

Target saturation

94–98%

Administer the initial oxygen dose until the vital signs are normal, then reduce oxygen dose and aim for target saturation within the range of **94–98%** as per table below.

Condition	Initial dose	Method of administration

● Cardiac arrest or resuscitation:
  – basic life support
  – advanced life support
  – foreign body airway obstruction
  – traumatic cardiac arrest
  – maternal resuscitation.
● Carbon monoxide poisoning.
	Maximum dose until the vital signs are normal	Bag-valve-mask

NOTE– Some oxygen saturation monitors cannot differentiate between carboxyhaemoglobin and oxyhaemoglobin owing to carbon monoxide poisoning.		

● Major trauma:
  – abdominal trauma
  – burns and scalds
  – electrocution
  – head trauma
  – limb trauma
  – neck and back trauma (spinal)
  – pelvic trauma
  – the immersion incident
  – thoracic trauma
  – trauma in pregnancy.
● Anaphylaxis
● Major pulmonary haemorrhage
● Sepsis (e.g. meningococcal septicemia)
● Shock
	15 litres per minute	Reservoir mask (non-rebreathe mask)

● Active convulsion ● Hypothermia	Administer 15 litres per minute until a reliable SpO_2 measurement can be obtained and the adjust oxygen flow to aim for target saturation within the range of **94–98%**	Reservoir mask (non-rebreathe mask)

Oxygen

Table 6.8 – Moderate levels of supplemental oxygen for adults with serious illnesses if the patient is hypoxaemic

Target saturation

94–98%

Administer the initial oxygen dose until a reliable SpO_2 measurement is available, then adjust oxygen flow to aim for target saturation within the range of **94–98%** as per the table below.

Condition	INITIAL DOSE	Method of administration
● Acute hypoxaemia (cause not yet diagnosed) ● Deterioration of lung fibrosis or other interstitial lung disease ● Acute asthma ● Acute heart failure ● Pneumonia ● Lung cancer ● Postoperative breathlessness ● Pulmonary embolism ● Pleural effusions ● Pneumothorax ● Severe anaemia ● Sickle cell crisis	**SpO_2 <85%** 10–15 litres per minute	Reservoir mask (non-rebreathe mask)
	SpO_2 ≥85–93% 2–6 litres per minute	Nasal cannulae
	SpO_2 ≥85–93% 5–10 litres per minute	Simple face mask

Table 6.9 – Controlled or low-dose supplemental oxygen for adults with COPD and other conditions requiring controlled or low-dose oxygen therapy

Target saturation

88–92%

Administer the initial oxygen dose until a reliable SpO_2 measurement is available, then adjust oxygen flow to aim for target saturation within the range of **88–92%** or **prespecified range** detailed on the patient's alert card, as per the table below.

Condition	Initial dose	Method of administration
● Chronic obstructive pulmonary disease (COPD) ● Exacerbation of cystic fibrosis	4 litres per minute	28% Venturi mask or patient's own mask
	NB If respiratory rate is >30 breaths/min using Venturi mask set flow rate to 50% above the minimum specified for the mask.	
● Chronic neuromuscular disorders ● Chest wall disorders ● Morbid obesity (body mass index >40 kg/m²)	4 litres per minute	28% Venturi mask or patient's own mask
NB If the oxygen saturation remains below 88% change to simple face mask.	5–10 litres per minute	Simple face mask
NB Critical illness **AND** COPD/or other risk factors for hypercapnia.	If a patient with COPD or other risk factors for hypercapnia sustains or develops critical illness/injury ensure the same target saturations as indicated in Table 6.7.	

6 Drugs SECTION

Oxygen

Table 6.10 – No supplemental oxygen required for adults with these conditions unless the patient is hypoxaemic but patients should be monitored closely

Target saturation

94–98%

If hypoxaemic (SpO₂ <94%) administer the initial oxygen dose, then adjust oxygen flow to aim for target saturation within the range of **94–98%**, as per table below.

Condition	Initial dose	Method of administration

● Myocardial infarction and acute coronary syndromes
● Stroke
● Cardiac rhythm disturbance
● Non-traumatic chest pain/discomfort
● Implantable cardioverter defibrillator firing
● Pregnancy and obstetric emergencies:
  – birth imminent
  – haemorrhage during pregnancy
  – pregnancy induced hypertension
  – vaginal bleeding.
● Abdominal pain
● Headache
● Hyperventilation syndrome or dysfunctional breathing
● Most poisonings and drug overdoses (refer to **Table 6.7** for **carbon monoxide poisioning** and special cases below for **paraquat poisioning**)
● Metabolic and renal disorders
● Acute and sub-acute neurological and muscular conditions producing muscle weakness (assess the need for assisted ventilation if **SpO₂ <94%**)
● Post convulsion
● Gastrointestinal bleeds
● Glycaemic emergencies
● Heat exhaustion/heat stroke
	SpO₂ <85%
	10–15 litres per minute
		Reservoir mask (non-rebreathe mask)

	SpO₂ ≥85–93% 2–6 litres per minute	Nasal cannulae
	SpO₂ ≥85–93% 5–10 litres per minute	Simple face mask

SPECIAL CASES
● Poisoning with paraquat

> **NOTE** – patients with paraquat poisoning may be harmed by supplemental oxygen so avoid oxygen unless the patient is hypoxaemic. Target saturation 88–92%.

SECTION
6
Drugs

Oxygen

Table 6.7 – Critical illnesses in adults requiring HIGH levels of supplemental oxygen

- Cardiac arrest or resuscitation:
  - basic life support
  - advanced life support
  - foreign body airway obstruction
  - traumatic cardiac arrest
  - maternal resuscitation.
- Major trauma:
  - abdominal trauma
  - burns and scalds
  - electrocution
  - head trauma
  - limb trauma
  - neck and back trauma (spinal)
  - pelvic trauma
  - the immersion incident
  - thoracic trauma
  - trauma in pregnancy.
- Active convulsion
- Anaphylaxis
- Carbon monoxide poisoning
- Hypothermia
- Major pulmonary haemorrhage
- Sepsis (e.g. meningococcal septicaemia)
- Shock

Table 6.8 – Serious illnesses in adults requiring MODERATE levels of supplemental oxygen if hypoxaemic

- Acute hypoxaemia
- Deterioration of lung fibrosis or other interstitial lung disease
- Acute asthma
- Acute heart failure
- Pneumonia
- Lung cancer
- Postoperative breathlessness
- Pulmonary embolism
- Pleural effusions
- Pneumothorax
- Severe anaemia
- Sickle cell crisis

Table 6.9 – COPD and other conditions in adults requiring CONTROLLED OR LOW-DOSE supplemental oxygen

- Chronic obstructive pulmonary disease (COPD)
- Exacerbation of cystic fibrosis
- Chronic neuromuscular disorders
- Chest wall disorders
- Morbid obesity (body mass index >40 kg/m^2)

Table 6.10 – Conditions in adults NOT requiring supplemental oxygen unless the patient is hypoxaemic

- Myocardial infarction and acute coronary syndromes
- Stroke
- Cardiac rhythm disturbance
- Non-traumatic chest pain/discomfort
- Implantable cardioverter defibrillator firing
- Pregnancy and obstetric emergencies:
  - birth imminent
  - haemorrhage during pregnancy
  - pregnancy induced hypertension
  - vaginal bleeding.
- Abdominal pain
- Headache
- Hyperventilation syndrome or dysfunctional breathing
- Most poisonings and drug overdoses (except carbon monoxide poisoning)
- Metabolic and renal disorders
- Acute and sub-acute neurological and muscular conditions producing muscle weakness
- Post convulsion
- Gastrointestinal bleeds
- Glycaemic emergencies
- Heat exhaustion/heat stroke

Special cases:
- Paraquat poisoning

Oxygen

Is the patient in CARDIAC and/or RESPIRATORY ARREST or in need of VENTILATORY SUPPORT?

— YES → Administer the maximum dose of oxygen via a bag-valve-mask until the vital signs are normal, then aim for target saturation within the range of **94–98%**

↓ NO

Do you know or suspect CARBON MONOXIDE poisoning?

— YES → Administer maximum dose of oxygen via a reservoir mask

↓ NO

Do you know or suspect a critical illness requiring HIGH levels of oxygen? Refer to Table 6.7

— YES → Is SpO$_2$ ≥94% and are the vital signs normal?
- NO → Administer 15 l/min of oxygen via a reservoir mask until the vital signs are normal, then aim for target saturation within the range of **94–98%**
- YES → Monitor SpO$_2$ and if the saturation falls below **94%** administer oxygen to maintain a saturation within the range of **94–98%**

↓ NO

Do you know or suspect a condition requiring CONTROLLED OR LOW–DOSE levels of oxygen? Refer to Table 6.9

— YES → Is SpO$_2$ ≥88%?
- NO → Administer 4 l/min of oxygen via a 28% Venturi mask or patient's own mask to aim for target saturation within the range of **88–92%**
- YES → Monitor SpO$_2$ and if the saturation falls below **88%** administer oxygen to maintain a saturation within the range of **88–92%**

↓ NO

> Patients with **PARAQUAT** poisoning may be harmed by supplemental oxygen so avoid oxygen unless the patient is hypoxic

Do you know or suspect PARAQUAT poisoning?

— YES → Is SpO$_2$ ≥88%?
- NO → SpO$_2$ <**85%** administer 15 l/min of oxygen via a reservoir mask SpO$_2$ **85–87%** administer 2–6 l/min via nasal cannulae or 5–10 l/min of oxygen via a simple face mask. Aim for target saturation within the range of **88–92%**
- YES → Monitor SpO$_2$ and if the saturation falls below 88% administer oxygen to maintain a saturation within the range of **88–92%**

↓ NO

Do you know or suspect a serious illness requiring MODERATE levels oxygen? Refer to Table 6.8

— YES → Is SpO$_2$ ≥94%?
- NO → SpO$_2$ <**85%** administer 10–15 l/min of oxygen via a reservoir mask. SpO$_2$ **85–93%** administer 2–6 l/min via nasal cannulae or 5–10 l/min of oxygen via a simple face mask. Aim for target saturation within the range of **94–98%**
- YES → Monitor SpO$_2$ and if the saturation falls below 94% administer oxygen to maintain a saturation within the range of **94–98%**

↓ NO

Other conditions NOT requiring oxygen unless hypoxaemic? Refer to Table 6.10

— YES → Is SpO$_2$ ≥94%?
- NO → SpO$_2$ <**85%** administer 10–15 l/min of oxygen via a reservoir mask. SpO$_2$ **85–93%** administer 2–6 l/min via nasal cannulae or 5–10 l/min of oxygen via a simple face mask. Aim for target saturation within the range of **94–98%**
- YES → Monitor SpO$_2$ and if the saturation falls below 94% administer oxygen to maintain a saturation within the range of **94–98%**

Figure 6.1 – Administration of supplemental oxygen algorithm.

SECTION **6** Drugs

Presentation

Both oral and intravenous preparations are available.

Oral

Paracetamol solutions/suspensions:

- **Infant paracetamol suspension** (120 milligrams in 5 ml), used from 3 months to 5 years.
- **Paracetamol 6 plus suspension** (250 milligrams in 5 ml), used from 5 years of age upwards.

Paracetamol tablets

- 500 milligram tablets.

Intravenous

- Bottle containing paracetamol 1 gram in 100 ml (10 mg/ml) for intravenous infusion.

Indications

Relief of mild to moderate pain and/or high temperature. Oral administration only. IV route is not appropriate for this indication.

As part of a balanced analgesic regimen for severe pain (IV paracetamol is effective in reducing opioid requirements while improving analgesic efficacy). Only use IV paracetamol for severe pain or if contra-indication to opiates.

Actions

Analgesic (pain relieving) and antipyretic (temperature reducing) drug.

Contra-indications

Known paracetamol allergy.

Do **NOT** give further paracetamol if a paracetamol containing product (e.g. Calpol, co-codamol) has already been given within the last 4 hours or if the maximum cumulative daily dose has been given already.

Side Effects

Side effects are extremely rare; occasionally intravenous paracetamol may cause may cause systemic hypotension if administered too rapidly.

Additional Information

A febrile child should not be left at home except where:

- a full assessment has been carried out,

and

- the child has no apparent serious underlying illness,

and

- the child has a defined clinical pathway for reassessment and follow up, with the full consent of the parent (or carer).

Any IV paracetamol that remains within the giving set can be flushed using 0.9% saline. Take care to ensure that air does not become entrained into the giving set; if there is air in the giving set ensure that it does not run into the patient with further fluids. Ambulance clinicians should strictly adhere to the administration procedure as set out by their Trust to minimise this risk.

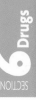

Paracetamol

Dosage and Administration

NB Ensure:
1. Paracetamol has not been taken within the previous 4 hours.
2. The correct paracetamol containing solution/suspension for the patients's age is being used, that is 'infant paracetamol suspension' for age groups 0–5 years: 'paracetamol 6 plus suspension' for ages 6 years and over.

Route: Oral – infant paracetamol suspension.

AGE	INITIAL DOSE	REPEAT DOSE	DOSE INTERVAL	CONCENTRATION	VOLUME	MAXIMUM DOSE
Adult	N/A	N/A	N/A	N/A	N/A	N/A
11 years	N/A	N/A	N/A	N/A	N/A	N/A
10 years	N/A	N/A	N/A	N/A	N/A	N/A
9 years	N/A	N/A	N/A	N/A	N/A	N/A
8 years	N/A	N/A	N/A	N/A	N/A	N/A
7 years	N/A	N/A	N/A	N/A	N/A	N/A
6 years	N/A	N/A	N/A	N/A	N/A	N/A
5 years	240 milligrams	240 milligrams	4–6 hours	120 milligrams in 5 ml	10 ml	960 milligrams in 24 hours
4 years	240 milligrams	240 milligrams	4–6 hours	120 milligrams in 5 ml	10 ml	960 milligrams in 24 hours
3 years	180 milligrams	180 milligrams	4–6 hours	120 milligrams in 5 ml	7.5 ml	720 milligrams in 24 hours
2 years	180 milligrams	180 milligrams	4–6 hours	120 milligrams in 5 ml	7.5 ml	720 milligrams in 24 hours
18 months	120 milligrams	120 milligrams	4–6 hours	120 milligrams in 5 ml	5 ml	480 milligrams in 24 hours
12 months	120 milligrams	120 milligrams	4–6 hours	120 milligrams in 5 ml	5 ml	480 milligrams in 24 hours
9 months	120 milligrams	120 milligrams	4–6 hours	120 milligrams in 5 ml	5 ml	480 milligrams in 24 hours
6 months	120 milligrams	120 milligrams	4–6 hours	120 milligrams in 5 ml	5 ml	480 milligrams in 24 hours
3 months	60 milligrams	60 milligrams	4–6 hours	120 milligrams in 5 ml	2.5 ml	240 milligrams in 24 hours
1 month	N/A	N/A	N/A	N/A	N/A	N/A
Birth	N/A	N/A	N/A	N/A	N/A	N/A

SECTION
6
Drugs

Paracetamol

NB Ensure:
1. Paracetamol has not been taken within the previous 4 hours.
2. The correct paracetamol containing solution/suspension for the patients's age is being used, that is 'infant paracetamol suspension' for age groups 0–5 years: 'paracetamol 6 plus suspension' for ages 6 years and over.

Route: Oral – paracetamol 6 plus suspension.

AGE	INITIAL DOSE	REPEAT DOSE	DOSE INTERVAL	CONCENTRATION	VOLUME	MAXIMUM DOSE
12 years – Adult	1 gram	1 gram	4–6 hours	250 milligrams in 5 ml	20 ml	4 grams in 24 hours
11 years	500 milligrams	500 milligrams	4–6 hours	250 milligrams in 5 ml	10 ml	2 grams in 24 hours
10 years	500 milligrams	500 milligrams	4–6 hours	250 milligrams in 5 ml	10 ml	2 grams in 24 hours
9 years	375 milligrams	375 milligrams	4–6 hours	250 milligrams in 5 ml	7.5 ml	1.5 grams in 24 hours
8 years	375 milligrams	375 milligrams	4–6 hours	250 milligrams in 5 ml	7.5 ml	1.5 grams in 24 hours
7 years	250 milligrams	250 milligrams	4–6 hours	250 milligrams in 5 ml	5 ml	1 gram in 24 hours
6 years	250 milligrams	250 milligrams	4–6 hours	250 milligrams in 5 ml	5 ml	1 gram in 24 hours
5 years	N/A	N/A	N/A	N/A	N/A	N/A
4 years	N/A	N/A	N/A	N/A	N/A	N/A
3 years	N/A	N/A	N/A	N/A	N/A	N/A
2 years	N/A	N/A	N/A	N/A	N/A	N/A
18 months	N/A	N/A	N/A	N/A	N/A	N/A
12 months	N/A	N/A	N/A	N/A	N/A	N/A
9 months	N/A	N/A	N/A	N/A	N/A	N/A
6 months	N/A	N/A	N/A	N/A	N/A	N/A
3 months	N/A	N/A	N/A	N/A	N/A	N/A
1 month	N/A	N/A	N/A	N/A	N/A	N/A
Birth	N/A	N/A	N/A	N/A	N/A	N/A

Route: Oral – tablet.

AGE	INITIAL DOSE	REPEAT DOSE	DOSE INTERVAL	CONCENTRATION	VOLUME	MAXIMUM DOSE
12 years – Adult	1 gram	1 gram	4–6 hours	500 milligrams per tablet	2 tablets	4 grams in 24 hours

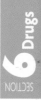

Paracetamol

NB Ensure:
Paracetamol has not been taken within the previous 4 hours. IV paracetamol to be administered for severe pain only. Do not administer IV for control of fever. Use oral preparation.

Route: Intravenous infusion; typically given over 5–10 minutes.

AGE	INITIAL DOSE	REPEAT DOSE	DOSE INTERVAL	CONCENTRATION	VOLUME	MAXIMUM DOSE
12 years – Adult	1 gram	1 gram	4–6 hours	10 milligrams in 1 ml	100 ml	4 grams in 24 hours
11 years	500 milligrams	500 milligrams	4–6 hours	10 milligrams in 1 ml	50 ml	2 grams in 24 hours
10 years	500 milligrams	500 milligrams	4–6 hours	10 milligrams in 1 ml	50 ml	2 grams in 24 hours
9 years	500 milligrams	500 milligrams	4–6 hours	10 milligrams in 1 ml	50 ml	2 grams in 24 hours
8 years	300 milligrams	300 milligrams	4–6 hours	10 milligrams in 1 ml	30 ml	1.2 grams in 24 hours
7 years	300 milligrams	300 milligrams	4–6 hours	10 milligrams in 1 ml	30 ml	1.2 grams in 24 hours
6 years	300 milligrams	300 milligrams	4–6 hours	10 milligrams in 1 ml	30 ml	1.2 grams in 24 hours
5 years	250 milligrams	250 milligrams	4–6 hours	10 milligrams in 1 ml	25 ml	1 gram in 24 hours
4 years	250 milligrams	250 milligrams	4–6 hours	10 milligrams in 1 ml	25 ml	1 gram in 24 hours
3 years	250 milligrams	250 milligrams	4–6 hours	10 milligrams in 1 ml	25 ml	1 gram in 24 hours
2 years	150 milligrams	150 milligrams	4–6 hours	10 milligrams in 1 ml	15 ml	600 milligrams in 24 hours
18 months	150 milligrams	150 milligrams	4–6 hours	10 milligrams in 1 ml	15 ml	600 milligrams in 24 hours
12 months	150 milligrams	150 milligrams	4–6 hours	10 milligrams in 1 ml	15 ml	600 milligrams in 24 hours
9 months	50 milligrams	50 milligrams	4–6 hours	10 milligrams in 1 ml	5 ml	200 milligrams in 24 hours
6 months	50 milligrams	50 milligrams	4–6 hours	10 milligrams in 1 ml	5 ml	200 milligrams in 24 hours
3 months	N/A	N/A	N/A	N/A	N/A	N/A
1 month	N/A	N/A	N/A	N/A	N/A	N/A
Birth	N/A	N/A	N/A	N/A	N/A	N/A

Presentation

Vials of **reteplase** 10 units for reconstitution with 10 ml water for injection.

NOTE: Whilst the strength of thrombolytics is traditionally expressed in 'units', these units are unique to each particular drug and are **NOT** interchangeable.

Indications

Acute ST segment elevation MI (STEMI) 12 hours of symptom onset where primary percutaneous coronary intervention (PPCI) is **NOT** readily available.

Ensure patient fulfils the criteria for drug administration following the model checklist (below). Variation of these criteria is justifiable at local level with agreement of appropriate key stakeholders (e.g. cardiac network, or in the context of an approved clinical trial).

Contra-Indications

See checklist.

Actions

Activates the fibrinolytic system, inducing the breaking up of intravascular thrombi and emboli.

Side Effects

Bleeding:

- major – seek medical advice and transport to hospital rapidly

- minor (e.g. at injection sites) – use local pressure.

Arrhythmias – these are usually benign in the form of transient idioventricular rhythms and usually require no special treatment. Treat ventricular fibrillation (VF) as a complication of myocardial infarction (MI) with standard protocols; bradycardia with atropine as required.

Anaphylaxis – extremely rare (0.1%) with third generation bolus agents.

Hypotension – often responds to laying the patient flat.

Additional Information

PPCI is now the dominant reperfusion treatment and should be used where available; patients with STEMI will be taken direct to a specialist cardiac centre instead of receiving thrombolysis (**refer to acute coronary syndrome guideline**). Local guidelines should be followed.

'**Time is muscle!**' Do not delay transportation to hospital if difficulties arise whilst setting up the equipment or establishing IV access. Qualified single responders should administer a thrombolytic if indicated while awaiting arrival of an ambulance.

In All Cases

Ensure a defibrillator is immediately available at all times.

Monitor conscious level, pulse, blood pressure and cardiac rhythm during and following injections. Manage complications (associated with the acute MI) as they occur using standard protocols. The main early adverse event associated with thrombolysis is bleeding, which should be managed according to standard protocols.

AT HOSPITAL – emphasise the need to commence a heparin infusion in accordance with local protocols – to reduce the risk of re-infarction.

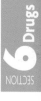

Reteplase

Thrombolysis Checklist

Is primary PCI available?

- **YES** – undertake a **TIME CRITICAL** transfer to PPCI capable hospital.
- **NO** – ask the patient the questions listed below, to determine whether they are suitable to receive thrombolysis.

Assessment Questions	Yes	No
Has the patient suffered a haemorrhagic stroke or stroke of unknown origin at any time?	☐	☐
Has the patient suffered a transient ischaemic attack in the preceding 6 months?	☐	☐
Has the patient suffered a central nervous system trauma or neoplasm?	☐	☐
Has the patient had recent trauma, surgery or head injury within the preceding 3 weeks?	☐	☐
Has the patient suffered from gastrointestinal bleeding (within the last month)?	☐	☐
Has the patient a known bleeding disorder?	☐	☐
Do you suspect aortic dissection?	☐	☐
Has the patient a non-compressible puncture (e.g. liver biopsy, lumbar puncture)?	☐	☐
Is the patient taking oral anticoagulant therapy (e.g. warfarin)?	☐	☐
Is the patient pregnant or within 1 week post-partum?	☐	☐
Is the patient's systolic blood pressure >180 mmHg and/or diastolic blood pressure >110 mmHg?	☐	☐
Is the patient suffering from advanced liver disease?	☐	☐
Is the patient suffering from active peptic ulcer?	☐	☐

If the patient answers **YES TO ANY** of the above questions, thrombolysis **IS NOT** indicated; seek advice.

If the patient answers **NO TO ALL** of the above questions and thrombolysis is indicated, refer to the dosage and administration table.

Dosage and Administration

RETEPLASE

1. Administer a bolus of intravenous injection un-fractionated heparin before the first dose of reteplase (refer to heparin guideline). Flush the cannula well with saline **OR** use a separate cannula to administer reteplase as the two agents are physically incompatible.

2. Note the time the first dose is administered.

3. Administer the second dose 30 minutes after the first.

4. **AT HOSPITAL** – It is essential that the care of the patient is handed over as soon as possible to a member of hospital staff qualified to administer the second bolus (if not already given) and commence a heparin infusion.

Route: Intravenous bolus injections separated by 30 minutes.

AGE	INITIAL DOSE	REPEAT DOSE	DOSE INTERVAL	CONCENTRATION	VOLUME	MAXIMUM DOSE
≥18	First dose 10 units	NONE	N/A	10 units in 10 ml	10 ml	10 units
	Second dose 10 units	NONE	N/A	10 units in 10 ml	10 ml	10 units

Salbutamol [870]

Presentation

Nebules containing salbutamol 2.5 milligrams/2.5 ml or 5 milligrams/2.5 ml.

Indications

Acute asthma attack where normal inhaler therapy has failed to relieve symptoms.

Expiratory wheezing associated with allergy, anaphylaxis, smoke inhalation or other lower airway cause.

Exacerbation of chronic obstructive pulmonary disease (COPD).

Shortness of breath in patients with severe breathing difficulty due to left ventricular failure (secondary treatment).

Actions

Salbutamol is a selective beta2 adrenoreceptor stimulant drug. This has a relaxant effect on the smooth muscle in the medium and smaller airways, which are in spasm in acute asthma attacks. If given by nebuliser, especially if oxygen powered, its smooth-muscle relaxing action, combined with the airway moistening effect of nebulisation, can relieve the attack rapidly.

Contra-Indications

None in the emergency situation.

Cautions

Salbutamol should be used with care in patients with:

- Hypertension.
- Angina.
- Overactive thyroid.
- Late pregnancy (can relax uterus).
- Severe hypertension may occur in patients on beta-blockers and half doses should be used unless there is profound hypotension.

If COPD is a possibility limit nebulisation to 6 minutes.

Side Effects

Tremor (shaking).

Tachycardia.

Palpitations.

Headache.

Feeling of tension.

Peripheral vasodilatation.

Muscle cramps.

Rash.

Additional Information

In acute severe or life-threatening asthma, ipratropium should be given after the first dose of salbutamol. In acute asthma or COPD unresponsive to salbutamol alone, a single dose of ipratropium may be given after salbutamol.

Salbutamol often provides initial relief. In more severe attacks, however, the use of steroids by injection or orally and further nebuliser therapy will be required. Do not be lulled into a false sense of security by an initial improvement after salbutamol nebulisation.

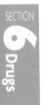
SECTION
6
Drugs

Salbutamol

Dosage and Administration

- **In life-threatening or acute severe asthma:** undertake a **TIME CRITICAL** transfer to the **NEAREST SUITABLE RECEIVING HOSPITAL** and provide nebulisation en-route.
- If COPD is a possibility limit nebulisation to 6 minutes.
- The pulse rate in children may exceed 140 after significant doses of salbutamol; this is not usually of any clinical significance and should not usually preclude further use of the drug.
- Repeat doses should be discontinued if the side effects are becoming significant (e.g. tremors, tachycardia >140 beats per minute in adults) – this is a clinical decision by the ambulance clinician.

Route: Nebulised with 6–8 litres per minute of oxygen.

AGE	INITIAL DOSE	REPEAT DOSE	DOSE INTERVAL	CONCENTRATION	VOLUME	MAXIMUM DOSE
Adult	5 milligrams	5 milligrams	5 minutes	2.5 milligrams in 2.5 ml	5 ml	No limit
11 years	5 milligrams	5 milligrams	5 minutes	2.5 milligrams in 2.5 ml	5 ml	No limit
10 years	5 milligrams	5 milligrams	5 minutes	2.5 milligrams in 2.5 ml	5 ml	No limit
9 years	5 milligrams	5 milligrams	5 minutes	2.5 milligrams in 2.5 ml	5 ml	No limit
8 years	5 milligrams	5 milligrams	5 minutes	2.5 milligrams in 2.5 ml	5 ml	No limit
7 years	5 milligrams	5 milligrams	5 minutes	2.5 milligrams in 2.5 ml	5 ml	No limit
6 years	5 milligrams	5 milligrams	5 minutes	2.5 milligrams in 2.5 ml	5 ml	No limit
5 years	2.5 milligrams	2.5 milligrams	5 minutes	2.5 milligrams in 2.5 ml	2.5 ml	No limit
4 years	2.5 milligrams	2.5 milligrams	5 minutes	2.5 milligrams in 2.5 ml	2.5 ml	No limit
3 years	2.5 milligrams	2.5 milligrams	5 minutes	2.5 milligrams in 2.5 ml	2.5 ml	No limit
2 years	2.5 milligrams	2.5 milligrams	5 minutes	2.5 milligrams in 2.5 ml	2.5 ml	No limit
18 months	2.5 milligrams	2.5 milligrams	5 minutes	2.5 milligrams in 2.5 ml	2.5 ml	No limit
12 months	2.5 milligrams	2.5 milligrams	5 minutes	2.5 milligrams in 2.5 ml	2.5 ml	No limit
9 months	2.5 milligrams	2.5 milligrams	5 minutes	2.5 milligrams in 2.5 ml	2.5 ml	No limit
6 months	2.5 milligrams	2.5 milligrams	5 minutes	2.5 milligrams in 2.5 ml	2.5 ml	No limit
3 months	2.5 milligrams	2.5 milligrams	5 minutes	2.5 milligrams in 2.5 ml	2.5 ml	No limit
1 month	2.5 milligrams	2.5 milligrams	5 minutes	2.5 milligrams in 2.5 ml	2.5 ml	No limit
Birth	N/A	N/A	N/A	N/A	N/A	N/A

Salbutamol

Route: Nebulised with 6–8 litres per minute of oxygen.

AGE	INITIAL DOSE	REPEAT DOSE	DOSE INTERVAL	CONCENTRATION	VOLUME	MAXIMUM DOSE
Adult	5 milligrams	5 milligrams	5 minutes	5 milligrams in 2.5 ml	2.5 ml	No limit
11 years	5 milligrams	5 milligrams	5 minutes	5 milligrams in 2.5 ml	2.5 ml	No limit
10 years	5 milligrams	5 milligrams	5 minutes	5 milligrams in 2.5 ml	2.5 ml	No limit
9 years	5 milligrams	5 milligrams	5 minutes	5 milligrams in 2.5 ml	2.5 ml	No limit
8 years	5 milligrams	5 milligrams	5 minutes	5 milligrams in 2.5 ml	2.5 ml	No limit
7 years	5 milligrams	5 milligrams	5 minutes	5 milligrams in 2.5 ml	2.5 ml	No limit
6 years	5 milligrams	5 milligrams	5 minutes	5 milligrams in 2.5 ml	2.5 ml	No limit
5 years	2.5 milligrams	2.5 milligrams	5 minutes	5 milligrams in 2.5 ml	1.25 ml	No limit
4 years	2.5 milligrams	2.5 milligrams	5 minutes	5 milligrams in 2.5 ml	1.25 ml	No limit
3 years	2.5 milligrams	2.5 milligrams	5 minutes	5 milligrams in 2.5 ml	1.25 ml	No limit
2 years	2.5 milligrams	2.5 milligrams	5 minutes	5 milligrams in 2.5 ml	1.25 ml	No limit
18 months	2.5 milligrams	2.5 milligrams	5 minutes	5 milligrams in 2.5 ml	1.25 ml	No limit
12 months	2.5 milligrams	2.5 milligrams	5 minutes	5 milligrams in 2.5 ml	1.25 ml	No limit
9 months	2.5 milligrams	2.5 milligrams	5 minutes	5 milligrams in 2.5 ml	1.25 ml	No limit
6 months	2.5 milligrams	2.5 milligrams	5 minutes	5 milligrams in 2.5 ml	1.25 ml	No limit
3 months	2.5 milligrams	2.5 milligrams	5 minutes	5 milligrams in 2.5 ml	1.25 ml	No limit
1 month	2.5 milligrams	2.5 milligrams	5 minutes	5 milligrams in 2.5 ml	1.25 ml	No limit
Birth	N/A	N/A	N/A	N/A	N/A	N/A

0.9% Sodium Chloride

Presentation

100 ml, 250 ml, 500 ml and 1,000 ml packs of sodium chloride intravenous infusion 0.9%.

5 ml and 10 ml ampoules for use as flushes.

5 ml and 10 ml pre-loaded syringes for use as flushes.

Indications

Adult fluid therapy

- Medical conditions without haemorrhage.
- Medical conditions with haemorrhage.
- Trauma related haemorrhage.
- Burns.
- Limb crush injury.

Child fluid therapy

- Medical conditions.
- Trauma related haemorrhage.
- Burns.

Flush

- As a flush to confirm patency of an intravenous or intraosseous cannula.
- As a flush following drug administration.

Dosage and Administration

Route: Intravenous or intraosseous for **ALL** conditions.

FLUSH

Actions

Increases vascular fluid volume which consequently raises cardiac output and improves perfusion.

Contra-indications

None.

Side Effects

Over-infusion may precipitate pulmonary oedema and cause breathlessness.

Additional Information

Fluid replacement in cases of dehydration should occur over hours; rapid fluid replacement is seldom indicated; refer to intravascular fluid therapy guidelines.

AGE	INITIAL DOSE	REPEAT DOSE	DOSE INTERVAL	CONCEN-TRATION	VOLUME	MAXIMUM DOSE
Adult	2 ml – 5 ml	2 ml – 5 ml	PRN	0.9%	2 – 5 ml	N/A
Adult	10 ml – 20 ml (if infusing glucose)	10 ml – 20 ml (if infusing glucose)	PRN	0.9%	10 – 20 ml	N/A
5 – 11 years	2 ml – 5 ml	2 ml – 5 ml	PRN	0.9%	2 – 5 ml	N/A
5 – 11 years	5 ml – 10 ml (if infusing glucose)	5 ml – 10 ml (if infusing glucose)	PRN	0.9%	5 – 10 ml	N/A
Birth – <5 years	2 ml	2 ml	PRN	0.9%	2 ml	N/A
Birth – <5 years	2 ml – 5 ml (if infusing glucose)	2 ml – 5ml (if infusing glucose)	PRN	0.9%	2 – 5 ml	N/A

0.9% Sodium Chloride

ADULT MEDICAL EMERGENCIES

General medical conditions without haemorrhage: Anaphylaxis, hyperglycaemic ketoacidosis, dehydration[a]

AGE	INITIAL DOSE	REPEAT DOSE	DOSE INTERVAL	CONCENTRATION	VOLUME	MAXIMUM DOSE
Adult	250 ml	250 ml	PRN	0.9%	250 ml	2 litres

[a] In cases of dehydration fluid replacement should usually occur over hours.

Sepsis: Clinical signs of infection **AND** systolic BP<90 mmHg **AND** tachypnoea

AGE	INITIAL DOSE	REPEAT DOSE	DOSE INTERVAL	CONCENTRATION	VOLUME	MAXIMUM DOSE
Adult	1 litre	1 litre	30 minutes	0.9%	1 litre	2 litres

Medical conditions with haemorrhage: Systolic BP<90 mmHg and signs of poor perfusion

AGE	INITIAL DOSE	REPEAT DOSE	DOSE INTERVAL	CONCENTRATION	VOLUME	MAXIMUM DOSE
Adult	250 ml	250 ml	PRN	0.9%	250 ml	2 litres

ADULT TRAUMA EMERGENCIES

Blunt trauma, head trauma or penetrating limb trauma: Systolic BP<90 mmHg and signs of poor perfusion

AGE	INITIAL DOSE	REPEAT DOSE	DOSE INTERVAL	CONCENTRATION	VOLUME	MAXIMUM DOSE
Adult	250 ml	250 ml	PRN	0.9%	250 ml	2 litres

Penetrating torso trauma: Systolic BP<60 mmHg and signs of poor perfusion

AGE	INITIAL DOSE	REPEAT DOSE	DOSE INTERVAL	CONCENTRATION	VOLUME	MAXIMUM DOSE
Adult	250 ml	250 ml	PRN	0.9%	250 ml	2 litres

Burns:

- Total body surface area (TBSA): between 15% and 25% and time to hospital is greater than 30 minutes
- TBSA: more than 25%

AGE	INITIAL DOSE	REPEAT DOSE	DOSE INTERVAL	CONCENTRATION	VOLUME	MAXIMUM DOSE
Adult	1 litre	NONE	N/A	0.9%	1 litre	1 litre

Limb crush injury

AGE	INITIAL DOSE	REPEAT DOSE	DOSE INTERVAL	CONCENTRATION	VOLUME	MAXIMUM DOSE
Adult	2 litres	NONE	N/A	0.9%	2 litres	2 litres

NB Manage crush injury of the torso as per blunt trauma.

0.9% Sodium Chloride

MEDICAL EMERGENCIES IN CHILDREN (20 ml/kg)

NB Exceptions: cardiac failure, renal failure, diabetic ketoacidosis (see following).

AGE	INITIAL DOSE	REPEAT DOSE	DOSE INTERVAL	CONCENTRATION	VOLUME	MAXIMUM DOSE
11 years	500 ml	500 ml	PRN	0.9%	500 ml	1,000 ml
10 years	500 ml	500 ml	PRN	0.9%	500 ml	1,000 ml
9 years	500 ml	500 ml	PRN	0.9%	500 ml	1,000 ml
8 years	500 ml	500 ml	PRN	0.9%	500 ml	1,000 ml
7 years	460 ml	460 ml	PRN	0.9%	460 ml	920 ml
6 years	420 ml	420 ml	PRN	0.9%	420 ml	840 ml
5 years	380 ml	380 ml	PRN	0.9%	380 ml	760 ml
4 years	320 ml	320 ml	PRN	0.9%	320 ml	640 ml
3 years	280 ml	280 ml	PRN	0.9%	280 ml	560 ml
2 years	240 ml	240 ml	PRN	0.9%	240 ml	480 ml
18 months	220 ml	220 ml	PRN	0.9%	220 ml	440 ml
12 months	200 ml	200 ml	PRN	0.9%	200 ml	400 ml
9 months	180 ml	180 ml	PRN	0.9%	180 ml	360 ml
6 months	160 ml	160 ml	PRN	0.9%	160 ml	320 ml
3 months	120 ml	120 ml	PRN	0.9%	120 ml	240 ml
1 month	90 ml	90 ml	PRN	0.9%	90 ml	180 ml
Birth	70 ml	70 ml	PRN	0.9%	70 ml	140 ml

0.9% Sodium Chloride

MEDICAL EMERGENCIES IN CHILDREN

Heart failure or renal failure (10 ml/kg)

AGE	INITIAL DOSE	REPEAT DOSE	DOSE INTERVAL	CONCENTRATION	VOLUME	MAXIMUM DOSE
11 years	350 ml	350 ml	PRN	0.9%	350 ml	1000 ml
10 years	320 ml	320 ml	PRN	0.9%	320 ml	1000 ml
9 years	290 ml	290 ml	PRN	0.9%	290 ml	1000 ml
8 years	250 ml	250 ml	PRN	0.9%	250 ml	1000 ml
7 years	230 ml	230 ml	PRN	0.9%	230 ml	920 ml
6 years	210 ml	210 ml	PRN	0.9%	210 ml	840 ml
5 years	190 ml	190 ml	PRN	0.9%	190 ml	760 ml
4 years	160 ml	160 ml	PRN	0.9%	160 ml	640 ml
3 years	140 ml	140 ml	PRN	0.9%	140 ml	560 ml
2 years	120 ml	120 ml	PRN	0.9%	120 ml	480 ml
18 months	110 ml	110 ml	PRN	0.9%	110 ml	440 ml
12 months	100 ml	100 ml	PRN	0.9%	100 ml	400 ml
9 months	90 ml	90 ml	PRN	0.9%	90 ml	360 ml
6 months	80 ml	80 ml	PRN	0.9%	80 ml	320 ml
3 months	60 ml	60 ml	PRN	0.9%	60 ml	240 ml
1 month	45 ml	45 ml	PRN	0.9%	45 ml	180 ml
Birth	35 ml	35 ml	PRN	0.9%	35 ml	140 ml

0.9% Sodium Chloride

MEDICAL EMERGENCIES IN CHILDREN

Diabetic ketoacidosis (10 ml/kg) administer **ONCE** only over 15 minutes.

AGE	INITIAL DOSE	REPEAT DOSE	DOSE INTERVAL	CONCENTRATION	VOLUME	MAXIMUM DOSE
11 years	350 ml	NONE	NA	0.9%	350 ml	350 ml
10 years	320 ml	NONE	NA	0.9%	320 ml	320 ml
9 years	290 ml	NONE	NA	0.9%	290 ml	290 ml
8 years	250 ml	NONE	NA	0.9%	250 ml	250 ml
7 years	230 ml	NONE	NA	0.9%	230 ml	230 ml
6 years	210 ml	NONE	NA	0.9%	210 ml	210 ml
5 years	190 ml	NONE	NA	0.9%	190 ml	190 ml
4 years	160 ml	NONE	NA	0.9%	160 ml	160 ml
3 years	140 ml	NONE	NA	0.9%	140 ml	140 ml
2 years	120 ml	NONE	NA	0.9%	120 ml	120 ml
18 months	110 ml	NONE	NA	0.9%	110 ml	110 ml
12 months	100 ml	NONE	NA	0.9%	100 ml	100 ml
9 months	90 ml	NONE	NA	0.9%	90 ml	90 ml
6 months	80 ml	NONE	NA	0.9%	80 ml	80 ml
3 months	60 ml	NONE	NA	0.9%	60 ml	60 ml
1 month	45 ml	NONE	NA	0.9%	45 ml	45 ml
Birth	35 ml	NONE	NA	0.9%	35 ml	35 ml

0.9% Sodium Chloride

TRAUMA EMERGENCIES IN CHILDREN (5 ml/kg)

NB Exceptions: burns.

AGE	INITIAL DOSE	REPEAT DOSE	DOSE INTERVAL	CONCENTRATION	VOLUME	MAXIMUM DOSE
11 years	175 ml	175 ml	PRN	0.9%	175 ml	1,000 ml
10 years	160 ml	160 ml	PRN	0.9%	160 ml	1,000 ml
9 years	145 ml	145 ml	PRN	0.9%	145 ml	1,000 ml
8 years	130 ml	130 ml	PRN	0.9%	130 ml	1,000 ml
7 years	115 ml	115 ml	PRN	0.9%	115 ml	920 ml
6 years	105 ml	105 ml	PRN	0.9%	105 ml	840 ml
5 years	95 ml	95 ml	PRN	0.9%	95 ml	760 ml
4 years	80 ml	80 ml	PRN	0.9%	80 ml	640 ml
3 years	70 ml	70 ml	PRN	0.9%	70 ml	560 ml
2 years	60 ml	60 ml	PRN	0.9%	60 ml	480 ml
18 months	55 ml	55 ml	PRN	0.9%	55 ml	440 ml
12 months	50 ml	50 ml	PRN	0.9%	50 ml	400 ml
9 months	45 ml	45 ml	PRN	0.9%	45 ml	360 ml
6 months	40 ml	40 ml	PRN	0.9%	40 ml	320 ml
3 months	30 ml	30 ml	PRN	0.9%	30 ml	240 ml
1 month	20 ml	20 ml	PRN	0.9%	20 ml	180 ml
Birth	20 ml	20 ml	PRN	0.9%	20 ml	140 ml

0.9% Sodium Chloride

Burns (10 ml/kg, given over 1 hour):

- TBSA: between 10% and 20% and time to hospital is greater than 30 minutes
- TBSA: more than 20%

AGE	INITIAL DOSE	REPEAT DOSE	DOSE INTERVAL	CONCENTRATION	VOLUME	MAXIMUM DOSE
11 years	350 ml	NONE	N/A	0.9%	350 ml	350 ml
10 years	320 ml	NONE	N/A	0.9%	320 ml	320 ml
9 years	290 ml	NONE	N/A	0.9%	290 ml	290 ml
8 years	250 ml	NONE	N/A	0.9%	250 ml	250 ml
7 years	230 ml	NONE	N/A	0.9%	230 ml	230 ml
6 years	210 ml	NONE	N/A	0.9%	210 ml	210 ml
5 years	190 ml	NONE	N/A	0.9%	190 ml	190 ml
4 years	160 ml	NONE	N/A	0.9%	160 ml	160 ml
3 years	140 ml	NONE	N/A	0.9%	140 ml	140 ml
2 years	120 ml	NONE	N/A	0.9%	120 ml	120 ml
18 months	110 ml	NONE	N/A	0.9%	110 ml	110 ml
12 months	100 ml	NONE	N/A	0.9%	100 ml	100 ml
9 months	90 ml	NONE	N/A	0.9%	90 ml	90 ml
6 months	80 ml	NONE	N/A	0.9%	80 ml	80 ml
3 months	60 ml	NONE	N/A	0.9%	60 ml	60 ml
1 month	45 ml	NONE	N/A	0.9%	45 ml	45 ml
Birth	35 ml	NONE	N/A	0.9%	35 ml	35 ml

Presentation

250 ml, 500 ml and 1,000 ml packs of compound sodium lactate intravenous infusion (also called Hartmann's solution for injection or Ringer's lactate solution for injection).

Indications

Blood and fluid loss, to correct hypovolaemia and improve tissue perfusion if sodium chloride 0.9% is **NOT** available.

Dehydration.

Actions

Increases vascular fluid volume which consequently raises cardiac output and improves perfusion.

Contra-Indications

Diabetic hyperglycaemic ketoacidotic coma, and precoma. NB Administer 0.9% sodium chloride intravenous infusion.

Neonates.

Cautions

Sodium lactate should not be used in limb crush injury when 0.9% sodium chloride is available.

Renal failure.

Liver failure.

Side Effects

Infusion of an excessive volume may overload the circulation and precipitate heart failure (increased breathlessness, wheezing and distended neck veins). Volume overload is unlikely if the patient is correctly assessed initially and it is very unlikely indeed if patient response is assessed after initial 250 ml infusion and then after each 250 ml of infusion. If there is evidence of this complication, the patient should be transported rapidly to nearest suitable receiving hospital whilst administering high-flow oxygen.

Do not administer further fluid.

Additional Information

Compound sodium lactate intravenous infusion contains mainly sodium, but also small amounts of potassium and lactate. It is useful for initial fluid replacement in cases of blood loss.

The volume of compound sodium lactate intravenous infusion needed is 3 times as great as the volume of blood loss. Sodium lactate has **NO** oxygen carrying capacity.

Dosage and Administration if sodium chloride 0.9% is NOT available.

Route: Intravenous or intraosseous for **ALL** conditions.

ADULT MEDICAL EMERGENCIES

General medical conditions without haemorrhage: anaphylaxis, dehydration[a]

NB Exception sodium lactate compound is contra-indicated in diabetic ketoacidosis – refer to sodium chloride 0.9% guideline.

AGE	INITIAL DOSE	REPEAT DOSE	DOSE INTERVAL	CONCENTRATION	VOLUME	MAXIMUM DOSE
Adult	250 ml	250 ml	PRN	Compound	250 ml	1 litre

Sepsis: Clinical signs of infection **AND** systolic BP<90 mmHg **AND** tachypnoea

AGE	INITIAL DOSE	REPEAT DOSE	DOSE INTERVAL	CONCENTRATION	VOLUME	MAXIMUM DOSE
Adult	1 litre	1 litre	30 minutes	Compound	1 litre	2 litres

[a] In cases of dehydration fluid replacement should usually occur over hours.

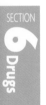

Sodium Lactate Compound (Hartmann's/Ringer's Lactate)

ADULT TRAUMA EMERGENCIES

Medical conditions with haemorrhage: Systolic BP<90 mmHg and signs of poor perfusion

AGE	INITIAL DOSE	REPEAT DOSE	DOSE INTERVAL	CONCENTRATION	VOLUME	MAXIMUM DOSE
Adult	250 ml	250 ml	PRN	Compound	250 ml	2 litres

Blunt trauma, head trauma or penetrating limb trauma: Systolic BP<90 mmHg and signs of poor perfusion

AGE	INITIAL DOSE	REPEAT DOSE	DOSE INTERVAL	CONCENTRATION	VOLUME	MAXIMUM DOSE
Adult	250 ml	250 ml	PRN	Compound	250 ml	2 litres

Penetrating torso trauma: Systolic BP<60 mmHg and signs of poor perfusion

AGE	INITIAL DOSE	REPEAT DOSE	DOSE INTERVAL	CONCENTRATION	VOLUME	MAXIMUM DOSE
Adult	250 ml	250 ml	PRN	Compound	250 ml	2 litres

Burns:

- TBSA: between 15% and 25% and time to hospital is greater than 30 minutes.
- TBSA: more than 25%.

AGE	INITIAL DOSE	REPEAT DOSE	DOSE INTERVAL	CONCENTRATION	VOLUME	MAXIMUM DOSE
Adult	1 litre	N/A	N/A	Compound	1 litre	1 litre

Limb crush injury

AGE	INITIAL DOSE	REPEAT DOSE	DOSE INTERVAL	CONCENTRATION	VOLUME	MAXIMUM DOSE
Adult	2 litres	N/A	N/A	Compound	2 litres	2 litres

NB Sodium chloride 0.9% is the fluid of choice in crush injury. NB Manage crush injury of the torso as per blunt trauma.

Sodium Lactate Compound (Hartmann's/Ringer's Lactate)

MEDICAL EMERGENCIES IN CHILDREN (20 ml/kg)

NB Exceptions heart failure, renal failure, liver failure, diabetic ketoacidosis (sodium lactate compound is contra-indicated in diabetic ketoacidosis – refer to sodium chloride 0.9% guideline).

AGE	INITIAL DOSE	REPEAT DOSE	DOSE INTERVAL	CONCENTRATION	VOLUME	MAXIMUM DOSE
11 years	500 ml	500 ml	PRN	Compound	500 ml	1 litre
10 years	500 ml	500 ml	PRN	Compound	500 ml	1 litre
9 years	500 ml	500 ml	PRN	Compound	500 ml	1 litre
8 years	500 ml	500 ml	PRN	Compound	500 ml	1 litre
7 years	460 ml	460 ml	PRN	Compound	460 ml	920 ml
6 years	420 ml	420 ml	PRN	Compound	420 ml	840 ml
5 years	380 ml	380 ml	PRN	Compound	380 ml	760 ml
4 years	320 ml	320 ml	PRN	Compound	320 ml	640 ml
3 years	280 ml	280 ml	PRN	Compound	280 ml	560 ml
2 years	240 ml	240 ml	PRN	Compound	240 ml	480 ml
18 months	220 ml	220 ml	PRN	Compound	220 ml	440 ml
12 months	200 ml	200 ml	PRN	Compound	200 ml	400 ml
9 months	180 ml	180 ml	PRN	Compound	180 ml	360 ml
6 months	160 ml	160 ml	PRN	Compound	160 ml	320 ml
3 months	120 ml	120 ml	PRN	Compound	120 ml	240 ml
1 month	90 ml	90 ml	PRN	Compound	90 ml	180 ml
Birth	N/A	N/A	N/A	N/A	N/A	N/A

Sodium Lactate Compound (Hartmann's/Ringer's Lactate)

Burns (10 ml/kg, given over 1 hour):

- TBSA: between 10% and 20% and time to hospital is greater than 30 minutes.
- TBSA: more than 20%.

AGE	INITIAL DOSE	REPEAT DOSE	DOSE INTERVAL	CONCENTRATION	VOLUME	MAXIMUM DOSE
11 years	350 ml	NONE	N/A	Compound	350 ml	350 ml
10 years	320 ml	NONE	N/A	Compound	320 ml	320 ml
9 years	290 ml	NONE	N/A	Compound	290 ml	290 ml
8 years	250 ml	NONE	N/A	Compound	250 ml	250 ml
7 years	230 ml	NONE	N/A	Compound	230 ml	230 ml
6 years	210 ml	NONE	N/A	Compound	210 ml	210 ml
5 years	190 ml	NONE	N/A	Compound	190 ml	190 ml
4 years	160 ml	NONE	N/A	Compound	160 ml	160 ml
3 years	140 ml	NONE	N/A	Compound	140 ml	140 ml
2 years	120 ml	NONE	N/A	Compound	120 ml	120 ml
18 months	110 ml	NONE	N/A	Compound	110 ml	110 ml
12 months	100 ml	NONE	N/A	Compound	100 ml	100 ml
9 months	90 ml	NONE	N/A	Compound	90 ml	90 ml
6 months	80 ml	NONE	N/A	Compound	80 ml	80 ml
3 months	60 ml	NONE	N/A	Compound	60 ml	60 ml
1 month	45 ml	NONE	N/A	Compound	45 ml	45 ml
Birth	N/A	N/A	N/A	N/A	N/A	N/A

Presentation

An ampoule containing ergometrine 500 micrograms and oxytocin 5 units in 1 ml.

Indications

Post-partum haemorrhage within 24 hours of delivery of the infant where bleeding from the uterus is uncontrollable by uterine massage.

Miscarriage with life-threatening bleeding and a confirmed diagnosis (e.g. where a patient has gone home with medical management and starts to bleed).

Actions

Stimulates contraction of the uterus.

Onset of action 7–10 minutes.

Contra-Indications

- Known hypersensitivity to syntometrine.
- Active labour.
- Severe cardiac, liver or kidney disease.
- Hypertension and severe pre-eclampsia.
- Possible multiple pregnancy/known or suspected fetus in utero.

Side Effects

- Nausea and vomiting.
- Abdominal pain.
- Headache.
- Hypertension and bradycardia.
- Chest pain and, rarely, anaphylactic reactions.

Additional Information

Syntometrine and misoprostol reduce bleeding from a pregnant uterus through different pathways; therefore if one drug has not been effective after 15 minutes, the other may be administered in addition.

Dosage and Administration

Route: Intramuscular.

AGE	INITIAL DOSE	REPEAT DOSE	DOSE INTERVAL	CONCENTRATION	VOLUME	MAXIMUM DOSE
Adult	500 micrograms of ergometrine and 5 units of oxytocin	**None**	N/A	500 micrograms of ergometrine and 5 units of oxytocin in 1 ml	1 ml	500 micrograms of ergometrine and 5 units of oxytocin

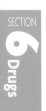

Presentation

Vials of **tenecteplase** 10,000 units for reconstitution with 10 ml water for injection, or 8,000 units for reconstitution with 8 ml water for injection.

NOTE: Whilst the strength of thrombolytics is traditionally expressed in 'units' these units are unique to each particular drug and are **NOT** interchangeable.

Indications

Acute ST segment elevation MI (STEMI) within 6 hours of symptom onset where primary percutaneous coronary intervention (PPCI) is **NOT** readily available.

Ensure patient fulfils the criteria for drug administration following the model checklist (below). Variation of these criteria is justifiable at local level with agreement of appropriate key stakeholders (e.g. cardiac network, or in the context of an approved clinical trial).

Contra-Indications

See checklist.

Actions

Activates the fibrinolytic system, inducing the breaking up of intravascular thrombi and emboli.

Side Effects

Bleeding:

- Major – seek medical advice and transport to hospital rapidly.

- Minor (e.g. at injection sites) – use local pressure.

Arrhythmias – these are usually benign in the form of transient idioventricular rhythms and usually require no special treatment. Treat ventricular fibrillation (VF) as a complication of myocardial infarction (MI) with standard protocols; bradycardia with atropine as required.

Anaphylaxis – extremely rare (0.1%) with third generation bolus agents.

Hypotension – often responds to laying the patient flat.

Additional Information

PPCI is now the dominant reperfusion treatment and should be used where available; patients with STEMI will be taken direct to a specialist cardiac centre instead of receiving thrombolysis (**refer to acute coronary syndrome guideline**). Local guidelines should be followed.

'Time is muscle!' Do not delay transportation to hospital if difficulties arise whilst setting up the equipment or establishing IV access. Qualified single responders should administer a thrombolytic if indicated while awaiting arrival of an ambulance.

In All Cases

Ensure a defibrillator is immediately available at all times.

Monitor conscious level, pulse, blood pressure and cardiac rhythm during and following injections. Manage complications (associated with the acute MI) as they occur using standard protocols. The main early adverse event associated with thrombolysis is bleeding, which should be managed according to standard guidelines.

AT HOSPITAL – emphasise the need to commence a heparin infusion in accordance with local guidelines – to reduce the risk of re-infarction.

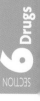

Tenecteplase

Thrombolysis Checklist

Is primary PCI available?

- **YES** – undertake a **TIME CRITICAL** transfer to PPCI capable hospital.
- **NO** – ask the patient the questions listed below, to determine whether they are suitable to receive thrombolysis.

Assessment Questions	Yes	No
Has the patient suffered a haemorrhagic stroke or stroke of unknown origin at any time?	☐	☐
Has the patient suffered a transient ischaemic attack in the preceding 6 months?	☐	☐
Has the patient suffered a central nervous system trauma or neoplasm?	☐	☐
Has the patient had recent trauma, surgery or head injury within the preceding 3 weeks?	☐	☐
Has the patient suffered from gastrointestinal bleeding (within the last month)?	☐	☐
Has the patient a known bleeding disorder?	☐	☐
Do you suspect aortic dissection?	☐	☐
Has the patient a non-compressible puncture (e.g. liver biopsy, lumbar puncture)?	☐	☐
Is the patient taking oral anticoagulant therapy (e.g. warfarin)?	☐	☐
Is the patient pregnant or within 1 week post-partum?	☐	☐
Is the patient's systolic blood pressure >180 mmHg and/or diastolic blood pressure >110 mmHg?	☐	☐
Is the patient suffering from advanced liver disease?	☐	☐
Is the patient suffering from active peptic ulcer?	☐	☐

If the patient answers **YES TO ANY** of the above questions, thrombolysis **IS NOT** indicated; seek advice.

If the patient answers **NO TO ALL** of the above questions and thrombolysis is indicated, refer to the dosage and administration table.

Tenecteplase

Dosage and Administration

1. Administer a bolus of intravenous injection of un-fractionated heparin before administration of tenecteplase (refer to heparin guideline). Flush the cannula well with saline.
2. **AT HOSPITAL** – It is essential that the care of the patient is handed over as soon as possible to a member of hospital staff qualified to administer a heparin infusion.

Route: Intravenous single bolus adjusted for patient weight.

AGE	WEIGHT	INITIAL DOSE	REPEAT DOSE	DOSE INTERVAL	CONCENTRATION	VOLUME	MAXIMUM DOSE
≥18	<60 kg (<9st 6lbs)	6,000 units	NONE	N/A	1,000 U/ml	6 ml	6,000 units
≥18	60–69 kg (9st 6lbs–10st 13lbs)	7,000 units	NONE	N/A	1,000 U/ml	7 ml	7,000 units
≥18	70–79 kg (11st–12st 7lbs)	8,000 units	NONE	N/A	1,000 U/ml	8 ml	8,000 units
≥18	80–90 kg (12st 8lbs–14st 2lbs)	9,000 units	NONE	N/A	1,000 U/ml	9 ml	9,000 units
≥18	>90 kg (>14st 2lbs)	10,000 units	NONE	N/A	1,000 U/ml	10 ml	10,000 units

Presentation

1 or 1.5 gram tubes of white semi-transparent gel.

Transparent occlusive dressing.

Indications

Where venepuncture may be required in a non-urgent situation, in individuals who are believed to have a fear of, or likely to become upset if undergoing venepuncture (usually children, some vulnerable adults or needle-phobic adults). Venepuncture includes intravenous injection, cannulation and obtaining venous blood.

Time of application should be noted and included in hand-over to the emergency department or other care facility.

Actions

Tetracaine 4% cream is a local anaesthetic agent, that has properties that allow it to penetrate intact skin, thus providing local anaesthesia to the area of skin with which it has been in contact.

Contra-Indications

DO NOT apply tetracaine in the following circumstances:

- The application of tetracaine should not take preference over life-saving or any other clinically urgent procedures.
- If the area being considered for anaesthesia will require venepuncture in less than 15 minutes.
- Known allergy to tetracaine cream, or any of its other constituents.
- Known allergy to the brand of transparent occlusive dressing.
- If the patient is allergic to other local anaesthetics.
- If the patient is pregnant or breastfeeding.
- If the patient is less than 1 month old.
- Avoid applying to open wounds, broken skin, lips, mouth, eyes, ears, anal or genital region, mucous membranes.

Cautions

Allergy to Elastoplast or other adhesive dressing – discuss risk/benefit with carer.

Side Effects

Expect mild vasodilatation over the treated area.

Occasionally local irritation may occur.

Additional Information

Although the application of tetracaine may not directly improve the quality of care experienced by the patient from the ambulance service, it is in line with good patient care, and its use will benefit the patient's subsequent management.

Tetracaine takes 30–40 minutes after application before the area will become numb and remain numb for 4–6 hours.

Sites of application should be based on local guidelines.

Tetracaine only needs refrigeration if it is unlikely to be used for a considerable time; therefore bulk stores should be kept refrigerated. Generally speaking, it does not require refrigeration in everyday use; however, tubes that are not refrigerated or used within 3 months should be discarded.

Special Precautions

Do not leave on for more than an hour.

Do not delay transfer to further care of TIME CRITICAL patients.

Dosage and Administration

- Apply one tube directly over a vein that looks as if it would support cannulation – refer to local care guideline.
- Do not rub the cream in.
- Place an occlusive dressing directly over the 'blob' of cream, taking care to completely surround the cream to ensure it does not leak out.
- Repeat the procedure in one similar, alternative site.
- **REMEMBER** to tell the receiving staff the time of application and location when handing the patient over.

Route: Topical.

AGE	INITIAL DOSE	REPEAT DOSE	DOSE INTERVAL	CONCENTRATION	VOLUME	MAXIMUM DOSE
>1 month	1–1.5 grams	N/A	N/A	4%	1 tube	N/A

SECTION **6** Drugs

Tranexamic Acid [875–879]

TXA

Presentation

Vial containing 500 mg tranexamic acid in 5 ml (100 mg/ml).

Indications

- Patients with **TIME CRITICAL** injury where significant internal/external haemorrhage is suspected.
- Injured patients fulfilling local Step 1 or Step 2 trauma triage protocol – **refer to Appendix in trauma emergencies overview (adults)**.

Actions

Tranexamic acid is an anti-fibrinolytic which reduces the breakdown of blood clot.

Contra-Indications

- Isolated head injury.
- Critical interventions required (if critical interventions leave insufficient time for TXA administration).
- Bleeding now stopped.

Side Effects

Rapid injection might rarely cause hypotension.

Additional Information

- There are good data that this treatment is safe and effective (giving a 9% reduction in the number of deaths in patients in the CRASH2 trial).
- There is no evidence about whether or not tranexamic acid is effective in patients with head injury; however, there is no evidence of harm.
- High dose regimes have been associated with convulsions; however, in the low dose regime recommended here, the benefit from giving TXA in trauma outweighs the risk of convulsions.
- Refer to local PGD for information on administration procedures.

Dosage and Administration

Route: Intravenous only – **administer SLOWLY over 10 minutes – can be given as 10 aliquots administered 1 minute apart.**

AGE	INITIAL DOSE	REPEAT DOSE	DOSE INTERVAL	CONCENTRATION	VOLUME	MAXIMUM DOSE
>12 years – Adult	1 gram	NONE	N/A	100 mg/ml	10 ml	1 g
11 years	500 mg	NONE	N/A	100 mg/ml	5 ml	500 mg
10 years	500 mg	NONE	N/A	100 mg/ml	5 ml	500 mg
9 years	450 mg	NONE	N/A	100 mg/ml	4.5 ml	450 mg
8 years	400 mg	NONE	N/A	100 mg/ml	4 ml	400 mg
7 years	350 mg	NONE	N/A	100 mg/ml	3.5 ml	350 mg
6 years	300 mg	NONE	N/A	100 mg/ml	3 ml	300 mg
5 years	300 mg	NONE	N/A	100 mg/ml	3 ml	300 mg
4 years	250 mg	NONE	N/A	100 mg/ml	2.5 ml	250 mg
3 years	200 mg	NONE	N/A	100 mg/ml	2 ml	200 mg
2 years	200 mg	NONE	N/A	100 mg/ml	2 ml	200 mg
18 months	150 mg	NONE	N/A	100 mg/ml	1.5 ml	150 mg
12 months	150 mg	NONE	N/A	100 mg/ml	1.5 ml	150 mg
9 months	150 mg	NONE	N/A	100 mg/ml	1.5 ml	150 mg
6 months	100 mg	NONE	N/A	100 mg/ml	1 ml	100 mg
3 months	100 mg	NONE	N/A	100 mg/ml	1 ml	100 mg
1 month	50 mg	NONE	N/A	100 mg/ml	0.5 ml	50 mg
Birth	50 mg	NONE	N/A	100 mg/ml	0.5 ml	50 mg

Intravascular Fluid Therapy (Adults)

1. Introduction [178, 682, 880–885]

- Despite a lack of evidence demonstrating any significant beneficial effects, pre-hospital fluid therapy has become an established practice.

- There is, however, a significant body of evidence that indicates that routine pre-hospital intravascular fluid therapy may, in fact, be detrimental.

- Adverse effects may be attributed to prolonged on-scene times delaying time to definitive surgical intervention, thrombus disruption, dilution of clotting factors and other coagulopathies.

2. Pathophysiology [880, 885, 886]

- The objective of fluid therapy is to improve end-organ perfusion and, as a consequence, oxygen delivery.

- By increasing the circulating volume, cardiac output and blood pressure are increased by the Bainbridge Reflex and Frank–Starling Law of the Heart.

- The speed with which a given fluid will produce its effect will largely be determined by how it is distributed throughout the body and how long it remains in the vascular space.

2.1 pH buffering

- Reduced perfusion leads to acidosis as a result of anaerobic metabolism producing lactic acid, phosphoric acids and unoxidised amino acids.

- This acidosis can depress cardiac function (negative inotropic effect) and cause arrhythmias.

2.2 Oxygen transport

- Crystalloid fluids currently used in the pre-hospital environment have no oxygen carrying capacity.

- However, the administration of fluids reduces blood viscosity which in turn may lead to improved peripheral blood flow and hence oxygen delivery.

2.3 Haemostasis

- In general, administration of fluid has a detrimental effect on haemostasis and a tendency to increase bleeding.

- The administration of fluid raises intravascular pressures and usually causes vasodilation, both of which may precipitate disruption of the primary haemostatic thrombus.

- Furthermore, supplemental administration of fluid reduces blood viscosity and dilutes clotting factors both of which can be detrimental to haemostatic mechanisms.

- Finally, in order to minimise hypothermia-induced coagulopathies, the use of cold fluids should be avoided if possible.

3. Haemorrhagic Emergencies [887–899]

- Haemorrhage may occur as a result of traumatic or medical aetiologies and may be classified as:
  - **apparent** (external) blood loss
  - **concealed** (internal) blood loss

- Current thinking suggests that fluids should **ONLY** be administered when there are signs of impaired major organ perfusion (refer to Table 6.11).

Table 6.11 – EARLY INDICATORS OF IMPAIRED MAJOR ORGAN PERFUSION

SIGNS	CAUSE
Tachypnoea	↑ Metabolic acidosis
Tachycardia	↓ Cardiac output
Hypotension	↓ Vascular volume
↓ Consciousness	↓ Cerebral perfusion

- Control of external haemorrhage must be achieved before administering fluids.

3.1 Trauma

3.1.1 Penetrating trauma to the trunk

- Penetrating trauma to the trunk carries the risk of significant disruption of major vessels that, due to their location, are not amenable to compression or other methods of haemorrhage control.

- As a consequence of this inability to control further bleeding, the general aim of fluid therapy is to maintain blood pressure at 60 mmHg systolic.

3.1.2 Penetrating trauma to the limbs

- Penetrating trauma to the limbs also carries a risk of significant disruption of major vessels; however, these vessels are both fewer and more amenable to compression or other methods of haemorrhage control.

- As a consequence of this ability to control further bleeding, the general aim of fluid therapy is to maintain blood pressure at 90 mmHg systolic.

3.1.3 Blunt trauma to trunk or limbs

- Blunt trauma to the trunk carries a lower risk of major vessel disruption; consequently, the trigger point for fluid administration is different from penetrating trauma.

- In cases of blunt trauma to the trunk or limbs, the aim of fluid therapy is to maintain blood pressure at 90 mmHg systolic.

3.1.4 Trauma to the head (all types)

- Significant head injury results in raised intracranial pressure (ICP) as cerebral tissues swell within the enclosed skull; to ensure adequate cerebral perfusion pressure (CPP) the body compensates and raises the mean arterial blood pressure (MAP).

$$CPP = MAP - ICP$$

- As a result of this compensatory mechanism, significant head injuries are usually associated with hypertension and **NOT** hypotension.

- Hypotension in the setting of significant head injury indicates not only significant blood loss but also **CRITICALLY IMPAIRED CEREBRAL PERFUSION.**

- In order to support cerebral perfusion the administration of fluids may be required.

- In the setting of significant head injury with hypotension, fluid therapy should be titrated to a systolic blood pressure of 90 mmHg.

- Hypertensive head injury does not normally require fluid therapy. Research concerning pre-hospital hypertonic saline has yet to demonstrate conclusive evidence of beneficial effect.

3.2 Medical conditions

- Principles of fluid therapy in medically related haemorrhage are fundamentally no different from those of blunt trauma.

- Generally, the aim of fluid therapy is to maintain systolic blood pressure at 90 mmHg.

- Medically related haemorrhage may also be complicated by vascular disease, coagulopathies or the presence of tumors.

3.3 Fluid therapy following haemorrhage

- **DO NOT** delay at scene to obtain vascular access or to commence fluid replacement; wherever possible obtain vascular access and administer fluid **EN-ROUTE TO HOSPITAL.**

- If the clinician determines that there is a definite need for fluid therapy they should obtain vascular access.

- Clinicians should attempt to gain intravenous access in the first instance; however, they may consider intraosseous access where intravenous access fails or is unlikely to be successful.

- Vascular access devices should be flushed with 5 ml of 0.9% sodium chloride for injection to confirm patency prior to administering large volumes of fluid.

- Once patent vascular access is confirmed, administer a single bolus of 250 ml of crystalloid (refer to Table 6.12).

- Where the need for intravascular fluid therapy is less certain, clinicians should still obtain vascular access and flush to confirm patency.

- **Do not connect any fluids to the cannula unless intravascular fluid therapy is indicated.**

NB The slow administration of fluids to keep a vein open (TKO/TKVO) should not be practised to avoid inadvertent excess fluid administration.

Table 6.12 – DOSAGES FOR FLUID THERAPY – HAEMORRHAGIC EMERGENCIES

INITIAL DOSE	REPEAT DOSE	REPEAT INTERVAL	MAXIMUM DOSE
250 ml	250 ml	PRN	2 litres

- Monitor the physiological response; re-assess perfusion, pulse, respiratory rate and blood pressure wherever possible.

- If these observations improve, suspend any further administration.

- If there is no improvement administer further 250 ml boluses, re-assessing for improvement after each fluid bolus (refer to Table 6.12).

- The maximum cumulative fluid dose is usually 2 litres (refer to Table 6.12).

- If the patient remains hypotensive despite repeated 250 ml boluses **OR** the patient is likely to remain on

scene for a considerable time (e.g. due to entrapment), request senior clinical support (according to local procedures).

3.4 Exceptions and special circumstances

3.4.1 Crush injury

- A crush injury is caused by direct compressive force on the body. Crush syndrome is the systemic manifestation of muscle cell damage resulting from pressure or crushing.

- The severity of the injury is related to both the magnitude of the compressing force, and the bulk of muscle affected, but not necessarily the duration for which the force has been applied.

- The pathophysiology of crush syndrome results from the leakiness of the cellular membranes as a consequence of pressure or stretching. Sodium, calcium and water leak through the cellular membrane into the muscle cell, trapping extracellular fluid inside the muscle cells. In addition to the influx of these elements into the cell, the cell releases potassium and other toxic substances such as myoglobin, phosphate and uric acid into the circulation.

- The end result of these events is hypotension, hyperkalaemia (which may precipitate cardiac arrest), hypocalcaemia, metabolic acidosis, compartment syndrome (due to swelling) and acute renal failure (ARF).

- If possible, fluid therapy should commence prior to extrication; however, extrication or transport **MUST NOT** be unnecessarily delayed in order to obtain intravenous access or to administer fluid.

- In crush injury of the limbs an initial fluid bolus of 2 litres of 0.9% sodium chloride should be administered (refer to Table 6.13).

- In crush injury of the torso follow blunt trauma fluid therapy practices (see 3.1.3).

- If possible, request senior clinical support to guide further therapy.

Table 6.13 – DOSAGES FOR FLUID THERAPY – CRUSH INJURY OF THE LIMBS

INITIAL DOSE	REPEAT DOSE	REPEAT INTERVAL	MAXIMUM DOSE
2 litres	NONE	N/A	2 litres

3.4.2 Obstetric emergencies

- Clinicians must remember that the gravid uterus may compress the inferior vena cava in a pregnant patient who is supine. Appropriate positioning of the patient, that is left lateral tilt or manual displacement of the gravid uterus must be considered to ensure adequate venous return before determining that a pregnant patient is in need of fluid resuscitation.

- Due to their increase in blood volume, the obstetric patient is able to tolerate far greater blood loss, up to 50%, before showing signs of hypovolaemia/shock.

- In obstetric patients, the uterus, and thus the fetus, will often become 'underperfused' **PRIOR** to the pregnant women showing outward signs of shock (i.e. becoming tachycardic or hypotensive).

- Signs of shock appear very late during pregnancy and hypotension is an extremely late sign.

- Clinicians should take frequent clinical observations and be vigilant for subtle changes that may indicate the onset of shock.

- Fluid replacement should aim to maintain a systolic blood pressure of 90 mmHg in obstetric patients who are bleeding.

4. Non-Haemorrhagic Emergencies

[725–726, 892–897, 900–910]

4.1 Trauma

- The loss of bodily fluids other than blood, as a result of trauma, is rare. Burn injuries are notable exceptions (see exceptions and special circumstances below).

4.2 Medical conditions

- Patients suffering medical emergencies may experience fluid loss as a result of dehydration (e.g. heat related illness, vomiting or diarrhoea) and/or redistribution of fluid from the vascular compartment (e.g. as a result of anaphylaxis).

- The volume of fluids lost to such processes can easily be underestimated.

- Such patients may be significantly dehydrated resulting in reduced fluid volumes in both the vascular and tissue compartments which has usually taken time to develop and will take time to correct.

- Rapid fluid replacement into the vascular compartment can compromise the cardiovascular system particularly where there is pre-existing cardiovascular disease and in the elderly.

- In cases of dehydration, fluid replacement should be aimed at gradual re-hydration over many hours rather than minutes. Oral electrolyte solutions may be an appropriate consideration in some patients (e.g. heat illness).

4.3 Fluid therapy

- **DO NOT** delay at scene to obtain vascular access or to provide fluid replacement; wherever possible obtain vascular access and administer fluid **EN-ROUTE TO HOSPITAL.**

- If the clinician determines that there is a definite need for fluid therapy, they should obtain vascular access.

- Clinicians should attempt to gain intravenous access in the first instance; however, they may consider intraosseous access where intravenous access fails or is unlikely to be successful.

- Vascular access devices should be flushed with 5 ml of 0.9% sodium chloride for injection to confirm patency prior to administering large volumes of fluid.

- Once patent vascular access is confirmed, administer a single bolus of 250 ml of crystalloid (refer to Table 6.14).

- Where the need for intravascular fluid therapy is less certain, clinicians should still obtain vascular access and flush to confirm patency.

- **Do not connect any fluids to the cannula unless intravascular fluid therapy is indicated.**

NB The slow administration of fluids to keep a vein open (TKO/TKVO) should not be practised to avoid inadvertent excess fluid administration.

Table 6.14 – DOSAGES FOR FLUID THERAPY			
INITIAL DOSE	**REPEAT DOSE**	**REPEAT INTERVAL**	**MAXIMUM DOSE**
250 ml	250 ml	PRN	2 litres

- Monitor the physiological response, re-assess perfusion, pulse, respiratory rate and blood pressure wherever possible.

- If these observations improve, suspend any further administration.

- If there is no improvement, administer further 250 ml boluses, reassessing for improvement after each fluid bolus (refer to Table 6.14).

- The maximum cumulative fluid dose is usually 2 litres (refer to Table 6.14).

- If the patient remains hypotensive despite repeated 250 ml boluses OR the patient is likely to remain on scene for a considerable time (e.g. due to extrication difficulties), request senior clinical support (according to local procedures).

4.4 Exceptions and special circumstances

4.4.1 Burns

Where burn surface area is:

- <15% do not administer fluid.

- ≥15 – <25% and time to hospital is greater than 30 minutes, then administer 1 litre sodium chloride 0.9% (refer to Table 6.15).

- ≥25% administer 1 litre sodium chloride 0.9% (refer to Table 6.15).

NB If fluid therapy is indicated **DO NOT** delay transfer to further care but continue fluid therapy en-route – stopping if practicable to insert the cannula.

- Care must be taken to ensure that elderly or heart failure patients are not over-infused.

- In order to minimise the risk of hypothermia, the use of cold fluids should be avoided if possible.

Table 6.15 – DOSAGES FOR FLUID THERAPY – BURNS			
INITIAL DOSE	**REPEAT DOSE**	**REPEAT INTERVAL**	**MAXIMUM DOSE**
1 litre over 1 hour	NONE[a]	N/A	1 litre

[a] Seek senior clinical input for prolonged delays

4.4.2 Sepsis

- Sepsis should be suspected in patients who have a history of infection, a systolic blood pressure below 90 mmHg and tachypnoea.

SECTION 6 Drugs

- Patients with sepsis will benefit from early fluid therapy and an appropriate hospital alert/information call.
- Intravascular fluid should be administered in cases of suspected sepsis (refer to Tables 6.16 and 6.17).

Table 6.16 – CLINICAL SIGNS OF SEPSIS

- History of infection
- Systolic blood pressure <90 mmHg
- Tachypnoea

- The presence of additional clinical signs helps to confirm the diagnosis (NB not all will be present).

Table 6.17 – ADDITIONAL CLINICAL SIGNS OF SEPSIS

Signs

- Body temperature less than 36°C
  OR
  Body temperature greater than 38°C
- Tachycardia
- Altered mental status
- Mottled skin
- Prolonged capillary refill (>2 seconds)

- Clinicians should administer 1 litre of sodium chloride 0.9%.

Table 6.18 – DOSAGES FOR FLUID THERAPY – SEPSIS

INITIAL DOSE	REPEAT DOSE	REPEAT INTERVAL	MAXIMUM DOSE
1 litre over 30 minutes	Repeat ONCE if still hypotensive	PRN	2 litres

KEY POINTS

Intravascular Fluid Therapy (Adults)

- **Current research shows little evidence to support the routine use of IV fluids in adult acute blood loss.**
- **Current thinking is that fluids should only be administered when major organ perfusion is impaired.**
- **DO NOT delay on scene for vascular access or fluid replacement; wherever possible obtain vascular access and administer fluid EN-ROUTE TO HOSPITAL stopping if practicable to insert the cannula.**

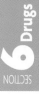

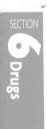

Systolic BP <60 mmHg **AND** signs of impaired major organ perfusion.
Infuse 250 ml **0.9% sodium chloride** and re-assess.
Maximum cumulative dose 2 litres

Systolic BP <90 mmHg **AND** signs of impaired major organ perfusion.
Infuse 250 ml **0.9% sodium chloride** and re-assess.
Maximum cumulative dose 2 litres

Administer 1 litre **0.9% sodium chloride** over 1 hour

NB If fluid therapy is indicated **DO NOT** delay transfer to further care but continue fluid therapy en-route – stopping if practicable to insert the cannula

Exceptions:
Limb crush injury – infuse 2 litres.
Sepsis – infuse 1 litre over 30 minutes (repeat **ONCE** if required)

Transfer to further care **<30 minutes** – do not administer fluid

Transfer to further care **>30 minutes** – administer 1 litre **0.9% sodium chloride** over 1 hour

Systolic BP <90 mmHg **AND** signs of impaired major organ perfusion.
Infuse 250 ml **0.9% sodium chloride** and re-assess.
Maximum cumulative dose 2 litres (in dehydration, fluid replacement over many hours)

Trunk

Head and limbs

Penetrating

Blunt

For example: GI bleed, aneurysm

Burn surface area **>25%**

Burn surface area **≥15 – ≤25%**

Burns

Trauma

Trauma

Medical

For example: anaphylaxis

Medical

Haemorrhagic

Non-haemorrhagic

Fluid Therapy

Figure 6.2 – Intravascular fluid therapy algorithm – adults

Intravascular Fluid Therapy (Children)

1. Introduction

- There has been no significant research in paediatric fluid administration in the literature and thus advice is dependent on that of adult studies and expert consensus.

2. Pathophysiology

- Although the basic pathophysiology is similar to adults, children have one very important difference. Their relatively healthy hearts and vasculature make the compensatory mechanisms very efficient. This means that only subtle signs of circulatory failure (shock) may be evident even in children with severe intravascular fluid depletion. When compensatory mechanisms start to fail, the child is in extremis and will deteriorate very quickly.

3. Assessment

- It is crucial that children with shock are treated before decompensation occurs whenever possible. There is no one sign that reliably dictates the state of shock a child may be in and a combination of all the markers of shock, along with an assessment of the mechanism of the shock (the history) must all be taken into account when deciding how shocked a child is.

- Blood pressure drops late in children for the reasons given above, and therefore is not a good indicator of the degree of volume depletion of the child. It is therefore of limited use in the pre-hospital setting, but if it is taken and found to be low (for the age of the child), this can be regarded as a pre-terminal sign.

- The following should be assessed:
  - pulse rate and volume
  - capillary refill measured on the forehead or sternum
  - respiratory rate
  - colour (pallor etc.)
  - cold peripheries
  - conscious level (AVPU) including drowsiness.

These must be considered as a whole in the light of what is known about the mechanism (i.e. volume of blood or fluid lost).

Only when all these are taken together can a rough estimate of the degree of shock be made. Each one of these is not reliable when measured on its own.

NB Children have compensatory physiological mechanisms that maintain "normal" blood pressures even in the face of significant blood loss; as a result, 'permissive hypotension' is neither recommended nor practiced in paediatric trauma. Small boluses (5 ml/kg) of fluid are administered and repeated (as needed) following frequent clinical reassessment (titrated against response/improvement) – see below.

NB There is **NO** evidence that the absence of the radial pulse correlates with the blood pressure or degree of shock in a consistent manner in children. Do not monitor the need for fluids against the presence of the radial pulse.

4. Management

For the management of burns and scalds see below and refer to Figure 6.3.

4.1 Medical causes of shock

It is usually difficult to measure volumes of fluid lost in children with medical causes of shock.

- 20 ml/kg is used as standard medical fluid replacement (equates to 25% of the child's blood volume).

- This can be given intravenously or intraosseously and is given as a bolus.

- The exact volume given must be documented.

- The child must be re-assessed after each bolus.

- It may be repeated once – total 40 ml/kg.

4.2 Exceptions

- Diabetic ketoacidosis (DKA). Children with DKA are very prone to cerebral oedema if given IV fluids and can die because of it. Children with renal failure and heart failure should also be treated with extreme caution. IV fluids should not be given unless there is significant shock (as opposed to dehydration) and only 10 ml/kg given. If there is no improvement following this, it may be repeated once (total 20 ml/kg) except in DKA where the dose is 10 ml/kg over 15 minutes. NB If these patients deteriorate during fluid administration, stop administering fluid immediately. If it is felt that further fluid will not wait until hospital, senior medical advice should be sought.

4.3 Trauma: hypovolaemic shock

- Fluid overload should be avoided. For ease and because all trauma patients should not be overloaded, it is not necessary to distinguish between compressible and non compressible haemorrhage.

- 5 ml/kg aliquots of fluid should be given.

- Re-assessment should be undertaken after each 5 ml/kg dose, using the signs described above.

- The 5 ml/kg dose can be repeated until the child is **significantly** improved. The vital signs (e.g. pulse) need not be normalised, but the child must be obviously more stable. There is no absolute upper dose.

- The child must be constantly re-assessed during transport.

- Clinical deterioration should be addressed with further 5 ml/kg fluid bolus(es), until the child improves clinically.

4.4 Burns

- Children lose fluids rapidly from severe burns and scalds and should have intravenous sodium chloride 0.9% started early.

- If the child has a >10% but <20% burn and the hospital time is more than 30 minutes, fluids should be started, and if greater than 20% burn fluid should be given regardless of the time to hospital.

Where burn surface area is:

- <10% do not administer fluid.

- ≥10 – <20% and time to hospital is greater than 30 minutes then administer **sodium chloride 0.9%** 10ml/kg over an hour.

- ≥20% administer **sodium chloride 0.9%** 10 ml/kg over an hour.

- The total dose must be calculated and given as regular, tiny portions of this to aim to have infused the correct amount over the hour.

- If fluid therapy is indicated **DO NOT** delay transfer to further care but continue fluid therapy en-route – stopping if practicable to insert the cannula.

- Vascular access also means analgesia can be administered.

KEY POINTS

Intravascular Fluid Therapy (Children)

- Children compensate well for shock.

- Once decompensated, they deteriorate very rapidly.

- All physiological signs must be taken in combination to diagnose shock.

- 20 ml/kg is the standard bolus for medically caused shock.

- 5 ml/kg is the standard bolus for traumatic shock.

- 10 ml/kg over 1 hour should be given to children with burns ≥20% and also to children with burns of ≥10 and <20% whose journey time will be more than 30 minutes. This procedure must not delay the time to hospital admission.

- Re-assessment after each bolus is vital to avoid fluid overload.

- Fluids should be used with extreme caution in DKA, renal failure and cardiac failure.

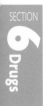

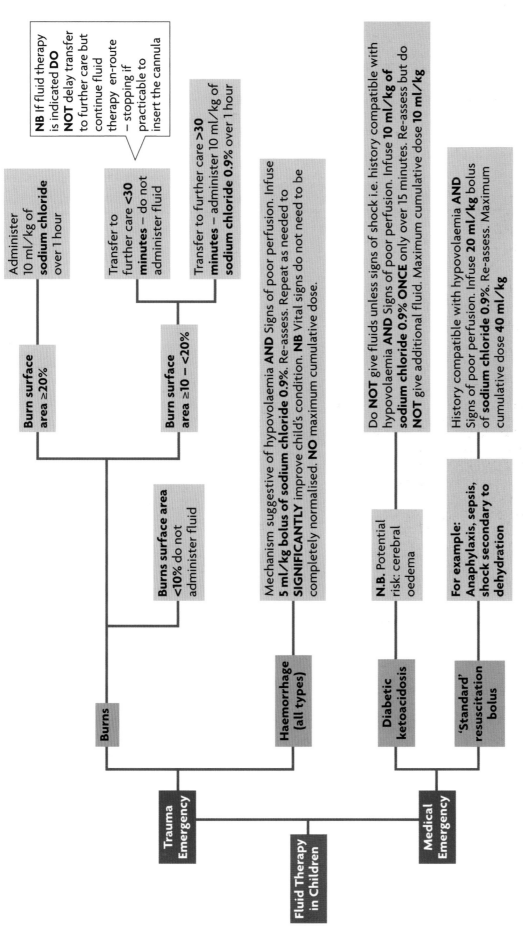

Figure 6.3 – Assessment and management of intravascular fluid therapy in children.

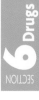

Fluid Therapy in Children

Trauma Emergency

Medical Emergency

Burns

Haemorrhage (all types)

Diabetic ketoacidosis

'Standard' resuscitation bolus

Burn surface area ≥20%

Burn surface area ≥10 – <20%

Burns surface area <10% do not administer fluid

N.B. Potential risk: cerebral oedema

For example: Anaphylaxis, sepsis, shock secondary to dehydration

Administer 10 ml/kg of **sodium chloride** over 1 hour

Transfer to further care <30 **minutes** – do not administer fluid

Transfer to further care >30 **minutes** – administer 10 ml/kg of **sodium chloride 0.9%** over 1 hour

NB If fluid therapy is indicated **DO NOT** delay transfer to further care but continue fluid therapy en-route – stopping if practicable to insert the cannula

Mechanism suggestive of hypovolaemia **AND** Signs of poor perfusion. Infuse **5 ml/kg bolus of sodium chloride 0.9%**. Re-assess. Repeat as needed to **SIGNIFICANTLY** improve child's condition. **NB** Vital signs do not need to be completely normalised. **NO** maximum cumulative dose.

Do **NOT** give fluids unless signs of shock i.e. history compatible with hypovolaemia **AND** Signs of poor perfusion. Infuse **10 ml/kg of sodium chloride 0.9% ONCE** only over 15 minutes. Re-assess but do **NOT** give additional fluid. Maximum cumulative dose 10 ml/kg

History compatible with hypovolaemia **AND** Signs of poor perfusion. Infuse **20 ml/kg bolus of sodium chloride 0.9%**. Re-assess. Maximum cumulative dose 40 ml/kg

Drugs

SECTION **6**

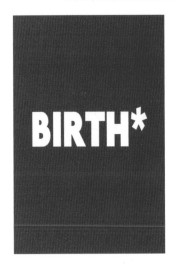

BIRTH*

Vital Signs

	GUIDE WEIGHT 3.5 kg		HEART RATE 110–160		RESPIRATION RATE 30–40		SYSTOLIC BLOOD PRESSURE 70–90

Airway Size by Type

OROPHARYNGEAL AIRWAY	LARYNGEAL MASK	I-GEL AIRWAY	ENDOTRACHEAL TUBE
000	1	1	Diameter: **3 mm**; Length: **10 cm**

Defibrillation – Cardiac Arrest

MANUAL	AUTOMATED EXTERNAL DEFIBRILLATOR
20 Joules	Where possible, use a manual defibrillator. If an AED is the only defibrillator available, it should be used (preferably using paediatric attenuation pads or else in paediatric mode).

Intravascular Fluid

FLUID	ROUTE	INITIAL DOSE	REPEAT DOSE	DOSE INTERVAL	CONCENTRATION	VOLUME	MAX DOSE
0.9% Sodium Chloride (5 ml/kg)	IV/IO	20 ml	20 ml	PRN	0.9%	20 ml	140 ml
0.9% Sodium Chloride (10 ml/kg)	IV/IO	35 ml	35 ml	PRN	0.9%	35 ml	140 ml
0.9% Sodium Chloride (20 ml/kg)	IV/IO	70 ml	70 ml	PRN	0.9%	70 ml	140 ml

Cardiac Arrest

DRUG	ROUTE	INITIAL DOSE	REPEAT DOSE	DOSE INTERVAL	CONCENTRATION	VOLUME	MAX DOSE
Adrenaline	IV/IO	35 micrograms	35 micrograms	3–5 minutes	1 milligram in 10 ml (1:10,000)	0.35 ml	No limit
Amiodarone	IV/IO	18 milligrams (After 3rd shock)	18 milligrams	After 5th shock	300 milligrams in 10 ml	0.6 ml	36 milligrams

Reversal of respiratory and central nervous system depression in a neonate following maternal opioid use during labour – single dose only

DRUG	ROUTE	INITIAL DOSE	REPEAT DOSE	DOSE INTERVAL	CONCENTRATION	VOLUME	MAX DOSE
Naloxone[ab] NB cautions	IM	200 micrograms	NONE	N/A	400 micrograms in 1 ml	0.5 ml	200 micrograms

* The Page for Age is provided for ease of use and quick look purposes. It is not a substitute for the information contained in the complete drugs guidelines or for sound clinical judgement.

[a] Reversal of respiratory arrest/extreme respiratory depression.

[b] Single dose for neonates where maternal opiates have been administered.

Quick Reference Table

DRUG	ROUTE	INITIAL DOSE	REPEAT DOSE	DOSE INTERVAL	CONCENTRATION	VOLUME	MAX DOSE
Adrenaline - anaphylaxis/asthma	IM	150 micrograms	150 micrograms	5 minutes	1 milligram in 1 ml (1:1,000)	0.15 ml	No limit
Benzylpenicillin (Penicillin G)	IV/IO	300 milligrams	NONE	N/A	600 milligrams dissolved in 9.6 ml water for injection	5 ml	300 milligrams
Benzylpenicillin (Penicillin G)	IM	300 milligrams	NONE	N/A	600 milligrams dissolved in 1.6 ml water for injection	1 ml	300 milligrams
Chlorphenamine	IV/IO/IM	N/A	N/A	N/A	N/A	N/A	N/A
Chlorphenamine	Oral (solution)	N/A	N/A	N/A	N/A	N/A	N/A
Chlorphenamine	Oral (tablet)	N/A	N/A	N/A	N/A	N/A	N/A
Dexamethasone - croup	Oral	N/A	N/A	N/A	N/A	N/A	N/A
Diazepam	IV/IO	1 milligram	NONE	N/A	10 milligrams in 2 ml	0.2 ml	1 milligram
Diazepam	Rectal (large dose)	2.5 milligrams	NONE	N/A	2.5 milligrams in 1.25 ml	1 × 2.5 milligram tube	2.5 milligrams
Diazepam	Rectal (small dose)	1.25 milligrams	NONE	N/A	2.5 milligrams in 1.25 ml	½ × 2.5 milligram tube	1.25 milligrams
Glucagon (Glucagen)	IM	100 micrograms	NONE	N/A	1 milligram per vial	0.1 vial	100 micrograms
Glucose 10%	IV	0.9 grams	0.9 grams	5 minutes	50 grams in 500 ml	9 ml	2.7 grams
Hydrocortisone	IV/IO/IM	10 milligrams	NONE	N/A	100 milligrams in 1 ml	0.1 ml	10 milligrams
Hydrocortisone	IV/IO/IM	10 milligrams	NONE	N/A	100 milligrams in 2 ml	0.2 ml	10 milligrams
Ibuprofen	Oral	N/A	N/A	N/A	N/A	N/A	N/A
Ipratropium Bromide (Atrovent) 250 micrograms in 1 ml	Neb	N/A	N/A	N/A	N/A	N/A	N/A
Ipratropium Bromide (Atrovent) 500 micrograms in 1 ml	Neb	N/A	N/A	N/A	N/A	N/A	N/A
Midazolam[c]	Buccal	See Epilepsy Passport	See Epilepsy Passport	10 mins	5 milligrams in 1 ml	See Epilepsy Passport	See Epilepsy Passport
Morphine Sulphate	IV/IO	N/A	N/A	N/A	N/A	N/A	N/A
Morphine Sulphate	Oral	N/A	N/A	N/A	N/A	N/A	N/A
Naloxone[ba] NB Cautions	IV/IO	40 micrograms	40 micrograms	3 minutes	400 micrograms in 1 ml	0.1 ml	440 micrograms
Naloxone[a] - initial dose	IM	40 micrograms	See repeat dose	3 minutes	400 micrograms in 1 ml	0.1 ml	See below
Naloxone[a] - repeat dose	IM	See initial dose	400 micrograms	3 minutes	400 micrograms in 1 ml	1 ml	440 micrograms
Ondansetron	IV/IO/IM	N/A	N/A	N/A	N/A	N/A	N/A
Paracetamol	Oral	N/A	N/A	N/A	N/A	N/A	N/A
Paracetamol	IV infusion/IO	N/A	N/A	N/A	N/A	N/A	N/A
Salbutamol 2.5 milligrams in 2.5 ml	Neb	N/A	N/A	N/A	N/A	N/A	N/A
Salbutamol 5 milligrams in 2.5 ml	Neb	N/A	N/A	N/A	N/A	N/A	N/A
Tranexamic Acid	IV	50 mg	NONE	N/A	100 mg/ml	0.5 ml	50 mg

Intramuscular naloxone is used to reverse respiratory and central nervous system depression in a neonate following maternal opioid use during labour. For specific indication, the dose is described in a separate box on the previous page.

Reversal of respiratory and central nervous system depression in a neonate following maternal opioid use during labour – single dose only.

Give the dose as prescribed in the child's individual treatment plan (the dosages described above reflect the recommended dosages for a child of this age).

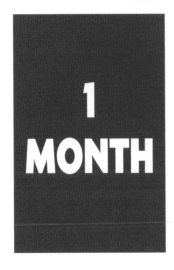

Vital Signs

	GUIDE WEIGHT 4.5 kg		HEART RATE 110–160		RESPIRATION RATE 30–40		SYSTOLIC BLOOD PRESSURE 70–90

Airway Size by Type

OROPHARYNGEAL AIRWAY	LARYNGEAL MASK	I-GEL AIRWAY	ENDOTRACHEAL TUBE
00	1	1	Diameter: **3 mm**; Length: **10 cm**

Defibrillation – Cardiac Arrest

MANUAL	AUTOMATED EXTERNAL DEFIBRILLATOR
20 Joules	Where possible, use a manual defibrillator. If an AED is the only defibrillator available, it should be used (preferably using paediatric attenuation pads or else in paediatric mode).

Intravascular Fluid

FLUID	ROUTE	INITIAL DOSE	REPEAT DOSE	DOSE INTERVAL	CONCENTRATION	VOLUME	MAX DOSE
0.9% Sodium Chloride (5 ml/kg)	IV/IO	20 ml	20 ml	PRN	0.9%	20 ml	180 ml
0.9% Sodium Chloride (10 ml/kg)	IV/IO	45 ml	45 ml	PRN	0.9%	45 ml	180 ml
0.9% Sodium Chloride (20 ml/kg)	IV/IO	90 ml	90 ml	PRN	0.9%	90 ml	180 ml

Cardiac Arrest

DRUG	ROUTE	INITIAL DOSE	REPEAT DOSE	DOSE INTERVAL	CONCENTRATION	VOLUME	MAX DOSE
Adrenaline	IV/IO	50 micrograms	50 micrograms	3–5 minutes	1 milligram in 10 ml (1:10,000)	0.5 ml	No limit
Amiodarone	IV/IO	25 milligrams (After 3rd shock)	25 milligrams	After 5th shock	300 milligrams in 10 ml	0.8 ml	50 milligrams

ick Reference Table

DRUG	ROUTE	INITIAL DOSE	REPEAT DOSE	DOSE INTERVAL	CONCENTRATION	VOLUME	MAX DOSE
Adrenaline - anaphylaxis/ asthma	IM	150 micrograms	150 micrograms	5 minutes	1 milligram in 1 ml (1:1,000)	0.15 ml	No limit
Benzylpenicillin (Penicillin G)	IV/IO	300 milligrams	NONE	N/A	600 milligrams dissolved in 9.6 ml water for injection	5 ml	300 milligrams
Benzylpenicillin (Penicillin G)	IM	300 milligrams	NONE	N/A	600 milligrams dissolved in 1.6 ml water for injection	1 ml	300 milligrams
Chlorphenamine	IV/IO/IM	N/A	N/A	N/A	N/A	N/A	N/A
Chlorphenamine	Oral (solution)	N/A	N/A	N/A	N/A	N/A	N/A
Chlorphenamine	Oral (tablet)	N/A	N/A	N/A	N/A	N/A	N/A
Dexamethasone - croup	Oral	1.9 milligrams	NONE	N/A	3.8 milligrams per ml	0.5 ml	1.9 milligrams
Diazepam	IV/IO	1.5 milligrams	NONE	N/A	10 milligrams in 2 ml	0.3 ml	1.5 milligrams
Diazepam	Rectal	5 milligrams	None	N/A	5 milligrams in 2.5 ml	1 × 5 milligram tube	5 milligrams
Glucagon (Glucagen)	IM	500 micrograms	NONE	N/A	1 milligram per vial	0.5 vial	500 micrograms
Glucose 10%	IV	1 gram	1 gram	5 minutes	50 grams in 500 ml	10 ml	3 grams
Hydrocortisone	IV/IO/IM	25 milligrams	NONE	N/A	100 milligrams in 1 ml	0.25 ml	25 milligrams
Hydrocortisone	IV/IO/IM	25 milligrams	NONE	N/A	100 milligrams in 2 ml	0.5 ml	25 milligrams
Ibuprofen	Oral	N/A	N/A	N/A	N/A	N/A	N/A
Ipratropium Bromide (Atrovent) 250 micrograms in 1 ml	Neb	125–250 micrograms	NONE	N/A	250 micrograms in 1 ml	0.5 ml–1 ml	125–250 micrograms
Ipratropium Bromide (Atrovent) 500 micrograms in 1 ml	Neb	125–250 micrograms	NONE	N/A	500 micrograms in 2 ml	0.5 ml–1 ml	125–250 micrograms
Midazolam[a]	Buccal	See Epilepsy Passport	See Epilepsy Passport	10 mins	5 milligrams in 1 ml	See Epilepsy Passport	See Epilepsy Passport
Morphine Sulphate	IV/IO	N/A	N/A	N/A	N/A	N/A	N/A
Morphine Sulphate	Oral	N/A	N/A	N/A	N/A	N/A	N/A
Naloxone NB cautions	IV/IO	40 micrograms	40 micrograms	3 minutes	400 micrograms in 1 ml	0.1 ml	440 micrograms
Naloxone - initial dose	IM	40 micrograms	See repeat dose	3 minutes	400 micrograms in 1 ml	0.1 ml	See below
Naloxone - repeat dose	IM	See initial dose	400 micrograms	3 minutes	400 micrograms in 1 ml	1 ml	440 micrograms
Ondansetron	IV/IO/IM	0.5 milligrams	NONE	N/A	2 milligrams in 1 ml	0.25 ml	0.5 milligrams
Paracetamol - Infant suspension	Oral	N/A	N/A	N/A	N/A	N/A	N/A
Paracetamol	IV infusion/IO	N/A	N/A	N/A	N/A	N/A	N/A
Salbutamol 2.5 milligrams in 2.5 ml	Neb	2.5 milligrams	2.5 milligrams	5 minutes	2.5 milligrams in 2.5 ml	2.5 ml	No limit
Salbutamol 5 milligrams in 2.5 ml	Neb	2.5 milligrams	2.5 milligrams	5 minutes	5 milligrams in 2.5 ml	1.25 ml	No limit
Tranexamic Acid	IV	50 mg	NONE	N/A	100 mg/ml	0.5 ml	50 mg

ive the dose as prescribed in the child's individual treatment plan/Epilepsy Passport (the dosages described above reflect the recommended dosages for a
d of this age).

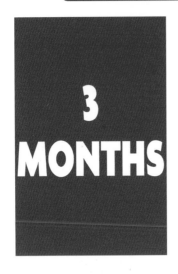

3 MONTHS

Vital Signs

GUIDE WEIGHT 6 kg	**HEART RATE** 110–160	**RESPIRATION RATE** 30–40	**SYSTOLIC BLOOD PRESSURE** 70–90

Airway Size by Type

OROPHARYNGEAL AIRWAY	LARYNGEAL MASK	I-GEL AIRWAY	ENDOTRACHEAL TUBE
00	1.5	1.5	Diameter: **3.5 mm**; Length: **11 cm**

Defibrillation – Cardiac Arrest

MANUAL	AUTOMATED EXTERNAL DEFIBRILLATOR
25 Joules	Where possible, use a manual defibrillator. If an AED is the only defibrillator available, it should be used (preferably using paediatric attenuation pads or else in paediatric mode).

Intravascular Fluid

FLUID	ROUTE	INITIAL DOSE	REPEAT DOSE	DOSE INTERVAL	CONCENTRATION	VOLUME	MAX DOSE
0.9% Sodium Chloride (5 ml/kg)	IV/IO	30 ml	30 ml	PRN	0.9%	30 ml	240 ml
0.9% Sodium Chloride (10 ml/kg)	IV/IO	60 ml	60 ml	PRN	0.9%	60 ml	240 ml
0.9% Sodium Chloride (20 ml/kg)	IV/IO	120 ml	120 ml	PRN	0.9%	120 ml	240 ml

Cardiac Arrest

DRUG	ROUTE	INITIAL DOSE	REPEAT DOSE	DOSE INTERVAL	CONCENTRATION	VOLUME	MAX DOSE
Adrenaline	IV/IO	60 micrograms	60 micrograms	3–5 minutes	1 milligram in 10 ml (1:10,000)	0.6 ml	No limit
Amiodarone	IV/IO	30 milligrams (After 3rd shock)	30 milligrams	After 5th shock	300 milligrams in 10 ml	1 ml	60 milligrams

Quick Reference Table

DRUG	ROUTE	INITIAL DOSE	REPEAT DOSE	DOSE INTERVAL	CONCENTRATION	VOLUME	MAX DOSE
Adrenaline - anaphylaxis/asthma	IM	150 micrograms	150 micrograms	5 minutes	1 milligram in 1 ml (1:1,000)	0.15 ml	No limit
Benzylpenicillin (Penicillin G)	IV/IO	300 milligrams	NONE	N/A	600 milligrams dissolved in 9.6 ml water for injection	5 ml	300 milligrams
Benzylpenicillin (Penicillin G)	IM	300 milligrams	NONE	N/A	600 milligrams dissolved in 1.6 ml water for injection	1 ml	300 milligrams
Chlorphenamine	IV/IO/IM	N/A	N/A	N/A	N/A	N/A	N/A
Chlorphenamine	Oral (solution)	N/A	N/A	N/A	N/A	N/A	N/A
Chlorphenamine	Oral (tablet)	N/A	N/A	N/A	N/A	N/A	N/A
Dexamethasone - croup	Oral	1.9 milligrams	NONE	N/A	3.8 milligrams per ml	0.5 ml	1.9 milligrams
Diazepam	IV/IO	2 milligrams	NONE	N/A	10 milligrams in 2 ml	0.4 ml	2 milligrams
Diazepam	Rectal	5 milligrams	None	N/A	5 milligrams in 2.5 ml	1 × 5 milligram tyube	5 milligrams
Glucagon (Glucagen)	IM	500 micrograms	NONE	N/A	1 milligram per vial	0.5 vial	500 micrograms
Glucose 10%	IV	1 gram	1 gram	5 minutes	50 grams in 500 ml	10 ml	3 grams
Hydrocortisone	IV/IO/IM	25 milligrams	NONE	N/A	100 milligrams in 1 ml	0.25 ml	25 milligrams
Hydrocortisone	IV/IO/IM	25 milligrams	NONE	N/A	100 milligrams in 2 ml	0.5 ml	25 milligrams
Ibuprofen	Oral	50 milligrams	50 milligrams	8 hours	100 milligrams in 5 ml	2.5 ml	150 milligrams per 24 hours
Ipratropium Bromide (Atrovent) 250 micrograms in 1 ml	Neb	125–250 micrograms	NONE	N/A	250 micrograms in 1 ml	0.5 ml–1 ml	125–250 micrograms
Ipratropium Bromide (Atrovent) 500 micrograms in 1 ml	Neb	125–250 micrograms	NONE	N/A	500 micrograms in 2 ml	0.5 ml–1 ml	125–250 micrograms
Midazolam[a]	Buccal	See Epilepsy Passport	See Epilepsy Passport	10 mins	5 milligrams in 1 ml	See Epilepsy Passport	See Epilepsy Passport
Morphine Sulphate	IV/IO	N/A	N/A	N/A	N/A	N/A	N/A
Morphine Sulphate	Oral	N/A	N/A	N/A	N/A	N/A	N/A
Naloxone NB cautions	IV/IO	60 micrograms	60 micrograms	3 minutes	400 micrograms in 1 ml	0.15 ml	660 micrograms
Naloxone - initial dose	IM	60 micrograms	See repeat dose	3 minutes	400 micrograms in 1 ml	0.15 ml	See below
Naloxone - repeat dose	IM	See initial dose	400 micrograms	3 minutes	400 micrograms in 1 ml	1 ml	460 micrograms
Ondansetron	IV/IO/IM	0.5 milligrams	NONE	N/A	2 milligrams in 1 ml	0.25 ml	0.5 milligrams
Paracetamol - Infant suspension	Oral	60 milligrams	60 milligrams	4–6 hours	120 milligrams in 5 ml	2.5 ml	240 milligrams in 24 hours
Paracetamol	IV infusion/IO	N/A	N/A	N/A	N/A	N/A	N/A
Salbutamol 2.5 milligrams in 2.5 ml	Neb	2.5 milligrams	2.5 milligrams	5 minutes	2.5 milligrams in 2.5 ml	2.5 ml	No limit
Salbutamol 5 milligrams in 2.5 ml	Neb	2.5 milligrams	2.5 milligrams	5 minutes	5 milligrams in 2.5 ml	1.25 ml	No limit
Tranexamic Acid	IV	100 mg	NONE	N/A	100 mg/ml	1 ml	100 mg

Give the dose as prescribed in the child's individual treatment plan/Epilepsy Passport (the dosages described above reflect the recommended dosages for a child of this age).

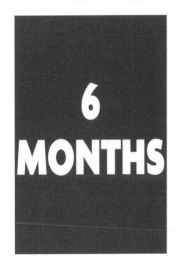

6 MONTHS

Vital Signs

	GUIDE WEIGHT 8 kg		HEART RATE 110–160		RESPIRATION RATE 30–40		SYSTOLIC BLOOD PRESSURE 70–90

Airway Size by Type

OROPHARYNGEAL AIRWAY	LARYNGEAL MASK	I-GEL AIRWAY	ENDOTRACHEAL TUBE
00	1.5	1.5	Diameter: **4 mm**; Length: **12 cm**

Defibrillation – Cardiac Arrest

MANUAL	AUTOMATED EXTERNAL DEFIBRILLATOR
40 Joules	Where possible, use a manual defibrillator. If an AED is the only defibrillator available, it should be used (preferably using paediatric attenuation pads or else in paediatric mode).

Intravascular Fluid

FLUID	ROUTE	INITIAL DOSE	REPEAT DOSE	DOSE INTERVAL	CONCENTRATION	VOLUME	MAX DOSE
0.9% Sodium Chloride (5 ml/kg)	IV/IO	40 ml	40 ml	PRN	0.9%	40 ml	320 ml
0.9% Sodium Chloride (10 ml/kg)	IV/IO	80 ml	80 ml	PRN	0.9%	80 ml	320 ml
0.9% Sodium Chloride (20 ml/kg)	IV/IO	160 ml	160 ml	PRN	0.9%	160 ml	320 ml

Cardiac Arrest

DRUG	ROUTE	INITIAL DOSE	REPEAT DOSE	DOSE INTERVAL	CONCENTRATION	VOLUME	MAX DOSE
Adrenaline	IV/IO	80 micrograms	80 micrograms	3–5 minutes	1 milligram in 10 ml (1:10,000)	0.8 ml	No limit
Amiodarone	IV/IO	40 milligrams (After 3rd shock)	40 milligrams	After 5th shock	300 milligrams in 10 ml	1.3 ml	80 milligrams

Quick Reference Table

DRUG	ROUTE	INITIAL DOSE	REPEAT DOSE	DOSE INTERVAL	CONCENTRATION	VOLUME	MAX DOSE
Adrenaline - anaphylaxis/asthma	IM	150 micrograms	150 micrograms	5 minutes	1 milligram in 1 ml (1:1,000)	0.15 ml	No limit
Benzylpenicillin (Penicillin G)	IV/IO	300 milligrams	NONE	N/A	600 milligrams dissolved in 9.6 ml water for injection	5 ml	300 milligrams
Benzylpenicillin (Penicillin G)	IM	300 milligrams	NONE	N/A	600 milligrams dissolved in 1.6 ml water for injection	1 ml	300 milligrams
Chlorphenamine	IV/IO/IM	N/A	N/A	N/A	N/A	N/A	N/A
Chlorphenamine	Oral (solution)	N/A	N/A	N/A	N/A	N/A	N/A
Chlorphenamine	Oral (tablet)	N/A	N/A	N/A	N/A	N/A	N/A
Dexamethasone - croup	Oral	1.9 milligrams	NONE	N/A	3.8 milligrams per ml	0.5 ml	1.9 milligrams
Diazepam	IV/IO	2.5 milligrams	NONE	N/A	10 milligrams in 2 ml	0.5 ml	2.5 milligrams
Diazepam	Rectal	5 milligrams	None	N/A	5 milligrams in 2.5 ml	1 × 5 milligram tube	5 milligrams
Glucagon (Glucagen)	IM	500 micrograms	NONE	N/A	1 milligram per vial	0.5 vial	500 micrograms
Glucose 10%	IV	1.5 grams	1.5 grams	5 minutes	50 grams in 500 ml	15 ml	4.5 grams
Hydrocortisone	IV/IO/IM	50 milligrams	NONE	N/A	100 milligrams in 1 ml	0.5 ml	50 milligrams
Hydrocortisone	IV/IO/IM	50 milligrams	NONE	N/A	100 milligrams in 2 ml	1 ml	50 milligrams
Ibuprofen	Oral	50 milligrams	50 milligrams	8 hours	100 milligrams in 5 ml	2.5 ml	150 milligrams per 24 hours
Ipratropium Bromide (Atrovent) 250 micrograms in 1 ml	Neb	125–250 micrograms	NONE	N/A	250 micrograms in 1 ml	0.5 ml–1 ml	125–250 micrograms
Ipratropium Bromide (Atrovent) 500 micrograms in 1 ml	Neb	125–250 micrograms	NONE	N/A	500 micrograms in 2 ml	0.5 ml–1 ml	125–250 micrograms
Midazolam[a]	Buccal	2.5 milligrams	2.5 milligrams	10 mins	5 milligrams in 1 ml	0.5 ml pre-filled syringe	5 milligrams
Morphine Sulphate	IV/IO	N/A	N/A	N/A	N/A	N/A	N/A
Morphine Sulphate	Oral	N/A	N/A	N/A	N/A	N/A	N/A
Naloxone NB cautions	IV/IO	80 micrograms	80 micrograms	3 minutes	400 micrograms in 1 ml	0.2 ml	880 micrograms
Naloxone - initial dose	IM	80 micrograms	See repeat dose	3 minutes	400 micrograms in 1 ml	0.2 ml	See below
Naloxone - repeat dose	IM	See initial dose	400 micrograms	3 minutes	400 micrograms in 1 ml	1 ml	480 micrograms
Ondansetron	IV/IO/IM	1 milligram	NONE	N/A	2 milligrams in 1 ml	0.5 ml	1 milligram
Paracetamol - Infant suspension	Oral	120 milligrams	120 milligrams	4–6 hours	120 milligrams in 5 ml	5 ml	480 milligrams in 24 hours
Paracetamol	IV infusion/IO	50 milligrams	50 milligrams	4–6 hours	10 milligrams in 1 ml	5 ml	200 milligrams in 24 hours
Salbutamol 2.5 milligrams in 2.5 ml	Neb	2.5 milligrams	2.5 milligrams	5 minutes	2.5 milligrams in 2.5 ml	2.5 ml	No limit
Salbutamol 5 milligrams in 2.5 ml	Neb	2.5 milligrams	2.5 milligrams	5 minutes	5 milligrams in 2.5 ml	1.25 ml	No limit
Tranexamic Acid	IV	100 mg	NONE	N/A	100 mg/ml	1 ml	100 mg

Give the dose as prescribed in the child's individual treatment plan/Epilepsy Passport (the dosages described above reflect the recommended dosages for a child of this age).

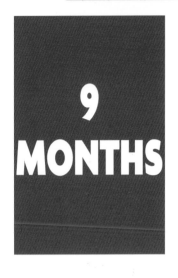

9 MONTHS

Vital Signs

	GUIDE WEIGHT 9 kg		HEART RATE 110–160		RESPIRATION RATE 30–40		SYSTOLIC BLOOD PRESSURE 70–90

Airway Size by Type

OROPHARYNGEAL AIRWAY	LARYNGEAL MASK	I-GEL AIRWAY	ENDOTRACHEAL TUBE
00	1.5	1.5	Diameter: **4 mm**; Length: **12 cm**

Defibrillation – Cardiac Arrest

MANUAL	AUTOMATED EXTERNAL DEFIBRILLATOR
40 Joules	Where possible, use a manual defibrillator. If an AED is the only defibrillator available, it should be used (preferably using paediatric attenuation pads or else in paediatric mode).

Intravascular Fluid

FLUID	ROUTE	INITIAL DOSE	REPEAT DOSE	DOSE INTERVAL	CONCENTRATION	VOLUME	MAX DOSE
0.9% Sodium Chloride (5 ml/kg)	IV/IO	45 ml	45 ml	PRN	0.9%	45 ml	360 ml
0.9% Sodium Chloride (10 ml/kg)	IV/IO	90 ml	90 ml	PRN	0.9%	90 ml	360 ml
0.9% Sodium Chloride (20 ml/kg)	IV/IO	180 ml	180 ml	PRN	0.9%	180 ml	360 ml

Cardiac Arrest

DRUG	ROUTE	INITIAL DOSE	REPEAT DOSE	DOSE INTERVAL	CONCENTRATION	VOLUME	MAX DOSE
Adrenaline	IV/IO	90 micrograms	90 micrograms	3–5 minutes	1 milligram in 10 ml (1:10,000)	0.9 ml	No limit
Amiodarone	IV/IO	45 milligrams (After 3rd shock)	45 milligrams	After 5th shock	300 milligrams in 10 ml	1.5 ml	90 milligrams

ick Reference Table

DRUG	ROUTE	INITIAL DOSE	REPEAT DOSE	DOSE INTERVAL	CONCENTRATION	VOLUME	MAX DOSE
Adrenaline - anaphylaxis/ asthma	IM	150 micrograms	150 micrograms	5 minutes	1 milligram in 1 ml (1:1,000)	0.15 ml	No limit
Benzylpenicillin (Penicillin G)	IV/IO	300 milligrams	NONE	N/A	600 milligrams dissolved in 9.6 ml water for injection	5 ml	300 milligrams
Benzylpenicillin (Penicillin G)	IM	300 milligrams	NONE	N/A	600 milligrams dissolved in 1.6 ml water for injection	1 ml	300 milligrams
Chlorphenamine	IV/IO/IM	N/A	N/A	N/A	N/A	N/A	N/A
Chlorphenamine	Oral (solution)	N/A	N/A	N/A	N/A	N/A	N/A
Chlorphenamine	Oral (tablet)	N/A	N/A	N/A	N/A	N/A	N/A
Dexamethasone - croup	Oral	1.9 milligrams	NONE	N/A	3.8 milligrams per ml	0.5 ml	1.9 milligrams
Diazepam	IV/IO	2.5 milligrams	NONE	N/A	10 milligrams in 2 ml	0.5 ml	2.5 milligrams
Diazepam	Rectal	5 milligrams	None	N/A	5 milligrams in 2.5 ml	1 × 5 milligram tube	5 milligrams
Glucagon (Glucagen)	IM	500 micrograms	NONE	N/A	1 milligram per vial	0.5 vial	500 micrograms
Glucose 10%	IV	2 grams	2 grams	5 minutes	50 grams in 500 ml	20 ml	6 grams
Hydrocortisone	IV/IO/IM	50 milligrams	NONE	N/A	100 milligrams in 1 ml	0.5 ml	50 milligrams
Hydrocortisone	IV/IO/IM	50 milligrams	NONE	N/A	100 milligrams in 2 ml	1 ml	50 milligrams
Ibuprofen	Oral	50 milligrams	50 milligrams	8 hours	100 milligrams in 5 ml	2.5 ml	150 milligrams per 24 hours
Ipratropium Bromide (Atrovent) 250 micrograms in 1 ml	Neb	125–250 micrograms	NONE	N/A	250 micrograms in 1 ml	0.5 ml–1 ml	125–250 micrograms
Ipratropium Bromide (Atrovent) 500 micrograms in 1 ml	Neb	125–250 micrograms	NONE	N/A	500 micrograms in 2 ml	0.5 ml–1 ml	125–250 micrograms
Midazolam[a]	Buccal	2.5 milligrams	2.5 milligrams	10 mins	5 milligrams in 1 ml	0.5 ml pre-filled syringe	5 milligrams
Morphine Sulphate	IV/IO	N/A	N/A	N/A	N/A	N/A	N/A
Morphine Sulphate	Oral	N/A	N/A	N/A	N/A	N/A	N/A
Naloxone NB cautions	IV/IO	80 micrograms	80 micrograms	3 minutes	400 micrograms in 1 ml	0.2 ml	880 micrograms
Naloxone - initial dose	IM	80 micrograms	See repeat dose	3 minutes	400 micrograms in 1 ml	0.2 ml	See below
Naloxone - repeat dose	IM	See initial dose	400 micrograms	3 minutes	400 micrograms in 1 ml	1 ml	480 micrograms
Ondansetron	IV/IO/IM	1 milligram	NONE	N/A	2 milligrams in 1 ml	0.5 ml	1 milligram
Paracetamol - Infant suspension	Oral	120 milligrams	120 milligrams	4–6 hours	120 milligrams in 5 ml	5 ml	480 milligrams in 24 hours
Paracetamol	IV infusion/IO	50 milligrams	50 milligrams	4–6 hours	10 milligrams in 1 ml	5 ml	200 milligrams in 24 hours
Salbutamol 2.5 milligrams in 2.5 ml	Neb	2.5 milligrams	2.5 milligrams	5 minutes	2.5 milligrams in 2.5 ml	2.5 ml	No limit
Salbutamol 5 milligrams in 2.5 ml	Neb	2.5 milligrams	2.5 milligrams	5 minutes	5 milligrams in 2.5 ml	1.25 ml	No limit
Tranexamic Acid	IV	150 mg	NONE	N/A	100 mg/ml	1.5 ml	150 mg

ive the dose as prescribed in the child's individual treatment plan/Epilepsy Passport (the dosages described above reflect the recommended dosages for a
d of this age).

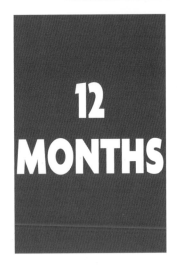

Vital Signs

GUIDE WEIGHT 10 kg	**HEART RATE** 110–150	**RESPIRATION RATE** 25–35	**SYSTOLIC BLOOD PRESSURE** 80–95

Airway Size by Type

OROPHARYNGEAL AIRWAY	LARYNGEAL MASK	I-GEL AIRWAY	ENDOTRACHEAL TUBE
00 OR 0	1.5	1.5 OR 2	Diameter: **4.5 mm**; Length: **13 cm**

Defibrillation – Cardiac Arrest

MANUAL	AUTOMATED EXTERNAL DEFIBRILLATOR
40 Joules	A standard AED (either with paediatric attenuation pads or else in paediatric mode) can be used. If paediatric pads are not available, standard adult pads can be used (but must not overlap).

Intravascular Fluid

FLUID	ROUTE	INITIAL DOSE	REPEAT DOSE	DOSE INTERVAL	CONCENTRATION	VOLUME	MAX DOSE
0.9% Sodium Chloride (5 ml/kg)	IV/IO	50 ml	50 ml	PRN	0.9%	50 ml	400 ml
0.9% Sodium Chloride (10 ml/kg)	IV/IO	100 ml	100 ml	PRN	0.9%	100 ml	400 ml
0.9% Sodium Chloride (20 ml/kg)	IV/IO	200 ml	200 ml	PRN	0.9%	200 ml	400 ml

Cardiac Arrest

DRUG	ROUTE	INITIAL DOSE	REPEAT DOSE	DOSE INTERVAL	CONCENTRATION	VOLUME	MAX DOSE
Adrenaline	IV/IO	100 micrograms	100 micrograms	3–5 minutes	1 milligram in 10 ml (1:10,000)	1 ml	No limit
Amiodarone	IV/IO	50 milligrams (After 3rd shock)	50 milligrams	After 5th shock	300 milligrams in 10 ml	1.7 ml	100 milligrams

ick Reference Table

DRUG	ROUTE	INITIAL DOSE	REPEAT DOSE	DOSE INTERVAL	CONCENTRATION	VOLUME	MAX DOSE
Adrenaline - anaphylaxis/ asthma	IM	150 micrograms	150 micrograms	5 minutes	1 milligram in 1 ml (1:1,000)	0.15 ml	No limit
Benzylpenicillin (Penicillin G)	IV/IO	600 milligrams	NONE	N/A	600 milligrams dissolved in 9.6 ml water for injection	10 ml	600 milligrams
Benzylpenicillin (Penicillin G)	IM	600 milligrams	NONE	N/A	600 milligrams dissolved in 1.6 ml water for injection	2 ml	600 milligrams
Chlorphenamine	IV/IO/IM	2.5 milligrams	NONE	N/A	10 milligrams in 1 ml	0.25 ml	2.5 milligrams
Chlorphenamine	Oral (solution)	1 milligram	NONE	N/A	2 milligrams in 5 ml	2.5 ml	1 milligram
Chlorphenamine	Oral (tablet)	1 milligram	NONE	N/A	4 milligrams per tablet	¼ of one tablet	1 milligram
Dexamethasone - croup	Oral	1.9 milligrams	NONE	N/A	3.8 milligrams per ml	0.5 ml	1.9 milligrams
Diazepam	IV/IO	3 milligrams	NONE	N/A	10 milligrams in 2 ml	0.6 ml	3 milligrams
Diazepam	Rectal	5 milligrams	None	N/A	5 milligrams in 2.5 ml	1 × 5 milligram tube	5 milligrams
Glucagon (Glucagen)	IM	500 micrograms	NONE	N/A	1 milligram per vial	0.5 vial	500 micrograms
Glucose 10%	IV	2 grams	2 grams	5 minutes	50 grams in 500 ml	20 ml	6 grams
Hydrocortisone	IV/IO/IM	50 milligrams	NONE	N/A	100 milligrams in 1 ml	0.5 ml	50 milligrams
Hydrocortisone	IV/IO/IM	50 milligrams	NONE	N/A	100 milligrams in 2 ml	1 ml	50 milligrams
Ibuprofen	Oral	100 milligrams	100 milligrams	8 hours	100 milligrams in 5 ml	5 ml	300 milligrams per 24 hours
Ipratropium Bromide (Atrovent) 250 micrograms in 1 ml	Neb	125–250 micrograms	NONE	N/A	250 micrograms in 1 ml	0.5–1 ml	125–250 micrograms
Ipratropium Bromide (Atrovent) 500 micrograms in 1 ml	Neb	125–250 micrograms	NONE	N/A	500 micrograms in 2 ml	0.5–1 ml	125–250 micrograms
Midazolam[a]	Buccal	5 milligrams	5 milligrams	10 mins	5 milligrams in 1 ml	1 ml pre-filled syringe	10 milligrams
Morphine Sulphate	IV/IO	1 milligram	1 milligram	5 minutes	10 milligrams in 10 ml	1 ml	2 milligrams
Morphine Sulphate	Oral	2 milligrams	NONE	N/A	10 milligrams in 5 ml	1 ml	2 milligrams
Naloxone NB cautions	IV/IO	100 micrograms	100 micrograms	3 minutes	400 micrograms in 1 ml	0.25 ml	1,100 micrograms
Naloxone - initial dose	IM	100 micrograms	See repeat dose	3 minutes	400 micrograms in 1 ml	0.25 ml	See below
Naloxone - repeat dose	IM	See initial dose	400 micrograms	3 minutes	400 micrograms in 1 ml	1 ml	500 micrograms
Ondansetron	IV/IO/IM	1 milligram	NONE	N/A	2 milligrams in 1 ml	0.5 ml	1 milligram
Paracetamol - Infant suspension	Oral	120 milligrams	120 milligrams	4–6 hours	120 milligrams in 5 ml	5 ml	480 milligrams in 24 hours
Paracetamol	IV infusion/IO	150 milligrams	150 milligrams	4–6 hours	10 milligrams in 1 ml	15 ml	600 milligrams in 24 hours
Salbutamol 2.5 milligrams in 2.5 ml	Neb	2.5 milligrams	2.5 milligrams	5 minutes	2.5 milligrams in 2.5 ml	2.5 ml	No limit
Salbutamol 5 milligrams in 2.5 ml	Neb	2.5 milligrams	2.5 milligrams	5 minutes	5 milligrams in 2.5 ml	1.25 ml	No limit
Tranexamic Acid	IV	150 mg	NONE	N/A	100 mg/ml	1.5 ml	150 mg

ive the dose as prescribed in the child's individual treatment plan/Epilepsy Passport (the dosages described above reflect the recommended dosages for a d of this age).

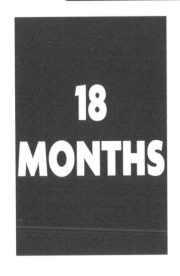

18 MONTHS

Vital Signs

GUIDE WEIGHT 11 kg	HEART RATE 110–150	RESPIRATION RATE 25–35	SYSTOLIC BLOOD PRESSURE 80–95

Airway Size by Type

OROPHARYNGEAL AIRWAY	LARYNGEAL MASK	I-GEL AIRWAY	ENDOTRACHEAL TUBE
00 OR 0	2	1.5 OR 2	Diameter: **4.5 mm**; Length: **13 cm**

Defibrillation – Cardiac Arrest

MANUAL	AUTOMATED EXTERNAL DEFIBRILLATOR
50 Joules	A standard AED (either with paediatric attenuation pads or else in paediatric mode) can be used. If paediatric pads are not available, standard adult pads can be used (but must not overlap).

Intravascular Fluid

FLUID	ROUTE	INITIAL DOSE	REPEAT DOSE	DOSE INTERVAL	CONCENTRATION	VOLUME	MAX DOSE
0.9% Sodium Chloride (5 ml/kg)	IV/IO	55 ml	55 ml	PRN	0.9%	55 ml	440 ml
0.9% Sodium Chloride (10 ml/kg)	IV/IO	110 ml	110 ml	PRN	0.9%	110 ml	440 ml
0.9% Sodium Chloride (20 ml/kg)	IV/IO	220 ml	220 ml	PRN	0.9%	220 ml	440 ml

Cardiac Arrest

DRUG	ROUTE	INITIAL DOSE	REPEAT DOSE	DOSE INTERVAL	CONCENTRATION	VOLUME	MAX DOSE
Adrenaline	IV/IO	110 micrograms	110 micrograms	3–5 minutes	1 milligram in 10 ml (1:10,000)	1.1 ml	No limit
Amiodarone	IV/IO	55 milligrams (After 3rd shock)	55 milligrams	After 5th shock	300 milligrams in 10 ml	1.8 ml	110 milligrams

ick Reference Table

DRUG	ROUTE	INITIAL DOSE	REPEAT DOSE	DOSE INTERVAL	CONCENTRATION	VOLUME	MAX DOSE
Adrenaline - anaphylaxis/ asthma	IM	150 micrograms	150 micrograms	5 minutes	1 milligram in 1 ml (1:1,000)	0.15 ml	No limit
Benzylpenicillin (Penicillin G)	IV/IO	600 milligrams	NONE	N/A	600 milligrams dissolved in 9.6 ml water for injection	10 ml	600 milligrams
Benzylpenicillin (Penicillin G)	IM	600 milligrams	NONE	N/A	600 milligrams dissolved in 1.6 ml water for injection	2 ml	600 milligrams
Chlorphenamine	IV/IO/IM	2.5 milligrams	NONE	N/A	10 milligrams in 1 ml	0.25 ml	2.5 milligrams
Chlorphenamine	Oral (solution)	1 milligram	NONE	N/A	2 milligrams in 5 ml	2.5 ml	1 milligram
Chlorphenamine	Oral (tablet)	1 milligram	NONE	N/A	4 milligrams per tablet	$\frac{1}{4}$ of one tablet	1 milligram
Dexamethasone - croup	Oral	3.8 milligrams	NONE	N/A	3.8 milligrams per ml	1 ml	3.8 milligrams
Diazepam	IV/IO	3.5 milligrams	NONE	N/A	10 milligrams in 2 ml	0.7 ml	3.5 milligrams
Diazepam	Rectal	5 milligrams	NONE	N/A	5 milligrams in 2.5 ml	1 × 5 milligram tube	5 milligrams
Glucagon (Glucagen)	IM	500 micrograms	NONE	N/A	1 milligram per vial	0.5 vial	500 micrograms
Glucose 10%	IV	2 grams	2 grams	5 minutes	50 grams in 500 ml	20 ml	6 grams
Hydrocortisone	IV/IO/IM	50 milligrams	NONE	N/A	100 milligrams in 1 ml	0.5 ml	50 milligrams
Hydrocortisone	IV/IO/IM	50 milligrams	NONE	N/A	100 milligrams in 2 ml	1 ml	50 milligrams
Ibuprofen	Oral	100 milligrams	100 milligrams	8 hours	100 milligrams in 5 ml	5 ml	300 milligrams per 24 hours
Ipratropium Bromide (Atrovent) 250 micrograms in 1 ml	Neb	250 micrograms	NONE	N/A	250 micrograms in 1 ml	1 ml	250 micrograms
Ipratropium Bromide (Atrovent) 500 micrograms in 1 ml	Neb	250 micrograms	NONE	N/A	500 micrograms in 2 ml	1 ml	250 micrograms
Midazolam[a]	Buccal	5 milligrams	5 milligrams	10 mins	5 milligrams in 1 ml	1 ml pre-filled syringe	10 milligrams
Morphine Sulphate	IV/IO	1 milligram	1 milligram	5 minutes	10 milligrams in 10 ml	1 ml	2 milligrams
Morphine Sulphate	Oral	2 milligrams	NONE	N/A	10 milligrams in 5 ml	1 ml	2 milligrams
Naloxone NB cautions	IV/IO	120 micrograms	120 micrograms	3 minutes	400 micrograms in 1 ml	0.3 ml	1,320 micrograms
Naloxone - initial dose	IM	120 micrograms	See repeat dose	3 minutes	400 micrograms in 1 ml	0.3 ml	See below
Naloxone - repeat dose	IM	See initial dose	400 micrograms	3 minutes	400 micrograms in 1 ml	1 ml	520 micrograms
Ondansetron	IV/IO/IM	1 milligram	NONE	N/A	2 milligrams in 1 ml	0.5 ml	1 milligram
Paracetamol - Infant suspension	Oral	120 milligrams	120 milligrams	4–6 hours	120 milligrams in 5 ml	5 ml	480 milligrams in 24 hours
Paracetamol	IV infusion/IO	150 milligrams	150 milligrams	4–6 hours	10 milligrams in 1 ml	15 ml	600 milligrams in 24 hours
Salbutamol 2.5 milligrams in 2.5 ml	Neb	2.5 milligrams	2.5 milligrams	5 minutes	2.5 milligrams in 2.5 ml	2.5 ml	No limit
Salbutamol 5 milligrams in 2.5 ml	Neb	2.5 milligrams	2.5 milligrams	5 minutes	5 milligrams in 2.5 ml	1.25 ml	No limit
Tranexamic Acid	IV	150 mg	NONE	N/A	100 mg/ml	1.5 ml	150 mg

ive the dose as prescribed in the child's individual treatment plan/Epilepsy Passport (the dosages described above reflect the recommended dosages for a d of this age).

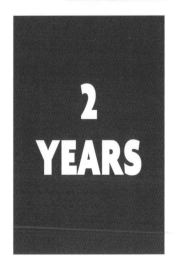

2 YEARS

Vital Signs

GUIDE WEIGHT 12 kg	**HEART RATE** 95–140	**RESPIRATION RATE** 25–30	**SYSTOLIC BLOOD PRESSURE** 80–100

Airway Size by Type

OROPHARYNGEAL AIRWAY	LARYNGEAL MASK	I-GEL AIRWAY	ENDOTRACHEAL TUBE
0 OR 1	2	1.5 OR 2	Diameter: **5 mm**; Length: **14 cm**

Defibrillation – Cardiac Arrest

MANUAL	AUTOMATED EXTERNAL DEFIBRILLATOR
50 Joules	A standard AED (either with paediatric attenuation pads or else in paediatric mode) can be used. If paediatric pads are not available, standard adult pads can be used (but must not overlap).

Intravascular Fluid

FLUID	ROUTE	INITIAL DOSE	REPEAT DOSE	DOSE INTERVAL	CONCENTRATION	VOLUME	MAX DOSE
0.9% Sodium Chloride (5 ml/kg)	IV/IO	60 ml	60 ml	PRN	0.9%	60 ml	480 ml
0.9% Sodium Chloride (10 ml/kg)	IV/IO	120 ml	120 ml	PRN	0.9%	120 ml	480 ml
0.9% Sodium Chloride (20 ml/kg)	IV/IO	240 ml	240 ml	PRN	0.9%	240 ml	480 ml

Cardiac Arrest

DRUG	ROUTE	INITIAL DOSE	REPEAT DOSE	DOSE INTERVAL	CONCENTRATION	VOLUME	MAX DOSE
Adrenaline	IV/IO	120 micrograms	120 micrograms	3–5 minutes	1 milligram in 10 ml (1:10,000)	1.2 ml	No limit
Amiodarone	IV/IO	60 milligrams (After 3rd shock)	60 milligrams	After 5th shock	300 milligrams in 10 ml	2 ml	120 milligrams

ʼick Reference Table

DRUG	ROUTE	INITIAL DOSE	REPEAT DOSE	DOSE INTERVAL	CONCENTRATION	VOLUME	MAX DOSE
Adrenaline - anaphylaxis/asthma	IM	150 micrograms	150 micrograms	5 minutes	1 milligram in 1 ml (1:1,000)	0.15 ml	No limit
Benzylpenicillin (Penicillin G)	IV/IO	600 milligrams	NONE	N/A	600 milligrams dissolved in 9.6 ml water for injection	10 ml	600 milligrams
Benzylpenicillin (Penicillin G)	IM	600 milligrams	NONE	N/A	600 milligrams dissolved in 1.6 ml water for injection	2 ml	600 milligrams
Chlorphenamine	IV/IO/IM	2.5 milligrams	NONE	N/A	10 milligrams in 1 ml	0.25 ml	2.5 milligrams
Chlorphenamine	Oral (solution)	1 milligram	NONE	N/A	2 milligrams in 5 ml	2.5 ml	1 milligram
Chlorphenamine	Oral (tablet)	1 milligram	NONE	N/A	4 milligrams per tablet	¼ of one tablet	1 milligram
Dexamethasone - croup	Oral	3.8 milligrams	NONE	N/A	3.8 milligrams per ml	1 ml	3.8 milligrams
Diazepam	IV/IO	3.5 milligrams	NONE	N/A	10 milligrams in 2 ml	0.7 ml	3.5 milligrams
Diazepam	Rectal (large dose)	10 milligrams	NONE	N/A	10 milligrams in 2.5 ml	1 × 10 milligram tube	10 milligrams
Diazepam	Rectal (small dose)	5 milligrams	NONE	N/A	5 milligrams in 2.5 ml	1 × 5 milligram tube	5 milligrams
Glucagon (Glucagen)	IM	500 micrograms	NONE	N/A	1 milligram per vial	0.5 vial	500 micrograms
Glucose 10%	IV	2.5 grams	2.5 grams	5 minutes	50 grams in 500 ml	25 ml	7.5 grams
Hydrocortisone	IV/IO/IM	50 milligrams	NONE	N/A	100 milligrams in 1 ml	0.5 ml	50 milligrams
Hydrocortisone	IV/IO/IM	50 milligrams	NONE	N/A	100 milligrams in 2 ml	1 ml	50 milligrams
Ibuprofen	Oral	100 milligrams	100 milligrams	8 hours	100 milligrams in 5 ml	5 ml	300 milligrams per 24 hours
Ipratropium Bromide (Atrovent) 250 micrograms in 1 ml	Neb	250 micrograms	NONE	N/A	250 micrograms in 1 ml	1 ml	250 micrograms
Ipratropium Bromide (Atrovent) 500 micrograms in 1 ml	Neb	250 micrograms	NONE	N/A	500 micrograms in 2 ml	1 ml	250 micrograms
Midazolam[a]	Buccal	5 milligrams	5 milligrams	10 mins	5 milligrams in 1 ml	1 ml pre-filled syringe	10 milligrams
Morphine Sulphate	IV/IO	1 milligram	1 milligram	5 minutes	10 milligrams in 10 ml	1 ml	2 milligrams
Morphine Sulphate	Oral	2 milligrams	NONE	N/A	10 milligrams in 5 ml	1 ml	2 milligrams
Naloxone NB cautions	IV/IO	120 micrograms	120 micrograms	3 minutes	400 micrograms in 1 ml	0.3 ml	1,320 micrograms
Naloxone - initial dose	IM	120 micrograms	See repeat dose	3 minutes	400 micrograms in 1 ml	0.3 ml	See below
Naloxone - repeat dose	IM	See initial dose	400 micrograms	3 minutes	400 micrograms in 1 ml	1 ml	520 micrograms
Ondansetron	IV/IO/IM	1 milligram	NONE	N/A	2 milligrams in 1 ml	0.5 ml	1 milligram
Paracetamol - Infant suspension	Oral	180 milligrams	180 milligrams	4–6 hours	120 milligrams in 5 ml	7.5 ml	720 milligrams in 24 hours
Paracetamol	IV infusion/IO	150 milligrams	150 milligrams	4–6 hours	10 milligrams in 1 ml	15 ml	600 milligrams in 24 hours
Salbutamol 2.5 milligrams in 2.5 ml	Neb	2.5 milligrams	2.5 milligrams	5 minutes	2.5 milligrams in 2.5 ml	2.5 ml	No limit
Salbutamol 5 milligrams in 2.5 ml	Neb	2.5 milligrams	2.5 milligrams	5 minutes	5 milligrams in 2.5 ml	1.25 ml	No limit
Tranexamic Acid	IV	200 mg	NONE	N/A	100 mg/ml	2 ml	200 mg

ʼive the dose as prescribed in the child's individual treatment plan/Epilepsy Passport (the dosages described above reflect the recommended dosages for a ᵈd of this age).

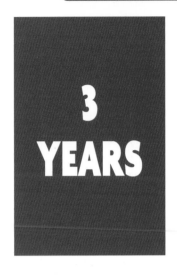

3 YEARS

Vital Signs

	GUIDE WEIGHT 14 kg		HEART RATE 95–140		RESPIRATION RATE 25–30		SYSTOLIC BLOOD PRESSURE 80–100

Airway Size by Type

OROPHARYNGEAL AIRWAY	LARYNGEAL MASK	I-GEL AIRWAY	ENDOTRACHEAL TUBE
1	2	2	Diameter: **5 mm**; Length: **14 cm**

Defibrillation – Cardiac Arrest

MANUAL	AUTOMATED EXTERNAL DEFIBRILLATOR
60 Joules	A standard AED (either with paediatric attenuation pads or else in paediatric mode) can be used. If paediatric pads are not available, standard adult pads can be used (but must not overlap).

Intravascular Fluid

FLUID	ROUTE	INITIAL DOSE	REPEAT DOSE	DOSE INTERVAL	CONCENTRATION	VOLUME	MAX DOSE
0.9% Sodium Chloride (5 ml/kg)	IV/IO	70 ml	70 ml	PRN	0.9%	70 ml	560 ml
0.9% Sodium Chloride (10 ml/kg)	IV/IO	140 ml	140 ml	PRN	0.9%	140 ml	560 ml
0.9% Sodium Chloride (20 ml/kg)	IV/IO	280 ml	280 ml	PRN	0.9%	280 ml	560 ml

Cardiac Arrest

DRUG	ROUTE	INITIAL DOSE	REPEAT DOSE	DOSE INTERVAL	CONCENTRATION	VOLUME	MAX DOSE
Adrenaline	IV/IO	140 micrograms	140 micrograms	3–5 minutes	1 milligram in 10 ml (1:10,000)	1.4 ml	No limit
Amiodarone	IV/IO	70 milligrams (After 3rd shock)	70 milligrams	After 5th shock	300 milligrams in 10 ml	2.3 ml	140 milligrams

ick Reference Table

DRUG	ROUTE	INITIAL DOSE	REPEAT DOSE	DOSE INTERVAL	CONCENTRATION	VOLUME	MAX DOSE
Adrenaline - anaphylaxis/asthma	IM	150 micrograms	150 micrograms	5 minutes	1 milligram in 1 ml (1:1,000)	0.15 ml	No limit
Benzylpenicillin (Penicillin G)	IV/IO	600 milligrams	NONE	N/A	600 milligrams dissolved in 9.6 ml water for injection	10 ml	600 milligrams
Benzylpenicillin (Penicillin G)	IM	600 milligrams	NONE	N/A	600 milligrams dissolved in 1.6 ml water for injection	2 ml	600 milligrams
Chlorphenamine	IV/IO/IM	2.5 milligrams	NONE	N/A	10 milligrams in 1 ml	0.25 ml	2.5 milligrams
Chlorphenamine	Oral (solution)	1 milligram	NONE	N/A	2 milligrams in 5 ml	2.5 ml	1 milligram
Chlorphenamine	Oral (tablet)	1 milligram	NONE	N/A	4 milligrams per tablet	¼ of one tablet	1 milligram
Dexamethasone - croup	Oral	3.8 milligrams	NONE	N/A	3.8 milligrams per ml	1 ml	3.8 milligrams
Diazepam	IV/IO	4.5 milligrams	NONE	N/A	10 milligrams in 2 ml	0.9 ml	4.5 milligrams
Diazepam	Rectal (large dose)	10 milligrams	NONE	N/A	10 milligrams in 2.5 ml	1 × 10 milligram tube	10 milligrams
Diazepam	Rectal (small dose)	5 milligrams	NONE	N/A	5 milligrams in 2.5 ml	1 × 5 milligram tube	5 milligrams
Glucagon (Glucagen)	IM	500 micrograms	NONE	N/A	1 milligram per vial	0.5 vial	500 micrograms
Glucose 10%	IV	3 grams	3 grams	5 minutes	50 grams in 500 ml	30 ml	9 grams
Hydrocortisone	IV/IO/IM	50 milligrams	NONE	N/A	100 milligrams in 1 ml	0.5 ml	50 milligrams
Hydrocortisone	IV/IO/IM	50 milligrams	NONE	N/A	100 milligrams in 2 ml	1 ml	50 milligrams
Ibuprofen	Oral	100 milligrams	100 milligrams	8 hours	100 milligrams in 5 ml	5 ml	300 milligrams per 24 hours
Ipratropium Bromide (Atrovent) 250 micrograms in 1 ml	Neb	250 micrograms	NONE	N/A	250 micrograms in 1 ml	1 ml	250 micrograms
Ipratropium Bromide (Atrovent) 500 micrograms in 1 ml	Neb	250 micrograms	NONE	N/A	500 micrograms in 2 ml	1 ml	250 micrograms
Midazolam[a]	Buccal	5 milligrams	5 milligrams	10 mins	5 milligrams in 1 ml	1 ml pre-filled syringe	10 milligrams
Morphine Sulphate	IV/IO	1.5 milligrams	1.5 milligrams	5 minutes	10 milligrams in 10 ml	1.5 ml	3 milligrams
Morphine Sulphate	Oral	3 milligrams	NONE	N/A	10 milligrams in 5 ml	1.5 ml	3 milligrams
Naloxone NB cautions	IV/IO	160 micrograms	160 micrograms	3 minutes	400 micrograms in 1 ml	0.4 ml	1,760 micrograms
Naloxone - initial dose	IM	160 micrograms	See repeat dose	3 minutes	400 micrograms in 1 ml	0.4 ml	See below
Naloxone - repeat dose	IM	See initial dose	400 micrograms	3 minutes	400 micrograms in 1 ml	1 ml	560 micrograms
Ondansetron	IV/IO/IM	1.5 milligrams	NONE	N/A	2 milligrams in 1 ml	0.75 ml	1.5 milligrams
Paracetamol - Infant suspension	Oral	180 milligrams	180 milligrams	4–6 hours	120 milligrams in 5 ml	7.5 ml	720 milligrams in 24 hours
Paracetamol	IV infusion/IO	250 milligrams	250 milligrams	4–6 hours	10 milligrams in 1 ml	25 ml	1 gram in 24 hours
Salbutamol 2.5 milligrams in 2.5 ml	Neb	2.5 milligrams	2.5 milligrams	5 minutes	2.5 milligrams in 2.5 ml	2.5 ml	No limit
Salbutamol 5 milligrams in 2.5 ml	Neb	2.5 milligrams	2.5 milligrams	5 minutes	5 milligrams in 2.5 ml	1.25 ml	No limit
Tranexamic Acid	IV	200 mg	NONE	N/A	100 mg/ml	2 ml	200 mg

Give the dose as prescribed in the child's individual treatment plan/Epilepsy Passport (the dosages described above reflect the recommended dosages for a d of this age).

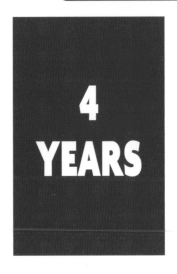

Vital Signs

GUIDE WEIGHT 16 kg	HEART RATE 95–140	RESPIRATION RATE 25–30	SYSTOLIC BLOOD PRESSURE 80–100

Airway Size by Type

OROPHARYNGEAL AIRWAY	LARYNGEAL MASK	I-GEL AIRWAY	ENDOTRACHEAL TUBE
1	2	2	Diameter: **5 mm**; Length: **15 cm**

Defibrillation – Cardiac Arrest

MANUAL	AUTOMATED EXTERNAL DEFIBRILLATOR
70 Joules	A standard AED (either with paediatric attenuation pads or else in paediatric mode) can be used. If paediatric pads are not available, standard adult pads can be used (but must not overlap).

Intravascular Fluid

FLUID	ROUTE	INITIAL DOSE	REPEAT DOSE	DOSE INTERVAL	CONCENTRATION	VOLUME	MAX DOSE
0.9% Sodium Chloride (5 ml/kg)	IV/IO	80 ml	80 ml	PRN	0.9%	80 ml	640 ml
0.9% Sodium Chloride (10 ml/kg)	IV/IO	160 ml	160 ml	PRN	0.9%	160 ml	640 ml
0.9% Sodium Chloride (20 ml/kg)	IV/IO	320 ml	320 ml	PRN	0.9%	320 ml	640 ml

Cardiac Arrest

DRUG	ROUTE	INITIAL DOSE	REPEAT DOSE	DOSE INTERVAL	CONCENTRATION	VOLUME	MAX DOSE
Adrenaline	IV/IO	160 micrograms	160 micrograms	3–5 minutes	1 milligram in 10 ml (1:10,000)	1.6 ml	No limit
Amiodarone	IV/IO	80 milligrams (After 3rd shock)	80 milligrams	After 5th shock	300 milligrams in 10 ml	2.7 ml	160 milligrams

ick Reference Table

DRUG	ROUTE	INITIAL DOSE	REPEAT DOSE	DOSE INTERVAL	CONCENTRATION	VOLUME	MAX DOSE
Adrenaline - anaphylaxis/asthma	IM	150 micrograms	150 micrograms	5 minutes	1 milligram in 1 ml (1:1,000)	0.15 ml	No limit
Benzylpenicillin (Penicillin G)	IV/IO	600 milligrams	NONE	N/A	600 milligrams dissolved in 9.6 ml water for injection	10 ml	600 milligrams
Benzylpenicillin (Penicillin G)	IM	600 milligrams	NONE	N/A	600 milligrams dissolved in 1.6 ml water for injection	2 ml	600 milligrams
Chlorphenamine	IV/IO/IM	2.5 milligrams	NONE	N/A	10 milligrams in 1 ml	0.25 ml	2.5 milligrams
Chlorphenamine	Oral (solution)	1 milligram	NONE	N/A	2 milligrams in 5 ml	2.5 ml	1 milligram
Chlorphenamine	Oral (tablet)	1 milligram	NONE	N/A	4 milligrams per tablet	$\frac{1}{4}$ of one tablet	1 milligram
Dexamethasone - croup	Oral	3.8 milligrams	NONE	N/A	3.8 milligrams per ml	1 ml	3.8 milligrams
Diazepam	IV/IO	5 milligrams	NONE	N/A	10 milligrams in 2 ml	1 ml	5 milligrams
Diazepam	Rectal (large dose)	10 milligrams	NONE	N/A	10 milligrams in 2.5 ml	1 × 10 milligram tube	10 milligrams
Diazepam	Rectal (small dose)	5 milligrams	NONE	N/A	5 milligrams in 2.5 ml	1 × 5 milligram tube	5 milligrams
Glucagon (Glucagen)	IM	500 micrograms	NONE	N/A	1 milligram per vial	0.5 vial	500 micrograms
Glucose 10%	IV	3 grams	3 grams	5 minutes	50 grams in 500 ml	30 ml	9 grams
Hydrocortisone	IV/IO/IM	50 milligrams	NONE	N/A	100 milligrams in 1 ml	0.5 ml	50 milligrams
Hydrocortisone	IV/IO/IM	50 milligrams	NONE	N/A	100 milligrams in 2 ml	1 ml	50 milligrams
Ibuprofen	Oral	150 milligrams	150 milligrams	8 hours	100 milligrams in 5 ml	7.5 ml	450 milligrams per 24 hours
Ipratropium Bromide (Atrovent) 250 micrograms in 1 ml	Neb	250 micrograms	NONE	N/A	250 micrograms in 1 ml	1 ml	250 micrograms
Ipratropium Bromide (Atrovent) 500 micrograms in 1 ml	Neb	250 micrograms	NONE	N/A	500 micrograms in 2 ml	1 ml	250 micrograms
Midazolam[a]	Buccal	5 milligrams	5 milligrams	10 mins	5 milligrams in 1 ml	1 ml pre-filled syringe	10 milligrams
Morphine Sulphate	IV/IO	1.5 milligrams	1.5 milligrams	5 minutes	10 milligrams in 10 ml	1.5 ml	3 milligrams
Morphine Sulphate	Oral	3 milligrams	NONE	N/A	10 milligrams in 5 ml	1.5 ml	3 milligrams
Naloxone NB cautions	IV/IO	160 micrograms	160 micrograms	3 minutes	400 micrograms in 1 ml	0.4 ml	1,760 micrograms
Naloxone - initial dose	IM	160 micrograms	See repeat dose	3 minutes	400 micrograms in 1 ml	0.4 ml	See below
Naloxone - repeat dose	IM	See initial dose	400 micrograms	3 minutes	400 micrograms in 1 ml	1 ml	560 micrograms
Ondansetron	IV/IO/IM	1.5 milligrams	NONE	N/A	2 milligrams in 1 ml	0.75 ml	1.5 milligrams
Paracetamol - Infant suspension	Oral	240 milligrams	240 milligrams	4–6 hours	120 milligrams in 5 ml	10 ml	960 milligrams in 24 hours
Paracetamol	IV infusion/IO	250 milligrams	250 milligrams	4–6 hours	10 milligrams in 1 ml	25 ml	1 gram in 24 hours
Salbutamol 2.5 milligrams in 2.5 ml	Neb	2.5 milligrams	2.5 milligrams	5 minutes	2.5 milligrams in 2.5 ml	2.5 ml	No limit
Salbutamol 5 milligrams in 2.5 ml	Neb	2.5 milligrams	2.5 milligrams	5 minutes	5 milligrams in 2.5 ml	1.25 ml	No limit
Tranexamic Acid	IV	250 mg	NONE	N/A	100 mg/ml	2.5 ml	250 mg

ive the dose as prescribed in the child's individual treatment plan/Epilepsy Passport (the dosages described above reflect the recommended dosages for a
d of this age).

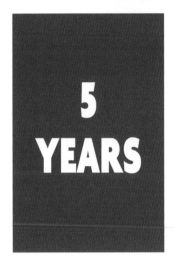

5 YEARS

Vital Signs

GUIDE WEIGHT 19 kg	HEART RATE 80–120	RESPIRATION RATE 20–25	SYSTOLIC BLOOD PRESSURE 90–100

Airway Size by Type

OROPHARYNGEAL AIRWAY	LARYNGEAL MASK	I-GEL AIRWAY	ENDOTRACHEAL TUBE
1	2	2	Diameter: **5.5 mm**; Length: **15 cm**

Defibrillation – Cardiac Arrest

MANUAL	AUTOMATED EXTERNAL DEFIBRILLATOR
80 Joules	A standard AED (either with paediatric attenuation pads or else in paediatric mode) can be used. If paediatric pads are not available, standard adult pads can be used (but must not overlap).

Intravascular Fluid

FLUID	ROUTE	INITIAL DOSE	REPEAT DOSE	DOSE INTERVAL	CONCENTRATION	VOLUME	MAX DOSE
0.9% Sodium Chloride (5 ml/kg)	IV/IO	95 ml	95 ml	PRN	0.9%	95 ml	760 ml
0.9% Sodium Chloride (10 ml/kg)	IV/IO	190 ml	190 ml	PRN	0.9%	190 ml	760 ml
0.9% Sodium Chloride (20 ml/kg)	IV/IO	380 ml	380 ml	PRN	0.9%	380 ml	760 ml

Cardiac Arrest

DRUG	ROUTE	INITIAL DOSE	REPEAT DOSE	DOSE INTERVAL	CONCENTRATION	VOLUME	MAX DOSE
Adrenaline	IV/IO	190 micrograms	190 micrograms	3–5 minutes	1 milligram in 10 ml (1:10,000)	1.9 ml	No limit
Amiodarone	IV/IO	100 milligrams (After 3rd shock)	100 milligrams	After 5th shock	300 milligrams in 10 ml	3.3 ml	200 milligrams

ick Reference Table

DRUG	ROUTE	INITIAL DOSE	REPEAT DOSE	DOSE INTERVAL	CONCENTRATION	VOLUME	MAX DOSE
Adrenaline - anaphylaxis/ asthma	IM	150 micrograms	150 micrograms	5 minutes	1 milligram in 1 ml (1:1,000)	0.15 ml	No limit
Benzylpenicillin (Penicillin G)	IV/IO	600 milligrams	NONE	N/A	600 milligrams dissolved in 9.6 ml water for injection	10 ml	600 milligrams
Benzylpenicillin (Penicillin G)	IM	600 milligrams	NONE	N/A	600 milligrams dissolved in 1.6 ml water for injection	2 ml	600 milligrams
Chlorphenamine	IV/IO/IM	2.5 milligrams	NONE	N/A	10 milligrams in 1 ml	0.25 ml	2.5 milligrams
Chlorphenamine	Oral (solution)	1 milligram	NONE	N/A	2 milligrams in 5 ml	2.5 ml	1 milligram
Chlorphenamine	Oral (tablet)	1 milligram	NONE	N/A	4 milligrams per tablet	¼ of one tablet	1 milligram
Dexamethasone - croup	Oral	3.8 milligrams	NONE	N/A	3.8 milligrams per ml	1 ml	3.8 milligrams
Diazepam	IV/IO	6 milligrams	NONE	N/A	10 milligrams in 2 ml	1.2 ml	6 milligrams
Diazepam	Rectal (large dose)	10 milligrams	NONE	N/A	10 milligrams in 2.5 ml	1 × 10 milligram tube	10 milligrams
Diazepam	Rectal (small dose)	5 milligrams	NONE	N/A	5 milligrams in 2.5 ml	1 × 5 milligram tube	5 milligrams
Glucagon (Glucagen)	IM	500 micrograms	NONE	N/A	1 milligram per vial	0.5 vial	500 micrograms
Glucose 10%	IV	4 grams	4 grams	5 minutes	50 grams in 500 ml	40 ml	12 grams
Hydrocortisone	IV/IO/IM	50 milligrams	NONE	N/A	100 milligrams in 1 ml	0.5 ml	50 milligrams
Hydrocortisone	IV/IO/IM	50 milligrams	NONE	N/A	100 milligrams in 2 ml	1 ml	50 milligrams
Ibuprofen	Oral	150 milligrams	150 milligrams	8 hours	100 milligrams in 5 ml	7.5 ml	450 milligrams per 24 hours
Ipratropium Bromide (Atrovent) 250 micrograms in 1 ml	Neb	250 micrograms	NONE	N/A	250 micrograms in 1 ml	1 ml	250 micrograms
Ipratropium Bromide (Atrovent) 500 micrograms in 1 ml	Neb	250 micrograms	NONE	N/A	500 micrograms in 2 ml	1 ml	250 micrograms
Midazolam[a]	Buccal	7.5 milligrams	7.5 milligrams	10 mins	5 milligrams in 1 ml	1.5 ml pre-filled syringe	15 milligrams
Morphine Sulphate	IV/IO	2 milligrams	2 milligrams	5 minutes	10 milligrams in 10 ml	2 ml	4 milligrams
Morphine Sulphate	Oral	4 milligrams	NONE	N/A	10 milligrams in 5 ml	2 ml	4 milligrams
Naloxone NB cautions	IV/IO	200 micrograms	200 micrograms	3 minutes	400 micrograms in 1 ml	0.5 ml	2,200 micrograms
Naloxone - initial dose	IM	200 micrograms	See repeat dose	3 minutes	400 micrograms in 1 ml	0.5 ml	See below
Naloxone - repeat dose	IM	See initial dose	400 micrograms	3 minutes	400 micrograms in 1 ml	1 ml	600 micrograms
Ondansetron	IV/IO/IM	2 milligrams	NONE	N/A	2 milligrams in 1 ml	1 ml	2 milligrams
Paracetamol - Infant suspension	Oral	240 milligrams	240 milligrams	4–6 hours	120 milligrams in 5 ml	10 ml	960 milligrams in 24 hours
Paracetamol	IV infusion/IO	250 milligrams	250 milligrams	4–6 hours	10 milligrams in 1 ml	25 ml	1 gram in 24 hours
Salbutamol 2.5 milligrams in 2.5 ml	Neb	2.5 milligrams	2.5 milligrams	5 minutes	2.5 milligrams in 2.5 ml	2.5 ml	No limit
Salbutamol 5 milligrams in 2.5 ml	Neb	2.5 milligrams	2.5 milligrams	5 minutes	5 milligrams in 2.5 ml	1.25 ml	No limit
Tranexamic Acid	IV	300 mg	NONE	N/A	100 mg/ml	3 ml	300 mg

ive the dose as prescribed in the child's individual treatment plan/Epilepsy Passport (the dosages described above reflect the recommended dosages for a d of this age).

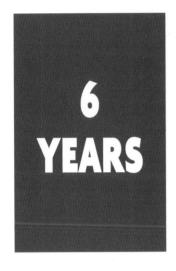

6 YEARS

Vital Signs

 GUIDE WEIGHT 21 kg **HEART RATE** 80–120 **RESPIRATION RATE** 20–25 **SYSTOLIC BLOOD PRESSURE** 80–110

Airway Size by Type

OROPHARYNGEAL AIRWAY	LARYNGEAL MASK	I-GEL AIRWAY	ENDOTRACHEAL TUBE
1	2.5	2	Diameter: **6 mm**; Length: **16 cm**

Defibrillation – Cardiac Arrest

MANUAL	AUTOMATED EXTERNAL DEFIBRILLATOR
80 Joules	A standard AED (either with paediatric attenuation pads or else in paediatric mode) can be used. If paediatric pads are not available, standard adult pads can be used (but must not overlap).

Intravascular Fluid

FLUID	ROUTE	INITIAL DOSE	REPEAT DOSE	DOSE INTERVAL	CONCENTRATION	VOLUME	MAX DOSE
0.9% Sodium Chloride (5 ml/kg)	IV/IO	105 ml	105 ml	PRN	0.9%	105 ml	840 ml
0.9% Sodium Chloride (10 ml/kg)	IV/IO	210 ml	210 ml	PRN	0.9%	210 ml	840 ml
0.9% Sodium Chloride (20 ml/kg)	IV/IO	420 ml	420 ml	PRN	0.9%	420 ml	840 ml

Cardiac Arrest

DRUG	ROUTE	INITIAL DOSE	REPEAT DOSE	DOSE INTERVAL	CONCENTRATION	VOLUME	MAX DOSE
Adrenaline	IV/IO	210 micrograms	210 micrograms	3–5 minutes	1 milligram in 10 ml (1:10,000)	2.1 ml	No limit
Amiodarone	IV/IO	100 milligrams (After 3rd shock)	100 milligrams	After 5th shock	300 milligrams in 10 ml	3.3 ml	200 milligrams

ick Reference Table

DRUG	ROUTE	INITIAL DOSE	REPEAT DOSE	DOSE INTERVAL	CONCENTRATION	VOLUME	MAX DOSE
Adrenaline - anaphylaxis/asthma	IM	300 micrograms	300 micrograms	5 minutes	1 milligram in 1 ml (1:1,000)	0.3 ml	No limit
Benzylpenicillin (Penicillin G)	IV/IO	600 milligrams	NONE	N/A	600 milligrams dissolved in 9.6 ml water for injection	10 ml	600 milligrams
Benzylpenicillin (Penicillin G)	IM	600 milligrams	NONE	N/A	600 milligrams dissolved in 1.6 ml water for injection	2 ml	600 milligrams
Chlorphenamine	IV/IO/IM	5–10 milligrams	NONE	N/A	10 milligrams in 1 ml	0.5–1 ml	5–10 milligrams
Chlorphenamine	Oral (solution)	2 milligrams	NONE	N/A	2 milligrams in 5 ml	5 ml	2 milligrams
Chlorphenamine	Oral (tablet)	2 milligrams	NONE	N/A	4 milligrams per tablet	½ of one tablet	2 milligrams
Dexamethasone - croup	Oral	3.8 milligrams	NONE	N/A	3.8 milligrams per ml	1 ml	3.8 milligrams
Diazepam	IV/IO	6.5 milligrams	NONE	N/A	10 milligrams in 2 ml	1.3 ml	6.5 milligrams
Diazepam	Rectal (large dose)	10 milligrams	NONE	N/A	10 milligrams in 2.5 ml	1 × 10 milligram tube	10 milligrams
Diazepam	Rectal (small dose)	5 milligrams	NONE	N/A	5 milligrams in 2.5 ml	1 × 5 milligram tube	5 milligrams
Glucagon (Glucagen)	IM	500 micrograms	NONE	N/A	1 milligram per vial	0.5 vial	500 micrograms
Glucose 10%	IV	4 grams	4 grams	5 minutes	50 grams in 500 ml	40 ml	12 grams
Hydrocortisone	IV/IO/IM	100 milligrams	NONE	N/A	100 milligrams in 1 ml	1 ml	100 milligrams
Hydrocortisone	IV/IO/IM	100 milligrams	NONE	N/A	100 milligrams in 2 ml	2 ml	100 milligrams
Ibuprofen	Oral	150 milligrams	150 milligrams	8 hours	100 milligrams in 5 ml	7.5 ml	450 milligrams per 24 hours
Ipratropium Bromide (Atrovent) 250 micrograms in 1 ml	Neb	250 micrograms	NONE	N/A	250 micrograms in 1 ml	1 ml	250 micrograms
Ipratropium Bromide (Atrovent) 500 micrograms in 1 ml	Neb	250 micrograms	NONE	N/A	500 micrograms in 2 ml	1 ml	250 micrograms
Midazolam[a]	Buccal	7.5 milligrams	7.5 milligrams	10 mins	5 milligrams in 1 ml	1.5 ml pre-filled syringe	15 milligrams
Morphine Sulphate	IV/IO	2 milligrams	2 milligrams	5 minutes	10 milligrams in 10 ml	2 ml	4 milligrams
Morphine Sulphate	Oral	4 milligrams	NONE	N/A	10 milligrams in 5 ml	2 ml	4 milligrams
Naloxone NB cautions	IV/IO	200 micrograms	200 micrograms	3 minutes	400 micrograms in 1 ml	0.5 ml	2,200 micrograms
Naloxone - initial dose	IM	200 micrograms	See repeat dose	3 minutes	400 micrograms in 1 ml	0.5 ml	See below
Naloxone - repeat dose	IM	See initial dose	400 micrograms	3 minutes	400 micrograms in 1 ml	1 ml	600 micrograms
Ondansetron	IV/IO/IM	2 milligrams	NONE	N/A	2 milligrams in 1 ml	1 ml	2 milligrams
Paracetamol - six plus suspension	Oral	250 milligrams	250 milligrams	4–6 hours	250 milligrams in 5 ml	5 ml	1 gram in 24 hours
Paracetamol	IV infusion/IO	300 milligrams	300 milligrams	4–6 hours	10 milligrams in 1 ml	30 ml	1.2 grams in 24 hours
Salbutamol 2.5 milligrams in 2.5 ml	Neb	5 milligrams	5 milligrams	5 minutes	2.5 milligrams in 2.5 ml	5 ml	No limit
Salbutamol 5 milligrams in 2.5 ml	Neb	5 milligrams	5 milligrams	5 minutes	5 milligrams in 2.5 ml	2.5 ml	No limit
Tranexamic Acid	IV	300 mg	NONE	N/A	100 mg/ml	3 ml	300 mg

ive the dose as prescribed in the child's individual treatment plan/Epilepsy Passport (the dosages described above reflect the recommended dosages for a d of this age).

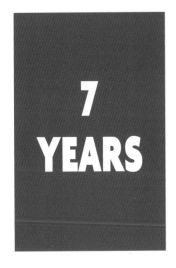

7 YEARS

Vital Signs

GUIDE WEIGHT 23 kg	**HEART RATE** 80–120	**RESPIRATION RATE** 20–25	**SYSTOLIC BLOOD PRESSURE** 90–110

Airway Size by Type

OROPHARYNGEAL AIRWAY	LARYNGEAL MASK	I-GEL AIRWAY	ENDOTRACHEAL TUBE
1 OR 2	2.5	2	Diameter: **6 mm**; Length: **16 cm**

Defibrillation – Cardiac Arrest

MANUAL	AUTOMATED EXTERNAL DEFIBRILLATOR
100 Joules	A standard AED (either with paediatric attenuation pads or else in paediatric mode) can be used. If paediatric pads are not available, standard adult pads can be used (but must not overlap).

Intravascular Fluid

FLUID	ROUTE	INITIAL DOSE	REPEAT DOSE	DOSE INTERVAL	CONCENTRATION	VOLUME	MAX DOSE
0.9% Sodium Chloride (5 ml/kg)	IV/IO	115 ml	115 ml	PRN	0.9%	115 ml	920 ml
0.9% Sodium Chloride (10 ml/kg)	IV/IO	230 ml	230 ml	PRN	0.9%	230 ml	920 ml
0.9% Sodium Chloride (20 ml/kg)	IV/IO	460 ml	460 ml	PRN	0.9%	460 ml	920 ml

Cardiac Arrest

DRUG	ROUTE	INITIAL DOSE	REPEAT DOSE	DOSE INTERVAL	CONCENTRATION	VOLUME	MAX DOSE
Adrenaline	IV/IO	230 micrograms	230 micrograms	3–5 minutes	1 milligram in 10 ml (1:10,000)	2.3 ml	No limit
Amiodarone	IV/IO	120 milligrams (After 3rd shock)	120 milligrams	After 5th shock	300 milligrams in 10 ml	4 ml	240 milligrams

Quick Reference Table

DRUG	ROUTE	INITIAL DOSE	REPEAT DOSE	DOSE INTERVAL	CONCENTRATION	VOLUME	MAX DOSE
Adrenaline - anaphylaxis/ asthma	IM	300 micrograms	300 micrograms	5 minutes	1 milligram in 1 ml (1:1,000)	0.3 ml	No limit
Benzylpenicillin (Penicillin G)	IV/IO	600 milligrams	NONE	N/A	600 milligrams dissolved in 9.6 ml water for injection	10 ml	600 milligrams
Benzylpenicillin (Penicillin G)	IM	600 milligrams	NONE	N/A	600 milligrams dissolved in 1.6 ml water for injection	2 ml	600 milligrams
Chlorphenamine	IV/IO/IM	5–10 milligrams	NONE	N/A	10 milligrams in 1 ml	0.5 ml–1 ml	5–10 milligrams
Chlorphenamine	Oral (solution)	2 milligrams	NONE	N/A	2 milligrams in 5 ml	5 ml	2 milligrams
Chlorphenamine	Oral (tablet)	2 milligrams	NONE	N/A	4 milligrams per tablet	½ of one tablet	2 milligrams
Dexamethasone - croup	Oral	N/A	N/A	N/A	N/A	N/A	N/A
Diazepam	IV/IO	7 milligrams	NONE	N/A	10 milligrams in 2 ml	1.4 ml	7 milligrams
Diazepam	Rectal (large dose)	10 milligrams	NONE	N/A	10 milligrams in 2.5 ml	1 × 10 milligram tube	10 milligrams
Diazepam	Rectal (small dose)	5 milligrams	NONE	N/A	5 milligrams in 2.5 ml	1 × 5 milligram tube	5 milligrams
Glucagon (Glucagen)	IM	500 micrograms	NONE	N/A	1 milligram per vial	0.5 vial	500 micrograms
Glucose 10%	IV	5 grams	5 grams	5 minutes	50 grams in 500 ml	50 ml	15 grams
Hydrocortisone	IV/IO/IM	100 milligrams	NONE	N/A	100 milligrams in 1 ml	1 ml	100 milligrams
Hydrocortisone	IV/IO/IM	100 milligrams	NONE	N/A	100 milligrams in 2 ml	2 ml	100 milligrams
Ibuprofen	Oral	200 milligrams	200 milligrams	8 hours	100 milligrams in 5 ml	10 ml	600 milligrams per 24 hours
Ipratropium Bromide (Atrovent) 250 micrograms in 1 ml	Neb	250 micrograms	NONE	N/A	250 micrograms in 1 ml	1 ml	250 micrograms
Ipratropium Bromide (Atrovent) 500 micrograms in 1 ml	Neb	250 micrograms	NONE	N/A	500 micrograms in 2 ml	1 ml	250 micrograms
Midazolam[a]	Buccal	7.5 milligrams	7.5 milligrams	10 mins	5 milligrams in 1 ml	1.5 ml pre-filled syringe	15 milligrams
Morphine Sulphate	IV/IO	2.5 milligrams	2.5 milligrams	5 minutes	10 milligrams in 10 ml	2.5 ml	5 milligrams
Morphine Sulphate	Oral	5 milligrams	NONE	N/A	10 milligrams in 5 ml	2.5 ml	5 milligrams
Naloxone NB cautions	IV/IO	240 micrograms	240 micrograms	3 minutes	400 micrograms in 1 ml	0.6 ml	2,640 micrograms
Naloxone - initial dose	IM	240 micrograms	See repeat dose	3 minutes	400 micrograms in 1 ml	0.6 ml	See below
Naloxone - repeat dose	IM	See initial dose	400 micrograms	3 minutes	400 micrograms in 1 ml	1 ml	640 micrograms
Ondansetron	IV/IO/IM	2.5 milligrams	NONE	N/A	2 milligrams in 1 ml	1.3 ml	2.5 milligrams
Paracetamol - six plus suspension	Oral	250 milligrams	250 milligrams	4–6 hours	250 milligrams in 5 ml	5 ml	1 gram in 24 hours
Paracetamol	IV infusion/IO	300 milligrams	300 milligrams	4–6 hours	10 milligrams in 1 ml	30 ml	1.2 grams in 24 hours
Salbutamol 2.5 milligrams in 2.5 ml	Neb	5 milligrams	5 milligrams	5 minutes	2.5 milligrams in 2.5 ml	5 ml	No limit
Salbutamol 5 milligrams in 2.5 ml	Neb	5 milligrams	5 milligrams	5 minutes	5 milligrams in 2.5 ml	2.5 ml	No limit
Tranexamic Acid	IV	350 mg	NONE	N/A	100 mg/ml	3.5 ml	350 mg

ive the dose as prescribed in the child's individual treatment plan/Epilepsy Passport (the dosages described above reflect the recommended dosages for a d of this age).

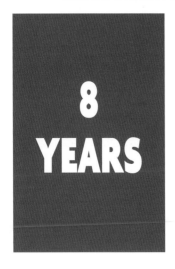

8 YEARS

Vital Signs

	GUIDE WEIGHT		HEART RATE		RESPIRATION RATE		SYSTOLIC BLOOD PRESSURE
	26 kg		80–120		20–25		90–110

Airway Size by Type

OROPHARYNGEAL AIRWAY	LARYNGEAL MASK	I-GEL AIRWAY	ENDOTRACHEAL TUBE
1 OR 2	2.5	2.5	Diameter: **6.5 mm**; Length: **17 cm**

Defibrillation – Cardiac Arrest

MANUAL	AUTOMATED EXTERNAL DEFIBRILLATOR
100 Joules	A standard AED (either with paediatric attenuation pads or else in paediatric mode) can be used. If paediatric pads are not available, standard adult pads can be used (but must not overlap).

Intravascular Fluid

FLUID	ROUTE	INITIAL DOSE	REPEAT DOSE	DOSE INTERVAL	CONCENTRATION	VOLUME	MAX DOSE
0.9% Sodium Chloride (5 ml/kg)	IV/IO	130 ml	130 ml	PRN	0.9%	130 ml	1,000 ml
0.9% Sodium Chloride (10 ml/kg)	IV/IO	250 ml	250 ml	PRN	0.9%	250 ml	1,000 ml
0.9% Sodium Chloride (20 ml/kg)	IV/IO	500 ml	500 ml	PRN	0.9%	500 ml	1,000 ml

Cardiac Arrest

DRUG	ROUTE	INITIAL DOSE	REPEAT DOSE	DOSE INTERVAL	CONCENTRATION	VOLUME	MAX DOSE
Adrenaline	IV/IO	260 micrograms	260 micrograms	3–5 minutes	1 milligram in 10 ml (1:10,000)	2.6 ml	No limit
Amiodarone	IV/IO	130 milligrams (After 3rd shock)	130 milligrams	After 5th shock	300 milligrams in 10 ml	4.3 ml	260 milligrams

Quick Reference Table

DRUG	ROUTE	INITIAL DOSE	REPEAT DOSE	DOSE INTERVAL	CONCENTRATION	VOLUME	MAX DOSE
Adrenaline - anaphylaxis/asthma	IM	300 micrograms	300 micrograms	5 minutes	1 milligram in 1 ml (1:1,000)	0.3 ml	No limit
Benzylpenicillin (Penicillin G)	IV/IO	600 milligrams	NONE	N/A	600 milligrams dissolved in 9.6 ml water for injection	10 ml	600 milligrams
Benzylpenicillin (Penicillin G)	IM	600 milligrams	NONE	N/A	600 milligrams dissolved in 1.6 ml water for injection	2 ml	600 milligrams
Chlorphenamine	IV/IO/IM	5–10 milligrams	NONE	N/A	10 milligrams in 1 ml	0.5–1 ml	5–10 milligrams
Chlorphenamine	Oral (solution)	2 milligrams	NONE	N/A	2 milligrams in 5 ml	5 ml	2 milligrams
Chlorphenamine	Oral (tablet)	2 milligrams	NONE	N/A	4 milligrams per tablet	½ of one tablet	2 milligrams
Dexamethasone - croup	Oral	N/A	N/A	N/A	N/A	N/A	N/A
Diazepam	IV/IO	8 milligrams	NONE	N/A	10 milligrams in 2 ml	1.6 ml	8 milligrams
Diazepam	Rectal (large dose)	10 milligrams	NONE	N/A	10 milligrams in 2.5 ml	1 × 10 milligram tube	10 milligrams
Diazepam	Rectal (small dose)	5 milligrams	NONE	N/A	5 milligrams in 2.5 ml	1 × 5 milligram tube	5 milligrams
Glucagon (Glucagen)	IM	1 milligram	NONE	N/A	1 milligram per vial	1 vial	1 milligram
Glucose 10%	IV	5 grams	5 grams	5 minutes	50 grams in 500 ml	50 ml	15 grams
Hydrocortisone	IV/IO/IM	100 milligrams	NONE	N/A	100 milligrams in 1 ml	1 ml	100 milligrams
Hydrocortisone	IV/IO/IM	100 milligrams	NONE	N/A	100 milligrams in 2 ml	2 ml	100 milligrams
Ibuprofen	Oral	200 milligrams	200 milligrams	8 hours	100 milligrams in 5 ml	10 ml	600 milligrams per 24 hours
Ipratropium Bromide (Atrovent) 250 micrograms in 1 ml	Neb	250 micrograms	NONE	N/A	250 micrograms in 1 ml	1 ml	250 micrograms
Ipratropium Bromide (Atrovent) 500 micrograms in 1 ml	Neb	250 micrograms	NONE	N/A	500 micrograms in 2 ml	1 ml	250 micrograms
Midazolam[a]	Buccal	7.5 milligrams	7.5 milligrams	10 mins	5 milligrams in 1 ml	1.5 ml pre-filled syringe	15 milligrams
Morphine Sulphate	IV/IO	2.5 milligrams	2.5 milligrams	5 minutes	10 milligrams in 10 ml	2.5 ml	5 milligrams
Morphine Sulphate	Oral	5 milligrams	NONE	N/A	10 milligrams in 5 ml	2.5 ml	5 milligrams
Naloxone NB cautions	IV/IO	280 micrograms	280 micrograms	3 minutes	400 micrograms in 1 ml	0.7 ml	3,080 micrograms
Naloxone - initial dose	IM	280 micrograms	See repeat dose	3 minutes	400 micrograms in 1 ml	0.7 ml	See below
Naloxone - repeat dose	IM	See initial dose	400 micrograms	3 minutes	400 micrograms in 1 ml	1 ml	680 micrograms
Ondansetron	IV/IO/IM	2.5 milligrams	NONE	N/A	2 milligrams in 1 ml	1.3 ml	2.5 milligrams
Paracetamol - six plus suspension	Oral	375 milligrams	375 milligrams	4–6 hours	250 milligrams in 5 ml	7.5 ml	1.5 grams in 24 hours
Paracetamol	IV infusion/IO	300 milligrams	300 milligrams	4–6 hours	10 milligrams in 1 ml	30 ml	1.2 grams in 24 hours
Salbutamol 2.5 milligrams in 2.5 ml	Neb	5 milligrams	5 milligrams	5 minutes	2.5 milligrams in 2.5 ml	5 ml	No limit
Salbutamol 5 milligrams in 2.5 ml	Neb	5 milligrams	5 milligrams	5 minutes	5 milligrams in 2.5 ml	2.5 ml	No limit
Tranexamic Acid	IV	400 mg	NONE	N/A	100 mg/ml	4 ml	400 mg

Give the dose as prescribed in the child's individual treatment plan/Epilepsy Passport (the dosages described above reflect the recommended dosages for a child of this age).

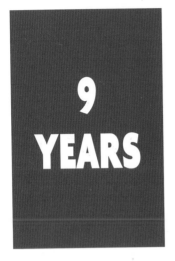

9 YEARS

Vital Signs

GUIDE WEIGHT 29 kg	**HEART RATE** 80–120	**RESPIRATION RATE** 20–25	**SYSTOLIC BLOOD PRESSURE** 90–110

Airway Size by Type

OROPHARYNGEAL AIRWAY	LARYNGEAL MASK	I-GEL AIRWAY	ENDOTRACHEAL TUBE
1 OR 2	2.5	2.5	Diameter: **6.5 mm**; Length: **17 cm**

Defibrillation – Cardiac Arrest

MANUAL	AUTOMATED EXTERNAL DEFIBRILLATOR
120 Joules	A standard AED can be used (without the need for paediatric attenuation pads).

Intravascular Fluid

FLUID	ROUTE	INITIAL DOSE	REPEAT DOSE	DOSE INTERVAL	CONCENTRATION	VOLUME	MAX DOSE
0.9% Sodium Chloride (5 ml/kg)	IV/IO	145 ml	145 ml	PRN	0.9%	145 ml	1,000 ml
0.9% Sodium Chloride (10 ml/kg)	IV/IO	290 ml	290 ml	PRN	0.9%	290 ml	1,000 ml
0.9% Sodium Chloride (20 ml/kg)	IV/IO	500 ml	500 ml	PRN	0.9%	500 ml	1,000 ml

Cardiac Arrest

DRUG	ROUTE	INITIAL DOSE	REPEAT DOSE	DOSE INTERVAL	CONCENTRATION	VOLUME	MAX DOSE
Adrenaline	IV/IO	300 micrograms	300 micrograms	3–5 minutes	1 milligram in 10 ml (1:10,000)	3 ml	No limit
Amiodarone	IV/IO	150 milligrams (After 3rd shock)	150 milligrams	After 5th shock	300 milligrams in 10 ml	5 ml	300 milligrams

ick Reference Table

DRUG	ROUTE	INITIAL DOSE	REPEAT DOSE	DOSE INTERVAL	CONCENTRATION	VOLUME	MAX DOSE
Adrenaline - anaphylaxis/ asthma	IM	300 micrograms	300 micrograms	5 minutes	1 milligram in 1 ml (1:1,000)	0.3 ml	No limit
Benzylpenicillin (Penicillin G)	IV/IO	600 milligrams	NONE	N/A	600 milligrams dissolved in 9.6 ml water for injection	10 ml	600 milligrams
Benzylpenicillin (Penicillin G)	IM	600 milligrams	NONE	N/A	600 milligrams dissolved in 1.6 ml water for injection	2 ml	600 milligrams
Chlorphenamine	IV/IO/IM	5–10 milligrams	NONE	N/A	10 milligrams in 1 ml	0.5 ml–1 ml	5–10 milligrams
Chlorphenamine	Oral (solution)	2 milligrams	NONE	N/A	2 milligrams in 5 ml	5 ml	2 milligrams
Chlorphenamine	Oral (tablet)	2 milligrams	NONE	N/A	4 milligrams per tablet	½ of one tablet	2 milligrams
Dexamethasone - croup	Oral	N/A	N/A	N/A	N/A	N/A	N/A
Diazepam	IV/IO	9 milligrams	NONE	N/A	10 milligrams in 2 ml	1.8 ml	9 milligrams
Diazepam	Rectal (large dose)	10 milligrams	NONE	N/A	10 milligrams in 2.5 ml	1 × 10 milligram tube	10 milligrams
Diazepam	Rectal (small dose)	5 milligrams	NONE	N/A	5 milligrams in 2.5 ml	1 × 5 milligram tube	5 milligrams
Glucagon (Glucagen)	IM	1 milligram	NONE	N/A	1 milligram per vial	1 vial	1 milligram
Glucose 10%	IV	6 grams	6 grams	5 minutes	50 grams in 500 ml	60 ml	18 grams
Hydrocortisone	IV/IO/IM	100 milligrams	NONE	N/A	100 milligrams in 1 ml	1 ml	100 milligrams
Hydrocortisone	IV/IO/IM	100 milligrams	NONE	N/A	100 milligrams in 2 ml	2 ml	100 milligrams
Ibuprofen	Oral	200 milligrams	200 milligrams	8 hours	100 milligrams in 5 ml	10 ml	600 milligrams per 24 hours
Ipratropium Bromide (Atrovent) 250 micrograms in 1 ml	Neb	250 micrograms	NONE	N/A	250 micrograms in 1 ml	1 ml	250 micrograms
Ipratropium Bromide (Atrovent) 500 micrograms in 1 ml	Neb	250 micrograms	NONE	N/A	500 micrograms in 2 ml	1 ml	250 micrograms
Midazolam[a]	Buccal	7.5 milligrams	7.5 milligrams	10 mins	5 milligrams in 1 ml	1.5 ml pre-filled syringe	15 milligrams
Morphine Sulphate	IV/IO	3 milligrams	3 milligrams	5 minutes	10 milligrams in 10 ml	3 ml	6 milligrams
Morphine Sulphate	Oral	6 milligrams	NONE	N/A	10 milligrams in 5 ml	3 ml	6 milligrams
Naloxone NB cautions	IV/IO	280 micrograms	280 micrograms	3 minutes	400 micrograms in 1 ml	0.7 ml	3,080 micrograms
Naloxone - initial dose	IM	280 micrograms	See repeat dose	3 minutes	400 micrograms in 1 ml	0.7 ml	See below
Naloxone - repeat dose	IM	See initial dose	400 micrograms	3 minutes	400 micrograms in 1 ml	1 ml	680 micrograms
Ondansetron	IV/IO/IM	3 milligrams	NONE	N/A	2 milligrams in 1 ml	1.5 ml	3 milligrams
Paracetamol - six plus suspension	Oral	375 milligrams	375 milligrams	4–6 hours	250 milligrams in 5 ml	7.5 ml	1.5 grams in 24 hours
Paracetamol	IV infusion/IO	500 milligrams	500 milligrams	4–6 hours	10 milligrams in 1 ml	50 ml	2 grams in 24 hours
Salbutamol 2.5 milligrams in 2.5 ml	Neb	5 milligrams	5 milligrams	5 minutes	2.5 milligrams in 2.5 ml	5 ml	No limit
Salbutamol 5 milligrams in 2.5 ml	Neb	5 milligrams	5 milligrams	5 minutes	5 milligrams in 2.5 ml	2.5 ml	No limit
Tranexamic Acid	IV	450 mg	NONE	N/A	100 mg/ml	4.5 ml	450 mg

ive the dose as prescribed in the child's individual treatment plan/Epilepsy Passport (the dosages described above reflect the recommended dosages for a d of this age).

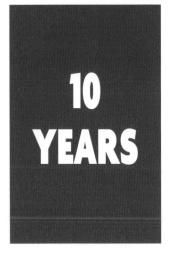

10 YEARS

Vital Signs

GUIDE WEIGHT 32 kg	**HEART RATE** 80–120	**RESPIRATION RATE** 20–25	**SYSTOLIC BLOOD PRESSURE** 90–110

Airway Size by Type

OROPHARYNGEAL AIRWAY	LARYNGEAL MASK	I-GEL AIRWAY	ENDOTRACHEAL TUBE
2 OR 3	3	2.5 OR 3	Diameter: **7 mm**; Length: **18 cm**

Defibrillation – Cardiac Arrest

MANUAL	AUTOMATED EXTERNAL DEFIBRILLATOR
130 Joules	A standard AED can be used (without the need for paediatric attenuation pads).

Intravascular Fluid

FLUID	ROUTE	INITIAL DOSE	REPEAT DOSE	DOSE INTERVAL	CONCENTRATION	VOLUME	MAX DOSE
0.9% Sodium Chloride (5 ml/kg)	IV/IO	160 ml	160 ml	PRN	0.9%	160 ml	1,000 ml
0.9% Sodium Chloride (10 ml/kg)	IV/IO	320 ml	320 ml	PRN	0.9%	320 ml	1,000 ml
0.9% Sodium Chloride (20 ml/kg)	IV/IO	500 ml	500 ml	PRN	0.9%	500 ml	1,000 ml

Cardiac Arrest

DRUG	ROUTE	INITIAL DOSE	REPEAT DOSE	DOSE INTERVAL	CONCENTRATION	VOLUME	MAX DOSE
Adrenaline	IV/IO	320 micrograms	320 micrograms	3–5 minutes	1 milligram in 10 ml (1:10,000)	3.2 ml	No limit
Amiodarone	IV/IO	160 milligrams (After 3rd shock)	160 milligrams	After 5th shock	300 milligrams in 10 ml	5.3 ml	320 milligrams

March 2016

Quick Reference Table

DRUG	ROUTE	INITIAL DOSE	REPEAT DOSE	DOSE INTERVAL	CONCENTRATION	VOLUME	MAX DOSE
Adrenaline - anaphylaxis/asthma	IM	300 micrograms	300 micrograms	5 minutes	1 milligram in 1 ml (1:1,000)	0.3 ml	No limit
Benzylpenicillin (Penicillin G)	IV/IO	1.2 grams	NONE	N/A	1.2 grams dissolved in 19.2 ml water for injection	20 ml	1.2 grams
Benzylpenicillin (Penicillin G)	IM	1.2 grams	NONE	N/A	1.2 grams dissolved in 3.2 ml water for injection	4 ml	1.2 grams
Chlorphenamine	IV/IO/IM	5–10 milligrams	NONE	N/A	10 milligrams in 1 ml	0.5–1 ml	5–10 milligrams
Chlorphenamine	Oral (solution)	2 milligrams	NONE	N/A	2 milligrams in 5 ml	5 ml	2 milligrams
Chlorphenamine	Oral (tablet)	2 milligrams	NONE	N/A	4 milligrams per tablet	½ of one tablet	2 milligrams
Dexamethasone - croup	Oral	N/A	N/A	N/A	N/A	N/A	N/A
Diazepam	IV/IO	10 milligrams	NONE	N/A	10 milligrams in 2 ml	2 ml	10 milligrams
Diazepam	Rectal (large dose)	10 milligrams	NONE	N/A	10 milligrams in 2.5 ml	1 × 10 milligram tube	10 milligrams
Diazepam	Rectal (small dose)	5 milligrams	NONE	N/A	5 milligrams in 2.5 ml	1 × 5 milligram tube	5 milligrams
Glucagon (Glucagen)	IM	1 milligram	NONE	N/A	1 milligram per vial	1 vial	1 milligram
Glucose 10%	IV	6.5 grams	6.5 grams	5 minutes	50 grams in 500 ml	65 ml	19.5 grams
Hydrocortisone	IV/IO/IM	100 milligrams	NONE	N/A	100 milligrams in 1 ml	1 ml	100 milligrams
Hydrocortisone	IV/IO/IM	100 milligrams	NONE	N/A	100 milligrams in 2 ml	2 ml	100 milligrams
Ibuprofen	Oral	300 milligrams	300 milligrams	8 hours	100 milligrams in 5 ml	15 ml	900 milligrams per 24 hours
Ipratropium Bromide (Atrovent) 250 micrograms in 1 ml	Neb	250 micrograms	NONE	N/A	250 micrograms in 1 ml	1 ml	250 micrograms
Ipratropium Bromide (Atrovent) 500 micrograms in 1 ml	Neb	250 micrograms	NONE	N/A	500 micrograms in 2 ml	1 ml	250 micrograms
Midazolam[a]	Buccal	10 milligrams	10 milligrams	10 mins	5 milligrams in 1 ml	2 ml pre-filled syringe	20 milligrams
Morphine Sulphate	IV/IO	3 milligrams	3 milligrams	5 minutes	10 milligrams in 10 ml	3 ml	6 milligrams
Morphine Sulphate	Oral	6 milligrams	NONE	N/A	10 milligrams in 5 ml	3 ml	6 milligrams
Naloxone NB cautions	IV/IO	320 micrograms	320 micrograms	3 minutes	400 micrograms in 1 ml	0.8 ml	3,520 micrograms
Naloxone - initial dose	IM	320 micrograms	See repeat dose	3 minutes	400 micrograms in 1 ml	0.8 ml	See below
Naloxone - repeat dose	IM	See initial dose	400 micrograms	3 minutes	400 micrograms in 1 ml	1 ml	720 micrograms
Ondansetron	IV/IO/IM	3 milligrams	NONE	N/A	2 milligrams in 1 ml	1.5 ml	3 milligrams
Paracetamol - six plus suspension	Oral	500 milligrams	500 milligrams	4–6 hours	250 milligrams in 5 ml	10 ml	2 grams in 24 hours
Paracetamol	IV infusion/IO	500 milligrams	500 milligrams	4–6 hours	10 milligrams in 1 ml	50 ml	2 grams in 24 hours
Salbutamol 2.5 milligrams in 2.5 ml	Neb	5 milligrams	5 milligrams	5 minutes	2.5 milligrams in 2.5 ml	5 ml	No limit
Salbutamol 5 milligrams in 2.5 ml	Neb	5 milligrams	5 milligrams	5 minutes	5 milligrams in 2.5 ml	2.5 ml	No limit
Tranexamic Acid	IV	500 mg	NONE	N/A	100 mg/ml	5 ml	500 mg

Give the dose as prescribed in the child's individual treatment plan/Epilepsy Passport (the dosages described above reflect the recommended dosages for a child of this age).

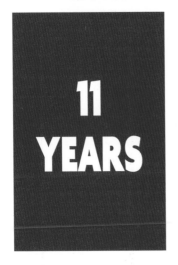

11 YEARS

Vital Signs

GUIDE WEIGHT 35 kg	HEART RATE 80–120	RESPIRATION RATE 20–25	SYSTOLIC BLOOD PRESSURE 90–110

Airway Size by Type

OROPHARYNGEAL AIRWAY	LARYNGEAL MASK	I-GEL AIRWAY	ENDOTRACHEAL TUBE
2 OR 3	3	2.5 OR 3	Diameter: **7 mm**; Length: **18 cm**

Defibrillation – Cardiac Arrest

MANUAL	AUTOMATED EXTERNAL DEFIBRILLATOR
140 Joules	A standard AED can be used (without the need for paediatric attenuation pads).

Intravascular Fluid

FLUID	ROUTE	INITIAL DOSE	REPEAT DOSE	DOSE INTERVAL	CONCENTRATION	VOLUME	MAX DOSE
0.9% Sodium Chloride (5 ml/kg)	IV/IO	175 ml	175 ml	PRN	0.9%	175 ml	1,000 ml
0.9% Sodium Chloride (10 ml/kg)	IV/IO	350 ml	350 ml	PRN	0.9%	350 ml	1,000 ml
0.9% Sodium Chloride (20 ml/kg)	IV/IO	500 ml	500 ml	PRN	0.9%	500 ml	1,000 ml

Cardiac Arrest

DRUG	ROUTE	INITIAL DOSE	REPEAT DOSE	DOSE INTERVAL	CONCENTRATION	VOLUME	MAX DOSE
Adrenaline	IV/IO	350 micrograms	350 micrograms	3–5 minutes	1 milligram in 10 ml (1:10,000)	3.5 ml	No limit
Amiodarone	IV/IO	180 milligrams (After 3rd shock)	180 milligrams	After 5th shock	300 milligrams in 10 ml	6 ml	360 milligrams

March 2016

Quick Reference Table

DRUG	ROUTE	INITIAL DOSE	REPEAT DOSE	DOSE INTERVAL	CONCENTRATION	VOLUME	MAX DOSE
Adrenaline - anaphylaxis/ asthma	IM	300 micrograms	300 micrograms	5 minutes	1 milligram in 1 ml (1:1,000)	0.3 ml	No limit
Benzylpenicillin (Penicillin G)	IV/IO	1.2 grams	NONE	N/A	1.2 grams dissolved in 19.2 ml water for injection	20 ml	1.2 grams
Benzylpenicillin (Penicillin G)	IM	1.2 grams	NONE	N/A	1.2 grams dissolved in 3.2 ml water for injection	4 ml	1.2 grams
Chlorphenamine	IV/IO/IM	5–10 milligrams	NONE	N/A	10 milligrams in 1 ml	0.5–1 ml	5–10 milligrams
Chlorphenamine	Oral (solution)	2 milligrams	NONE	N/A	2 milligrams in 5 ml	5 ml	2 milligrams
Chlorphenamine	Oral (tablet)	2 milligrams	NONE	N/A	4 milligrams per tablet	½ of one tablet	2 milligrams
Dexamethasone - croup	Oral	N/A	N/A	N/A	N/A	N/A	N/A
Diazepam	IV/IO	10 milligrams	NONE	N/A	10 milligrams in 2 ml	2 ml	10 milligrams
Diazepam	Rectal (large dose)	10 milligrams	NONE	N/A	10 milligrams in 2.5 ml	1 × 10 milligram tube	10 milligrams
Diazepam	Rectal (small dose)	5 milligrams	NONE	N/A	5 milligrams in 2.5 ml	1 × 5 milligram tube	5 milligrams
Glucagon (Glucagen)	IM	1 milligram	NONE	N/A	1 milligram per vial	1 vial	1 milligram
Glucose 10%	IV	7 grams	7 grams	5 minutes	50 grams in 500 ml	70 ml	21 grams
Hydrocortisone	IV/IO/IM	100 milligrams	NONE	N/A	100 milligrams in 1 ml	1 ml	100 milligrams
Hydrocortisone	IV/IO/IM	100 milligrams	NONE	N/A	100 milligrams in 2 ml	2 ml	100 milligrams
Ibuprofen	Oral	300 milligrams	300 milligrams	8 hours	100 milligrams in 5 ml	15 ml	900 milligrams per 24 hours
Ipratropium Bromide (Atrovent) 250 micrograms in 1 ml	Neb	250 micrograms	NONE	N/A	250 micrograms in 1 ml	1 ml	250 micrograms
Ipratropium Bromide (Atrovent) 500 micrograms in 1 ml	Neb	250 micrograms	NONE	N/A	500 micrograms in 2 ml	1 ml	250 micrograms
Midazolam[a]	Buccal	10 milligrams	10 milligrams	10 mins	5 milligrams in 1 ml	2 ml pre-filled syringe	20 milligrams
Morphine Sulphate	IV/IO	3.5 milligrams	3.5 milligrams	5 minutes	10 milligrams in 10 ml	3.5 ml	7 milligrams
Morphine Sulphate	Oral	7 milligrams	NONE	N/A	10 milligrams in 5 ml	3.5 ml	7 milligrams
Naloxone NB cautions	IV/IO	350 micrograms	350 micrograms	3 minutes	400 micrograms in 1 ml	0.9 ml	3,850 micrograms
Naloxone - initial dose	IM	350 micrograms	See repeat dose	3 minutes	400 micrograms in 1 ml	0.9 ml	See below
Naloxone - repeat dose	IM	See initial dose	400 micrograms	3 minutes	400 micrograms in 1 ml	1 ml	750 micrograms
Ondansetron	IV/IO/IM	3 milligrams	NONE	N/A	2 milligrams in 1 ml	1.5 ml	3 milligrams
Paracetamol - six plus suspension	Oral	500 milligrams	500 milligrams	4–6 hours	250 milligrams in 5 ml	10 ml	2 grams in 24 hours
Paracetamol	IV infusion/IO	500 milligrams	500 milligrams	4–6 hours	10 milligrams in 1 ml	50 ml	2 grams in 24 hours
Salbutamol 2.5 milligrams in 2.5 ml	Neb	5 milligrams	5 milligrams	5 minutes	2.5 milligrams in 2.5 ml	5 ml	No limit
Salbutamol 5 milligrams in 2.5 ml	Neb	5 milligrams	5 milligrams	5 minutes	5 milligrams in 2.5 ml	2.5 ml	No limit
Tranexamic Acid	IV	500 mg	NONE	N/A	100 mg/ml	5 ml	500 mg

a Give the dose as prescribed in the child's individual treatment plan/Epilepsy Passport (the dosages described above reflect the recommended dosages for a child of this age).

7

Special Situations

Special Situations

Major Incident Management   437

Chemical, Biological, Radiological,
Nuclear and Explosive Incidents   438

Atropine (CBRNE)   447

Ciprofloxacin (CBRNE)   453

Dicobalt Edetate (CBRNE)   454

Doxycycline (CBRNE)   455

Obidoxime Chloride (CBRNE)   456

Potassium Iodate (CBRNE)   457

Pralidoxime Mesylate (CBRNE)   458

Incapacitating Agents   459

Major Incident Management

Safety First

Carry out a dynamic risk assessment and undertake measures to preserve your own safety, and where possible, that of the patient, bystanders, and other rescuers. Safety is a dynamic process and needs to be continually re-assessed throughout the incident.

- Be alert to the incident surroundings in addition to the incident.

- Appropriate personal protective equipment must be worn – this may include:
  - helmets
  - eye protection
  - high visibility apparel
  - overalls
  - waterproofs
  - gloves
  - boots
  - identity cards.

- Consider the resources required to manage the major incident.

- Consider the possibility of a major chemical, biological, radiological, nuclear or explosive (CBRNE) incident (**refer to CBRNE guideline**).

- Provide an early situation report using the '**METHANE**' report format (refer to Table 7.1).

- Check the scene for other patients who are not immediately or easily visible, for example, patients ejected from vehicles during an RTC.

Table 7.1 – METHANE REPORT FORMAT

M	Major incident standby or declared
E	Exact location of incident
T	Type of incident
H	Hazards (present and potential)
A	Access and egress routes
N	Number, severity and type of casualties
E	Emergency services present on scene and further resources required

Section 7 Special Situations

Chemical, Biological, Radiological, Nuclear and Explosive Incidents

1. Introduction

- Chemical, biological, radiological and nuclear (CBRN) incidents present unique difficulties for ambulance services.

- CBRN incidents may also be associated with explosions and therefore the terminology has changed to CBRN**E** in recognition of this.

- Explosions can be accidental or terrorist related, taking place in industrial or community settings.

- The cause of the explosion will determine the explosive force; this together with the environment and distance from the source will determine the nature of the injuries sustained (refer to Table 7.2).

- Confined space explosions usually cause more severe injury due to confinement of the blast and resultant barotrauma. This has nothing to do with structural collapse, which mitigates some of the blast injury effects by absorbing energy. Reflection of the blast wave from the walls and ceiling may also exaggerate the effects of barotrauma.

The materials involved in CBRNE incidents are all very different; they present four main types of hazard, depending on the physical properties and characteristics of the agent released:

1. contact hazard
2. inhalation hazard
3. injection hazard
4. ingestion hazard.

1. **Contact hazards** – are created by chemical, biological or radioactive agents that can be absorbed into the skin. These agents can be in solid, liquid or vapour form. Most biological agents do not pose contact hazards, unless the skin is cut or abraded.
2. **Inhalation hazards** – are created by vapour, aerosols or contaminated dust that can be inhaled into the lungs.
3. **Injection hazards** – result from chemical, biological or radiological agents being absorbed into open wounds (injected) – either by the agent moving from the injection scene into the blood stream or being injected directly into a vein or artery.

Table 7.2 – MECHANISMS OF INJURY AND RELATED INJURIES

Phase	Cause	Area affected/Injuries
Primary	Injuries caused by the interaction of the blast (shock) wave with the patient's body.	**Area affected:** ● gas-containing organs – barotrauma. **Injuries:** ● pulmonary bleeding, pneumothorax ● air emboli ● perforation of the GI tract ● burns. NB Death may occur in absence of any outward signs.
Secondary	Injuries caused by flying fragments/debris blown against the patient.	**Area affected:** ● body surface ● skeletal system. **Injuries:** ● lacerations ● fractures ● burns.[a] NB Some fragments may be human tissue (i.e. suicide bombers).
Tertiary	Injuries caused by the patient being blown against an object due to the blast wind (dynamic overpressure).	**Area affected:** ● area of impact or referred energy. **Injuries:** ● lacerations ● fractures.
Quaternary	All explosion-related injuries, illnesses or diseases not due to primary, secondary or tertiary mechanisms.	**Area affected:** ● body surface ● skeletal system. **Injuries:** ● burns[a] ● crush ● toxic chemical injury.

[a] Burns following an explosion may be superficial flash burns confined to exposed skin, typically the face and hands. Full thickness burns may also be seen in patients close to the point of explosion.

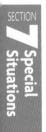

4. **Ingestion hazards** – result from chemical, biological or radiological agents being ingested.

In addition, radioactive agents present a significant additional hazard because of the radiation they emit from radioactive material, vapours or liquids. Exposure may result from explosion, fire damage or direct radiation effects.

Suspect package(s)/material(s)

- If you are called to, or identify, a suspect package/material, alert ambulance control to call the police.
- Isolate the package/material and do not open, move or handle.

Personal protective equipment (PPE)

- PPE is designed to protect you, the patient and other patients and colleagues from contamination and from other hazards, but only if selected, worn and discarded correctly.
- Specially trained staff will wear appropriate PPE; advice will be provided at the time to ambulance clinicians by Public Health experts, Ambulance Trust Medical Director and Hazardous Area Response Teams (HART) Medical Advisors.
- Appropriate PPE may include:
  - simple face masks
  - gloves and aprons
  - gas tight chemical suits with breathing apparatus
  - CR1 police style overalls with respirator
  - PRPS (powered respirator protective suits).

Decontamination – will be managed by HART, Special Operations Response Team (SORT) and Fire Service colleagues (refer to Figure 7.1).

STEP 1	STEP 2	STEP 3
RINSE	**WIPE**	**RINSE**
Gently wash affected areas with soapy water (0.9% saline for open wounds and eyes): this dilutes the contaminant and removes particles and water based chemicals.	Wipe affected area gently but thoroughly with sponge or soft brush or washcloth: this removes organic chemical and petrochemicals.	Gently rinse affected areas.

Figure 7.1 – Decontamination technique.

The equipment necessary for decontamination will be provided by the HART/SORT/Fire Service.

Incident identification – Consider whether this is or potentially is a CBRNE incident – refer to Figure 7.2, Table 7.3, Table 7.4 and Appendix 1.

- On identification or if you have a high suspicion of a CBRNE incident, advise Ambulance Control using the METHANE report protocol (refer to Table 7.3).

STEP 1	STEP 2	STEP 3
One collapsed casualty: • approach using normal procedures • CBRN contamination unlikely.	**Two collapsed casualties at one location:** • CBRN contamination possible • approach with caution • if CBRN possible or suspected follow the advice for STEP 3.	**Three or more collapsed casualties at one location:** • CBRN contamination possible • DO NOT approach the scene – CBRN contamination likely.

Figure 7.2 – Identification of CBRNE incident and approach.

Table 7.3 – METHANE REPORT PROTOCOL

M	**My call sign,** or name and appointment. Major incident, **STANDBY** or **DECLARED**.
E	**Exact location** – where possible, map reference.
T	**Type of incident** – for example chemical, explosion, road traffic collision (RTC).
H	**Hazards** – present and potential.
A	**Access** – best routes for access and egress to scene and rendezvous point(s) (RVP).
N	**Number of casualties** – approximate numbers and types of casualties (**T[a]1, T2, T3, DEAD** and whether contaminated).
E	**Emergency services report** – on emergency services already on scene and if further services required.

[a] In this guideline the letter 'T' stands for triage, but in some documents 'P' may be used, which stands for priority; these terms are interchangeable.

2. Assessment and Management

For the assessment and management of unspecified CBRNE incidents refer to Figure 7.3.

3. Additional Information

CBRNE detection

- There are a wide range of products available to aid with the detection of chemical and radiological incidents. Detection of the agent will be undertaken by the Fire Service, HART or emergency department staff as appropriate.
- Emergency departments (ED) have been supplied with Toxi-Boxes (toxicological analytical sampling kits). These are to be used for toxicological sampling.
- When provided, electronic personal dosimeters (EPD) or other personal monitors should be worn to give advance notice of other hazards that may not have been identified.

Chemical, Biological, Radiological, Nuclear and Explosive Incidents

Risk Assessment

Hazard Assessment

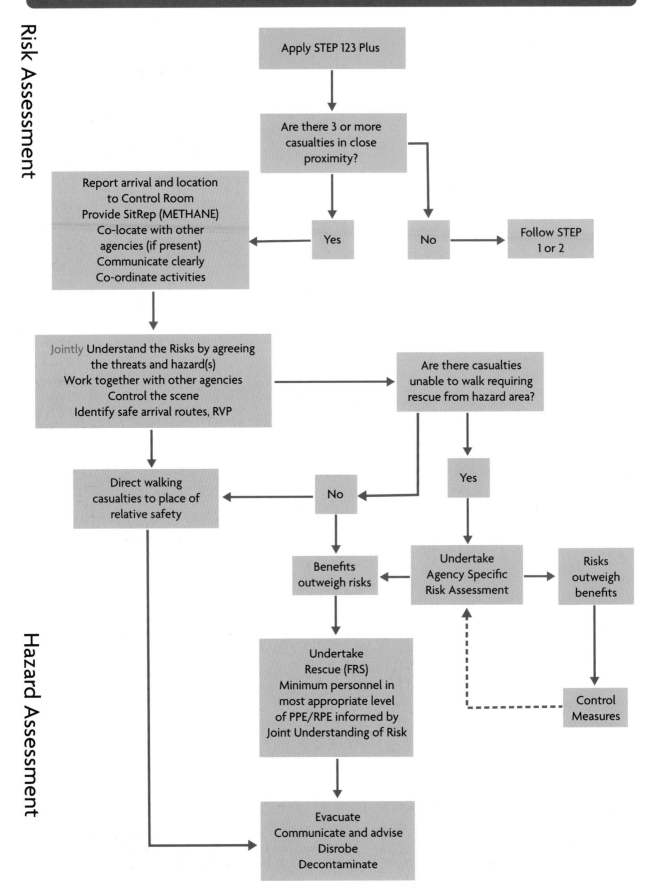

Apply STEP 123 Plus

Are there 3 or more casualties in close proximity?

Yes

No

Follow STEP 1 or 2

Report arrival and location to Control Room
Provide SitRep (METHANE)
Co-locate with other agencies (if present)
Communicate clearly
Co-ordinate activities

Jointly Understand the Risks by agreeing the threats and hazard(s)
Work together with other agencies
Control the scene
Identify safe arrival routes, RVP

Are there casualties unable to walk requiring rescue from hazard area?

Yes

No

Direct walking casualties to place of relative safety

Benefits outweigh risks

Undertake Agency Specific Risk Assessment

Risks outweigh benefits

Undertake Rescue (FRS)
Minimum personnel in most appropriate level of PPE/RPE informed by Joint Understanding of Risk

Control Measures

Evacuate
Communicate and advise
Disrobe
Decontaminate

Figure 7.3 – General management for an unspecified CBRNE incident.
Reproduced with permission from National Ambulance Resilience Unit (NARU)

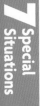

SECTION
7 Special
Situations

Table 7.4 – INCEDENT DESCRIPTIONS[a]

Incident	Characteristics	Casualties	Decontamination
Chemical – Refer to Appendix 1	• Rapid action producing mass casualties. • Persistent liquid contact and downwind vapour hazards. • Casualties can contaminate first responders. • Decontamination will probably be necessary and needs to start quickly. • Most effective in confined spaces where there are lots of people.	• Mass casualties at scene. • Rapid onset of symptoms/signs. • Rapid treatment is essential.	• Wear PPE as appropriate. • Most contamination will be on clothing **which should be removed as soon as possible**. • Skin must be decontaminated rapidly – **wet decontamination is advised**. Where possible get contaminated patients out of doors to prevent ongoing further exposure from off gassing. (Chemical evaporation from clothing, etc, producing further chemical exposure.)
Biological	• Slow action producing mass casualties over time. • Could go undetected until people become ill and attend their GP or emergency departments. • Potential for epidemic with some diseases. • The need for decontamination will depend on agent used. • Deliberate releases are most effective in confined spaces where there are lots of people.	• Unlikely to be any casualties at the scene. • Window for treatment in first 12–24 hours. • Cannot tell who has been exposed. • First casualties will start to appear 2–3 days later. • It may be very difficult to be sure the incident is over. • Recommended prophylaxis for potential biological agents will be available as advised by incident officers.	• Wear PPE as appropriate. • Washing skin and clothing should be effective.
Radiological	• Few immediate casualties. • **Some may have blast injuries.** • Need to monitor those present for contamination. • Persistent radiation hazard. • Persistent contact and downwind hazards. • Casualties can contaminate first responders.	• Few casualties at scene. • Damage is dosage related and cumulative. • Casualties will become ill over a period of days to weeks. • Casualties will need reassurance. • Most contamination on clothing. • Skin must be decontaminated rapidly.	• Wear PPE as appropriate. • Decontamination will be necessary **and needs to start quickly with removal of clothing and wet decontamination**.
Nuclear	There are two types of deliberate release involving radiological substances: 1. 'Dirty Bomb' – explosive device delivering radioactive material. 2. Exposure to radioactive material deliberately left in a public place.	There are three classic symptoms of radiation sickness: 1. Vomiting 2. Diarrhoea 3. Skin burns.	• Wear PPE as appropriate.

[a] Specific advice will be available to the ambulance service on specific measure(s) required.

• Most EDs have access to RAM GENE-1 (combined dose-rate/contamination monitors) monitoring equipment to screen patients for radioactive contaminants.

Specific treatments for CBRNE

• In extreme circumstances you may be asked to administer specific antidotes and drugs for CBRNE. This will be on the instructions of your Ambulance Service Medical Director who will take advice from the Public Health Service –refer to specific CBRNE drug guidelines as instructed.

• You may be asked to assist in taking samples for toxicological or biological analysis. You will receive directions from your Ambulance Service Medical Director.

Table 7.5 – CONDITIONS ASSOCIATED WITH AGENTS

Disease/agent	Chlorine/ irritant gases	Mustard/ vesicants	Riot control agents	Ricin/abrin – toxalbumins	Phosgene	Nerve agents/ organo- phosphate	Hydrogen cyanide/ cyanogens
Exposure – skin							
Vesicant		●					
Irritant	●	●	●		●		
Corrosive	●				●		
Erythema or redness	●	●	●				
Blisters		●	●				
Sweating						●	
Fasiculations							
Muscle paralysis						●	
Itching		●					
Burns or frostbite	●				●		
Exposure – eyes							
Lacrimation	●	●	●		●	●	
Stinging/burning	●		●			●	
Blepharospasm	●	●	●		●		
Periorbital oedema		●					●
Blurred vision			●			●	
Blindness		●					
Corneal ulceration/clouding		●	●				
Burns or frostbite	●				●		
Airway							
Salivation			●			●	
Runny nose			●			●	
Bronchospasm	●	●	●		●	●	
Breathing							
Throat pain			●				
Cough	●	●		●	●	●	●
Choking	●						●
Chest pain	●				●		
Chest tightness	●		●	●	●		●
Laryngospasm					●		
Wheezing	●				●	●	
Dyspnoea	●	●	●	●	●	●	●
Increased respiration	●						
Hoarseness/loss of voice		●	●				
Respiratory arrest				●		●	●
Pseudomembrane		●					
Pneumonitis/pneumonia	●	●			●		
Pulmonary oedema	●	●	●	●	●	●	●

Table 7.5 – CONDITIONS ASSOCIATED WITH AGENTS – *continued*

Disease/agent	Chlorine/ irritant gases	Mustard/ vesicants	Riot control agents	Ricin/abrin – toxalbumins	Phosgene	Nerve agents/ organo- phosphate	Hydrogen cyanide/ cyanogens
Circulation/cardiac							
Arrhythmias		●			●	●	
Cardiac arrest	●					●	●
Hypotension				●	●		●
Hypoxia	●				●		
Headache				●		●	●
Cyanosis							●
Dehydration				●			
Hypovolaemic shock				●			
Disability							
Pinpoint pupils						●	●
Fixed dilated pupils							●
Confusion/agitation						●	●
Dizziness						●	●
Miosis						●	
Convulsions				●		●	●
Arthralgia				●			
Myalgia				●			
CNS depression		●				●	
Unconscious						●	●
Other							
Fever		●		●			
Nausea	●	●			●		●
Vomiting	●	●		●	●	●	●
Diarrhoea		●		●		●	●
GI bleeding				●			
Abdominal pain				●			
Faecal/urinary incontinence						●	

KEY POINTS

Chemical, Biological, Radiological, Nuclear and Explosive Incidents
● CBRN incidents may also be associated with explosions – the new terminology is CBRNE.
● Make an early METHANE call once a chemical incident is identified.
● Do not enter the scene unless protected in appropriate PPE and trained to do so.
● Encourage walking casualties to disrobe and self-decontaminate where possible.
● If ambulance clinicians become contaminated they are considered to be patients.

7 Special Situations
SECTION

CPNI
Centre for the Protection
of National Infrastructure

NaCTSO
National Counter Terrorism Security Office

DO NOT TOUCH!

Overleaf is a list of chemicals which are precursors for home made explosives (HMEs). Many of these chemicals are also used in the manufacture of illicit drugs and are additionally marked with a smiley face symbol. ☺ A small number of the drugs precursors are controlled under various pieces of drugs legislation and these also feature a key symbol. ⚷

DO NOT assume that any packaging or labelling is correct or corresponds to the contents of the container. Treat any unidentified substances with caution.

REMEMBER: Chemicals may present a multitude of hazards, some of which may not be immediately apparent.

All of these chemicals have a legitimate use, HOWEVER, if you encounter;

- any of the listed chemicals
- any combinations of the listed chemicals
- any potential laboratory equipment such as glassware, scales, funnels, filter papers etc, either dedicated or improvised,

in unusual or suspicious circumstances you should;

For suspected explosives related activity, inform your CT section and your CTSA, or your relevant agency contact immediately on; (insert number)...

For suspected illicit drugs manufacture contact;
Serious Organised Crime Agency (SOCA)
Chemical Control Team (CCT) on 020 7238 2426 or
Hazardous Environment Search Team (HEST) (24hr) on 0870 496 0093 and ask for the 'HEST Operations Manager'.

Produced jointly by the NaCTSO and CPNI.

OCTOBER 2011

DO NOT TOUCH!

INCLUDING ANYTHING WHICH MAY BE ON THE FLOOR!

☺		Acetic Acid	CH_3COOH
☺	⚷	Acetone	C_3H_6O / CH_3COCH_3
☺		Alcohol (Ethanol, Methanol)	C_2H_5OH / CH_3CH_2OH or CH_3OH
☺		Ammonium Nitrate	NH_4NO_3
☺		Anything Chlorate / Perchlorate	$NaClO_3$ / $KClO_3$ or $NaClO_4$ / $KClO_4$ / NH_4ClO_4
☺		Anything Nitrate	KNO_3 / $NaNO_3$
		Calcium Hypochlorite	$Ca(OCl)_2$
☺		Citric Acid	$C_6H_8O_7$
		Ethylene Glycol	$C_2H_6O_2$ / $HOCH_2CH_2OH$
		Glycerine	$C_3H_8O_3$
☺		Hexamine	$C_6H_{12}N_4$
☺	⚷	Hydrochloric Acid	HCl
☺		Hydrogen Peroxide	H_2O_2
		Lead Nitrate	$Pb(NO_3)_2$
☺		Mercury	Hg
☺	⚷	Methyl Ethyl Ketone	C_4H_8O / $CH_3COCH_2CH_3$
☺		Nitric Acid	HNO_3
☺		Nitrobenzene	$C_6H_5NO_2$
☺		Nitromethane	CH_3NO_2
		Pentaerythritol	$C_5H_{12}O_4$ / $C(CH_2OH)_4$
☺	⚷	Potassium Permanganate	$KMnO_4$
☺		Powdered Metals (Aluminium (Al) Magnesium (Mg) Magnalium (Al/Mg) Zinc (Zn))	
		Sodium Azide	NaN_3
☺		Sulphur	S
☺	⚷	Sulphuric Acid	H_2SO_4
☺		Urea	CH_4N_2O / $CO(NH_2)_2$

Appendix 1 – Chemical Incident[a]

In the case of a chemical incident – **DO NOT TOUCH** any of the chemicals, including anything which may be on the floor.

Do not assume that any packaging or labelling is correct and treat any unidentified substance with caution.

Do not assume the only hazard is explosive. There may be other health and safety hazards present from a variety of sources.

All of these chemicals have a legitimate use. **HOWEVER,** if you come across:

- Any of the listed chemicals
- Any combinations of the listed chemicals
- Any potential laboratory equipment such as flasks, scales, funnels, filter papers etc

in unusual or suspicious circumstances you should inform Ambulance Control **IMMEDIATELY**.

[a] Produced by the National Counter Terrorism Security Office/ ACPOS.

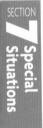

SECTION 7 Special Situations

Appendix 2

CBRNE (SPECIAL AGENT) TRIAGE SIEVE: For use before and during decontamination.

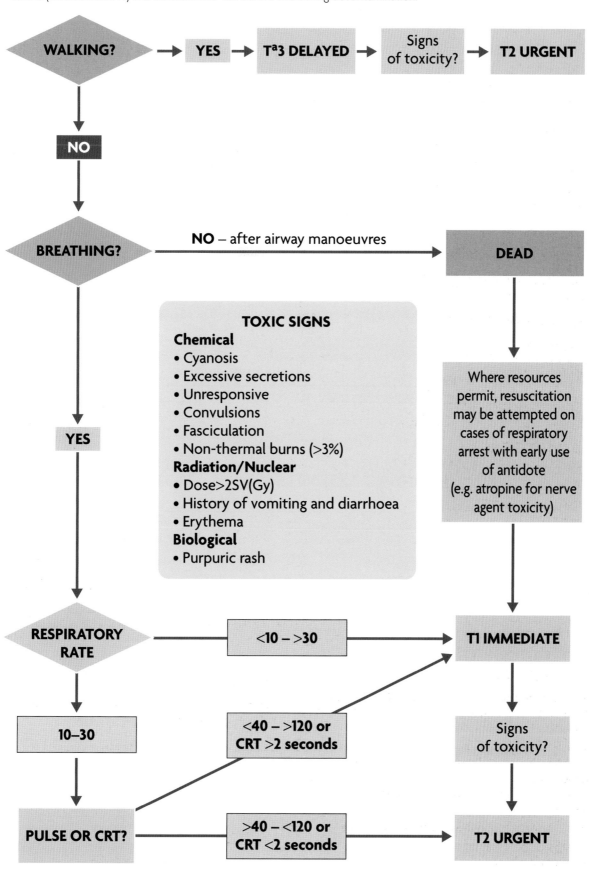

TOXIC SIGNS

Chemical
- Cyanosis
- Excessive secretions
- Unresponsive
- Convulsions
- Fasciculation
- Non-thermal burns (>3%)

Radiation/Nuclear
- Dose>2SV(Gy)
- History of vomiting and diarrhoea
- Erythema

Biological
- Purpuric rash

Where resources permit, resuscitation may be attempted on cases of respiratory arrest with early use of antidote (e.g. atropine for nerve agent toxicity)

[a] In this guideline the letter 'T' stands for triage, but in some documents 'P' may be used, which stands for priority; these terms are interchangeable.

7 Special Situations SECTION

Appendix 3

CBRNE SORT (for use after decontamination).

RESPIRATION		
	10–29 per minute	+4
	>30 per minute	+2
	>30 per minute + cyanosis	+0
	≤9 per minute	+0
	RESPIRATORY ARREST	**Immediate or expectant**

HEART RATE		
	60–100 per minute	+4
	40–59 OR 101–120 per minute	+2
	<40 per minute + cyanosis	+0
	>120 per minute	+0
	CARDIAC ARREST	**DEAD**

SYSTOLIC BLOOD PRESSURE		
	≥90 mmHg	+4
	70–89 mmHg	+3
	50–69 mmHg	+2
	1–49 mmHg	+1
	CARDIAC ARREST	**DEAD**

GLASGOW COMA SCALE		
	13–15	+4
	9–12	+3
	6–8	+2
	4–5	+1
	3 OR CONVULSIONS	**+0**

FASCICULATION		
	None	+4
	Local/intermittent	+2
	General/continuous	+0
	Flaccidity	+0

BIOLOGICAL RADIOLOGICAL		
	If purpuric rash	−2
	If vomiting, diarrhoea, erythema or dose >2Sv	−2

TOTAL SCORE OUT OF 20 [   ]

EVACUATION SCORE		EVACUATION PRIORITY
20	DELAYED	T3
18–19	URGENT	T2
0–17	IMMEDIATE	T1

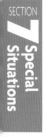

Presentation

- Pre-filled syringe containing 1 milligram atropine in 5 ml.
- Pre-filled syringe containing 1 milligram atropine in 10 ml.
- Pre-filled syringe containing 3 milligrams atropine in 10 ml.
- An ampoule containing 600 micrograms in 1 ml.
- Nerve agent antidote kit (NAAK) containing 2 milligrams of atropine sulphate.

Indications

Organophosphate (OP) poisoning.

Adults and children with a clinical diagnosis of poisoning by OP nerve agents, as an adjunct to maintenance of oxygenation.

Atropine should be administered for confirmed OP poisoning, or where features of OP poisoning develop. Clinical diagnosis of nerve agent poisoning (see below) is suggested by the characteristic features of nerve agent poisoning, associated with a history of possible exposure. Clinical features must include one or more of the following: bronchorrhoea, bronchospasm, severe bradycardia (<40 bpm).

Actions

Reduction or elimination of bronchorrhoea and bronchospasm in nerve agent poisoning.

Contra-Indications

Hypersensitivity to atropine sulphate or excipients in nerve agent poisoning.

Cautions

There are no other absolute criteria for the exclusion from administration of atropine in the treatment of OP poisoning, as the consequences of not instituting prompt treatment in poisoned patients will usually outweigh the risks associated with treatment. However, caution needs to be administered in the following:

- Patients with ulcerative colitis.
- Patients with risk of urinary retention.
- Patients with glaucoma.
- Patients with conditions characterised by tachycardia (e.g. thyrotoxicosis, heart failure).
- Patients with myasthenia gravis.

Side Effects

Reactions are mostly dose related and usually reversible and include:

- Loss of visual accommodation
- Photophobia
- Arrhythmias, transient bradycardia followed by tachycardia
- Palpitations
- Difficulty in micturition.

Additional Information

Toxic doses may cause CNS stimulation manifesting as restlessness, confusion, ataxia, lack of coordination, hallucinations and delirium. In severe intoxication CNS stimulation may give way to CNS depression, coma, circulatory and respiratory failure and death.

Characteristic features of nerve agent poisoning:

- Miosis, excess secretions (e.g. lacrimation and bronchorrhoea).
- Respiratory difficulty (e.g. bronchospasm or respiratory depression).
- Altered consciousness, convulsions, together with a history of possible exposure.

SECTION **7** Special Situations

Atropine (CBRNE)

Dosage and Administration

Nerve agent poisoning

- Atropine must only be administered after the patient is adequately oxygenated.
- In organophosphate poisoning there is no maximum dose and large doses (e.g. 20 milligrams) may be required to achieve atropinisation.[a]
- **When administering atropine via the intramuscular route:** administering large volumes intramuscularly could lead to poor absorption and/or tissue damage, therefore administer the smallest volume possible and divide where necessary and practicable. Vary the site of injection for repeated doses; appropriate sites include: buttock (gluteus maximus), thigh (vastus lateralis), lateral hip (gluteus medius) and upper arm (deltoid).

Route: Intramuscular.

AGE	INITIAL DOSE	REPEAT DOSE	DOSE INTERVAL	CONCENTRATION	VOLUME	MAXIMUM DOSE
≥12 years – adult	2 milligrams	2 milligrams	5 minutes	2 milligrams per auto-injector	0.7 ml automatically delivered	No limit
11 years	2 milligrams	2 milligrams	5 minutes	2 milligrams per auto-injector	0.7 ml automatically delivered	No limit
10 years	2 milligrams	2 milligrams	5 minutes	2 milligrams per auto-injector	0.7 ml automatically delivered	No limit
9 years	2 milligrams	2 milligrams	5 minutes	2 milligrams per auto-injector	0.7 ml automatically delivered	No limit
8 years	2 milligrams	2 milligrams	5 minutes	2 milligrams per auto-injector	0.7 ml automatically delivered	No limit

NB See charts on following pages for doses for children <8 years.

[a] **Signs of atropinisation include:** dry skin and mouth and an absence of bradycardia (e.g. heart rate adult ≥80; heart rate child ≥100 bpm). NB DO NOT rely on reversal of pinpoint pupils as a guide to atropinisation.

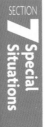

Atropine (CBRNE)

Route: Intravenous/intraosseous/intramuscular (as appropriate).

AGE	INITIAL DOSE	REPEAT DOSE	DOSE INTERVAL	CONCENTRATION	VOLUME	MAXIMUM DOSE
≥12 years – adult	2 milligrams	2 milligrams	5 minutes	1 milligram in 5 ml	10 ml	No limit
11 years	2 milligrams	2 milligrams	5 minutes	1 milligram in 5 ml	10 ml	No limit
10 years	2 milligrams	2 milligrams	5 minutes	1 milligram in 5 ml	10 ml	No limit
9 years	2 milligrams	2 milligrams	5 minutes	1 milligram in 5 ml	10 ml	No limit
8 years	2 milligrams	2 milligrams	5 minutes	1 milligram in 5 ml	10 ml	No limit
7 years	600 micrograms	600 micrograms	5 minutes	1 milligram in 5 ml	3 ml	No limit
6 years	600 micrograms	600 micrograms	5 minutes	1 milligram in 5 ml	3 ml	No limit
5 years	600 micrograms	600 micrograms	5 minutes	1 milligram in 5 ml	3 ml	No limit
4 years	600 micrograms	600 micrograms	5 minutes	1 milligram in 5 ml	3 ml	No limit
3 years	600 micrograms	600 micrograms	5 minutes	1 milligram in 5 ml	3 ml	No limit
2 years	600 micrograms	600 micrograms	5 minutes	1 milligram in 5 ml	3 ml	No limit
18 months	600 micrograms	600 micrograms	5 minutes	1 milligram in 5 ml	3 ml	No limit
12 months	600 micrograms	600 micrograms	5 minutes	1 milligram in 5 ml	3 ml	No limit
9 months	200 micrograms	200 micrograms	5 minutes	1 milligram in 5 ml	1 ml	No limit
6 months	200 micrograms	200 micrograms	5 minutes	1 milligram in 5 ml	1 ml	No limit
3 months	200 micrograms	200 micrograms	5 minutes	1 milligram in 5 ml	1 ml	No limit
1 month	200 micrograms	200 micrograms	5 minutes	1 milligram in 5 ml	1 ml	No limit
Birth	200 micrograms	200 micrograms	5 minutes	1 milligram in 5 ml	1 ml	No limit

Atropine (CBRNE)

Route: Intravenous/intraosseous/intramuscular (administer the smallest volume possible and divide where necessary and practicable).

AGE	INITIAL DOSE	REPEAT DOSE	DOSE INTERVAL	CONCENTRATION	VOLUME	MAXIMUM DOSE
≥12 years – adult	2 milligrams	2 milligrams	5 minutes	1 milligram in 10 ml	20 ml	No limit
11 years	2 milligrams	2 milligrams	5 minutes	1 milligram in 10 ml	20 ml	No limit
10 years	2 milligrams	2 milligrams	5 minutes	1 milligram in 10 ml	20 ml	No limit
9 years	2 milligrams	2 milligrams	5 minutes	1 milligram in 10 ml	20 ml	No limit
8 years	2 milligrams	2 milligrams	5 minutes	1 milligram in 10 ml	20 ml	No limit
7 years	600 micrograms	600 micrograms	5 minutes	1 milligram in 10 ml	6 ml	No limit
6 years	600 micrograms	600 micrograms	5 minutes	1 milligram in 10 ml	6 ml	No limit
5 years	600 micrograms	600 micrograms	5 minutes	1 milligram in 10 ml	6 ml	No limit
4 years	600 micrograms	600 micrograms	5 minutes	1 milligram in 10 ml	6 ml	No limit
3 years	600 micrograms	600 micrograms	5 minutes	1 milligram in 10 ml	6 ml	No limit
2 years	600 micrograms	600 micrograms	5 minutes	1 milligram in 10 ml	6 ml	No limit
18 months	600 micrograms	600 micrograms	5 minutes	1 milligram in 10 ml	6 ml	No limit
12 months	600 micrograms	600 micrograms	5 minutes	1 milligram in 10 ml	6 ml	No limit
9 months	200 micrograms	200 micrograms	5 minutes	1 milligram in 10 ml	2 ml	No limit
6 months	200 micrograms	200 micrograms	5 minutes	1 milligram in 10 ml	2 ml	No limit
3 months	200 micrograms	200 micrograms	5 minutes	1 milligram in 10 ml	2 ml	No limit
1 month	200 micrograms	200 micrograms	5 minutes	1 milligram in 10 ml	2 ml	No limit
Birth	200 micrograms	200 micrograms	5 minutes	1 milligram in 10 ml	2 ml	No limit

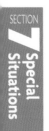

Atropine (CBRNE)

Route: Intravenous/intraosseous/intramuscular (as appropriate).

AGE	INITIAL DOSE	REPEAT DOSE	DOSE INTERVAL	CONCENTRATION	VOLUME	MAXIMUM DOSE
≥12 years – adult	2 milligrams	2 milligrams	5 minutes	3 milligrams in 10 ml	6.7 ml	No limit
11 years	2 milligrams	2 milligrams	5 minutes	3 milligrams in 10 ml	6.7 ml	No limit
10 years	2 milligrams	2 milligrams	5 minutes	3 milligrams in 10 ml	6.7 ml	No limit
9 years	2 milligrams	2 milligrams	5 minutes	3 milligrams in 10 ml	6.7 ml	No limit
8 years	2 milligrams	2 milligrams	5 minutes	3 milligrams in 10 ml	6.7 ml	No limit
7 years	600 micrograms	600 micrograms	5 minutes	3 milligrams in 10 ml	2 ml	No limit
6 years	600 micrograms	600 micrograms	5 minutes	3 milligrams in 10 ml	2 ml	No limit
5 years	600 micrograms	600 micrograms	5 minutes	3 milligrams in 10 ml	2 ml	No limit
4 years	600 micrograms	600 micrograms	5 minutes	3 milligrams in 10 ml	2 ml	No limit
3 years	600 micrograms	600 micrograms	5 minutes	3 milligrams in 10 ml	2 ml	No limit
2 years	600 micrograms	600 micrograms	5 minutes	3 milligrams in 10 ml	2 ml	No limit
18 months	600 micrograms	600 micrograms	5 minutes	3 milligrams in 10 ml	2 ml	No limit
12 months	600 micrograms	600 micrograms	5 minutes	3 milligrams in 10 ml	2 ml	No limit
9 months	200 micrograms	200 micrograms	5 minutes	3 milligrams in 10 ml	0.6 ml	No limit
6 months	200 micrograms	200 micrograms	5 minutes	3 milligrams in 10 ml	0.6 ml	No limit
3 months	200 micrograms	200 micrograms	5 minutes	3 milligrams in 10 ml	0.6 ml	No limit
1 month	200 micrograms	200 micrograms	5 minutes	3 milligrams in 10 ml	0.6 ml	No limit
Birth	200 micrograms	200 micrograms	5 minutes	3 milligrams in 10 ml	0.6 ml	No limit

Atropine (CBRNE)

Route: Intravenous/intraosseous/intramuscular.

AGE	INITIAL DOSE	REPEAT DOSE	DOSE INTERVAL	CONCENTRATION	VOLUME	MAXIMUM DOSE
≥12 years – adult	2 milligrams	2 milligrams	5 minutes	600 micrograms in 1 ml	3.3 ml	No limit
11 years	2 milligrams	2 milligrams	5 minutes	600 micrograms in 1 ml	3.3 ml	No limit
10 years	2 milligrams	2 milligrams	5 minutes	600 micrograms in 1 ml	3.3 ml	No limit
9 years	2 milligrams	2 milligrams	5 minutes	600 micrograms in 1 ml	3.3 ml	No limit
8 years	2 milligrams	2 milligrams	5 minutes	600 micrograms in 1 ml	3.3 ml	No limit
7 years	600 micrograms	600 micrograms	5 minutes	600 micrograms in 1 ml	1 ml	No limit
6 years	600 micrograms	600 micrograms	5 minutes	600 micrograms in 1 ml	1 ml	No limit
5 years	600 micrograms	600 micrograms	5 minutes	600 micrograms in 1 ml	1 ml	No limit
4 years	600 micrograms	600 micrograms	5 minutes	600 micrograms in 1 ml	1 ml	No limit
3 years	600 micrograms	600 micrograms	5 minutes	600 micrograms in 1 ml	1 ml	No limit
2 years	600 micrograms	600 micrograms	5 minutes	600 micrograms in 1 ml	1 ml	No limit
18 months	600 micrograms	600 micrograms	5 minutes	600 micrograms in 1 ml	1 ml	No limit
12 months	600 micrograms	600 micrograms	5 minutes	600 micrograms in 1 ml	1 ml	No limit
9 months	200 micrograms	200 micrograms	5 minutes	600 micrograms in 1 ml	0.3 ml	No limit
6 months	200 micrograms	200 micrograms	5 minutes	600 micrograms in 1 ml	0.3 ml	No limit
3 months	200 micrograms	200 micrograms	5 minutes	600 micrograms in 1 ml	0.3 ml	No limit
1 month	200 micrograms	200 micrograms	5 minutes	600 micrograms in 1 ml	0.3 ml	No limit
Birth	200 micrograms	200 micrograms	5 minutes	600 micrograms in 1 ml	0.3 ml	No limit

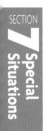

Presentation

500 milligrams ciprofloxacin (as hydrochloride) in tablet form.

Indications

Patients who have been exposed to a known or suspected biological agent:

- Anthrax – (licensed indication).
- Plague.
- Tularaemia.
- Other biological agent.

Dispensed on the instruction of the public health advice or Medical Director.

Actions

Antibiotic active against Gram-positive and Gram-negative bacteria.

Prophylaxis against these potentially life-threatening conditions.

Contra-Indications

Known hypersensitivity to ciprofloxacin or other quinolones (seek further guidance if contra-indicated).

Cautions

In the following cases the benefits of using ciprofloxacin to prevent the onset of disease outweigh the potential risks of the drug:

- Growing adolescents.
- Pregnancy and nursing mothers. **NOTE** nursing mothers should not breastfeed during treatment with ciprofloxacin.

- Older patients.

Seek medical advice for patients with:

- Epilepsy or a history of central nervous system disorders.
- A family history of or actual defects in glucose-6-phosphate dehydrogenase (G6PD).
- Severe renal impairment.
- Patients taking any of the following medication:
  - corticosteroid therapy
  - phenytoin
  - theophylline
  - anticoagulants including warfarin.
- NSAIDs.
- Ciclosporin.
- Glibenclamide.
- Probenecid.

Side Effects

Nausea, vomiting, dyspepsia, abdominal pain, diarrhoea (rarely antibiotic associated colitis), headache, restlessness, rash, renal disturbances, blurred vision, dizziness and pruritis.

Increases in liver enzymes, arthralgia, myalgia, leucopenia, thrombocytopenia also reported.

Tendon inflammation[a] and rupture may occur with ciprofloxacin. Such reactions have been observed particularly in older patients and in those treated concurrently with corticosteroids.

[a] At the first sign of pain or inflammation, patients taking quinolones should discontinue the treatment and rest the affected limb until tendon symptoms have resolved.

Dosage and Administration

NOTE: The initial treatment for adults is one tablet to be taken twice daily for 3 days until laboratory results are known. The dose and course of treatment may be amended and the medical director will advise.

AGE	INITIAL DOSE	REPEAT DOSE	DOSE INTERVAL	CONCENTRATION	TABLET	MAXIMUM DOSE
Adult	500 milligrams	Given in secondary care	N/A	500 milligrams per tablet	1 tablet	500 milligrams
< 12 years	10/30 milligrams/kilogram	Given in secondary care	N/A	500 milligrams per tablet	-	1 dose

Special Situations

SECTION 7

Presentation

Each 20 ml ampoule contains 300 mg (15 mg/ml) dicobalt edetate.

Indications

Adults and children with a clinical diagnosis of severe poisoning with hydrogen cyanide, or cyanide salts; in the presence of respiratory depression, and impaired consciousness (e.g. Glasgow Coma Score <8).

NB Dicobalt edetate can be toxic in the absence of cyanide ions – **IT MUST ONLY BE GIVEN WHEN POISONING IS SEVERE.**

Cyanide is rapidly detoxified in the body. Any casualty who is fully conscious and breathing normally more than five minutes after removal from exposure of hydrogen cyanide will recover spontaneously and does **NOT** require treatment with an antidote.

Dispensed on the instruction of the Health Protection Agency or Medical Director.

Actions

Chelating agent to diminish the effects of cyanide poisoning.

Contra-Indications

Hypersensitivity to dicobalt edetate.

There are no other absolute criteria for the exclusion from administration of dicobalt edetate as the consequences of not instituting prompt treatment in severely poisoned patients will usually outweigh the risks associated with treatment.

Cautions

ONLY TO BE ADMINISTERED WHEN POISONING IS SEVERE (i.e. coma, respiratory depression <9 and apparent cyanosis).

Side Effects

The initial effects of dicobalt edetate are vomiting, a fall in blood pressure and compensatory tachycardia.

Signs and symptoms may be due to cobalt toxicity or to an anaphylactic type reaction (**refer to anaphylaxis guidelines**), which may be severe.

Facial, laryngeal and pulmonary oedema, vomiting, chest pain, sweating, hypotension, cardiac irregularities and rashes may occur.

Anaphylaxis should be treated in the usual way.

Dosage and Administration

NOTE:

- Administer oxygen.
- Follow administration by an intravenous infusion of 250 ml 10% glucose (refer to glucose 10% guideline) in adults.
- Children receive 12.5 ml of 10% glucose for each 1 ml (15 mg) of dicobalt edetate.

Route: Intravenous injection at a regular rate over 1 minute.

AGE	INITIAL DOSE	REPEAT DOSE	DOSE INTERVAL	CONCENTRATION	VOLUME	MAXIMUM DOSE
Adult	300 milligrams	300 milligrams	30 minutes if no improvement	15 milligrams per ml	20 ml	600 milligrams
Children	7.5 milligrams/kilogram	7.5 mg/kg	30 minutes if no improvement	15 milligrams per ml	0.5 ml/kg	15 mg/kg

Adults

The dose required is related to the quantity of cyanide absorbed into the body. If the patient shows an inadequate response, a second 300 mg dose of dicobalt edetate may be administered followed by a further 250 ml intravenous infusion of 10% (500g/l) glucose (refer to glucose 10% guideline).

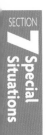

Presentation

100 milligram of doxycycline in capsules.

Indications

Patients who have been exposed to a known or suspected biological agent:

- Anthrax (licensed indication).
- Plague.
- Tularaemia.
- Other biological agent.

Actions

Prophylaxis against potentially life-threatening biological agents.

Contra-Indications

Known hypersensitivity to doxycycline or other tetracyclines.

Children under 12 years **UNLESS** specifically recommended by a medical advisor.

Cautions

Doxycycline is not usually recommended for use in pregnant women. In this case the benefits of using doxycycline to prevent the onset of disease outweigh the potential risks of the drug. Adverse effects on developing teeth and bones are dose related. Therefore, doxycycline may be used for a short course of therapy (7–14 days) prior to the 6th month of pregnancy. Nursing mothers should not breastfeed during treatment with doxycycline.

Obtain medical advice for patients with the following conditions/medications:

- Women more than 6 months pregnant.
- Patient with any exclusion criteria.
- Systemic lupus erythematosus.
- Patient declines treatment.
- Hepatic impairment.
- Porphyria.

- Myasthenia gravis.
- Achorhydria.
- Ciclosporin.
- Retinoids (isotretinoin, acitretin, tretinoin).
- Anticoagulants (e.g. warfarin).
- Antiepileptics (e.g. carbamazepine, phenytoin).
- Oral contraceptives.
- Antacids.
- Sucralfate.
- Barbiturates.
- Penicillins.

Advise the patient to sit upright, swallow the capsule whole with plenty of water.

Side Effects

Nausea, vomiting, diarrhoea, dysphagia, oesophageal irritation, hypersensitivity reactions (including rash, exfoliative dermatitis, urticaria, angioedema, anaphylaxis, pericarditis), headache and vision disturbances may indicate benign intracranial hypertension, hepatotoxicity, pancreatitis and antibiotic-associated colitis.

Rarely photosensitivity, blood dyscrasias.

Dosage and Administration

NOTE: The initial treatment for adults is one tablet to be taken twice daily for 3 days until laboratory results are known.

Route: Oral.

AGE	INITIAL DOSE	REPEAT DOSE	DOSE INTERVAL	CONCENTRATION	VOLUME	MAXIMUM DOSE
All ages	100 milligrams	100 milligrams	12 hours	100 milligrams per capsule	1 capsule	200 milligrams per 24 hours

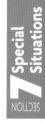

Obidoxime Chloride (CBRNE)

Presentation

Obidoxime chloride (Toxogonin), 250 mg ampoules, 250 mg per ml, for intravenous injection.

Indications

An adjunct to atropine in the treatment of organophosphorus (OP) poisoning by nerve agents.

Adults and children with a clinical diagnosis of poisoning by organophosphorus (OP) nerve agents, as an adjunct to maintenance of oxygenation and atropine administration.

Characteristic features of nerve agent poisoning include miosis, excess secretions (e.g. lacrimation and bronchorrhoea), respiratory difficulty (e.g. bronchospasm or respiratory depression), altered consciousness, and convulsions, together with a history of possible exposure.

Dispensed on the instruction of the Health Protection Agency or Medical Director.

Actions

Binds to organophosphate thus restoring enzyme function.

Contra-Indications

Hypersensitivity to obidoxime or excipients.

NOTE: There are no other absolute criteria for the exclusion from administration of obidoxime chloride, as the consequences of not instituting prompt treatment in poisoned patients will often outweigh the risks associated with treatment.

Cautions

Patients with impaired renal function.

Patients with myasthenia gravis.

Side Effects

Sensation of heat or flushing of the face 5–10 minutes after injection lasting several hours, pain at the injection site, numbness of the face, dry mouth, mild to moderate hypertension and tachycardia.

Patients with organophosphorus poisoning treated with obidoxime have developed abnormal liver function tests and renal impairment.

Dosage and Administration

NOTE: Only administer after oxygenation (refer to oxygen guideline) and atropinisation (refer to atropine guideline) of the patient.

Route: Intravenous injection. If necessary obidoxime chloride may be diluted with 0.9% saline for IV injection.

AGE	INITIAL DOSE	REPEAT DOSE	DOSE INTERVAL	CONCENTRATION	VOLUME	MAXIMUM DOSE
Adult	250 milligrams	250 milligrams	2 hourly	250 milligrams in 1 ml	1 ml	1 g
Children	2 mg/kg	2 mg/kg	2 hourly	250 milligrams in 1 ml	-	4 mg/kg

Severe poisoning in children

In cases of severe poisoning 2 milligrams/per kilogram body weight may be administered slowly every 2 hours, until clinical recovery is achieved and maintained.

NOTE: Undertake a medical review after second and third dose.

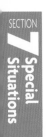

Presentation

Potassium iodate 85 milligram tablets (50 mg equivalent mass of iodine).

Indications

Known, expected or suspected exposure to radioactive iodine, at or above a level judged appropriate by a Director of Public Health (or delegate).

On the direction of a Director of Public Health (or delegate) or Ambulance Service Medical Director.

Actions

One treatment will provide protection for 24 hours.

Contra-Indications

Iodine sensitivity.

Hypocomplementaemic vasculitis.

Dermatitis herpetiformis.

Cautions

Pregnancy.

Hypothyroidism.

Side Effects

Allergic reactions, usually mild nausea, vomiting and skin rash.

Relapse of thyrotoxicosis.

Iodine-induced hyperthyroidism.

Additional Information

Priority should be given to young children (under the age of 10 years).

Pregnant and nursing mothers should receive the normal adult treatment.

It is not necessary to exclude those with previously treated or active thyroid disease.

Dosage and Administration

On the instructions of the Director of Public Health (or delegate) administer a single treatment of potassium iodate.

NOTE: Dose should be taken immediately.

Route: Oral – may be broken up and stirred into a drink or mixed with a small quantity of food to ease swallowing.

AGE	INITIAL DOSE Equivalent Mass of Iodine (mg)	REPEAT DOSE	DOSE INTERVAL	CONCENTRATION	TABLET	MAXIMUM DOSE
Birth – <1 month	12.5 milligrams	NONE	N/A	50 equivalent mass of iodine	$\frac{1}{4}$ tablet	$\frac{1}{4}$ tablet
1 month – <3 years	25 milligrams	NONE	N/A	50 equivalent mass of iodine	$\frac{1}{2}$ tablet	$\frac{1}{2}$ tablet
3–12 years	50 milligrams	NONE	N/A	50 equivalent mass of iodine	1 tablet	1 tablet
>12 years	100 milligrams	NONE	N/A	50 equivalent mass of iodine	2 tablets	2 tablets

Special Situations

SECTION 7

Presentation

A 5 ml ampoule containing 1 gram of pralidoxime.

Indications

Adults and children with a clinical diagnosis of poisoning by organophosphorus (OP) nerve agents, as an adjunct to maintenance of oxygenation and atropine administration.

Characteristic features of nerve agent poisoning include miosis, excess secretions (e.g. lacrimation and bronchorrhoea), respiratory difficulty (e.g. bronchospasm or respiratory depression), altered consciousness and convulsions, together with a history of possible exposure.

Actions

An antidote for poisoning with organophosphates.

Contra-Indications

Hypersensitivity to pralidoxime or excipients.

There are no other absolute criteria for the exclusion from administration of pralidoxime mesylate, as the consequences of not instituting prompt treatment in poisoned patients will usually outweigh the risks associated with treatment.

Cautions

Patients with impaired renal function.

Patients with myasthenia gravis.

Side Effects

Drowsiness, dizziness, visual disturbances, nausea, tachycardia, headache, hyperventilation and muscular weakness.

Large doses may cause transient neuromuscular blockade.

Dosage and Administration

NOTE: Pralidoxime must only be administered after oxygenation and atropinisation of the patient.

Route: Intravenous – slowly over 5–10 minutes.

AGE	INITIAL DOSE	REPEAT DOSE	DOSE INTERVAL	CONCENTRATION	TABLETS	MAXIMUM DOSE
Adult	2 grams	30 mg/kg	4 hourly	200 milligrams in 1 ml	20 ml	12 grams per 24 hours

Route: Intravenous – slowly over 5–10 minutes.

AGE	INITIAL DOSE	REPEAT DOSE	DOSE INTERVAL	CONCENTRATION	TABLETS	MAXIMUM DOSE
Children	30 milligrams/kg	30 mg/kg	4 hourly	200 milligrams in 1 ml	20 ml	12 grams per 24 hours

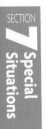

1. Introduction

- The deployment of incapacitating agents on individuals and/or groups can lead to conditions requiring pre-hospital care.
- The aim of this guideline is to support clinical decision making for the management of patients following the deployment of:
  - Conducted Electrical Weapon (CEW) for example TASER®, and stun guns.
  - Incapacitant sprays.
  - Projectiles.
  - Batons.
- Not all patients exposed to incapacitating agents will require hospital assessment; however, all patients should undergo a primary assessment.

⚠ **Safety first** – carry out a dynamic risk assessment; continually re-assess throughout the incident.

i. Conducted Electrical Weapon (CEW)

- Conducted Electrical Weapons (CWE) are battery operated hand-held devices which deliver up to 50,000 volts of electricity, in rapid pulses, via two barbed electrodes (refer to Figure 7.4).

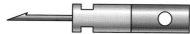

Figure 7.4 – CEW barb. Reproduction of CEW barb image by kind permission of TASER International.

- The barbs are designed to stick into skin or clothes, and connect to the device by fine long copper wires, or via two probes directly applied to the skin or clothes.
- Firing the weapon results in pain and a loss of voluntary control of muscles. These devices are currently in use by all police forces in the United Kingdom.

⚠ Before touching the patient ensure the wires are disconnected from the device; the wires break easily by cutting with scissors.

⚠ There is an increased risk of combustion if a CWE is deployed after the deployment of incapacitant sprays or following contact with flammable liquids such as petrol.

2. Assessment and Management (CEW)

- Most people incapacitated with an CEW do not require hospital assessment; however, patients should undergo a primary survey especially assessing for the presence of:
  - neck and back injuries
  - secondary injuries
  - cardiac symptoms
  - excited delirium
  - attached electrodes.
- For the assessment and management of symptoms, conditions and injuries following deployment of CEW refer to Table 7.6.

Table 7.6 – ASSESSMENT AND MANAGEMENT following

The Deployment of a Conducted Electrical Weapon (CEW)

PRIMARY EFFECTS

EFFECT	ASSESSMENT/MANAGEMENT
PAIN	**For specific guidance refer to the guidelines for:** ● **Management of pain in adults.** ● **Management of pain in children.**
Electrode attachment: ● The electrodes vary in length and have a 'fish hook' type end which is designed to stick to clothes and into the skin. NB Although the lengths of the barbs may vary, the management principles remain the same.	**Electrode removal:** 1. Slightly stretch the skin around the electrode and pull sharply on the electrode. 2. Dispose of the electrode as contaminated waste. 3. Clean the area with an alcohol/antiseptic wipe. 4. Cover the site with a dressing (e.g. a plaster). 5. Advise tetanus booster within 72 hours if not covered for tetanus. NB If the electrode cannot be removed at the first attempt or breaks during attempted removal, leave in situ and transfer to further care. DO NOT attempt to remove the electrode if it is: ● Attached to skin where blood vessels are close to the skin surface (e.g. neck and groin). ● Attached to one or both eye(s). ● Attached to the face. ● Attached to the genitalia. ● Attached to the mouth, throat or if the electrode has been swallowed. ● Firmly embedded in the scalp. ● Embedded in a joint (e.g. finger). ● Broken. **In these circumstances** – cut the wire close to the electrode leaving approximately 4 cm attached to the electrode and transfer to further care.

Special Situations

7 SECTION

Incapacitating Agents

Table 7.6 – ASSESSMENT AND MANAGEMENT following

The Deployment of a Conducted Electrical Weapon (CEW) *continued*

PRIMARY EFFECTS

EFFECT	ASSESSMENT/MANAGEMENT
Burns: ● Superficial burns are likely around the area where the electrode attached to the skin and electricity was delivered. ● Burns may also occur if a CWE is deployed after the deployment of incapacitant sprays or following contact with flammable liquids such as petrol.	**For specific guidance refer to the guidelines for:** ● **Management of pain in adults.** ● **Management of pain in children.**
Cardiac conditions/ symptoms: ● Cardiac conditions have been reported following the deployment of a CEW, including increases in heart rate, cardiac rhythm disturbance and cardiac arrest.	ECGs are not routinely necessary; however, always undertake a 12-lead ECG, and monitor blood pressure and oxygen saturation for patents: ● Complaining of chest pain. ● With cardiac symptoms (e.g. tachycardia, bradycardia). ● With significant cardiac history (e.g. angina, arrhythmias or a myocardial infarction). ● Fitted with pacemakers or cardioverter defibrillator. ● **Cardiac arrhythmia: Refer to the cardiac rhythm disturbance guidelines** for specific guidance. ● **Cardiac arrest: Refer to the appropriate resuscitation guidelines**.
Convulsions: ● The deployment of a CEW may trigger a convulsion or epileptic fit.	**For specific guidance refer to the guidelines for:** ● **Convulsions in adults.** ● **Convulsions in children.**
Obstetric and gynaecological conditions: Spontaneous abortion has been reported following the deployment of CWE.	● **Refer to the appropriate obstetric and gynaecological guidelines.**
Soft tissue injury/injuries: ● Contusions ● Tendon damage ● Abrasions ● Lacerations ● Puncture wounds	**Abrasions, lacerations and puncture wounds:** 1. Clean the area with an alcohol/antiseptic wipe. 2. Cover the site with a dressing (e.g. a plaster). 3. Advise tetanus booster within 72 hours if not covered for tetanus. **Contusions, damage to ligament and tendons:** These injuries should be managed accordingly.
Head injury: ● Head injuries and loss of consciousness may also result from intracranial penetration of an electrode.	**For specific guidance refer to the guidelines for:** ● **Head trauma**. ● **Altered level of consciousness.**

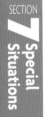

Table 7.6 – ASSESSMENT AND MANAGEMENT following

The Deployment of a Conducted Electrical Weapon (CEW) *continued*

SECONDARY EFFECTS

EFFECT	ASSESSMENT/MANAGEMENT
Head, neck and back injuries, contusions, abrasions and lacerations: ● The powerful muscular contractions caused by the deployment of a CEW may result in thoracolumbar fractures. ● The loss of voluntary control of the muscles caused by the deployment of a CEW may result in falls, leading to injuries of the head, neck and back, contusions, abrasions, lacerations, ligament and tendon injury, etc.	**For specific guidance refer to the guidelines for:** ● **Head trauma.** ● **Altered level of consciousness.** ● **Neck and back trauma.** **Contusions, abrasions, lacerations, ligament and tendon injury:** Manage as per soft tissue injuries above.

COINCIDENTAL EFFECTS

Injuries and conditions unrelated to CEW deployment: ● Injuries and or conditions may be sustained or develop that are unrelated to the deployment of a CEW, for example, as the result of a physical struggle, the consumption of drugs and of physical exhaustion.	Assess and manage coincidental injuries as per condition, cognisant of the effects of drugs, dehydration or exhaustion.
NB Excited delirium:	A CEW may be deployed on people in an aroused state which is sometimes described as 'excited delirium'. People in this state may be at a greater risk of collapse, arrhythmias and sudden death following deployment of a CEW – undertake a **TIME CRITICAL** transfer and provide an alert/information call. The signs of excited delirium include: bizarre behaviour, physical aggression against people and objects, ripping off clothing, being under the influence of drugs or alcohol, abnormal physical strength and reduced perception of pain. NB A doctor may be required to administer rapid tranquilisation; assistance from the police may also be required.

ii. Incapacitant sprays

● Incapacitant sprays/peripheral chemosensory irritants (PCSIs) such as pepper spray (oleoresin, capsicum, pelargonic acid, vanillylamide) and CS spray 2-chlorobenzalmalononitrile (O-chlorobenzylidene malononitrile) are prepared with methyl isobutyl ketone (MIBK).

● The sprays cause irritation (burning sensation) when in contact with exposed skin and mucus membranes including eye, nose, and mouth and respiratory tract causing lacrimation, rhinorrhoea, sialorrhoea, disorientation, dizziness, breathing difficulties, coughing, vomiting.

⚠ Try not to enter a contaminated or closed environment.

3. Assessment and Management (Incapacitant Sprays)

● Most people exposed to incapacitant sprays do not require hospital assessment.

● For the assessment and management of symptoms, and conditions following deployment of incapacitant sprays refer to Table 7.7.

iii. Projectiles

● Projectiles such as plastic or rubber bullets or bean bags can cause sudden death (after strikes to the head, chest and abdomen), dislocations, fractures, joint damage, ligaments and tendons, haemorrhage and

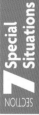

Section 7 Special Situations

haematoma, compartment syndrome, splenic rupture, subcapsular liver/haematoma, pneumothorax/ haemothorax, pentrating injuries to thorax, abdomen, eye, arm, leg, blood vessels.

4. Assessment and Management (Projectiles)

For the assessment and management of symptoms refer to Table 7.8.

iv. Batons

- Baton strikes can cause dislocations, fractures, joint damage, ligaments and tendons, haemorrhage and haematoma, compartment syndrome and death.

- Baton strikes to limbs will typically cause 'tramline bruising'; this is of no significant concern unless there is evidence of underlying fracture or neuromuscular condition.

5. Assessment and Management (Batons)

- For the assessment and management of symptoms refer to Table 7.9.

Table 7.7 – ASSESSMENT AND MANAGEMENT following

The Deployment of Incapacitant Sprays

PRIMARY EFFECTS

EFFECT	ASSESSMENT/MANAGEMENT
Lacrimation, rhinorrhoea, sialorrhoea, dizziness, coughing and vomiting	<ul><li>Move the patient away from the source of the contamination.</li><li>Expose to fresh air.</li><li>For patients with heavy contamination of the skin and eyes irrigate with tap water.</li><li>If symptoms persist for longer than 15 minutes transfer to further care.</li></ul>
Breathing difficulties	For specific guidance **refer to the guideline for**: ● **Dyspnoea**.

Table 7.8 – ASSESSMENT AND MANAGEMENT following

The Deployment of Projectiles

PRIMARY EFFECTS

EFFECT	ASSESSMENT/MANAGEMENT
Head injuries and loss of consciousness	For specific guidance refer to the guidelines for: ● **Head trauma**. ● **Altered level of consciousness**.
Chest injuries	For specific guidance **refer to the guidelines for**: ● **Thoracic trauma**.
Abdominal injuries	For specific guidance **refer to the guidelines for**: ● **Abdominal trauma**.

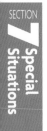

Table 7.9 – ASSESSMENT AND MANAGEMENT following

The Deployment of Batons

PRIMARY EFFECTS

EFFECT	ASSESSMENT/MANAGEMENT
Dislocations, fractures, joint damage, ligaments and tendons	For specific guidance refer to the guidelines for: ● **Trauma emergencies in adults – overview.** ● **Trauma emergencies in children – overview.**
Haemorrhage and haematoma, compartment syndrome	For specific guidance refer to the guidelines for: ● **Trauma emergencies in adults – overview.** ● **Trauma emergencies in children – overview.**

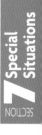

anti-emetic agents
    child analgesia 12
    and oral morphine 9
anti-histamine, use in anaphylaxis 80
antipsychotics 103
antipyretics 131
anxiety 105
anxiolytics 102
appendicitis 85
approved mental health professionals 103
Asperger's syndrome 104
    'Hospital Passport' 104
aspirin
    actions 311
    additional information 311
    cautions 311
    contra-indication in children 311
    contra-indications 311
    dosage and administration 311
    indications 311
    presentation 311
    side effects 311
asthma (adults)
    acute severe 157
    assessment 158
    assessment and management 159-160
    dyspnoea 97
    features of severity 157
    incidence 157
    inhaled medication 158
    introduction 157
    ipratropium bromide 80
    key points 159
    less severe attacks 158
    life-threatening 157
    management 158
    moderate exacerbation 157
    nebulised salbutamol 158
    pathophysiology 157
    peak expiratory flow rate 158
    preventer steroid inhalers 158
    reliever inhalers 158
    severity and outcome 157
    time critical 157
    wheezing 157
asthma (children) 202
    assessment and management 202, 204-205
    features of severity 202
    key points 203
    life-threatening 202
    management 202
    medication 202

    moderate exacerbation 202
    pathophysiology 202
    peak expiratory flow rate 202-203
    severe 202
    severity and outcome 202
asthma, resuscitation and
    acute severe 80
    adrenaline 81
    and anaphylaxis 80
    cardiac arrest 80-81
    food allergy and 80
    hydrocortisone 80
    introduction 80
    ipratropium bromide 80
    key points 81
    risk factors 80
    salbutamol 80
    symptoms and signs 81
    tracheal intubation 81
    treatment 80
asystole
    assessment and management 90
    risk of 89
ATMIST format handover 224
atropine
    actions 312
    additional information 312
    contra-indications 312
    dosage and administration 312
    indications 312
    presentation 312
    side effects 312
atropine (CBRNE)
    actions 447
    additional information 447
    cautions 447
    contra-indications 447
    dosage and administration 448-451
    indications 447
    presentation 447
    side effects 447
autism 104
automated external defibrillators (AEDs) 51, 72
'AVPU' score 125, 149, 232, 278

basic life support (BLS) (adult)
    assessment and management 50
    defibrillation 50-51
    introduction 50
    key points 51
    resuscitation in confined spaces 51
    support sequence 51

Index

basic life support (BLS) (child)
  airway management 62
  assessment and management 64-65
  bag-mask ventilation 62
  general principles 62
  hypothermia 62
  introduction 62
  key points 65
  resuscitation 62
batons 462
  effects of deployment of 463
benzodiazepines 102, 206
  poisoning 189
benzylpenicillin (penicillin G)
  actions 315
  additional information 315
  contra-indications 315
  dosage and administration 315
  indications 315
  in meningococcal septicaemia 150
  presentation 315
beta-blockers poisoning 189
bilevel positive airways pressure (BiPAP) 178
bradycardia
  assessment and management 90
  child trauma 231
  children 125-126
  definition 89
  immersion and drowning 271
'breakthrough' pain, end of life care 12, 28
breathlessness, severe 117
bronchiolitis, children 134
bronchitis 157
bronchoconstriction 80
bruising, mobile babies and toddlers 18
buccal drug route 304
burns
  dressings as pain relief 12
  Intravascular Fluid Therapy (Adults) 394
  pain management in adults 9
burns and scalds (adults)
  airway burns 262
  assessment and management 262, 264
  chemical 262
  electrical 262
  introduction 262
  key points 264
  Lund and Browder chart 262
  non-accidental 262
  severity 262
  thermal 262
  Wallace's Rule of Nines 262

burns and scalds (children)
  abusive burns 18, 265
  airway burns 265
  assessment and management 265, 267
  chemical 265
  electrical 265
  introduction 265
  intravascular fluid therapy 397
  key points 267
  Lund and Browder chart 265
  mobile babies and toddlers 18
  non-accidental 265
  severity 265
  thermal 265

cadaveric spasm (instant rigor mortis) 47
calcium-channel blockers poisoning 188
capillary refill, children 125
capnography, and tracheal intubation 39
carbon monoxide poisoning 188
cardiac arrest
  and anaphylaxis 80
  in asthma 80-81
  and child convulsions 206
  children 124
  in drowning 77
  heart rhythms 52
  maternal resuscitation 60
  in pregnancy 60
  in obstetrics 277
  and opioid overdose 79
cardiac arrest, traumatic
  assessment and management 44-45
  causes of 44
  introduction 44
  pre-hospital fluids 44
  reversible causes 44
  tranexamic acid 44
cardiac chest pain 117
cardiac rhythm disturbance
  acute myocardial ischaemia or infarction 89
  adverse signs and symptoms 89
  asystole 89-90
  bradycardia 89-90
  introduction 89
  key points 90
  principles of treatment 89
  tachycardia 89, 91
cardiogenic shock 117
cardiopulmonary resuscitation (CPR)
  capnography and 39
  and cardiac arrest 52

children 32-33
drowning 46, 77, 271
end of life care and 46
hypothermia and 143
obstetrics 277
and recognition of life extinct 46
and tracheal intubation 39
see also asthma, resuscitation and; pregnancy,
    resuscitation in
chemical, biological, radiological, nuclear and explosive
    incidents (CBRNE)
    assessment and management 439-440
    biological incident 441
    chemical incident 441, 444
    conditions associated with agents 443
    contact hazards 438
    decontamination 439
    detection 439
    incident identification 439
    ingestion hazards 439
    inhalation hazards 438
    injection hazards 438
    introduction 438
    key points 443
    mechanisms of injury and related injuries 438
    nuclear incident 441
    personal protective equipment 439
    radioactive agents 439
    radiological incident 441
    specific treatments 441
    suspect packages/materials 439
    triage sieve 445-446
chemical exposure, individual 80
    background 79
    hydrogen sulphide 79
    key points 79
    recognition of life extinct 79
    rescue principles 79
    risk assessment 79
    specialist help 79
chest pain/discomfort, non-traumatic
    acute coronary syndrome 152
    assessment and management 122-123
    causes of 122
    indigestion type pain 122
    incidence 122
    introduction 122
    key points 122
    muscular type pain 122
    pleuritic type pain 122
    severity and outcome 122
    suggested myocardial ischaemia 122
    suggested stable angina 122

types of 122, 152
child and adolescent mental health services (CAMHS) 103
Child Death Detective Inspector 34
children
    age definitions 62
    blood pressure 125
    child protection concerns 128
    circulatory system 125-126
    and cultural difference 19
    differences and challenges 129
    heart rate 125, 131, 231
    major and minor illnesses 129
    mental state 125
    normal physiological values 133
    normal respiratory rates 124
    pulse volume 125
    respiratory system 125-126
    skin colour 125
children, death of (SUDICA)
    care of family 32
    communication with other agencies 32
    conditions associated with 34
    detection of pulse 32
    documentation 32
    importance of attitude 33
    introduction 32
    multi-agency approach 32
    objectives 32
    procedure 34
    resuscitation 32-33
    support for ambulance technicians 33
    transfer of infant 33
children, minor illnesses
    assessment and management 129
    introduction 129
    key points 129
    'major' and 'minor' 129
    paediatric considerations 129
children, safeguarding
    bruising 17
    duty of care 16
    fractures 17
    'in need' 16
    introduction 16
    non-accidental injury 17
    non-mobile babies 17
    recognition of abuse 16
    significant harm 16
    suspicions of abuse 17
Children Act 1989 16
chlorphenamine (piriton)
    actions 317

Index

cautions 317
contra-indications 317
dosage and administration 317
indications 317
presentation 317
side effects 317
chronic obstructive pulmonary disease (COPD)
acute exacerbation 161-162
assessment and management 161, 163-164
conditions with similar features 161
dyspnoea 97
incidence 161
introduction 161
key points 162
pathophysiology 161
severity and outcome 161
signs and symptoms 161
cigarette burns, mobile babies and toddlers 18
ciprofloxacin (CBRNE)
actions 453
cautions 453
contra-indications 453
dosage and administration 453
indications 453
presentation 453
side effects 453
clopidogrel
actions 320
cautions 320
contra-indications 320
dosage and administration 320
indications 320
presentation 320
side effects 320
cocaine poisoning 190
coma 92, 94
community psychiatric nurses (CPN) 103
conducted electrical weapons (CWE) 459, 461
confidentiality see patient confidentiality
consent
and confidentiality 6
inability to 6
and public interest 6
continuous positive airway pressure (CPAP) 178
convulsions (adults)
assessment and management 165, 167-168
eclamptic 165, 296
epileptic 165
febrile 165
key points 165
pathophysiology 165
severity and outcome 165

convulsions (children)
assessment and management 206, 208-209
benzodiazepine in 206
common causes 206
convulsive status epilepticus 206
diazepam 207
hospital transfer 207
hypoglycaemia 206
incidence 206
introduction 206
key points 207
medication 210
meningococcal septicaemia 206
midazolam 207
risk of cardiac arrest 206
severity and outcome 206
and underlying condition 206
cosmetics poisoning 185
cough mixtures 136
coughing, and foreign body airway obstruction 74
croup, children
assessment 134
incidence 134
introduction 134
management 135
Modified Taussig Score 134-135
ominous signs 135
pathophysiology 134
referral pathway 135
severity and outcome 135
steroids 135
crush injury 393
cyanide poisoning 189
cyanosis 125

defibrillation
advanced life support (adult) 52
advanced life support (child) 70
and cardiac arrest 52
dehydration, and diabetic ketoacidosis 174, 217
dementia 104
dementia passports 104
Deprivation of Liberty Safeguards (DoLS) 114
dexamethasone
actions 321
additional information 321
cautions 321
contra-indications 321
dosage and administration 321
indications 321
oral 135
presentation 321

side effects 321

diabetes mellitus (DM)

in children 216

hyperglycaemia 215

hypoglycaemia 215

diabetic ketoacidosis (DKA)

assessment and management 172, 217

assessment and management (children) 215-216, 397

and dehydration 174, 217

signs and symptoms 217

diamorphine 9, 12

diarrhoea, bloody 211

diazepam

actions 322

additional information 322

cautions 322

and children 322

contra-indications 322

convulsions in children 207

dosage and administration 323

indications 322

presentation 322

side effects 322

dicobalt edetate (CBRNE)

actions 454

cautions 454

contra-indications 454

dosage and administration 454

indications 454

presentation 454

side effects 454

dihydrocodeine poisoning 188

diltiazem poisoning 188

disability – recognition of potential central neurological failure (children) 125

floppiness (hypotonia) 126

posture 126

pupils 126

response to painful stimulus 125

stiffness (hypertonia) 126

disseminated intravascular coagulation (DIC) 293

diverticular disease 86, 170

DNACPR (Do Not Attempt Cardio- Pulmonary Resuscitation) 46

doxycycline (CBRNE)

actions 455

cautions 455

contra-indications 455

dosage and administration 455

indications 455

side effects 455

drowning

cardiac arrest 77

chest compressions 77

definition of 271

general principles 77

hypothermia and drug protocols 77

introduction 77

key points 78

resuscitation effort 77

risk assessment 78

spinal injury 77

water rescue 77

drowsiness, children 125

drugs, allergic reactions to 155, 200

drugs overview

common abbreviations 303

documentation 303

drug codes 304, 307

drug routes 304-305

introduction 303

key points 304

non-parenteral routes 304

parenteral routes 304

prescribing terms 303

safety aspects 303

dyspnoea

acute coronary syndrome 97

acute heart failure 97

anaphylaxis 97

assessment and management 96, 99

asthma 97

causes of 96

chronic obstructive pulmonary disease 97

definition of 96

differential diagnosis 97

foreign body airway obstruction 97

incidence 96

introduction 96

key points 99

pathophysiology 96

pneumonia 97

pneumothorax 97

pulmonary embolism 97

severity and outcome 96

E.coli (*Escherichia coli*) 211

eclampsia

assessment and management 297

incidence 296

introduction 296

pathophysiology 297

risk factors 297

severity and outcome 296

ecstacy (MDMA) poisoning 192

ectopic pregnancy/ruptured ectopic pregnancy 292
    risk factors 292
    symptoms 86, 292
electrical injuries
    adults 268
    assessment and management 268-269, 9999
    burns 268
    cardiac arrhythmia 268
    children 268
    incidence 268
    introduction 268
    key points 268
    lightning 268
    muscular paralysis 268
    pathophysiology 268
    pregnancy 268
    severity and outcome 268
    trauma 268
end of life care
    assessment 28
    breakthrough pain 29
    care pathways 26
    'good death' 26
    introduction 26
    medical assessment 28
    metastatic spinal cord compression 26
    neutropenic sepsis 27
    if not expected to die within 72 hours 26
    pain management 28-29, 45
    pain management, self-assessment 28
    patient centred approach 29
    pharmacological approach 29
    psychological assessment 29
    and resuscitation 46
    reversible emergencies 26
    severity and outcome 26
    sociological assessment 29
    superior vein compression 27
    WHO analgesic ladder 29
    WHO step-care approach 28
entonox
    actions 326
    additional information 326
    analgesia in children 9, 11-12
    cautions 326
    contra-indications 326
    dosage and administration 326
    indications 326
    inhalational analgesia 9, 12
    and intravenous morphine 9
    presentation 326
    side effects 326

entrapments, use of ketamine 10
epiglottitis 126
epilepsy passport 206
ethanol poisoning 188
    in children 219
European Convention on Human Rights 114
explosions 438

factitious or induced illness, mobile babies and toddlers 18
FAST test for stroke/TIA 198-199
febrile convulsions (FC) 206
febrile illness (children)
    AMBER criteria 132
    antipyretic 131
    assessment 130
    convulsions 130
    dehydration 131
    disproportionate tachycardia 131
    examination 130
    fever 130
    fluid intake 130
    heart rate 131
    herpes simplex encephalitis 131
    incidence 130
    introduction 130
    Kawasaki's disease 131
    key points 132
    management 131
    measurement of temperature 130
    meningitis 131
    meningococcal septicaemia 131
    pneumonia 131
    primary survey 130
    RED criterial 131
    referral pathway 131
    'safety netting' 132
    septic arthritis/osteomyelitis 131
    serious bacterial infections 130
    severity and outcome 130
    source and severity 131
    tachycardia 131
    tachypnoea 131
    'Traffic Light' assessment 131, 133
    urinary tract infection 131
fentanyl, intra-nasal 9
fever 130
finger bruising, non-mobile babies 18
fire service, disclosure of information to 5
FLACC scale 11, 15
flushing of skin, children 125
foods, allergic reactions to 155, 200
foreign body airway obstruction (FBAO) (adult)

assessment and management 58-59

general signs 58

introduction 58

key points 59

foreign body airway obstruction (FBAO) (child)

abdominal thrusts, child over one year 74

algorithm 76

assessment and management 75, 80

back blows, child over one year 74

back blows, infants 74

chest and abdominal thrusts 74

chest thrusts for infants 74

dyspnoea 97

general management principles 74

general signs 74

inhalation of 202

introduction 74

key points 75

reassessment after chest or abdominal thrusts 74

fractures

of femur 13

mobile babies and toddlers 18

in non-mobile babies 17

splintage as pain relief 9, 12

types of 242

frenulum, torn, in non-mobile babies 17

furosemide

actions 327

additional information 327

cautions 327

contra-indications 327

dosage and administration 327

indications 327

presentation 327

side effects 327

gastritis 105, 169

gastroenteritis 86

gastroenteritis (children)

assessment 211

dehydration 211-213

differential diagnosis 211

examination 211

information for parents and carers 212

introduction 211

key points 214

management 211

nutritional considerations 212

pathophysiology 211

red flag symptoms 212

referral pathway 212

'safety netting' 212

severity and outcome 211

shock 213

stool samples 211

gastrointestinal (GI) bleeding

assessment and management 170-171

differential diagnosis 170

diverticular disease 170

gastritis 169

haematemesis 169

haemorrhoids 170

incidence 169

inflammatory bowel disease 170

introduction 169

key points 170

lower gastrointestinal bleeding 169

Mallory–Weiss tears 169

melaena 169

mortality 169

oesophageal varices 169

oesophagitis 169

pathophysiology 169

peptic ulcers 169

severity and outcome 169

tumour 169-170

upper gastrointestinal bleeding 169

Glasgow Coma Scale 128

assessment for acute stroke 198

modification for under 4s 128

as time-critical emergency 117

in traumatic brain injury 238

glucagon (glucagen)

actions 328

additional information 328

cautions 328

contra-indications 328

dosage and administration 329

indications 328

presentation 328

side effects 328

glucose 10%

actions 330

additional information 330

cautions 330

contra-indications 330

dosage and administration 330

indications 330

presentation 330

side effects 330

glucose 40% Oral Gel

actions 331

additional information 331

cautions 331

contra-indications 331

dosage and administration 331

indications 331

presentation 331

side effects 331

glycaemic emergencies (adults) 175

diabetic ketoacidosis (DKA) 172

hyperglycaemia 172, 174

hypoglycaemia 172-173

key points 174

normal blood glucose levels 172

glycaemic emergencies (children)

hyperglycaemia 215

hypoglycaemia 215

introduction 215

key points 217

glyceryl trinitrate (GTN, Suscard)

actions 332

contra-indications 332

dosage and administration 332

indications 332

presentation 332

side effects 332

greenstick fractures, non-mobile babies 17

haemolytic anaemia 146

haemorrhage

adult trauma 228

catastrophic 229

in pelvic trauma 252

time-critical 117

haemorrhage in pregnancy

assessment and management 292-293

key points 294

post-partum 287

haemorrhagic rash 149

haemorrhoids 170

head injury *see* traumatic brain injury (TBI)

headache

assessment and management 101

history of 100

incidence 100

introduction 100

key points 101

primary 100

rapid deterioration of patient 100

red flag signs and symptoms 100

secondary 100

severity and outcome 100

SOCRATES in pain management 100

heart failure

assessment and management 176, 178-179

bilevel positive airways pressure 178

clinical indicators 178

continuous positive airway pressure 178

diamorphine 178

furosemide 178

incidence 176

introduction 176

jugular venous pressure and 178

key points 178

left ventricular failure 176

morphine and 178

pathophysiology 176

positive pressure ventilation 178

right ventricular failure 176

risk factors 176

salbutamol and 178

severity and outcome 176

signs and symptoms 176

therapies 178

use of GTN 178

heat related illness

assessment and management 138-139

continuum of conditions 137

factors 137

features 137

heat exhaustion 137

heat stress 137

heat stroke 137

introduction 137

key points 138

pathophysiology 138

HEMS services in head injury 239

heparin

actions 333

additional information 333

contra-indications 333

dosage and administration 333

indications 333

presentation 333

side effects 333

herpes simplex encephalitis 131

household products poisoning 185

hydrocortisone

actions 334

in anaphylaxis 80

in asthma 80

cautions 334

contra-indications 334

dosage and administration 334

indications 334

presentation 334

side effects 334

hydrogen sulphide 79

hyperglycaemia (adults)

    assessment and management 172, 174

    signs and symptoms 174

hyperglycaemia (children) 215

    diabetes mellitus 215

    symptoms 215

hypersalivation, and ketamine 10, 13

hypertonic saline (HTS) 240

hyperventilation syndrome (HVS)

    anxiety and agitation 140

    assessment and management 140-142

    breathing 140

    definition of 140

    electrolyte imbalance 140

    and hypocapnia 140

    incidence 140

    introduction 140

    key points 140

    pathophysiology 140

    severity and outcome 140

    signs and symptoms 140

hypocapnia 140

hypoglycaemia (adults) 172

    and altered consciousness 232

    assessment and management 172-173

    definition of 172

    diabetes mellitus 215

    risk factors 172

    signs and symptoms 172, 215

    symptoms similar to stroke 198

hypoglycaemia (children) 215

    assessment and management 215-216

    convulsions 206

    definition in children 215

    in newborn 288-289

    risk factors 215

hypoperfusion, and traumatic cardiac arrest 44

hypostasis 47

hypotension

    children 125

    obstetrics and gynaecology emergencies 277

    as time critical 117

    traumatic brain injury 238

hypothermia

    acute (immersion hypothermia) 77, 143, 271

    assessment and management 144-145

    basic life support (children) 62

    chronic 143

    clinical stages 144

    definition of 143

    diagnosis 143

incidence 143

introduction 143

key points 145

and large burns 12

in newborn 288

pathophysiology 143

preterm delivery 289

resuscitation 143

risk factors 143

severity and outcome 143

subacute (exhaustion hypothermia) 143

and traumatic brain injury 238

hypotonia 126

hypovolaemia

    drowning 77

    meningococcal meningitis and septicaemia 150

    obstetrics and gynaecology emergencies 277

    and traumatic cardiac arrest 44

hypoxia

    and cardiac arrest 44, 124

    children 125

    immersion and drowning 271

    thoracic trauma 255

ibruprofen

    actions 338

    cautions 338

    contra-indications 338

    dosage and administration 339

    indications 338

    oral analgesia 9

    pain management children 12

    pre-hospital analgesic drugs children 11

    presentation 338

    side effects 338

immersion, definition of 271

immersion and drowning

    airway and breathing 271

    aquatic rescue 271

    assessment and management 273

    bradycardia 271

    chest compression 271

    discontinuing resuscitative efforts 273

    exacerbating factors 271

    hypercapnia 271

    hypothermia 271

    hypoxia 271

    incidence 271

    intravascular fluid therapy 271

    introduction 271

    key points 273

    laryngospasm 271

Index

neck and back trauma 271
    pathophysiology 271
    postural hypotension 271
    rescue and resuscitation 271
    risk assessment 271
    severity and outcome 271
    survival and submersion 273
    and trauma 271
implantable cardioverter defibrillator (ICD)
    assessment and management of patients fitted with 181, 183-184
    ECG monitoring 181
    general principles 180
    introduction 180
    key points 182
    therapies 180
    usual location 180
incapacitant sprays 461
    effects of deployment of 462
incapacitating agents
    introduction 459
    key points 462
    risk assessment 459
inflammatory bowel disease 170
inhaled drug route 304
insect stings and bites, allergic reaction to 155, 200
interpreters 19-20
intestinal obstruction 86
intramuscular drug route 304
intranasal drug route 304
intraosseous drug route 304
intravascular fluid therapy (adults)
    algorithm 396
    burns 394
    crush injury 393
    dosage 394
    dosage haemorrhagic emergencies 393
    early indicators of impaired major organ perfusion 392
    following haemorrhage 393
    haemorrhagic emergencies, medical 393
    haemorrhagic emergencies, traumatic 392
    haemostasis 392
    introduction 392
    key points 395
    medical conditions 394
    non-haemorrhagic emergencies 394
    obstetric emergencies 393
    oxygen transport 392
    pathophysiology 392
    pH buffering 392
    sepsis 394-395
    trauma 392, 394

intravascular fluid therapy (children)
    assessment and management 397, 399
    burns 397
    diabetic ketoacidosis 397
    introduction 397
    key points 398
    management 397
    medical causes of shock 397
    pathophysiology 397
    traumatic causes of shock 397
intravenous drug route 304
intussusception, abdominal pain 86
IPAP Suicide Risk Assessment 104, 108-110
ipratropium bromide (atrovent)
    actions 340
    cautions 340
    contra-indications 340
    dosage and administration 340
    indications 340
    presentation 340
    side effects 340
iron poisoning 189
    in children 219

Kawasaki's disease 131
ketamine 10, 13
    airway management 10
    analgesia (children) 11

learning disability 104
limb trauma
    amputations/partial amputations 242
    assessment and management 243, 245
    blood loss 242
    closed fracture 242
    comminuted fracture 242
    compartment syndrome 242
    compound fracture (open) 242
    degloving 242
    dislocations 242
    greenstick fractures 242
    incidence 242
    ischaemia 242
    introduction 242
    key points 243
    neck of femur fractures 242
    pain management 242
    pathophysiology 242
    severity and outcome 242
    spiral or oblique fractures 242
    splinting 242-243
    traction splinting 242
    transverse fractures 242

Index

types of 242

local authorities, disclosure of information to 5

LSD (lysergic acid) poisoning 193

major incident management
METHANE report format 437
risk assessment 437

Mallory–Weiss tears 169

mastoiditis 135

maternal resuscitation
assessment and management of cardiac arrest 60
cardiorespiratory collapse 60
introduction 60
key points 61
modifications for cardiac arrest in pregnancy 60
pathophysiology of cardiac arrest 60

media, disclosure of information to 6

medical emergencies (adults)
additional information sources 120
assessment and management 119
Glasgow Coma Scale 121
introduction 117
key points 121
patient assessment 117
primary survey 117
secondary survey 120
secondary survey abdomen 120
secondary survey chest 120
secondary survey head 120
secondary survey limbs 120
time-critical features and conditions 117

medical emergencies (children)
accessory muscle use and breathing 124
adequate oxygenation 126
agitation 125
airway management 124, 126
arrest of external haemorrhage 127
aspiration, foreign body removal 126
assessment 124
blood glucose measurement 127
blood pressure 125
bradycardia 125-126
breathing management 124, 126
cannulation 127
capillary refill 125
cardiac arrest 124
circulation management 127
circulatory inadequacy 125
cyanosis 125
diabetic ketoacidosis 127
disability assessment and management 125, 127
drowsiness 125

effect of neurological impairment 126
effects of respiratory inadequacy 125
endotracheal intubation 126
fluid administration 127
flushing of skin 125
grunting and breathing 124
heart rate 125
hyperventilation 127
hypotension 125
hypoxia 125
information, value of 127
introduction 124
key points 128
management 126
manual extension manoeuvres 126
mental state 125
nasopharyngeal airway 126
needle cricothyroidotomy 126
oropharyngeal airway 126
pallor 125
primary assessment 124
pulse oximetry and breathing 125
pulse volume 125
re-assessment ABCD 126
recession and breathing 124
respiratory rate 124-125
shock 125, 127
skin colour 125
stridor 124
summary 127
tachycardia 125
tachypnoea 125
wheezing 124

'MedicAlert®' type jewellery 117, 120, 155, 200

meningitis 131

meningococcal disease
early presentation in children 129
symptoms 131
and URTIs 136
and tachycardia 131

meningococcal meningitis and septicaemia
airway 149
assessment 149
'AVPU' disability score 149
breathing 149
circulation 149
clinical findings 149
decreasing consciousness 150
examination 149
fluid therapy 150
'Glass' or 'Tumbler' test 149
incidence 149

introduction 149

key points 150

management 150-151

oxygen administration 150

rash 149

risk of infection to ambulance personnel 150

severity and outcome 149

time critical transfer 149

meningococcal septicaemia

and convulsions 206

as febrile illness 131

non-blanching rash 150

time-critical transfer 149

mental capacity, definition of 111

Mental Capacity Act 2005 (MCA) 111

Advance Decisions to Refuse Treatment 112, 115

alcohol 113

assessment 112-113

'Best Interest Assessors' 114

best interests 114

Court Deputies 116

Court of Protection 115

helping to make decisions 112

Independent Mental Capacity Advocates 116

Lasting Power of Attorney 115

legal context 111

presumption of capacity 111-112

principles 111

protection from liability of staff 113

record keeping 114

responsibilities under 111

safeguards 115

and self-harm 112

transfer and continuing care 25, 115

use of restraint 114-115

mental disorder

acute psychosis 106

anxiety 105

Asperger's syndrome 104

assessment 105

autism 104

communication 105

de-escalation 105

dementia 104

introduction 111

IPAP Suicide Risk Assessment 108-109

key points 107

learning disability 104

management 104

pathways to referral 106

prevalence 102

psychotropic drugs 102-103

risk factors 102

self-harm 105

vulnerability 102

WHO definition 102

Mental Health Service 111

mental health services for older people (MHSOP) 103

mental health, key workers 103

metaphyseal fractures, non-mobile babies 17

metastatic spinal cord compression

background 26

management 27

signs and symptoms 27

METHANE report format 439

metoclopramide (maxolon)

actions 342

additional information 342

anti-emetic agent 9

cautions 12, 342

contra-indications 12, 342

dosage and administration 342

indications 342

presentation 342

side effects 342

midazolam in children's convulsions 207

midazolam in traumatic brain injury 239

adverse effects 240

background 239

cautions 239-240

contra-indications 239

indications 239

key considerations 240

preparation and dosage 242

type 239

midazolam, buccal, patient's own

actions 345

additional information 345

contra-indications 345

dosage and administration 345

indications 345

presentation 345

side effects 345

miscarriage

'cervical shock' 292

incidence 292

pathophysiology 292

risk factors 292

symptoms 292

misoprostol

actions 346

additional information 346

contra-indications 346

dosage and administration 346

indications 346
presentation 346
side effects 346
Modified Taussig Score 134-135
monoamine oxidase inhibitors (MAOs) 103
monocular visual loss, sudden 198
morphine sulphate
actions 347
additional information 347
analgesia (adults) 9
analgesia (children) 11-12
breakthrough pain in end of life care 29
cautions 347
contra-indications 347
dosage and administration 348
indications 347
intra-nasal 9
intravenous 9
oral 9
presentation 347
side effects 347
special precautions 347
mouth, bleeding from, in non-mobile babies 17
Multi-Agency Public Protection Arrangements (MAPPA) 19
myocardial dysfunction, and post-cardiac-arrest syndrome 54
myocardial ischaemia 152
features of pain 152

naloxone hydrochloride (narcan)
actions 351
additional information 351
contra-indications 351
dosage and administration 352
indications 351
presentation 351
side effects 351
use in opioid overdose 9, 12, 79
National Service Framework for Children, Young People and Maternity Services 20
nebulisation of drugs 304
neck and back trauma *see* spinal cord injury (SCI)
neck stiffness 149
nerve gas poisoning
atropine administration 448
characteristic features 447
background 27
end of life care 27
management 27
signs and symptoms 27
newborn, care of 288
abdominal wall defects 289
APGAR score 288-290

assessment and management 289, 291
birth asphyxia 288
congenital abnormalities 289
early onset neonatal infection 289
hypoglycaemia 288-289
hypothermia 288-289
key points 290
neonatal jaundice 289
pathophysiology 288
preterm delivery 289
reasons in baby for transfer 288
reasons in mother for transfer 288
therapeutic hypothermia 288
newborn life support
assessment and management 66, 68-69
chest compressions 66
importance of warmth 66
introduction 66
keypoints 66
physiology 66
non-blanching rash 149-150

obidoxime chloride (CBRNE)
actions 456
cautions 456
contra-indications 456
dosage and administration 456
indications 456
presentation 456
severe poisoning in children 456
side effects 456
oblique fractures, non-mobile babies 17
obstetric and gynaecology emergencies
airway assessment 278
assessment 277
'AVPU' score 278
breathing assessment 278
cardiac arrest 277
circulation assessment 278
compression of inferior vena cava 277
disability 278
environment 278
evaluation of time critical 278
examination of vaginal area 278
fundus 278
glossary 279
hypotension 277
hypovolaemia 277
intravascular fluid therapy 393
introduction 277
key points 279
manual displacement of uterus 277

manual tilt 277
massive external haemorrhage 278
maternal resuscitation 60
pathophysiology 277
primary survey 277
resuscitation of mother 277
secondary survey 278
vaginal bleeding assessment 278
obstetrics
breech birth 285
abdominal pain 287
delivery complications 283
key points 287
malpresentation 287
maternal seizures 283
multiple births, delayed 287
normal delivery and complications 280
normal delivery assessment and management 282
placental abruption 284
post-partum haemorrhage 287
pre-term delivery 287
prolapsed umbilical cord 283
shoulder dystocia 287
oesophageal varices 169
oesophagitis 169
ondansetron
actions 355
additional information 355
anti-emetic agent 9
cautions 355
contra-indications 355
dosage and administration 356
indications 355
presentation 355
side effects 355
opiate use 120
side effects 355
poisoning 193
opioid overdose 120
key points 79
management in children 219
opioid antagonists 9, 12, 79
specific substances management 189
opioids
analgesia in adults 9
intra-nasal 9
oral drug route 304
organophosphate (OP) poisoning 447
characteristic features 447
orthochlorobenzalmalononitrile (CS gas) poisoning 189
overdose and poisoning (adults) 185
assessment and management 185, 187

and capacity 185
duty of care 185
illegal drugs 193
incidence 185
key points 185
overdose 185
pathophysiology 185
poisoning 185
severity and outcome 185
substance specific management 189
overdose and poisoning (children)
accidental 218
alcohol poisoning 218
assessment and management 218, 220
chemicals 218
common agents 218
cosmetics, poisoning 218
household products, poisoning 218
incidence 218
intentional 218
introduction 218
key points 218
non-accidental 218
overdose 218
paracetamol 219
pathophysiology 218
pharmaceutical agents 218
plants/fungi 218
poisoning 218
severity and outcome 218
specific substance management 219
types of 218
oxygen
actions 357
administration of supplemental 362
cautions 357
conditions not requiring 361
controlled/low dose supplemental 359, 361
contra-indications 357
dosage and administration 357
high levels supplemental 358, 361
indications 357
moderate levels supplemental 359, 361
monitoring without supplemental 360
presentation 357
side effects 357

pain, definition of 8
pain, musculo-skeletal 9
pain management in adults
analgesia 8
assessment 8

Index

balanced analgesia 10

break-through pain 9

distraction 9

dressings 9

end of life care 28-29, 45

non-pharmacological methods 9

pain scoring 8

pharmacological methods 9

psychological methods 9

splintage 9

treating cause 8

pain management in children 11

    analgesia 11

    appropriate training 13

    assessment 11

    behavioural clues 11

    distraction 12

    non-pharmacological methods 12

    pain scoring 11

    pharmacological methods 12

    psychological methods 12

    topical analgesia 12

pallor 125

paracetamol (acetaminophen) 9

    actions 363

    additional information 363

    for children 11-12

    contra-indications 363

    dosage and administration 364

    end of life care 29

    indications 363

    intravenous, children 12

    poisoning 189, 219

    presentation 363

    side effects 363

patient confidentiality

    anonymisation of information 5-6

    best practice 5

    and consent 6

    Data Protection Act 4

    and disclosure to fire service 5

    and disclosure to for commercial purposes 6

    and disclosure to local authorities 5

    and disclosure to media 6

    and disclosure to police 5

    and disclosure to Secretary of State 5

    electronic information 4

    information-sharing policy 5

    loss or lack of security 5

    NHS policy 4

    patient identifiable information 4

    protection of patient information 4

patient records, accuracy of 4

patient-held warning cards 120

Peak Expiratory Flow Rate Measurements (PEFR)

    asthma in children 202

    flow chart 203

pelvic inflammatory disease 86

pelvic ring disruptions 252

pelvic trauma, major

    assessment and management 253

    audit information 254

    children 253

    classification of injury 252

    haemorrhage 252

    and hypotension 253

    incidence 252

    introduction 252

    key points 254

    other injuries 252

    pathophysiology 252

    rectal injury 252

    referral pathway 253

    severity and outcome 252

    skeletal anatomy 252

    unstable fractures 252

    urogenital injury 252

    vascular injury 252

peptic ulcers 86, 169

peripheral oedema, and potential heart failure 178

peripheral vein thrombosis 194

personal health records, patient access to 5

pharmaceutical/recreational substances poisoning 185

photophobia 149

placenta praevia 292

placental abruption 292-293

plants/fungi, poisoning 185

pneumonia 97, 131, 136

    children 136

pneumothorax 97

poisoning *see* overdose and poisoning

poisoning, deliberate 18

police, disclosure of information to 5

police officers, and mental health team 103

positive pressure ventilation (NiPPV) 178

post-cardiac-arrest syndrome 54

potassium iodate (CBRNE)

    actions 457

    additional information 457

    cautions 457

    contra-indications 457

    dosage and administration 457

    indications 457

    presentation 457

side effects 457
pralidoxime mesylate (CBRNE)
actions 458
cautions 458
contra-indications 458
dosage and administration 458
indications 458
presentation 458
side effects 458
pre-eclampsia
assessment and management 295-296
pathophysiology 295
risk factors 295
severe 295-296
pregnancy
electrical injuries 268
haemorrhage 292
pregnancy-induced hypertension (PIH)
incidence 295
eclampsia 296-297
introduction 295
key points 297
mild/moderate eclampsia 296
pathophysiology 295
severe pre-eclampsia 296
severity and outcome 295
see also trauma in pregnancy
Pre-Hospital Major Trauma Triage Tool 227
prescription-only medicines (POMs) 303
primary percutaneous coronary intervention (PPCI) 152
projectiles 461-462
effects of deployment of 462
psychiatrists 103
psychologists 103
psychotropic drugs 102-103
pulmonary embolism (PE)
assessment and management 195-197
dyspnoea 97
incidence 194
introduction 194
key points 195
pathophysiology 194
and peripheral vein thrombosis 194
predisposing factors 194
severity and outcome 194
signs 194
symptoms 194
types 194
Wells Criteria 195
pulmonary oedema
drug administration 327
and heart failure 176

and potential heart failure/therapies 178

quinsy (peritonsillar abscess) 135

rape, definition of 22
recognition of life extinct (ROLE)
actions to be taken after verification of death 47, 49
by ambulance technicians 48
asystole 46
conditions unequivocally associated with death 46
confirmatory ECG 46
decapitation 46
decomposition/putrefaction 46
discontinuation of resuscitation 46
documentation 47
hemicorporectomy 46
hypostasis 46-47
incineration 46
individual chemical exposure 79
introduction 46
massive cranial and cerebral destruction 46
rigor mortis 46-47
rectal drug route 304
regional nerve blocks 13
research, anonymisation of information 6
respiratory illness (children)
antibiotics 135
asthma 134
bronchiolitis 134
croup 134-135
introduction 134
key points 136
non-conveyance 136
pneumonia 136
'safety netting' 136
steroids 135
typical duration 135
URTIs 135-136
resuscitation see cardio-pulmonary resuscitation
reteplase
actions 367
additional information 367
in all cases 367
contra-indications 367
dosage and administration 369
indications 367
presentation 367
side effects 367
thrombolysis checklist 368
return of spontaneous circulation (ROSC) 54, 56
rib fractures, non-mobile babies 17
rigor mortis 46-47
rohypnol 22

safeguarding (children)

allegations against ambulance staff 20

asylum-seeking children or refugees 19

children of travelling families 19

child as carer 19

child prostitution 19

children in Armed Forces 19

children living away from home 19

disabled children 19

emotional abuse 21

examples of types of abuse and neglect 21

factors in vulnerability 18

individuals posing risk 19

Multi-Agency Public Protection Arrangements 19

neglect 21

older children and adolescents 18

overdose and self-harm 18

parental factors in vulnerability 18-19

physical abuse 21

procedure 19-20

runaway children 19

sexual abuse 21-22

unmet needs 19

vulnerability to abuse 18

safeguarding (vulnerable adults)

accurate records 25

assessment 24

capacity to consent 25

definition of abuse 24

definition of vulnerable adult 24

discriminatory 25

duty of care 24

financial/material 25

incidence 24

Inter-Agency Adult Protection Procedures 24

introduction 24

management 25

neglect 25

physical abuse 24

potential sources of 24

psychological abuse 24

record of body language 25

rights of 24

sexual abuse 24

types of abuse 25

salbutamol

actions 370

additional information 370

in asthma 80

cautions 370

contra-indications 370

dosage and administration 371

indications 370

presentation 370

side effects 370

scalds, mobile babies and toddlers 18

SCENE incident management 223, 230

selective serotonin reuptake inhibitors (SSRIs) 102

self-harm

and mental capacity 113

and mental disorder 105

NICE definition 105

in older children 18

sepsis 131

clinical signs 395

intravascular fluid therapy (adults) 394-395

and tachycardia in children 131

as time-critical emergency 117

septic arthritis/osteomyelitis 131

septic shock, definition of

septicaemia 149

serotonin and noradrenaline reuptake inhibitors (SNRIs) 102

sexual assault

assessment and management of 23

definition of 22

further care 22

incidence 22

introduction 22

pathophysiology 22

serious, definition of 22

severity and outcome 22

treatment and management 23

vulnerable adults and children 22

shaking injuries, non-mobile babies 18

sickle cell crisis

analgesia 9

assessment and management 146-148

incidence 146

introduction 146

key points 146

pathophysiology 146

precipitating factors 146

severity and outcome 146

signs and symptoms 146

skull fractures, non-mobile babies 17

SOCRATES in pain management 8

sodium chloride 0.9%

actions 373

additional information 373

contra-indications 373

dosage and administration 373

indications 373

presentation 373

side effects 373

sodium lactate compound (Hartmann's/Ringer's lactate)

    actions 380

    additional information 380

    cautions 380

    contra-indications 380

    dosage and administration 380

    indications 380

    presentation 380

    side effects 380

spinal cord injury (SCI)

    airway management and immobilisation 39

    assessment and management 248, 250

    blunt trauma 248

    in children 248

    emergency extrication 248

    falls 246

    fatality in 246

    immobilisation 246-248, 251

    incidence 246

    introduction 246

    key points 250

    neurogenic shock 246

    odontoid peg fractures 246

    pathophysiology 246

    penetrating trauma 248

    restless/combative patients 247

    risk factors 246

    road traffic collisions 246

    severity and outcome 246

    spinal nerves 247

    spinal shock 246

    sporting injuries 246

    vomiting 247

spinal nerves 247

spiral fractures, non-mobile babies 17

ST segment elevation myocardial infarction (STEMI) 152

stab wounds 236

stable angina, features of pain 152

staff wellbeing and health

    continued learning 35

    good physical health 35

    helping others 35

    introduction 35

    relationships 35

    self-awareness 35

    stress and anxiety 35

status epilepticus 117, 165

stertorous breathing, and airway obstruction (children) 124

stridor

    and airway obstruction (children) 124

    croup (children) 134-135

stroke/transient ischaemic attack (TIA)

    assessment 198

    audit information 199

    FAST test 198-199

    Glasgow Coma Scale 198

    incidence 198

    introduction 198

    key points 199

    management 199

    pathophysiology 198

    referral pathway 199

    severity and outcome 198

    symptoms 198

    thrombolytic therapy 198

    time critical features 198

    transient ischaemic attack 198

strychnine poisoning 47

subcutaneous drug route 29, 304

sub-lingual drug route 304

submersion

    definition of 271

    and resuscitation 46

'sudden unexpected death in epilepsy' (SUDEP) 165

sudden unexpected death in infancy (SUDI) 32

sudden, unexpected death in infancy, children and adolescents (SUDICA) 32

    see also children, death of

suffocation, deliberate, mobile babies and toddlers 18

suicidal ideation 110

suicide attempts, and self-harm 105

suicide risk assessment IPAP 104, 108

    rationale for use of 104

superior vein compression

    background 27

    management 27

    signs and symptoms 27

support workers, mental health 103

supraglottic airways (children) 70

syntometrine (ergometrine)

    additional information 386

    contra-indications 386

    dosage and administration 386

    indications 386

    presentation 386

    side effects 386

tachycardia

    assessment and management 91

    broad complex 91

    child trauma 231

    children 125, 131

    febrile illness 131

    narrow complex 91

tachypnoea (children) 125, 131, 136

tenecteplase
    actions 387
    additional information 387
    in all cases 387
    contra-indications 387
    dosage and administration 389
    indications 387
    presentation 387
    side effects 387
    thrombolysis checklist 388

tension pneumothorax 44

tetanus 47

tetracaine
    actions 390
    additional information 390
    cautions 390
    contra-indications 390
    dosage and administration 390
    indications 390
    presentation 390
    side effects 390
    special precautions 390

tetracaine 4% gel 9, 11-12

third heart sound, and potential heart failure 178

thoracic trauma
    air embolism 259
    assessment and management 255, 257
    cardiac tamponade 259
    blunt trauma 255
    cardiac tamponade 255
    ECG rhythm disturbances 255
    flail chest 259
    hypoxia 255
    incidence 255
    introduction 255
    key points 255
    pathophysiology 255
    penetrating trauma 255
    pneumothorax 255
    severity and outcome 255
    surgical emphysema 259
    tension pneumothorax 259

thrombolytic therapy 198

tracheal intubation
    advanced life support (children) 70
    asthma 81

'Traffic Light' assessment tool 131, 133

tranexamic acid
    actions 391
    additional information 391
    contra-indications 391
    dosage and administration 391
    indications 391
    presentation 391
    side effects 391
    and traumatic cardiac arrest 44

transdermal drug route 304

transient ischaemic attack (TIA) 198
    FAST test 198-199
    incidence 198
    pathophysiology 198
    see also stroke/transient ischaemic attack

transient loss of consciousness (TLoC) 92
    assessment and management 92-93

transverse fractures, non-mobile babies 17

trauma (adults) 223
    abdomen assessment 226
    altered mental status 225
    assessment and management 225
    ATMIST format handover 224
    catastrophic haemorrhage 229
    chest assessment 226
    Glasgow Coma Scale 227
    haemorrhage 228
    head assessment 226
    incidence 223
    incident management 223
    key points 227
    limb assessment 226
    management overview 223
    neck assessment 226
    pain management 223
    pelvis assessment 226
    Pre-Hospital Major Trauma Triage Tool 227
    primary survey 223
    SCENE incident management 223
    secondary survey 224, 226
    severity and outcome 223
    trapped patient 226

trauma (children)
    airway assessment 230
    airway burns 230
    analgesia 232
    assessment 230
    'AVPU' score 232
    bradycardia 231
    breathing assessment 231
    catastrophic haemorrhage 230, 232, 234
    cervical spine assessment 231
    circulation assessment 231
    circulation management 232
    disability assessment 232
    disability management 232

Index

exposure 232

haemorrhage 233

hypoglycaemia and altered consciousness 232

incidence 230

introduction 230

key points 235

long bone fractures 232

oxygen administration 230

primary survey 230

SCENE incident management 230

secondary survey 232

tachycardia 231

ventilation 231

trauma in pregnancy

assessment and management 260

incidence 260

introduction 260

key points 261

mechanism 260

pathophysiology 260

severity and outcome 260

traumatic brain injury (TBI) 238

airway with C spine control 238

assessment and management 247

and brain hypoxia 238

breathing and ventilation 238

cautions for midazolam 239

circulation 238

disability 238

in the elderly 239

evacuation considerations 239

Glasgow Coma Scale 238

head position 238

hypertonic saline (HTS) 240

hypotension 238

hypothermia 238

midazolam in 239-240, 242

oxygen administration 238

pain and agitation 238

pain management 238

pharmacokinetics / pharmacodynamics 239

tricyclic antidepressants 103

poisoning in adults 189

poisoning in children 219

'tripod' posture, children 135

ulcerative colitis 170

upper respiratory tract infections (URTIs) (children) 135

assessment 135

breathing 135

GP prescribing strategy 135

hydration 135

incidence 135

management 135

referral pathway 136

typical duration 135

urinary tract infection (UTI) 86, 131

vaginal bleeding

assessment and management 298

incidence 298

introduction 298

key points 299

pathophysiology 298

severity and outcome 298

see also haemorrhage in pregnancy

venous thromboembolism (VTE) 194

ventilation

assisted and opioids 9

bag-mask 62

failing as time-critical 117

positive pressure 178

verapamil poisoning 189

Wells Criteria for pulmonary embolism 195

Wong–Baker faces Pain Rating Scale 11, 15

Notes

Notes

Notes

Notes

Notes

Notes

Notes

Notes

Notes